Neurological and Neurosurgical Intensive Care

Fourth Edition

Neurological and Neurosurgical Intensive Care

Fourth Edition

Allan H. Ropper, M.D.

Professor and Chairman of Neurology
Tufts University School of Medicine
Remondi Chief of Neurology
St. Elizabeth's Medical Center
Boston, Massachusetts

Daryl R. Gress, M.D.

NeuroCritical Care and Stroke
Lynchburg General Hospital
Lynchburg, Virginia

Michael N. Diringer, M.D.

Associate Professor of Neurology,
Neurosurgery, and Anesthesiology
Director, Neurology/Neurosurgery
Intensive Care Unit
Washington University School of Medicine
St. Louis, Missouri

Deborah M. Green, M.D.

Assistant Clinical Professor of
Medicine and Surgery
University of Hawaii School of Medicine
Staff Neurointensivist
Neuroscience Institute
The Queen's Medical Center
Honolulu, Hawaii

Stephan A. Mayer, M.D.

Associate Professor of Clinical Neurology
and Neurological Surgery
Columbia University College of
Physicians & Surgeons
Director, Neurological Intensive Care Unit
New York Presbyterian Hospital
Columbia–Presbyterian Medical Center
New York, New York

Thomas P. Bleck, M.D.

The Louise Nerancy
Eminent Scholar in Neurology and
Professor of Neurology, Neurological Surgery,
and Internal Medicine
Director, Neuroscience Intensive Care Unit
The University of Virginia
Charlottesville, Virginia

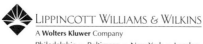

LIPPINCOTT WILLIAMS & WILKINS
A **Wolters Kluwer** Company

Philadelphia · Baltimore · New York · London
Buenos Aires · Hong Kong · Sydney · Tokyo

Acquisitions Editor: Charles W. Mitchell
Developmental Editor: Julia Seto
Production Editor: Jonathan Geffner
Manufacturing Manager: Benjamin Rivera
Cover Designer: Christine Jenny
Compositor: Lippincott Williams & Wilkins Desktop Division
Printer: Edwards Brothers

© 2004 by Lippincott Williams & Wilkins
227 East Washington Square
Philadelphia, PA 19106-3780 USA
LWW.com

Printed in the USA

Library of Congress Cataloging-in-Publication Data

Neurological and neurosurgical intensive care / Allan H. Ropper...[et al.]—4th. ed.
   p. ; cm.
  Includes bibliographical references and index.
  ISBN 0-7817-3196-8
   1. Neurological intensive care. 2. Surgical intensive care. I. Ropper, Allan H.
  [DNLM: 1. Nervous System Diseases—therapy. 2. Intensive Care Units.
  3. Intensive Care. 4. Neurosurgical Procedures. WL 100 N4944 2003]
  RC350.N4945 2003
  616.8′0428—dc21

                               2003047692

10 9 8 7 6 5 4 3 2 1

Contents

Preface

In the preface to the previous edition of *Neurological and Neurosurgical Intensive Care*, almost a decade ago, I commented that the field of neurological and neurosurgical intensive care had reached a maturity of sorts and was due for a rest. My colleagues and I were concerned that many of the major clinical problems relating to intracranial pressure and neuromuscular paralysis had been addressed to a reasonable degree, and perhaps the next level, a deeper understanding of the pathophysiology of the main diseases seen in the neurological intensive care unit (neuro-ICU), would be reached only via the laboratory. As usual, however, the progress of clinical medicine surprised and delighted, as a large number of new therapies and clinical insights from various trials and series clarified many previously opaque problems. This period of experience in the neuro-ICU, coinciding with the decade of the brain, occasions another edition of our text. The emphasis in the current revision is, much more than previously, on the details of therapeutics in critical care neurology.

The fourth edition also differs from the last three in that several close colleagues who are distinguished in the field and daily participants in their respective neuro-ICUs have written the book collectively. This affords the advantage of more uniformity of style than previous multi-authored editions and allows an authoritative voice regarding the main themes, all of which have been discussed among the authors. Furthermore, personal experience with difficult problems is expressed whenever there is a point of controversy or an approach that differs from published reports.

The continued progress of this branch of medicine requires that bright and ambitious young people continue to be attracted to the field. We hope that those neurologists, neurosurgeons, and anesthesia and the critical care physicians who are intrigued by the nervous system and its diseases (and who have an activist bent) will find the text exciting and that it will provide for them a basis for further study and clinical work. For established intensivists, neurologists, neurosurgeons, and emergency room physicians, the material presented is meant to serve as a guide for effective and thoughtful practice as synthesized by experienced neurointensivists.

Allan H. Ropper, M.D
June 2003

PART I

General Principles of Neurological Intensive Care

1

Introduction to Critical Care in Neurology and Neurosurgery

THE NATURE OF NEUROLOGICAL–NEUROSURGICAL INTENSIVE CARE

The specialized care of neurosurgical and neurological patients, which was virtually nonexistent as a specialty 20 years ago, has evolved to become one of the most popular components of neurology today. To appreciate the nature of this field and establish where it may be headed requires a description of the clinical practice and its constituent areas of medical knowledge, and a digression into the origins of neurological intensive care units (neuro-ICUs) as well as the medical–political and economic forces that have shaped them. In addition to previous versions of this book, a substantial number of texts, monographs, and review articles (1–12) have been devoted to the field (13–19), and most comprehensive textbooks of critical care include a chapter or more on neurological aspects. As important, the techniques of caring for critically ill neurological patients have been integrated into the mainstream of many neurology and neurosurgery training programs. In addition to the evolution of the field through courses, textbooks, and interest sections in various professional organizations, the notable inception in 2003 of the Neuro Critical Care Society and a corresponding journal has put the specialty on an equal footing with a number of other derivative fields in neurology and neurosurgery.

Neurologists, neurosurgeons, intensivists, and anesthesiologists have all influenced what has come to be known as neurological intensive care or neurological–neurosurgical critical care; "neuro-ICUs" or their equivalent have become commonplace in hospitals of all sizes. Initially, the development of neurological intensive care was driven by a need to house patients with neurological diseases in one area, and the desire to apply general ICU principles to their care. For the latter reason, many clinical practices have been adopted directly from the experiences in cardiopulmonary and postoperative intensive care, with special emphasis on those problems that are encountered in neurological diseases; for example, the mechanical respiratory failure that characterizes neuromuscular disease, autonomic changes that follow carotid endarterectomy, and nutritional requirements of patients with head injury.

However, the field of neurological and neurosurgical intensive care is mostly defined by a group of problems that derive from the acute aspects of diseases such as stroke, cerebral hemorrhage, brain and spinal cord injury, status epilepticus, encephalitis, generalized neuromuscular paralysis, brain tumors, and postoperative neurosurgical issues that are not addressed easily in a general ICU setting (Table 1.1). The care of these patients relates not only to understanding the neurological examination and knowledge of the course of these diseases, but also to certain physiologic changes in cerebral blood flow, intracranial

TABLE 1.1. *The approximate proportions of diagnoses in a typical neurological intensive care unit (ICU)*

Primary diagnosis	Admissions (percentage)
Postoperative tumor (all types)[a]	20%
Stroke or transient ischemic attack[b]	15%
Subarachnoid hemorrhage	12%
Head trauma (operative)[c]	11%
Cerebral hemorrhage (other than subarachnoid)	7%
Guillain–Barré syndrome	6%
Subdural hematoma (acute and chronic)	5%
Medical complication[d]	4%
Myasthenia gravis	4%
Interventional neuroradiology	3%
Spinal trauma	3%
Status epilepticus	3%
Postoperative laminectomy	2%
Postoperative AVM[e]	2%
Encephalitis	2%
Meningitis, brain abscess, acute global ischemia/carbon monoxide, brain tumor with raised intracranial pressure, epidural hematoma, giant carotid aneurysm	<1%

[a]Many admissions but ranked only eighth in total patient days in ICU.
[b]Including postoperative endarterectomy and stroke with brain swelling; excluding hemorrhage.
[c]Excluding isolated subdural or epidural hematoma or gunshot wounds.
[d]Primary gastrointestinal bleeding, pulmonary embolus, myocardial infarction with stable neurological state.
[e]AVM, arteriovenous malformation.

pressure, brain and neuromuscular electrical activity, electroencephalography and related techniques, ventilator mechanics, and so on, that have become the province of neurological intensive care. Despite this explicit description, defining the core knowledge of the field has proved somewhat difficult because of the diversity of clinical practices involved. From one limited perspective, it can be stated that the knowledge that underpins neurological intensive care is mainly a compilation of the acute aspects of most neurological illnesses, including those already mentioned. A broader perspective on the field would include a knowledge of all illnesses that risk brain loss or spinal cord function in which intervention might improve outcome, and those neurological illnesses that require intensive medical care and surveillance because of cerebral, respiratory, or cardiovascular dysfunction.

It is also accurate to say that all of the constituent specialties that have contributed to the field—neurology, neurosurgery, critical care,

and anesthesiology—have in turn been greatly altered by developments in neurological critical care. The neurological aspects of diseases in those fields have been delineated by critical care neurologists and neurosurgeons; and issues relating to neurological outcome and brain death have been greatly refined through experience in neuro-ICUs. One manifestation of this cross-fertilization has been the identification of several ubiquitous but previously unrecognized neurological manifestations of critical illness that are discussed in Chapter 11.

The rationale for the existence of neuro-ICUs is that a reduction in morbidity and mortality are anticipated from collecting acutely ill neurological patients in a geographic area of a hospital under the care of specially trained nurses and physician staff. In keeping with the model of other ICUs, it might be further anticipated that certain patients with neurological conditions will acquire delayed problems that can only be detected by close clinical observation and physiological monitoring and that these problems will benefit from special and rapid interventions, all of which are beyond the usual capabilities of a hospital ward. To the extent that the medical needs of such patients have reached a state of such complex and specialized nature that there is a requirement for specially trained individuals and unique types of technologic monitoring, the utility of a neuro-ICU no longer requires defending as it had in the past; only the details of various organizational models and health economics of these units are worth discussing.

These issues should not obscure the underlying differences between the neurological patient and other critically ill patients. Alterations in the functioning of the nervous system profoundly affect the human organism in ways that other systemic illnesses do not. Mobility, communication, and thought processes are dramatically changed, leaving patients extremely dependent on others to interpret and fulfill their needs. Similarly, families who are capable of conceptualizing most common somatic illnesses find it difficult to deal with a member who is neurologically impaired. Comforting family members is frequently to little avail, and lack of comprehension of neurological disease on the part of family may create guilt, anxiety, and fear beyond what is expected for other illnesses. The suddenness and severity of most catastrophic brain injuries preclude time for the family and others to express feelings to the patient and may produce an inordinate amount of later residual stress if not properly handled by unit staff. Behavioral alterations such as confusion, delirium, and aphasia greatly alter the image of patients as human beings and upset families more than even the most gruesome somatic illnesses. The handling of brain death cases and organ procurement for transplantation is an example that highlights special skills that must be cultivated in neuro-ICUs because of the delicacy and the frequency of this occurrence. The ability to guide patients, families, and others through these difficult periods distinguishes the care of the critically ill neurological patient from that of others.

Familiarity with these problems is paramount to maintaining the character of a successful neuro-ICU and breeds a kind of nursing staff that mixes the highly technical with the profoundly personal. Nurses of this nature are a unit's major sustaining resource. More than anything else, the work of neuro-ICUs in the next decade depends on a continued supply of qualified and motivated nurses. Invariably, all the unit staff (often including secretaries and coordinators) share the interests of neurologists and neurosurgeons in the most unique of all organs, the brain. This makes them patient but sharp observers of human behavior, and supportive friends.

THE NEUROINTENSIVIST

The neurocritical care physician is one of the few subspecialists who has been able to defragment the care of patients. This occurs when the clinician takes primary responsibility for the care of patients with serious neurological problems and combines knowledge and experience of these diseases with the diverse medical problems that derive from them and with traditional critical care skills. In addition, this individual brings skills in the application of certain modes of critical care that are unique to neurological disease, such as intracranial pressure (ICP) monitoring, electroencephalography, evoked potentials and their derivatives, and neuromuscular testing.

It goes without saying that the neurointensivist must have the leadership skills to establish and carry out clinical and administrative policies in a unit, work very closely with the nursing and other staff, and communicate if not mediate between the services that use a unit. Indeed, the perceived success of a unit depends as much on these roles as it does on the medical aptitude of the neurointensivist.

Furthermore, a number of specialized skills formerly embedded in the general practice of neurology (e.g., the management of patients with status epilepticus and metabolic encephalopathies) have informally accrued to neurological intensive care. Serious arrhythmias, cardiogenic and septic shock, hypoxic respiratory failure, and surgical complications requiring gastrointestinal or thoracic procedures are less common in the neuro-ICU than they are in the practice of general medical intensive care. Another difference between the medical–surgical ICU and the neuro-ICU is the difficulty in quantifying the effects of neurological disease, a problem that makes the effects of various therapies less certain. The generally poor outcome for many patients with severe brain or spinal injuries creates a sense of futility in comparison to medical intensive care; however, this fails to recognize that the goal is to prevent the numerous causes of secondary neurological deterioration and optimize neurological outcome in patients who might live productive lives when the crisis subsides.

The appropriate training for a neurointensivist has been a matter of some discussion but it converges on several items: direct experience with neurological and neurosurgical diseases, usually gained by residency, knowledge, and training in core critical care areas and techniques (including pulmonary and ventilator management, acute cardiovascular care, central and arterial pressure monitoring); a strong background in the general medical management of the typical secondary illnesses of severely ill patients (pneumonia, sepsis, pulmonary embolus, multitrauma, etc.); and special training with ICP monitoring and management. Almost always, a year or more of fellowship in a neuro-ICU is required and is ideally supplemented by a tour of training in a general or surgical ICU. The trainee should acquire some skill with arterial, venous, and pulmonary artery catheter insertion; the trainee should possess a thorough knowledge of waveform interpretation and troubleshooting of the devices at least. It is clear to the authors that training in the field of cerebrovascular disease, although addressing an integral part of critical care practice, does not equip an individual to run a neuro-ICU.

The matter of certification for neurological intensive care is also somewhat contentious and outside the scope of this text. The authors can only indicate that minimum standards for training have been suggested and someone experienced in the field should oversee the training of fellows who wish to pursue a career as neurointensivists. Until now, an organized specialty of neurological critical care had proved elusive. Neurosurgeons, anesthetist–intensivists, and neurologists have all attempted unsuccessfully to legitimize their subspecialty interests by seeking board certification in neurological intensive care (20–23). In 1985, the American Board of Neurological Surgeons tentatively considered an interspecialty certification in neurosurgical intensive care, and then reconsidered (24). The Society of Neurosurgical Anesthesia and Supportive Care (more than 1,000 members) has fostered clinical research in areas related to the neuro-ICU. A a subsection of Neurological Critical and Emergency Care of the American Academy of Neurology devoted to Intensive and Emergency Care has grown rapidly since its inception in 1988; it conducts courses and scientific and educational sessions, comparable to the evolution of rehabilitation and pain neurology among others, but has been so far unsuccessful in creating a board certification similar to pediatric neurology. This group has collected consensus guidelines on numerous clinical problems that are routinely handled by neurointensivists, given guidance on appropriate training, and held scientific sessions.

RUNNING A NEUROLOGICAL INTENSIVE CARE UNIT

Many of the political and strategic aspects of neurological intensive care have been mentioned already, but a few additional comments are justified (1). The interactions among neurological, neurosurgical, anesthesia, and other services often can be simplified by setting out clear goals for the existence of the unit. For example, there is an intrinsic competition for beds between critically ill neurological patients and postoperative neurosurgical cases. Cooperative planning by both services and clear admission criteria prevent disagreements and fragmentation of administration. The ideal unit serves the needs of the constituent services of course; however, ideally it also maintains a balance among types of patients, mixing patients who have neuromuscular diseases with those who have acute central nervous illnesses, and patients who have neurological problems with those who have neurosurgical diseases, so that expertise is maintained in each of these fields.

Medical and nursing leadership in a neuro-ICU should determine guidelines for admission, discharge, and standards of care for the most commonly encountered problems in each institution. The treatment of raised ICP and the handling of monitoring devices, management of respiratory failure, care of patients with subarachnoid hemorrhage, determination of brain death, nursing practices, responsibility of house staff and fellows and so on are best standardized; however, guidelines must be flexible enough to be altered according to each circumstance. Not at all surprisingly, a study has shown that ICUs coordinated by a director, and full-time house staff achieves better results than general ICU services (25).

Neuro-ICU nursing requires a high degree of proficiency in general neurology, critical care techniques, and knowledge of the special devices and medications used in the unit. One nurse generally cares for two critically ill patients. There may be, at times, a ratio of up to four patients per nurse, whereas some unstable patients may require a single nurse for limited periods of time.

THE ORIGINS OF NEUROLOGICAL INTENSIVE CARE UNITS

There are currently about 45 large neuro-ICUs in North American academic hospitals by informal count. There are several-fold this many smaller units in community and academic hospitals with active neurosurgical services, and more than 30 units of various sizes and configurations in Europe (particularly in Germany where the field has been quite ac-

tive). In many large institutions in the 1960s and 1970s, several beds or a large room was set aside on a general or neurology ward to care for patients who required frequent nursing care. In others, neurosurgical postoperative recovery services were shared with critical care patients who stayed longer than 1 day. These "informal ICUs" intersected with the progenitors of the modern ICU; namely, the respiratory units that flourished after the European poliomyelitis epidemic of the early 1950s; and later, the postoperative anesthesia wards for neurosurgical patients, and the general medical and surgical ICUs that evolved in most hospitals. Notable among the early units was Spalding and Crampton's at Radcliffe Infirmary (Fig. 1.1) and Ibsen's in Copenhagen that were devised mainly to deliver the then-novel care of mechanical ventilation. The evolution of general and respiratory intensive care has been summarized in Pontoppidan and colleagues (26). Other specialized inpatient services, particularly stroke and epilepsy units, also have had a significant influence on the practices and designs of neuro-ICUs over the years (see later).

One of the first large general academic neuro-ICUs in North America began in 1977 at the Massachusetts General Hospital, largely as a result of efforts of Nicholas Zervas of the neurosurgical department. It was run initially by a neurologist and a neuroanesthesiologist (Dr. Sean Kennedy, a previous editor of this book) with the close cooperation of a neurosurgeon, and began training fellows in 1980. Subsequently, units opened at Johns Hopkins, Columbia-Presbyterian, and elsewhere. Units focusing on head trauma opened in the 1970s in Miami, Richmond, and elsewhere in the United States and Europe; these gave great impetus to the use of ICP monitoring. Large units now are components of most sizable academic centers and are headed by a variety of individuals, with a recent inclination toward neurologists.

Nevertheless, the most common arrangement in general hospitals continues to be the transfer of critically ill patients to a medical or

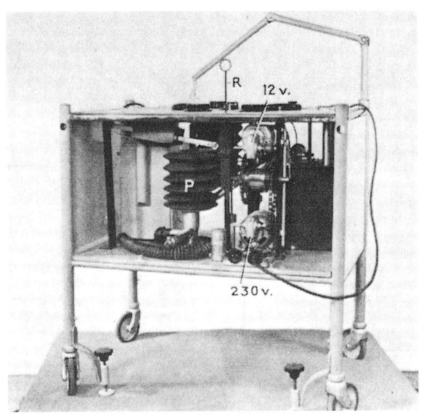

FIG. 1.1. Back of the Radcliffe positive–negative pressure respiration pump used by Russell, Schuster, Smith, and Spalding in their unit in the early 1950s. *P*, positive pressure bellows: The *black box* on the right is a humidifier and the *white box* on the left is a gas meter. (Photograph provided by J.M.K. Spalding and published with permission of surviving authors and *Lancet*. From: Russell WR, Schuster E, Smith AC, et al. Radcliffe respiration pumps. *Lancet* 1956:1:539–541, with permission.)

surgical ICU when there are insufficient numbers of patients to justify a separate neuro-ICU service. Even in the absence of a specialized unit, the clinical approaches and practices developed in neuro-ICUs have found applications in these units as well as in emergency wards, operating rooms, postoperative wards, and general neurological and neurosurgical services.

STROKE AND OTHER RELATED UNITS

Stroke units facilitate the work of investigative groups and may assist neurology services in applying high-quality standards to stroke patients, particularly if there is no geo-graphic neurology ward with specially trained nurses. In the right circumstances, they may be an important way for community hospitals to control the flow and use of resources for this large volume of patients.

There is an extensive literature on these stroke units and other similar "intermediate care units" (27). Some beds of this type are often appended to a neuro-ICU and are suitable for acute monitoring of neurological patients whose acuity does not require an ICU. Indeed, many stroke units serve as intermediate care units for other neurological patients, particularly those who are comatose or on ventilators. These beds also can be used for specialized stroke care and to facilitate clinical protocols (e.g., thrombolysis or interventional radiologic procedures) with more attention to procedure-specific details than can be accomplished on general wards (28). Undoubtedly they are the most practical place to carry out clinical investigation.

Published studies differ in their assessment of the value of stroke units. Most have shown a reduction in long-term hospitalization and fewer neurological deficits as a result of beginning therapy early (29), whereas others showed no such improvement (30,31). A 50% reduction in the cost of caring for stroke patients has been found without a difference in outcome, in a comparison of community and university hospitals (32); and reduced complications of stroke have been shown in one study but not in others. A controlled trial has provided perhaps the most convincing evidence that neurological outcome can be improved by a stroke unit (33).

ECONOMIC ASPECTS OF NEUROLOGICAL INTENSIVE CARE UNITS

Although it appears to neurologists and neurosurgeons that substantial benefits are derived from the presence of neurological ICUs, these advantages have proved difficult to quantitate, and depend in part on whether one's point of view is economic or medical. There is a general recognition that intensive care of any kind is expensive and patients with serious neurological diseases have poor outcomes in comparison to patients with mundane medical illnesses (e.g., gastrointestinal hemorrhage and myocardial infarction). The result in many instances is an unfavorable cost to outcome ratio for neurological cases, especially in comparison to medical ICUs. Any analysis of the value of neuro-ICUs is further complicated by the resources that must be devoted to postoperative care of neurosurgical patients. Units that fulfill this function are able to increase the productivity of neurosurgical departments and decompress postoperative wards and surgical ICUs, and to do so at relatively low cost compared to the costs of

longer-term care required by patients with illnesses such as stroke and neuromuscular paralysis.

Consequently, establishing the start-up and ongoing costs of a neuro-ICU is quite difficult and altered by the perspective taken. At the most basic administrative level, reflecting the conversation that often takes place when a new unit is contemplated, a business plan is constructed that takes the following into account. The profit considerations include: the prospect of attracting new patients to the institution, increased neurosurgical case flow, professional and hospital fee collection for special procedures (neurological procedures such as interpretation of electrophysiologic studies but also general critical care procedures such as line insertion), potential reductions in the number of nonintensive and other critical care beds on a neurological or neurosurgical floor, and the possibility of earlier discharge for some patients. The expense considerations include: the costs of an increased number of specially trained nurses, construction or alteration of hospital facilities, purchases of monitoring equipment, and so on. The artificiality of this type of cost accounting derives from the idiosyncrasies of current reimbursement schemes in the United States (diagnostic related groups, health maintenance organization payments, etc.) and sometimes from the cost limitations of European and other medical care systems; however, this way of analyzing the "cost-effectiveness" of neuro-ICUs currently is unavoidable. Moreover, extreme ambiguity is introduced when the financial expenditure is matched to the number of lives saved or preserved productivity of the workforce (as it often is), because no one can with remote accuracy make these calculations. As long as these methods are not confused with the value to the patients and gains for clinical research, rational arguments can be framed for and against building a new neuro-ICU or supporting an existing one. The neuro-ICU is not likely to be profitable on a strictly economic level, given current monetary policy in medical care. Most busy neuro-ICUs with which we are familiar break even or lose money in the current environment, but when viewed in the larger context of facilitating sophisticated neurosurgery, attracting tertiary admissions, and decompressing medical units, they may be profitable overall (34,45). As a Darwinian test of the overall monetary value of neuro-ICUs, one would think that if they were unprofitable (which they often are), hospital administrators would eschew them and accept some loss of patients, but the inability to service active neurology and neurosurgery programs uncovers another layer of complexity in judging the value of these units once they are viewed in a larger context.

It can be legitimately asked if every sizable and some smaller hospitals in the United States and elsewhere truly require such units or whether regional units are more sensible (of course, they are); however, in keeping with the duplication of services of almost every other technical hospital asset within geographical regions, the necessary fluidity of referral patterns across hospital systems and between neurology and neurosurgery departments, it is unlikely that this degree of rationality will prevail.

A related item regards the use of general ICUs to care for critically ill patients with neurological diseases. The costs of this approach vary depending on the specific configuration: assigned or floating bed allotments for different services, general ICU or specialist nurses, critical care or neurology/neurosurgery attending physicians, the proportion of postoperative neurosurgical patients, etc. It is not possible to judge the effectiveness of general ICUs for the care of neurological cases either clinically or monetarily. It can be said, nonetheless, that considerable existing patient volume in neurology and neurosurgical cases is required to legitimize building or converting to a neuro-ICU.

REFERENCES

1. Trubuhovich RV, ed. *Management of acute intracranial disasters. International anesthesiology clinics.* Vol. 17. Boston: Little, Brown, 1979.
2. Campkin TV, Turner JM. *Neurosurgical anesthesia and intensive care.* London: Butterworths, 1980.
3. Cottrell JE, Turndorf H. *Anesthesia and neurosurgery.* St. Louis: Mosby, 1980.
4. Green BA, Marshall LF, Gallagher TJ. *Intensive care for neurological trauma and disease.* New York: Academic Press, 1982.
5. Rogers MC, Traystsman RJ. *Neurological intensive care. Critical care clinics.* Philadelphia: WB Saunders, 1985.
6. Henning RJ, Jackson DL. *Handbook of critical care neurology and neurosurgery.* New York: Praeger, 1985.
7. Wirth FP, Ratcheson RA, eds. *Neurosurgical critical care.* Baltimore: Williams & Wilkins, 1987.
8. Grotta JC. *Management of the acutely ill neurological patient.* New York: Churchill Livingstone, 1993.
9. Andrews BT. *Neurosurgical intensive care.* New York: McGraw-Hill, 1993.
10. Hacke W. *NeuroCritical care.* Berlin: Springer-Verlag, 1994.
11. Wijdicks EFM. *The clinical practice of critical care neurology.* Philadelphia: Lippincott–Raven, 1997.
12. Ropper AH. *Critical care. Seminars in neurology.* New York: Thieme-Stratton, 1984.
13. Telleria-Diaz A. Intensive neurology. *Rev Neurol* 1998; 27:830–832.
14. Ropper AH. Neurological intensive care. In: Toole JF, Vinken PJ, Bruyn GW, et al, eds. *Handbook of clinical neurology.* Amsterdam: Elsevier, 1989:203–232.
15. Ropper AH. Neurological intensive care. *Ann Neurol* 1992;32:564–569.
16. Sundrani S. Neurological intensive care unit management and economic issues. *Neurol Clin* 1995;13: 679–693.
17. Bertram M, Schwarz S, Hacke W. Acute and critical care neurology. *Eur Neurol* 1997;38:155–166.
18. Schmutzhard E. New developments and perspectives of intensive neurology. *Wein Klin Wochen* 1999;111: 713–718.
19. Bolton CF, Young GB. The neurological consultation and neurological syndromes in the intensive care unit. *Ballieres Clin Neurol* 1996;5:645–671.
20. Correll JW, Becker GL, Countee RW. Intensive care of the patient with central nervous system disease. *Med Clin North Am* 1971;55:1233–1248.
21. Levin AB. Intensive care. In: Wilkins RK, Rengacherry SS, eds. *Neurosurgery.* New York: McGraw-Hill, 1985: 396–406.
22. Marsh ML, Marshall LF, Shapiro HM. Neuro-surgical intensive care. *Anesthesiology* 1977;47:149–163.
23. Snyder JV, Powner DJ, Grenvik A. Neurological intensive care. In: Cottrell JE, Turndorf H, eds. *Anesthesia in neurosurgery.* St. Louis: Mosby, 1980:322–360.
24. Kline DG, Mahaley MS. Recognition of special qualifications in neurological surgery. *J Neurosurg* 1986;64: 531–536.
25. Knaus WA, Draper EA, Wagner DP, et al. An evaluation of outcome from intensive care in major medical centers. *Ann Intern Med* 1986;104:410–418.
26. Pontoppidan H, Wilson RS, Rie MA, et al. Respiratory intensive care. *Anesthesiology* 1977;47:96–116.
27. Popovich J. Intermediate care units. Graded care options. *Chest* 1991;99:4–5.
28. Drake WE, Hamilton MJ, Carlssson M, et al. Acute stroke management and patient outcome. The value of neurovascular care units (NCU). *Stroke* 1973;4: 933–945.
29. Strand T, Asplund K, Eriksson S, et al. A nonintensive stroke unit reduces functional disability and the need for long-term hospitalization. *Stroke* 1985;16:29–34.

30. Pitney SF, Mance CJ. An evaluation of stroke intensive care: results in a municipal hospital. *Stroke* 1973;4: 737–741.

31. von Arbin M, Britton M, de Faire U, et al. A study of stroke patients treated in a nonintensive stroke unit or in medical wards. *Acta Med Scand* 1980;208:81–85.

32. Feigenson JS, Feigenson WD, Gitlow HS, et al. Outcome and cost for stroke patients in academic and community hospitals. *JAMA* 1978;240:1878–1880.

33. Indredavik B, Bakke F, Solberg R, et al. Benefit of a stroke unit: a randomized clinical trial. *Stroke* 1991;22: 1026–1031.

34. Bleck TP, Smith MC, Pierre-Louis SJC, et al. Neurologic complications of critical medical illness. *Crit Care Med* 1993;21:98–103.

35. Isensee LM, Weiner LJ, Hart RG. Neurologic disorders in a medical intensive care unit: a prospective survey. *J Crit Care* 1989;4:208–210.

2

Intracranial Physiology and Elevated Intracranial Pressure

An understanding of the physiologic changes that result from the addition of a mass to the intracranial vault is essential to the treatment of mass lesions and cerebral edema, and to the effective use of intracranial pressure monitoring devices. Much of this understanding has been derived from the clinical work of Lundberg and colleagues with head injury patients in the 1960s (Chapter 12) and experimental observations of mass effect in animals. Since then, this early work has been supplemented by systematic study in patients with head injury and massive brain swelling after cerebral infarction. It is not always clear how some of this work pertains to day-to-day basis decisions in an intensive care unit. Perhaps the largest problem has been the focus on manipulating physiologic variables without a clear understanding of how they may alter outcome; this often leads to physiologically desirable results but no improvement in outcome. Nonetheless, the following exposition gives a basis for sensibly managing all patients with cerebral masses.

The intracranial vault serves to protect the brain, provide it with nutrients, and remove waste products. Several unique physiologic aspects of the intracranial compartment are central to understanding the disturbances that occur in various pathologic states. In this chapter we review: (a) the components of the intracranial compartment [brain, cerebrospinal fluid (CSF), intravascular blood]; (b) the manner in which these components are perturbed in disease states and the resultant clinical signs; (c) the concept of intracranial hypertension and the mechanisms whereby it produces secondary injury; and (d) the monitoring of intracranial pressure.

CONTENTS OF THE CRANIAL CAVITY

The skull is a rigid, almost completely closed container filled with brain, blood, and CSF. The brain, including its intracellular and interstitial fluid, fills 80% to 90% of the skull; the remainder is approximately equally divided between blood and CSF. The essential tenet of intracranial bulk physiology is that expansion of one compartment occurs at the expense of the others (the Monro–Kellie doctrine).

Brain

The brain floats in the CSF under normal conditions. Dural reflections, which form the falx cerebri and tentorium, act to maintain the position of the brain. In addition, they create compartments that, in pathologic states, produce pressure differentials within the cranium. The brain consists of approximately 78% water, 80% to 85% of which is in the intracellular compartment (1); the remainder is in the interstitial compartment. These relative distributions of water become important when considering osmotic therapies that differentially affect the intracellular and interstitial water compartments.

Pathologic states that increase the water content of the brain generally increase its volume. Cell death, which is followed by an increase in osmolality caused by the breakdown of cellular elements, leads to a shift of fluid from the interstitial to the intracellular compartment ("cytotoxic edema") but causes no net change in brain volume. In contrast, disruption of the function of the blood–brain barrier (BBB) causes the overall water content of the brain to increase ("vasogenic edema"). These two mechanisms are operative to varying degrees in a wide variety of pathologic processes, including cerebral ischemia, trauma, and inflammation (1).

The brain, being virtually incompressible, is nonetheless capable of some degree of deformation as a consequence of pressure exerted by a mass within or external to it. Any further pressure causes the displacement of brain tissue, often into adjacent dural compartments, a circumstance called "herniation" by pathologists. These displacements correspond in some cases to particular clinical syndromes, as discussed in the following.

CEREBROSPINAL FLUID

Under normal conditions, the production of CSF is in dynamic equilibrium with its absorption. In the average adult there is 90 to 150 mL of CSF within the ventricular and subarachnoid spaces. The CSF volume in children (4 and 13 years of age) is 65 to 140 mL. Cerebrospinal fluid is produced at a rate of approximately 20 mL/h, originating predominantly in the choroid plexus (2). In addition, bulk flow of water from the interstitial fluid of the brain toward the lateral ventricles contributes to the CSF volume.

The production of CSF is depressed to a modest degree by elevated intracranial pressure (ICP), but it is usually unchanged in adults with most forms of hydrocephalus. Certain drugs, including acetazolamide (3), furosemide (4), and corticosteroids (5) are able to temporarily decrease CSF production in experimental and some clinical circumstances but they have no real clinical utility.

Choroid plexus papilloma is the only important cause of overproduction of CSF; hydrocephalus usually results.

Absorption of CSF into the venous system is less well understood. It appears that the arachnoid villi are the main sites for reabsorption. These structures act as one-way valves between the subarachnoid space and the superior sagittal sinus that open at a gradient of about 5 mm Hg. In addition, some CSF leaks out around spinal nerve roots. Reabsorption increases to a slight degree as ICP rises.

The natural bulk flow of CSF originates in the lateral ventricles, descends through the third and fourth ventricles to exit by the foramina of Luschka and Magendie at the medullary level, and then percolates upward via the brainstem basal subarachnoid cisterns through the perimesencephalic cisterns at the tentorial plane and over the convexity of the cerebral hemispheres to reach the arachnoid villi. The flow is driven by the slight pressure gradient that exists between the ventricles and the convexity subarachnoid space and appears to be facilitated by the pulsatile activity transmitted from the vascular system.

The flow of CSF can be disturbed in a number of ways to produce hydrocephalus. All hydrocephalus is essentially "obstructive" at some site in the ventricular or subarachnoid pathways (with the exception of CSF overproduction from choroid plexus papilloma). However, the term obstructive hydrocephalus has come to denote a blockage to flow within the ventricular system as occurs, for example, when intraventricular blood or a shift of brain tissue because a cerebral mass blocks the ventricles at any one of a number of locations. Subarachnoid blood, meningitis, and neoplastic infiltration obstruct the egress of CSF from the fourth ventricle or, more commonly, at the basal cisterns or over the cerebral convexity or arachnoidal reabsorption sites. The latter type of hydrocephalus has been called "communicating" (a misnomer), but rectifying the frequent misuse of these terms seems futile.

CEREBRAL BLOOD FLOW AND VOLUME

The blood within the cerebral vessels is the third constituent of the intracranial space. The volume of intracranial blood under normal conditions is determined primarily by cerebral blood flow (CBF) and the cerebral vascular tone (6,7). Conditions that raise CBF generally raise cerebral blood volume (CBV) and conditions that lower CBF also lower CBV.

A number of physiologic factors influence CBF and thus CBV, some locally and others globally. The main clinically relevant factors are regional cerebral metabolism, global cerebral perfusion pressure (CPP), and the tensions of blood oxygen and carbon dioxide. The ability to retain normal cerebral blood flow through inherent adjustments in cerebral vascular diameter (tone) of small penetrating arterioles is termed autoregulation, as discussed in the following.

METABOLISM AND CEREBRAL BLOOD FLOW

Because the brain generates high-energy phosphates through the oxidative metabolism of glucose and there is no storage of this substrate, cerebral metabolism ultimately is dependent on the continuous delivery of glucose and oxygen by the blood (8). This circumstance is unique to the brain, yet its metabolic needs are considerably higher than other organs. Thus, although the brain accounts for only 2% to 3% of body weight, it receives 15% to 20% of the cardiac output. In the normal adult, CBF is approximately 50 to 75 mL/100 g per minute in the gray matter where metabolic needs are highest, and about half that level in white matter. Under normal conditions CBF is tightly regulated to match the global and regional metabolic needs of the brain, the primary determinant of regional CBF being the metabolic requirement of the cerebral cortex (9,10). The mechanism of this coupling is complex and involves the local effects of several metabolic products [K^+, adenosine, adenosine triphosphate (ATP),

pH] as well as an incompletely understood neural regulation of vascular tone. The coupling provides for enhanced CBF in response to, or in anticipation of, cortical metabolic needs and is reflected by reduced flow in damaged or inactive areas.

As mentioned, factors that affect cerebral metabolism generally produce parallel changes in CBF. For example, fever and seizure activity correspondingly increase CBF, CBV, and ICP. Indeed, the most striking elevations in CBF are seen during seizures, in which maximal neuronal activity is elicited. However, CBF and cerebral metabolism may become uncoupled in pathologic states. The nature of this uncoupling is not fully understood but may reflect factors that have such profound effects on blood flow and metabolism as to overwhelm the normal relationship. In these situations CBF appears to be influenced by other factors such as perfusion pressure, PaO_2, arterial oxygen content (CaO_2), $PaCO_2$, and blood viscosity. All of these mechanisms are eclipsed in circumstances of greatly raised ICP, which ultimately reduces both CBF and CBV to levels that cause neuronal damage.

CEREBRAL PERFUSION PRESSURE AND AUTOREGULATION

Cerebral perfusion pressure is defined as the blood pressure gradient across the cerebral vasculature; it is an approximation that represents the difference between mean arterial pressure (MAP) at the entrance to the brain (Circle of Willis) and the venous pressure as its exits the skull. When ICP exceeds venous pressure, it replaces it in the calculation of CPP. For practical purposes, CPP is considered to be the mean arterial pressure (MAP) minus the mean ICP. When ICP and venous pressure are low, blood pressure is used to approximate CPP. Unless these measurements are made with the patient supine (in which case the brain and heart are at the same levels), all pressures can be referenced to head level, or appropriate account can be taken of the difference in altitude.

Cerebral blood flow remains constant over a fairly wide range of perfusion pressures in the absence of brain injury or other process that disrupts autoregulation (Fig. 2.1) (11–14). This allows the maintenance of constant brain perfusion over a similarly wide range of blood pressure and ICP changes. Autoregulation acts through changes in cerebrovascular resistance (CVR), specifically by altering the diameter of arterioles (12). As perfusion pressure falls, the arterioles apparently dilate to maintain CBF, thereby increasing CBV. Cerebral vasoconstriction occurs with increasing perfusion pressure, and CBF is maintained with a lower CBV. The upper and lower limits of autoregulation in healthy normotensive adults are approximately 50 and 150 mm Hg. Both the upper and lower limits of autoregulation are elevated in chronically hypertensive patients, but they tend to normalize with long-term blood pressure control (15). Although the limits of autoregulation are not known for children, autoregulation may be intact at lower absolute values of blood pressure in small children. Abrupt, pronounced elevations in blood pressures that ex-

ceed the upper limits of autoregulation result in increased CBF and when extreme, edema and hemorrhage. Outside the limits of autoregulation, CBF becomes passively dependent on changes in perfusion pressure. In this case, CBF and CBV fluctuate passively in the same direction.

Autoregulation is maintained through a combination of local myogenic control of arteriolar resistance and sympathetic neural activity. Sympathetic tone appears primarily to affect the upper and lower limits of autoregulation. Increased sympathetic activity during hypotension increases cerebrovascular tone and raises the threshold for blood pressure breakthrough (16). It should be noted that autoregulation may lag behind changes in blood pressure by 1 to 2 minutes, particularly in the damaged region of brain, allowing acute hypertension to raise ICP momentarily. Prolonged hypotension has been shown to impair autoregulation even after blood pressure has been restored (10,17).

Autoregulation is impaired or lost under a number of pathological states, including ischemic stroke and head injury (18–21). Per-

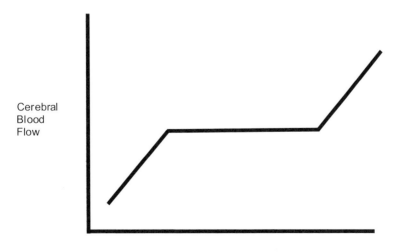

Cerebral
Blood
Flow

Cerebral Perfusion Pressure

FIG. 2.1. Cerebral perfusion pressure autoregulation curve for normotensive adults. Note that cerebral blood flow remains stable over a wide range of cerebral perfusion pressure but becomes pressure passive as the limits of autoregulation are exceeded at both extremes. This curve is shifted to the left in newborns and to the right in hypertensive adults.

haps of even greater importance, autoregulation is more effective in maintaining normal CBF when ICP is elevated than when blood pressure is reduced (22,23); restated, low perfusion pressure that results from systemic hypotension theoretically is a greater risk than the equivalent CPP that results from high ICP.

Oxygen Tension

The relationship between CBF and oxygen is best understood when considered in terms of arterial oxygen content (CaO_2) (Fig. 2.2). CaO_2 is measured as

$$1.34 \times ([\text{hemoglobin}] \times O_2 \text{ saturation}) + (PaO_2 \times 0.003)$$

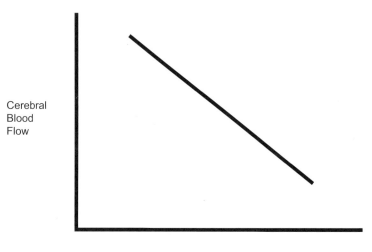

Arterial Oxygen Content

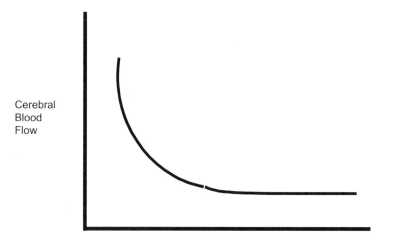

Arterial partial pressure of oxygen

FIG. 2.2. Relationship between arterial oxygen content and cerebral blood flow **(top)** and arterial partial pressure of oxygen and cerebral blood flow **(bottom).** See text for explanation.

The two components of this equation account for the oxygen that is bound to hemoglobin and O_2 dissolved in plasma, respectively. Because the amount of oxygen dissolved in plasma is small, practically speaking, CaO_2 is proportional to hemoglobin concentration times O_2 saturation. The relationship between CaO_2 and CBF is linear; thus, CBF rises dramatically with anemia (24). Because of the shape of the hemoglobin dissociation curve, CaO_2 changes little until PaO_2 falls below about 50 mm Hg; thus, CBF is constant within a wide range of arterial oxygen pressure (Fig. 2.1) (25,26).

Carbon Dioxide Tension

Cerebral blood flow is sensitive to arterial carbon dioxide pressure ($PaCO_2$) in the physiologic range of the latter (Fig. 2.3). There is a linear relationship between $PaCO_2$ and CBF for $PaCO_2$ between approximately 20 and 80 mm Hg (27–30). Lowering PCO_2 from 40 to 20 mm Hg reduces CBF by 40%, whereas raising PCO_2 to 80 mm Hg nearly doubles

CBF (31). When intracranial compliance is high, the added volume is buffered by CSF translocation. In states of poor compliance, marked elevations in ICP can result from even modest hypercarbia (32). It appears that carbon dioxide vascular reactivity is mediated by arteriolar and brain extracellular fluid hydrogen ion concentration (33). Cerebral blood flow is normally reduced for several hours after a single-step elevation in CSF pH, the same time required for correction of CSF alkalosis (34). Persistent hypercarbia in normal brain causes an elevation in CBF and ICP lasting less than 12 hours (35–37). Theoretically, profound hypocapnia could produce sufficient vasoconstriction to reduce blood flow below the level necessary to supply metabolic needs and cause ischemia. However, recent studies have challenged this assumption and suggest that short-term hyperventilation is probably safe (38), although it has not been shown to improve overall outcome. This ability of hypocarbia to reduce CBF and CBV and thereby to reduce ICP is the basis for therapeutic use of hyperventilation (Chapter 3).

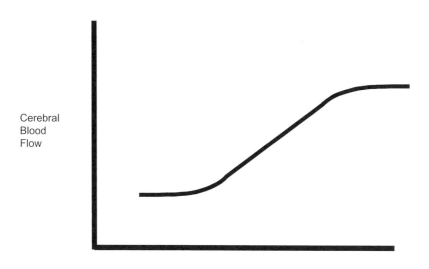

Cerebral
Blood
Flow

Arterial partial pressure of CO_2

FIG. 2.3. Relationship between arterial partial pressure of carbon dioxide and cerebral blood flow. Note that the relationship is essentially linear from a $PaCO_2$ of approximately 20 to 80 mm Hg.

Temperature

Cerebral blood flow in animals increases linearly as temperature rises to 42°C (39), whereas hypothermia reduces CBF approximately 6% for each degree centigrade (40). The variation in CBF is a response to increases and decreases in metabolism that occur in response to the change in temperature. The therapeutic use of hypothermia to treat ischemia or elevated intracranial pressure has been explored in the past and recently has elicited interest again (Chapter 3).

Blood Viscosity

Reducing hemoglobin concentration lowers blood viscosity and increases CBF (41–43). However, the effect on cerebral oxygen delivery is offset to some extent by a concomitant decrease in arterial oxygen content and thus a fall in oxygen delivery. Thus, there are circumstances where the rise in CBF compensates for the fall in arterial oxygen content and there is no net change in oxygen delivery to the brain (24). Other interventions designed to lower viscosity without reducing hemoglobin concentration, such as reducing fibrinogen concentration, may improve blood flow and oxygen delivery; however, this has yet to be established. The extent to which changes in blood viscosity influence ICP under pathologic conditions has not been studied extensively.

RELATIONSHIP BETWEEN CEREBRAL BLOOD FLOW AND CEREBRAL ISCHEMIA

Cerebral ischemia denotes the acute reduction in blood flow to a normally functioning brain to a degree that results in inadequate delivery of substrate to maintain normal metabolic function. Numerous studies have determined that the threshold for failure of neuronal function under normal conditions is a CBF of 18 to 20 mL/100 g per minute. The degree of blood flow reduction and its duration together ultimately determine the potential for neuronal damage; therefore, prolonged ischemia in the range of 20 to 25 mL/100 g per minute is capable of damaging neurons irrevocably (44). It is important to note that these thresholds of blood flow assume a condition of normal cerebral metabolism and are most useful when applied to acute ischemic stroke. Nevertheless, their utility is questionable in the presence of other factors that suppress cerebral metabolism. The relationship between blood flow and metabolism in such complex settings must be assessed, and ischemia should be considered a condition in which CBF falls to a point where it can no longer meet the lower metabolic needs of the brain; for example, ischemia does not occur at blood flows of 20 mL/100 g per minute when metabolism has been suppressed by barbiturates (45) or hypothermia (46) (Fig. 2.4).

One way to assess the relationship between CBF and metabolic demand is by measuring the oxygen extraction fraction (OEF) or the arteriovenous difference in oxygen content (a-vDO$_2$, the difference between arterial and cerebrovenous oxygen content). Under normal conditions, cerebral oxygen delivery exceeds the metabolic needs of the brain and the brain uses only 30% to 40% of the delivered oxygen (i.e., OEF 0.3 – 0.4). When CBF is reduced, more oxygen is extracted to meet the metabolic needs of the tissue. As CBF continues to fall, OEF rises until it is maximal, possibly as high as 90%. With extreme reductions in CBF, the rise in OEF no longer compensates for the fall in CBF, and cerebral energy failure occurs (47–50). The normal cellular biochemistry is disrupted as energy supply becomes insufficient as a result of an inadequate supply of oxygen. Interpreting the effects of ischemia is further complicated by a lack of clarity between levels of blood flow that lead to neuronal necrosis and lesser degrees of damage that set in motion cellular destructive processes now called apoptosis.

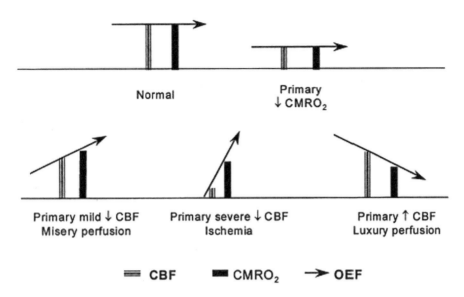

FIG. 2.4. Schematic representation of the relationship among cerebral blood flow (*CBF*), oxygen extraction fraction (*OEF*), and cerebral metabolic rate for oxygen (*CMRO₂*), during primary changes in CMRO₂ **(top)** and CBF **(bottom). Top:** Under normal circumstances, CBF and CMRO₂ are matched and the OEF is normal. If there is a primary reduction in CMRO₂, as observed in hypothermia or after administration of barbiturates, there is a secondary passive fall in CBF and OEF remains normal. **Bottom:** Situations in which there is a primary alteration in CBF. When there is a moderate reduction in CBF, OEF rises and CMRO₂ remains constant. This is referred to as misery perfusion. If the CBF falls further, OEF becomes maximal. Any further reduction in CBF results in a fall in CMRO₂ or ischemia. When CBF exceeds the metabolic needs, the OEF is low, a situation referred to as luxury perfusion. (From Diringer MN, Yundt K, Videen TO, et al. No reduction in cerebral metabolism with early moderate hyperventilation following severe traumatic brain injury. *J Neurosurg* 2000;92:7–13, with permission.)

THE INTRACRANIAL PRESSURE–VOLUME RELATIONSHIP

The idealized pressure–volume relationship of an incompressible substance filling a rigid container is depicted in Figure 2.5A. This relationship dictates that for any increase in the volume of such as system there is a proportional rise in pressure. As described, the skull and dura form a rigid and almost completely closed compartment that share many characteristics with such a system. For example, the cranium is filled largely with water (the brain is 78% water), which is incompressible. However, the pressure–volume relationship of the intracranial contents is influenced by shifts of tissue, CSF, and blood for which reason the actual relationship differs from the idealized one (Fig. 2.5B). Under normal conditions, a small increase in intracranial volume has little or no effect on pressure; as more volume is added, though, a threshold is reached beyond which further increases in volume lead to dramatic rises in pressure.

The nature of the intracranial pressure–volume relationship can be understood in terms of compliance (32,23). The system is compliant when the intracranial volume is relatively low (Point A in Fig. 2.5B)—it is able to tolerate the addition of more volume without an increase in pressure. The compartment becomes less compliant as the total intracranial

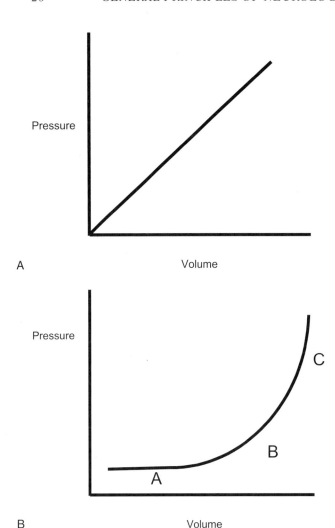

A

Pressure

Volume

B

Pressure

C

B

A

Volume

FIG. 2.5. A: Idealized pressure–volume relationship for a noncompressible substance in a rigid container. **B:** The pressure–volume relationship of the intracranial vault (see text for explanation).

volume rises (Point B in Figure 2.5B), and the addition of only a small volume leads to a modest rise in pressure. Compliance becomes low or absent at a certain point (Point C in Fig. 2.5B). Any additional volume beyond this point leads a substantial rise in pressure. These relationships define the "compliance curve," really a family of curves that approximate an exponential function.

Framed in mechanical terms, when compliance is high, the intracranial compartment is able to use compensatory mechanisms to prevent a rise in ICP. These mechanisms consist of reducing the intracranial volume by forcing CSF and venous blood out of the intracranial compartment into the spinal subarachnoid space and venous plexus, respectively. The shift of CSF out of the lateral ventricles is a well-recognized sign of "mass effect" on computed tomography (CT) scans that illustrates the compensatory movement of CSF out of the intracranial vault. Because there is only a finite amount of blood and CSF that can be displaced the compensatory mechanisms are eventually exhausted and the system can no longer adapt to added volume.

Adverse Consequences of Raised Intracranial Pressure

The consequences of elevated ICP generally have been attributed to ischemia. It should be emphasized, however, that most of the clinical consequences of a mass lesion are evident through constellations of clinical signs that are more a result of tissue shifts within the cranium than raised ICP per se (see the following). Nevertheless, greatly elevated ICP critically compromises cerebral perfusion and leads to global ischemia, which produces a vegetative state or brain death. The most common of these circumstances are diffuse traumatic edema, massive cerebral hemorrhage, and the progressive "malignant" edema that follows very large hemispheric infarctions. In contrast, the relatively high ICP associated with pseudotumor cerebri does not produce such dire consequences, suggesting that the absolute value is not always the critical factor in determining the consequences of raised ICP. In part, this is explained by the putative mechanism of pseudotumor, namely an increase in vascular pressures within the cranium but also as a result of the diffuse distribution of the pressure (see the following). Additionally, if a critical reduction in CPP were the only adverse consequence of high ICP, then artificially elevating blood pressure to restore CPP should prevent further injury. As mentioned, the equivalent perfusion pressure is apparently tolerated better if it is the result of raised ICP rather than hypotension, and the combination is particularly precarious.

Mass lesions are additionally harmful through a parallel mechanism that results from tissue shifts and local brain dysfunction. In the presence of a localized mass, the contour of the intracranial vault and its dural restrictions allows for a compartmentalization of pressures (pressure gradients across dural planes) that causes brain tissue to be displaced from one compartment to an adjacent one, thereby distorting brain structures at a distance from the mass. Radiographic signs of the progression of mass effect are readily evident on CT and magnetic resonance imaging (MRI). The specific signs are determined by the size and location of the mass. For example, basal ganglia hematomas progressively compress the ipsilateral lateral ventricle, displace the lateral ventricle to the contralateral hemisphere (septum pellucidum shift), produce horizontal shift of the diencephalon (pineal shift), obliterate the cisterns surrounding the midbrain, and finally cause protrusion of the medial temporal lobe downward through the tentorial opening (so-called transtentorial herniation). Frontal and occipital lesions produce more shift in the anterior–posterior direction and have less impact on diencephalic structures.

With enlargement of the mass lesion or expansion of surrounding edema, these tissue shifts eventually lead to herniations (Fig. 2.6). The main configurations of herniation are well known to neurologists: herniation of frontal white matter under the falx (subfalcial herniation), which may compress the contralateral anterior cerebral artery; the uncus of the temporal lobe can be forced through the tentorial opening into the perimesencephalic cisterns, thereby compressing the midbrain (uncal herniation); the cerebellar tonsils may be pushed through the foramen magnum (tonsillar herniation); and the downward movement of the entire supratentorial compartment produces central transtentorial herniation.

Classical descriptions ascribe a rostral-to-caudal progression of brainstem signs to downward displacement of brain tissue through the tentorial opening. Recently it has been proposed that the degree of horizontal shift of brain tissue is more reflective of the level of consciousness and that herniation is not always the proximate cause of coma. With acute lesions, horizontal displacement of the pineal gland of 3 to 6 mm from the midline is associated with drowsiness, 6 to 9 mm with stupor, and larger degrees with coma (51). These apparently conflicting concepts can be reconciled when considered in terms of the evolution of the brain distortion caused by a mass lesion. With moderate-sized lesions, the initial impact on level of consciousness may

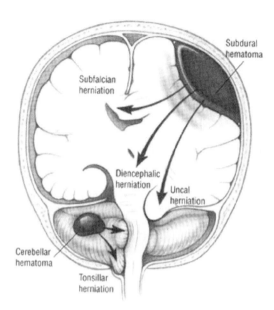

FIG. 2.6. Types of brain herniation. Different types of brain herniation caused by isolated areas of increased intracranial pressure. A mass (subdural in figure) located in the cerebral hemisphere may cause a shift of the intracranial contents past midline (subfalcial herniation). Uncal herniation results from a mass in one of the parietal, frontal, or temporal lobes creating pressure on the uncus of the temporal lobe, which then herniates through the tentorium. This can cause direct pressure on the underlying midbrain and third nerve, creating a unilateral dilated pupil. Cerebellar or tonsillar herniation can occur if a mass lesion (cerebellar hematoma in figure) develops in the cerebellum, causing compression of the medulla. This can cause a rapid deterioration in the patient with significant brainstem findings such as abnormal breathing, flexor or extensor posturing, impaired eye movements, hypertension, and bradycardia. Finally, central herniation (not shown) occurs if the tissue shifts are directed downward through the foramen magnum. These patients usually present with a global decline in level of consciousness and may have sixth nerve palsies. (From Deibert E, Diringer MN. Central nervous system hemorrhage and increased intracranial pressure. In: Wachter RM, Goldman L, Hollander H, eds. *Hospital medicine.* Philadelphia: Lippincott Williams & Wilkins, 2000:991–1003, with permission.)

result from horizontal shift of the upper brainstem and reticular activating system, all caused by translocation of tissue above the plane of the tentorial opening. As the lesion enlarges, these shifts progress to transtentorial herniation and there is a further progression of neurological signs.

Clinical Signs of a Cerebral Mass Lesion

The initial signs associated with a mass lesion are determined by the size and location of the lesion and the acuteness of its appearance. However, one of several fairly typical patterns emerges as cerebral lesions continue to enlarge. The classical descriptions of these signs, attributable to McNealy and Plum and then to Plum and Posner (52), were made through serial observations in patients during the final stages of an evolving mass lesion. They are constituted by alterations in pupil size and reactivity, eye movement, respiratory pattern, and motor signs. The goal of intervention for the purposes of this treatment-oriented book is to prevent these signs or slow their progression. Recognition of the effects of a mass lesion must occur before these signs have an opportunity to evolve.

Early detection of the progressive effects of a mass lesion is difficult. Subtle fluctuations in responsiveness may reflect worsening local signs from the mass, or may be the result of metabolic perturbations or even patient fatigue. Changes in the level of consciousness can result from medications, sleep deprivation, fever, infection, or metabolic disturbances. Elderly or demented patients are particularly prone to fluctuate in this manner. Many patients exhibit periodic decline in level of consciousness without apparent cause, which spontaneously resolves. These cyclical changes often are difficult to distinguish from true deterioration and complicate management. Intracranial pressure monitoring may provide an early guide to deterioration (see discussion further on), but progression even to the point of herniation can occur without elevated pressure depending on the location of the lesion and the ICP monitor.

This is especially true for temporal lobe lesions. Radiographic signs (compression of adjacent brain tissue, obliteration of brainstem cisterns, horizontal shift, ventricular enlargement) give critical information regarding the evolution of the mass, but repetitive imaging is logistically difficult. The most consistent radiologic feature associated with pupillary changes has been compression of both lateral perimesencephalic cisterns on CT scan (53). Thus, the clinician relies on an integration of clinical signs, laboratory values, ICP monitoring, and imaging studies. *Pupillary dilatation* is considered an indisputable sign of grave progression. It is the hallmark of "herniation" and is classically attributed to compression of the third nerve by the advancing uncus of the temporal lobe. However, some pathologic studies show no compression of the third nerve by the uncus, but rather stretching of the nerve over bony structures caused predominantly by horizontal movement of the midbrain, above the tentorium (54).

Systemic Hypertension as a Sign of Intracranial Hypertension and the Cushing Response (Reflex)

Hypertension that frequently accompanies intracranial catastrophes is caused by a generalized sympathoadrenal response at the time of the ictus or injury. In most instances, blood pressure gradually declines to premorbid levels over hours to days. This acute elevation in blood pressure is not predicated on the classic Cushing response, which is usually a late-stage phenomenon associated with markedly elevated ICP and herniation.

The features of the Cushing response are bradycardia, hypertension, and shallow breathing. Acute distortion of the lower brainstem and the firing of mechanoreceptors on the medullary surfaces appear to be the unifying mechanism in experimental work. The distortion is usually the result of a supratentorial mass. However, patients with evolving posterior fossa masses, such as cerebellar infarction, may exhibit similar features. Often

in that case the hypertension precedes bradycardia and may resemble the sympathoadrenal discharge of acute injury. A role for increased pressure that is transmitted to the medullary tegmentum via the ventricular system also has been proposed.

Plateau Waves of Lundberg

Several additional periodic and transient changes in ICP occur under pathologic conditions and, like the ICP pulse pressure, they are amplified when there is poor intracranial compliance (55). The most threatening elevations of this sort are "plateau waves," Lundberg "A-waves," to be distinguished from "B-waves" of the pulse and "C-waves" of respiration. They consist of 5- to 20-minute elevations in ICP, often to levels of 30 to 60 mm Hg, seemingly spontaneous but occasionally precipitated by stimulation such as tracheal suctioning (56). Plateau waves may coincide with headache, vomiting, and obtundation in the conscious patient with raised ICP. The unconscious patient may exhibit pupillary dilatation, systemic hypertension, bradycardia, and posturing during a plateau wave; or the waves may occur in the absence of any additional clinical signs (57). The origin of plateau waves is not entirely clear, but most experimental work relates them to cerebral vasodilation as a result of an abnormal sympathetic response of cerebral vessels. One series of observations suggests that they are incited by episodes of mild, often unnoticed, systemic hypotension that leads to cerebral vasodilatation and increased CBV (58).

NORMAL LEVELS OF INTRACRANIAL PRESSURE

Intracranial pressure in a supine individual normally is less than 10 mm Hg when measured at the level of the foramen of Monro (often referenced to the tragus of the ear) (59,60). When the head is elevated, ICP normally falls as CSF moves from the cranial to the spinal spaces. Intracranial pressure oscillates with the systemic arterial blood pressure and respiration, imparting both a ballistic waveform that follows the arterial pulse and a slower fluctuation with spontaneous or positive pressure ventilation (60). Maneuvers that increase central venous pressure (e.g., coughing and straining, congestive heart failure) increase ICP because valves do not effectively separate the cerebral venous system from the central venous system. Turning the head to the side can impair jugular venous drainage and increase ICP in circumstances of poor intracranial compliance.

The pressure is equally distributed throughout the craniospinal axis under normal conditions largely as a result of free communication of the CSF. Obstruction of this communication caused by mass lesions or tissue shifts commonly occurs at multiple levels; at communication points between the ventricles (Foramen of Monroe, cerebral aqueduct), at the outflow of CSF from the fourth ventricle (Foramina of Lusaka and Magendie), or within the extracerebral and spinal subarachnoid space. In addition, mass lesions commonly produce pressure gradients between compartments that are divided by dural reflections, the falx and tentorium. An intracranial pressure monitor gives information about pressure in one compartment that may not reflect the circumstances throughout the cranium. Pressure gradients between the two hemispheres as large as 15 mm Hg have been reported in the presence of unilateral mass lesions (61). (See discussion that follows regarding location of ICP monitors.)

REFERENCES

1. Fenstermacher JD. Flow of water and solutes across the blood-brain barrier. In: Dacey RG Jr., ed. *Trauma of the central nervous system.* New York: Raven Press, 1985:123–140.
2. Lyons MK, Meyer FB. Cerebrospinal fluid physiology and the management of increased intracranial pressure. *Mayo Clin Proc* 1990;65:684–707.
3. Rubin RC, Henderson ES, Ommaya AK, et al. The production of cerebrospinal fluid in man and its modification by acetazolamide. *J Neurosurg* 1966;25:430–436.
4. Clausen T, Bullock R. Medical treatment and neuroprotection in traumatic brain injury. *Curr Pharm Des* 2001; 7:1517–1532.
5. Shapiro HM. Intracranial hypertension: therapeutic and anesthetic considerations. *Anesthesiology* 1975;43: 445–471.
6. Mchedlishvili G. Pathogenetic role of circulatory factors in brain edema development. *Neurosurg Rev* 1988; 11:7–13.
7. Durward QJ, Del Maestro RF, Amacher AL, et al. The influence of systemic arterial pressure and intracranial pressure on the development of cerebral vasogenic edema. *J Neurosurg* 1983;59:803–809.
8. Siesjo BK, ed. *Brain energy metabolism.* New York: John Wiley & Sons, 1978.
9. Lassen NA, Christensen MS. Physiology of cerebral blood flow. *Br J Anaesthesiol* 1976;48:719–734.
10. Lassen NA, Agnoli A. Upper limits of autoregulation of cerebral blood flow on the pathogenesis of hypertensive encephalopathy. *Scand J Clin Lab Invest Suppl* 1972;30: 113–121.
11. Reed G, Devous M. Cerebral blood flow autoregulation and hypertension. *Am J Med Sci* 1985;289:37–44.
12. Paulson OB, Strandgaard S, Edvinsson L. Cerebral autoregulation. *Cerebrovasc Brain Metab Rev* 1990;2: 161–192.
13. Barry DI, Lassen NA. Cerebral blood flow autoregulation in hypertension and effects of antihypertensive drugs. *J Hypertens* 1984;2:S519–S526.
14. Aaslid R, Lindegaard KF, Sorteberg W, et al. Cerebral autoregulation dynamics in humans. *Stroke* 1989;20: 45–52.
15. Strandgaard S. Autoregulation of cerebral blood flow in hypertensive patients. *Circulation* 1976;53:720–727.
16. Bill A, Liner J, Linder M. Sympathetic effect on cerebral blood flow vessels in acute arterial hypertension. *Acta Physiol Scand* 1976;96:27A.
17. Bleyart AL, Sands PA, Safar P, et al. Augmentation of postischemic brain damage by intermittent hypertension. *Crit Care Med* 1980;8:41–47.
18. Bouma GJ, Muizelaar JP. Cerebral blood flow, cerebral blood volume, and cerebrovascular reactivity after severe head injury. [Review]. *J Neurotrauma* 1992;9: S333–348.
19. Bouma GJ, Muizelaar JP, Bandoh K, et al. Blood pressure and intracranial pressure-volume dynamics in severe head injury: relationship with cerebral blood flow. *J Neurosurg* 1992;77:15–19.
20. Nemoto EM, Snyder JV, Carroll RG, et al. Global ischemia in dogs: cerebrovascular CO_2 reactivity and autoregulation. *Stroke* 1975;6:425–431.
21. Strandgaard S, Paulson OB. Regulation of cerebral blood flow in health and disease. *J Cardiovasc Pharmacol* 1992;19:S89–S93.
22. Grubb RL, Raichle MW, Phelps ME, et al. Effects of increased intracranial pressure on cerebral blood volume blood flow and oxygen utilization in monkeys. *J Neurosurg* 1975;43:385–394.
23. Miller JD, Stanek A, Langfitt TW. Concepts of cerebral perfusion pressure and vascular compression during intracranial hypertension. *Prog Brain Res* 1972;35: 411–419.
24. Todd MM, Wu B, Warner DS. The hemispheric cerebrovascular response to hemodilution is attenuated by a focal cryogenic brain injury. *J Neurotrauma* 1994;11: 149–160.
25. Siesjo BK, Carlsson C, Hagerdal M, et al. Brain metabolism in the critically ill. *Crit Care Med* 1976;4: 283–294.

26. Siesjo BK. Hypoxia. In: *Brain energy metabolism.* New York: John Wiley & Sons, 1978:398–452.

27. Albrecht RF, Miletich DJ, Ruttle M. Cerebral effects of extended hyperventilation in unanesthetized goats. *Stroke* 1987;18:649–655.

28. Gulati SC, Sood SC, Bali IM, et al. Cerebral metabolism following brain injury. I. Acid-base and pO_2 changes. *Acta Neurochirurg* 1980;53:39–46.

29. Lassen NA, Christensen MS. Physiology of cerebral blood flow. *Br J Anaesthesiol* 1976;48:719–734.

30. Wilson DF, Pastuszko A, DiGiacomo JE, et al. Effect of hyperventilation on oxygenation of the brain cortex of newborn piglets. *J Appl Physiol* 1991;70:2691–2696.

31. Harper AM, Glass HI. Effect of alterations in arterial carbon dioxide tension on the blood flow though the cerebral cortex at normal and low arterial blood pressure. *J Neurol Neurosurg Psychiatry* 1965;28:449–462.

32. Leech P, Miller JD. Intracranial volume-pressure relationships during experimental brain compression in primates: effect of induced changes in systematic arterial pressure and cerebral blood flow. *J Neurol Neurosurg Psychiatry* 1974;37:1099–1104.

33. Koehler RC, Traystman RJ. Bicarbonate ion modulation of cerebral blood flow during hypoxia and hypercapnia. *Am J Physiol* 1982;243:H33–H40.

34. McDowall DG, Harper AM. CBF and CSF pH in the monkey during prolonged hypocapnia. *Scand J Clin Lab Invest Suppl* 1968;102:VIII:E.

35. Skinhoj E. CBF adaptation in man to chronic hypo and hypercapnia and its relation to CSF pH. *Scand J Clin Lab Invest Suppl* 1968;102:VIIIA.

36. Agnoli A. Adaptation of CBF during induced chronic normoxic respiratory acidosis. *Scand J Clin Lab Invest Suppl* 1968;102:VIIID.

37. Christensen MS, Paulson OB, Olesen J, et al. Cerebral apoplexy (stroke) treated with or without prolonged artificial hyperventilation: 1. Cerebral circulation, clinical course, and cause of death. *Stroke* 1973;4:568–619.

38. Diringer MN, Videen TO, Yundt K, et al. Regional cerebrovascular and metabolic effects of hyperventilation after severe traumatic brain injury. *J Neurosurg* 2002;96:103–108.

39. Clasen RA, Pandolfi I, Liang I, et al. Experimental study of relation of fever to cerebral edema. *J Neurosurg* 1974;41:516–558.

40. Carlsson A, Hagerdal M, Seisjo BK. The effect of hyperthermia upon oxygen consumption and upon organic phosphates glycolytic metabolites, citric acid cycle intermediates and associated amino acids in rat cerebral cortex. *J Neurochem* 1976;26:1001–1036.

41. Frewen TC, Sumabat WO, Han VK, et al. Effects of hyperventilation, hypothermia, and altered blood viscosity on cerebral blood flow, cross-brain oxygen extraction, and cerebral metabolic rate for oxygen in cats. *Crit Care Med* 1989;17:912–916.

42. Muizelaar JP, Wei EP, Kontos HA, et al. Mannitol causes compensatory cerebral vasoconstriction and vasodilation in response to blood viscosity changes. *J Neurosurg* 1983;59:822–828.

43. Muizelaar JP, Wei EP, Kontos HA, et al. Cerebral blood flow is regulated by changes in blood pressure and in blood viscosity alike. *Stroke* 1986;17:44–48.

44. Heiss WD, Rosner G. Functional recovery of cortical neurons as related to degree and duration of ischemia. *Ann Neurol* 1983;14:294–301.

45. Altman DI, Lich LL, Powers WJ. Brief inhalation method to measure cerebral oxygen extraction fraction with PET: accuracy determination under pathologic conditions. *J Nucl Med* 1991;32:1738–1741.

46. Frewen TC, Sumabat WO, Han VK, et al. Effects of hyperventilation, hypothermia, and altered blood viscosity on cerebral blood flow, cross-brain oxygen extraction, and cerebral metabolic rate for oxygen in cats. *Crit Care Med* 1989;17:912–916.

47. Carpenter DA, Grubb RL Jr, Tempel LW, et al. Cerebral oxygen metabolism after aneurysmal subarachnoid hemorrhage. *J Cereb Blood Flow Metab* 1991;11:837–844.

48. Powers WJ, Grubb RL Jr, Raichle ME. Physiologic responses to focal cerebral ischemia in humans. *Ann Neurol* 1984;16:546–552.

49. Powers WJ, Grubb RL Jr, Darriet D, et al. Cerebral blood flow and cerebral metabolic rate of oxygen requirements for cerebral function and viability in humans. *J Cereb Blood Flow Metab* 1985;5:600–608.

50. Carpenter DA, Grubb RL Jr, Powers WJ. Border zone hemodynamics in cerebrovascular disease. *Neurology* 1990;40:1587–1592.

51. Ropper AH. Lateral displacement of the brain and level of consciousness in patients with an acute hemispheral mass. *N Engl J Med* 1986;314:953–958.

52. Plum F, Posner JB. *The diagnosis of stupor and coma.* Philadelphia: FA Davis Comp., 1980.

53. Toutant SM, Klauber MR, Marshall LF, et al. Absent or compressed basal cisterns on first CT scan: ominous predictors of outcome in severe head injury. *J Neurosurg* 1984;61:691–694.

54. Ropper AH, Cole D, Louis DN. Clinicopathologic correlation in a case of pupillary dilation from cerebral hemorrhage. *Arch Neurol* 1991;48:1166–1169.

55. Nornes H, Aaslid R, Lindegaard KF. Intracranial pulse pressure dynamics in patients with intracranial hypertension. *Acta Neurochir (Wien)* 1977;38:177–186.

56. Hanlon K. Description and uses of intracranial pressure monitoring. *Heart Lung* 1976;5:277–282.

57. Bruce DA, Berman WA, Schut L. Cerebrospinal fluid pressure monitoring in children: physiology, pathology and clinical usefulness. *Adv Pediatr* 1977;24:233–290.

58. Rosner MJ, Becker DP. Origin and evolution of plateau waves. Experimental observations and a theoretical model. *J Neurosurg* 1984;60:312–324.

59. Beks JW. Increased intracranial pressure. *Clin Neurol Neurosurg* 1977;79:245–252.

60. Bradley KC. Cerebrospinal fluid pressure. *J Neurol Neurosurg Psychiatry* 1970;33:387–397.

61. Sahuquillo J, Poca MA, Arribas M, et al. Interhemispheric supratentorial intracranial pressure gradients in head-injured patients: are they clinically important? *J Neurosurg* 1999;90:16–26.

3

Management of Intracranial Hypertension and Mass Effect

For several decades, the management of intracranial hypertension has been a major focus of neurological and neurosurgical critical care. The concepts of intracranial pressure (ICP) monitoring and treatment were first developed in patients with head injuries and later applied to a wider range of disorders. The focus of ICP management has evolved over time. Initially, attention centered only on lowering ICP. Later ICP was treated in relation to blood pressure (BP) and cerebral perfusion pressure (CPP). In addition, the importance of pressure gradients within the intracranial vault that produce the tissue shifts and clinical deterioration discussed in Chapter 2 has been widely recognized.

The rationale for treating increased ICP or reduced CPP is based on the concept that either one eventually leads to cerebral hypoperfusion and global cerebral ischemia. Although this may be the case in the final stages of many disease processes, this concept leaves many questions unanswered. If critical reductions in CPP are the cause of ischemic damage why not raise BP to counteract the effects of elevated ICP? How can hyperventilation, which directly reduces cerebral blood flow (CBF), be useful in treating cerebral hypoperfusion? Why do treatments designed to lower ICP also reverse herniation syndromes that occur while ICP and CPP are normal? In the final analysis, although not questioning the deleterious effects of raised ICP, it has been difficult to prove that aggressive medical treatment improves outcome. Despite these polemic issues, few doubt that treatment of raised ICP in many circumstances is appropriate; it is the timing, method of monitoring, and specific treatments that are constantly under discussion.

The medical treatment of elevated ICP employs strategies that are designed to reduce the contents of the intracranial vault by reducing CSF, blood, and brain volume (largely water content). Surgical approaches remove the mass that is the proximate cause of raised ICP or decompress the cranium by removing a portion of the skull. These interventions treat both pressure gradients and tissue shifts. None of these interventions is used in isolation but rather in an integrated fashion designed to address the individual circumstances.

The physiology of the intracranial vault is reviewed in the previous chapter; this discussion of treatment builds on those principles. Each intervention is discussed individually and then an approach to combining them into an integrated treatment plan is presented. It is clear that the clinician is often faced with decisions for which there is insufficient evidence to indicate a clear course of action. The ultimate treatment plan often must be developed based on a combination of data, institutional bias, individual experience, and most importantly ongoing assessment of how the patient responds to any given intervention.

INDICATIONS FOR INTRACRANIAL PRESSURE MONITORING AND TREATMENT

The goal of intervention may be to reduce ICP, improve CPP, or mitigate the effects of tissue shifts. To meet the first two goals ICP monitoring is necessary in order to guide therapy. In the treatment of the parallel problem of intracranial tissue shifts, however, ICP monitoring is not necessary and may be falsely reassuring because clinical signs of herniation can develop while ICP remains normal (1,2). The response to treatment when dealing with tissue shifts only can be monitored with serial clinical examinations and imaging studies.

The value of ICP monitoring lies in its ability to reflect compromised cerebral perfusion, monitor for deterioration in difficult-to-assess patients, prevent iatrogenic elevations in ICP, provide prognostic information, and assess the response to treatment. Monitoring should be considered for any patient in whom it can be surmised that intracranial compliance is reduced and ICP might be elevated, and in processes known to be associated with delayed or progressive intracranial hypertension. Indications for ICP monitoring (Table 3.1) have been most studied in severe traumatic brain injury (TBI) and in which evidence-based guidelines have been published (3) and later revised (4–9).

These guidelines by their specific reference to traumatic lesions are of limited value in other diseases. The natural history of ICP changes in other conditions is not as well understood owing to a lack of data from routine ICP monitoring. In general, a Glasgow Coma Scale (GCS) score of 8 or less in the context of a large intracranial mass and radiographically observed tissue shifts has been used as an indication to instituting ICP monitoring because it is presumed that the degree of tissue shift reflected by a poor clinical state is likely be associated with increased ICP. Computed tomography (CT) signs that suggest (but by no means assure) the presence of elevated ICP include: obliteration of sulci of the cerebral hemisphere and, more sensitively, of the basal cisterns (10); tissue shifts across the midline; and hydrocephalus.

Another, albeit indirect indication for monitoring, arises when it becomes necessary to sedate a patient to a degree that limits neurological assessment or where an intervention may itself increase ICP (e.g., weaning of hyperventilation, general anesthesia for systemic surgery, etc.). In some circumstances the insertion of a ventricular catheter has therapeutic benefit by draining CSF while it is used for monitoring. Finally, ICP measurement can provide important prognostic information in certain conditions (11,12).

Medical and surgical measures to lower ICP are also effective in reducing tissue shifts and herniation. This statement is supported by the empiric observation that the clinical findings of herniation may improve, even if transiently, with these interventions and indeed, rapid improvement in these findings is the strongest indication of survival (13). These clinical improvements may be substantial and sustained as a recent observational study demonstrated (14). The mechanism responsible for clinical improvement is not entirely understood but is presumed to be the obvious one; namely, that the degree of tissue displacement and distortion is reduced.

TABLE 3.1. *Indications for intracranial pressure monitoring in severe head injury (Glasgow Coma Scale <9)*

Abnormal CT scan (hematoma, contusion, edema, compressed basal cisterns
Normal CT scan and two or more of the following:
  Age >40
  Unilateral or bilateral motor posturing
  Systolic blood pressure <90 mm Hg

From McDowell ME, Wolf AV, Steer A. Osmotic volumes of distribution. Idiogenic changes in osmotic pressure associated with administration of hypertonic solutions. *Am J Physiol* 1955;180:545–558, with permission.

For clinical purposes, ICP is usually measured in the supratentorial compartment. It also can be assessed from the lumbar subarachnoid space if free communication exists among brain compartments, but lumbar recordings may be inaccurate because of the distensibility of the spinal subarachnoid space. Continuous lumbar recording has found its main use in cases of pseudotumor cerebri. If intracranial mass lesions or noncommunicating hydrocephalus are present, this procedure, or course, can be dangerous and may result in the downward herniation of brain structures.

Practical Aspects of Intracranial Pressure Monitoring

Location

Invasive ICP monitoring devices can be placed in extradural, subdural, intraparenchymal, intraventricular, or intraspinal locations. Extradural and subdural devices are now infrequently used since the readings are not always reliable, primarily as a result of technical limitations of the devices. When the ventricles are of sufficient size many clinicians prefer the use of ventricular catheters because they provide the added ability to treat elevated ICP.

The decision about where to place an intraparenchymal device can be problematic. All other issues aside the preferred location is the right frontal lobe because it is felt that placing the catheter tip in that region does the least clinical ascertainable damage. However, when a mass lesion is present the issue is more complicated. It is not uncommon to measure a pressure gradient between the two hemispheres if monitors are placed bilaterally (15,16). There is little guidance in the literature and in most studies of ICP there was no consistent placement of monitors ipsilateral or contralateral to mass lesions. When using a monitor to define the ICP and CPP goals of therapy it is important to take into account whether the monitor is ipsilateral or contralateral to the mass lesion, and consider modifying treatment thresholds accordingly.

Types of Monitoring Devices, Their Advantages and Disadvantages

The gold standard for ICP measurement remains a ventricular catheter coupled to an external transducer through a continuous column of fluid in low compliance tubing. The setup is identical to those used for arterial and pulmonary artery pressure monitoring. (A similar apparatus also can be used to monitor pressure from the spinal subarachnoid space.) In the late 1970s and early 1980s a hollow bolt ("Richmond bolt" or screw) that was screwed into the skull and communicated directly with the subarachnoid space was popular but not always reliable. A number of more modern devices have been introduced in which the transducer is placed inside the skull and the pressure measurement transmitted to an electronic interface via a fiberoptic or electrical cable.

Each of these systems has inherent advantages and special problems. Fluid coupled systems allow the transducer to be rezeroed periodically after placement, thus avoiding inaccurate measurements owing to drift of the electromechanical transducer. This is not possible with implantable transducers, the only means of rezeroing and calibration being removal and reinsertion. (Drift was an important concern with earlier versions of implantable transducers and it was recommended that the devices be changed every few days; as the technology has improved this has become less of an issue.) Fluid coupled systems also require that the integrity of the fluid column be maintained in order to have accurate readings. The column must be contained within semirigid noncompliant tubing. Air bubbles within the column dampen the waveform and result in underestimation of the pressure. In addition, the catheter can become clogged with clot or debris, resulting in inaccurate readings. Implantable transducers do not suffer from these limitations but the older fiberoptic cables were subject to breakage and signal loss. The greatest drawback to fluid-coupled systems is the potential for infection that gains access to the cranium through the inner and outer surfaces of the connecting tubes.

Additionally, when using an external transducer it must be physically level with the site of the desired pressure measurement. Common locations include the vertex, brow, or tragus. The tragus is frequently chosen as an indicator of midventricular level. Any change in the height of the patient's head with respect to the transducer requires a repetition of the leveling process. Affixing the transducer to the side of the patient's head may avoid inaccuracies caused by changes in head height; however, head rotation then can introduce a similar error. With implantable systems, the transducer is zeroed to atmospheric pressure once, just prior to insertion and it is then placed in the compartment of interest. This arrangement allows for accurate pressure readings regardless of head position.

Complications

The two major complications of ICP monitoring are intracranial hemorrhage and infection. Both are extremely rare when using implantable transducers. The incidence of major hemorrhage with intraventricular catheters is on the order of 1% to 2% and has been attributed to coagulopathy or difficulty with catheter placement.

Intraventricular catheters carry a small but significant risk of ventriculitis, the reported incidence ranging from 4% to 10% (17,18). Many centers routinely administer antibiotics prior to placement of an intraventricular catheter (IVC) and continue to administer them in an attempt to prevent infection. The choice of agents varies widely, ranging from agents specifically directed at skin flora to broad-spectrum antibiotics. The efficacy of prophylactic antibiotics has not been established and recent nonrandomized controlled studies have failed to demonstrate any such benefit (19,20). Prophylactic antibiotics are usually not administered when implantable devices are inserted.

Several factors are thought to increase the risk of infection with the use of IVCs. Early on, it was identified that the duration of monitoring was the major risk factor and the infection rate was seen to rise exponentially after 5 to 7 days (17). More recent experience with use of catheters tunneled under the scalp has called this observation into question. Now it is common to leave catheters in place up to 2 to 3 weeks if they are carefully handled by experienced personnel. Another important risk factor for infection appears to be the number of times that the integrity of the system is violated, either inadvertently, or in order to sample the CSF or flush debris or clot through the tubing. Because the best means of monitoring for and identifying infection is through sampling CSF, this observation presents a dilemma. A compromise is reached in some centers by routinely sampling CSF every other day to monitor for infection, whereas others do so only in the presence of fever or if the catheter is to be left in place for a prolonged period of time. Interpretation of laboratory analysis of CSF samples to look for signs of ventriculitis can be difficult. Many patients have blood mixed in the CSF. In addition, there is often an inflammatory reaction to the catheter, blood in the CSF, or as part of the disease process that is difficult to distinguish from an inflammatory response to an infection. Therefore, the most useful components of the CSF analysis when evaluating for ventriculitis are the glucose concentration, Gram stain, and culture.

An IVC easily can become obstructed with clot in the presence of intraventricular hemorrhage. This situation is evident as a steady rise in ICP over hours, loss of the ballistic waveform, and an inability to drain CSF out of the catheter. Flushing the catheter with preservative-free saline frequently solves the problem, but infection risk is raised and reobstruction is common, especially in the presence of substantial amounts of intraventricular blood. The instillation of thrombolytic agents has been suggested in this situation but obviously carries the risk of recurrent hemorrhage. The safety and efficacy of this maneuver is currently under investigation (21,22). It is important to note that failure of CSF drainage in the setting of rising ICP also can result from poor catheter positioning, displacement of the catheter from the ventricular system because of tissue shifts or collapse of the ventricles from overdrainage. These possibilities can be evaluated through the use of imaging studies.

PHYSIOLOGIC APPROACHES TO THE TREATMENT OF RAISED INTRACRANIAL PRESSURE

Cerebral Perfusion Pressure

The initial goal of suspected or known intracranial hypertension is to insure that CPP is not compromised during the evaluation and initiation of treatment (Chapter 2). This holds particularly for avoidance of systemic hypotension, the adverse consequences of which have been best documented in head injury where systolic blood pressures below 90 mm Hg during the first several hours are associated with substantially worse outcome (23). (See also Chapter 12 for a discussion of the management of head injury.) It follows that overzealous treatment of systemic hypertension should be avoided in the setting of suspected intracranial hypertension.

The optimal CPP in the setting of elevated ICP is not known. Cerebral autoregulation maintains a nearly constant CBF over a CCP range of approximately 50 to 150 mm Hg in normal adults. As noted in Chapter 2, autoregulation is disrupted in a number of pathologic states, including stroke, head injury, and subarachnoid hemorrhage (24–27). The loss of autoregulation causes CBF to become pressure passive (i.e., CBF varies with CPP). The best data regarding the minimum tolerable CPP come again from TBI. Several studies have suggest improved outcome when CPP is maintained above 70 mm Hg (12,28,29). However, more recent studies using intermediate physiologic measurements such as CBF and brain tissue P_{O_2} have indicated that ad-

verse changes occur at a more conservative level of CPP below 50 to 60 mm Hg (3,31).

It is apparent from the preceding comments that the relationship between BP and ICP is complex. When autoregulation is preserved, systemic hypotension causes cerebrovascular vasodilation and an increase in CBV, which in turn can raise ICP if intracranial compliance is poor. Similarly, an elevation of BP produces cerebrovascular vasoconstriction, potentially reducing ICP through a decrease in blood volume. However, as noted, autoregulation is frequently disturbed following brain injuries (25–27); in these cases ICP may vary in parallel with BP. The recommendations for the clinicians can be summarized as a need for close attention to manipulations of BP and ICP because their interaction is potentially deleterious but at the same time unpredictable. As a general rule, extremes of BP are avoided but the precise limits of these extremes cannot be stated with confidence. It may be more appropriate not to manage BP in isolation but to manipulate BP to achieve a target CPP in the range of 60 to 80 mm Hg (see the following).

Intracranial Pressure Versus Cerebral Perfusion Pressure Management

From the preceding comments (and Chapter 2), controversy exists regarding the appropriate parameter to guide the management of patients with severe TBI, ICP, or CPP. In a randomized prospective trial CBF- and ICP-targeted management protocols were compared (32). The CBF-targeted protocol was designed to achieve optimal CBF, through treatment of elevated ICP and the elevation of BP to maintain a CPP greater than 70 mm Hg. The ICP-targeted protocol focused on control of ICP and did not raise BP unless CPP fell below 50 mm Hg. The CBF-targeted protocol reduced the frequency of oxygen desaturation in jugular venous blood samples (used in this study as a surrogate for cerebral ischemia), but there was no difference in neurological outcome. Interpretation of these results was confounded by a fivefold increase in the frequency of adult respiratory distress syndrome in the CBF-targeted protocol that offset any benefit in cerebral protection.

Other data suggest that a CPP of 50 mm Hg is adequate. When monitoring brain tissue Po_2 using commercially available probes, brain tissue oxygen pressure remains fairly steady until CPP falls below a threshold of 50 to 60 mm Hg (31,33). This also suggests that the CPP threshold below which cerebral oxygen delivery is compromised is closer to 50 than 70 mm Hg.

Many clinicians choose to modify treatment based on both ICP and CPP. In this approach, CPP is maintained above a threshold (approximately 60 mm Hg) at all times by raising BP and at the same time ICP is treated if it exceeds 20 to 25 mm Hg.

Threshold for Treatment of Raised Intracranial Pressure

The appropriate level for treatment of elevated ICP has been studied best in head injury; presumably, the same general principles apply to other conditions. Multivariate analysis of more than 1,000 severely injured patients has indicated that a high proportion of hourly ICP readings greater than 20 mm Hg is an independent predictor of poor outcome (12). It is recommended in the Guidelines for the Management of Severe TBI that active ICP treatment commence when ICP exceeds 20 to 25 mm Hg and that decisions about treatment of elevated ICP take into account serial clinical examinations and CPP (3).

The absolute value of the ICP or CPP should not be the only determinants of treatment. Mass effect with tissue shifts can compress the brainstem without necessarily elevating ICP. Indeed, clinical signs of herniation may occur in stroke patients before ICP becomes elevated (1,11). Similarly, herniation can occur with a normal ICP in TBI and ICH (2,34). Compression or obliteration of the basal cisterns is associated with poor outcome in head injury (35) and ICH (36) independent of ICP.

Patients who have a rapidly deteriorating neurological examination or clinical signs of herniation (dilated pupil and posturing)

should be empirically and aggressively treated while undergoing further diagnostic studies along with placement of an ICP monitor. Continued treatment for suspected increased ICP without a monitor or for minor tissue shifts should be undertaken with caution because no intervention is without risk.

GENERAL MEASURES FOR THE TREATMENT OF RAISED INTRACRANIAL PRESSURE

A number of routine medical and nursing interventions have a substantial impact on ICP. It is important that all personnel involved in the care of critically ill neurological and neurosurgical patients be thoroughly familiar with the principles that guide patient management and develop appropriate routine practices (Table 3.2). The following discussion ad-

TABLE 3.2. *Routine measures for patients at risk for intracranial hypertension*

Mechanical ventilation
  Premedicate for intubation *with* ultra–short-acting intravenous anesthetic agents
  Avoid hypoxia and hypercarbia
  Use PEEP as needed to maintain oxygenation
  Watch for CO_2 retention with sedation
  If suctioning of chest physiotherapy causes plateau waves, premedicate with intravenous lidocaine (0.5–1.0 mg/kg), thiopental (~1–3 mg/kg) or etomidate (~0.1–0.3 mg/kg)
Patient positioning
  Elevate head of bed—optimal height variable determine for each patient
  Avoid jugular compression
    Neck in neutral position
    Avoid constricting endotracheal tube and tracheostomy tube ties
Blood pressure
  Treat CPP below 60–70 mm Hg with vasopressors and correction of hypovolemia
  Avoid CPP >90–100 mm Hg—consider antihypertensives
Treat fever aggressively
Prophylactic anticonvulsants when appropriate
Fluid and electrolytes
  Avoid excessive free water, no hypotonic fluids
  Maintain normal volume status
  Encourage hyperosmolar state with 1.25%–3% saline and/or induce free water clearance with diuretics or mannitol

CPP, cerebral perfusion pressure; PEEP, positive end-expiratory pressure.

dresses the management of medical problems and intensive care unit interventions that impinge on ICP. This management is a prelude to the active treatments of raised ICP that are elaborated on in the next section.

Aspects of Respiratory Physiology and Intubation

The initiation and use of mechanical ventilation can raise ICP during intubation as a result of transiently inadequate oxygenation, CO_2 retention, coughing, use of positive end-expiratory pressure (PEEP) and during suctioning. The latter two maneuvers cause increased intrathoracic pressures to be transmitted to the cranial cavity through venous and CSF pathways.

Hypoxia and hypercarbia are potent cerebral vasodilators that can have profound effects on ICP, particularly when intracranial compliance is poor. Avoiding these detrimental circumstances requires constant assessment of respiratory status as well as careful attention to maneuvers that could raise P_{CO_2} or impair oxygenation, such as sedation, weaning mechanical ventilation, and suctioning. Continuous measurement of arterial oxygen saturation end expiratory carbon dioxide concentration is appropriate in virtually all circumstances of raised ICP.

Several factors conspire to raise ICP during intubation: hypoxia, hypercarbia, and direct tracheal stimulation (37). Etomidate is effective in blocking this reflex (38). Intravenous (i.v.) lidocaine (1.0 to 1.5 mg/kg) also has been recommended (39), although data supporting its use are lacking (40). In addition, short-acting i.v. anesthetic agents (thiopental 1 to 5 mg/kg or etomidate 0.1 to 0.5 mg/kg) also reduce brain metabolic rate and theoretically improve tolerance of a transient fall in CPP should it occur. Etomidate generally is preferred over thiopental because it is less likely to lower blood pressure.

The use of PEEP has long been a concern in patients with raised ICP. Although the pulmonary benefits of PEEP are clear, the risk, in terms of further elevation of ICP is largely theoretical for several reasons. Increases in PEEP and mean airway pressure certainly can be transmitted to the thoracic venous and CSF compartments and ultimately to the intracranial vault (41). The pressure transmitted from the airways and lungs to other thoracic structures depends on pulmonary compliance in large part. The effect on ICP is minimal in situations where high levels of PEEP are most likely to be used (a patient with stiff, poorly compliant lungs) (42,43). In most circumstances of serious respiratory failure combined with the presence of an intracranial mass, the detrimental effects of hypoxia almost always outweigh the theoretical risks of using higher levels of PEEP. Thus, it seems prudent not to forego its use simply because of raised ICP. Of course, direct measurement of ICP allows one to gauge the impact of PEEP and various other respiratory settings providing the means to optimize PEEP to achieve adequate oxygen saturation while avoiding a negative impact on ICP.

Coughing that arises spontaneously or in response to suctioning or chest physiotherapy is known to raise ICP momentarily by 30 to 40 mm Hg even in normal individuals (Fig. 3.1). In brain-injured patients coughing, or even tracheal manipulation without inducing a response, may cause a more sustained and greater rise (if compliance is poor), and may induce plateau waves that can markedly reduce CPP. One effective way to prevent stimulating a further rise in ICP is to suppress coughing with intermittent boluses of i.v. li-

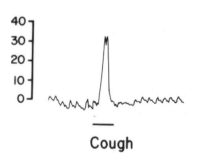

FIG. 3.1. Changes in intracranial pressure with cough.

docaine (0.5 to 1.0 mg/kg), thiopental (approximately 1 to 3 mg/kg), or etomidate (approximately 0.1 to 0.3 mg/kg), which are administered prior to suctioning or chest physiotherapy (44,45). Repeated doses must be used cautiously because they can lead to significant drug accumulation. Furthermore, completely blocking coughing may not be desirable because it may lead to the accumulation of pulmonary secretions, atelectasis, pneumonia, and an inability to effectively manage pulmonary infections. Brief hyperventilation with 100% oxygen before suctioning also may block the rise in ICP caused by tracheal manipulation (46–48).

Patient Positioning

The position of the head and neck influence ICP through a number of mechanisms. In particular, the height of the head relative to the heart influences intracranial arterial and venous pressures. Arterial pressure is reduced as a result of the work necessary to pump blood against gravity to the head and at the same time venous drainage is enhanced. It has been reported that ICP is generally lower when the head of the bed is elevated to 30 degrees compared to the horizontal position (49–51), but these results have been inconsistent. Another analysis has suggested that the optimal degree of head elevation varies from patient to patient and therefore should be determined for each individual (51). A recent study of patients with large stroke and edema found that both ICP and CPP were maximal when the patient was supine (52). They found that the rise in ICP was more than offset by the increase in perfusion pressure caused by the brain and heart being at the same level.

Perhaps more mundane is the problem of compression of the jugular veins by turning of the head or compressing the neck too tightly. Venous drainage can be impaired raising cerebrovenous pressure and ICP. Whether unilateral compression has an adverse effect that is more than transient is not known. On the other hand, compression of both jugular veins causes a slow and progressive rise in ICP that

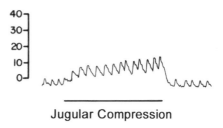

Jugular Compression

FIG. 3.2. Changes in intracranial pressure with jugular compression.

disappears rapidly when compression is released (Fig. 3.2). This response is so consistent that it may be used as a bedside test to assess the functioning of an intracranial ICP monitor (a variant of the Queckenstedt maneuver formerly used to detect spinal block). Therefore, it is imperative to avoid interventions that compress the jugular veins, such as securing an endotracheal or tracheostomy tube too tightly or inserting large catheters into the jugular veins.

Blood Pressure Control

Only broad guidelines can be offered here based on theoretical considerations of autoregulation, ICP, and CPP, as already discussed. If BP is "normal" but CPP is below 60 or 70 mm Hg, BP should be augmented. Raising BP in a euvolemic patient by using fluid infusion is slow, often ineffective, and can result in serious complications such as congestive heart failure, hyponatremia, and worsening of cerebral edema (32). The nature of the fluid used perhaps is of as much importance, as discussed in more detail in the following. The most rapid and consistent therapeutic hypertensive response can be achieved by the use of vasopressor agents such a phenylephrine or dopamine while administering moderate amounts of i.v. fluid (150 to 250 mL/h) if there is coexisting hypovolemia. In addition, several treatments for raised ICP can significantly lower BP through direct hypotensive (barbiturates, propofol) or diuretic (mannitol) effects. It is important to take measures to prevent these problems by replacing urinary losses when using mannitol, and to correct BP by administering vasopressors when faced with drug-induced hypotension.

There has been concern that the use of vasopressors may lead to cerebral vasoconstriction and consequently, cerebral hypoperfusion. When the blood–brain barrier (BBB) is intact, norepinephrine and phenylephrine do not appear to alter CBF (53), but the results are less clear when the barrier is disrupted. Despite this theoretical concern, our clinical experience suggests that vasopressors can be used almost with impunity in instances of raised ICP and that hypotension is to be avoided at all costs. A potential beneficial effect of vasopressors in aborting plateau waves has been discussed already (54).

On the opposite extreme, defining a safe upper limit for BP and CPP is as important and perhaps a more frequent clinical problem in the hours after hemorrhage and stroke. Cerebral edema and hemorrhage may result when the autoregulatory range is exceeded (approximately 150 mm Hg in normotensive adults). Furthermore, autoregulation may be impaired following brain injury, thereby lowering its upper limit (i.e., CBF may rise to extreme levels at modestly elevated levels of blood pressure). Moderate degrees of hypertension are known to worsen edema following brain trauma (55); therefore, caution in allowing hypertension is warranted. Consequently, it is probably prudent to keep CPP less than 90 to 100 mm Hg when elevating BP with vasopressors. If CPP spontaneously exceeds this level, antihypertensive medications should be administered.

Fever

As temperature rises, so does cerebral metabolism and oxygen requirements (56). Hyperthermia also increases CO_2 production and, if mechanical ventilation is not adjusted appropriately in sedated patients, this can lead to hypercarbia and an increase in ICP. Elevated temperature worsens ischemic damage in experimental animals and, conversely, hypothermia is protective (57,58). In clinical work it has been found that fever is an inde-

pendent predictor of poor outcome in patients with ischemic stroke (59–63). Thus, although control of fever has yet to be shown to improve outcome in circumstances of raised ICP, it seems prudent to take measures to reduce it; antipyretics are routinely administered to febrile patients with CNS insults. Unfortunately, agents such as acetaminophen and surface cooling with air blankets often are ineffective in reducing fever (64). Anecdotal experience suggests that other antipyretics such as ibuprofen may be more effective, but they carry a small risk of bleeding. The use of indomethacin as an antipyretic is appealing because it independently lowers CBF and ICP in head-injured patients (65,66). Recently introduced intravascular cooling devices appear to be highly effective in controlling fever. They operate by circulating cooled saline through a central venous catheter, thereby directly cooling the blood.

The Effect of Seizures on Intracranial Pressure

Even in the absence of overt convulsive activity, seizures profoundly increase cerebral metabolic activity, CBF, and CBV, which can lead to a rise in ICP (55). Although there are sparse data to support their routine use, anticonvulsants are often administered to patients at risk for seizures, including those with traumatic brain injury (3), subarachnoid hemorrhage (67), and intracerebral hemorrhage (ICH) involving cortical structures (68). Phenytoin is generally preferred because it can be administered parenterally and is rarely sedating. A second nonsedating parenteral anticonvulsant, valproic acid, is now available, but experience is limited.

Management of Fluids and Osmolality

Over the years there has been a considerable evolution regarding the appropriate fluid management for patients with elevated ICP. For some time, the dogma had been "dryer is better." Fluids were severely restricted and diuretics were administered to the point of inducing renal insufficiency and sometimes hypotension. Over the past decade, as the desirability of maintaining adequate CPP has become apparent, emphasis has shifted toward avoiding dehydration and administering fluids to maintain BP and thus improve CPP while avoiding serum hyposmolarity (see the following). In parallel, our understanding of the mechanisms responsible for hyponatremia, and the approach to its treatment has changed also. For many years hyponatremia was attributed routinely to the syndrome of inappropriate secretion of antidiuretic hormone (SIADH) and treated by fluid restriction. Overall fluid restriction has fallen out of favor with the growing recognition that "cerebral salt wasting" owing to natriuresis was another cause of hyponatremia and the understanding that SIADH can be effectively managed by restricting free water, but not limiting isotonic fluids (69).

When assessing the impact of fluid management on ICP, it is important to consider separately the effects of osmolality and intravascular volume. As the osmolality of the extracellular fluid (ECF) falls, there is an obligatory movement of water into the intracellular compartment, causing cells to expand. This swelling has more of an impact on the brain than other organs because the brain is enclosed in a rigid container. The result is an increase in brain volume and, if intracranial compliance is poor, raised ICP. For this reason, low osmolality should be avoided or rapidly corrected if it develops in patients at risk for elevated ICP.

Limiting the intake of free water is the most practical way to prevent a decline in serum osmolality. Even in the presence of SIADH, restriction of free water can limit or prevent hypo-osmolality. It should be emphasized that virtually all fluids normally taken orally are essentially free water. Other potential sources of free water should be minimized, including hypotonic tube feedings, medications mixed in D_5W, and nasogastric tube flushes with water. The fluids that are permissible in these circumstances are discussed in the following.

A rise in extracellular osmolality causes water to move out of cells and they shrink. This situation, however, is not static. If a hyperosmolar state is maintained, brain cells are believed to raise their intracellular osmolality, in part by increasing intracellular potassium and small proteins. The total rise in osmolality, however, is greater than can be accounted for by measured particles, and the remaining osmols are referred to as "idiogenic osmoles" that act to draw water inward and return the cell size to normal over a period of a few days (70). At this point, any fall in extracellular osmolality results in cellular swelling and rebound cerebral edema. Therefore, it is essential to lower osmolality very slowly over several days in patients who have a sustained rise in serum osmolality.

Changes in ECF volume also can impact brain volume and thus ICP, but to a much lesser degree. Because the brain is mostly made up of intracellular space, large changes in ECF volume are required in order to have any significant impact on cerebral edema (71). Such changes in ECF volume could easily lead to hypovolemia and hypotension, and reduce cerebral perfusion; thus, they not felt to be a useful clinical intervention. Excessive fluid administration could promote cerebral edema through similar mechanisms.

The current approach in patients at risk for elevated ICP or brain tissue shifts (prior to the administration of osmotic dehydrating agents discussed in detail in the following) is to maintain a state of euvolemia with somewhat elevated osmolality. This can be achieved by limiting the administration of free water, administration of sufficient isotonic or slightly hypertonic (1.25% to 2.0% saline) fluids to replace urinary losses, bearing in mind that some free water will be lost through the respiratory system and by diaphoresis.

MEDICAL MANAGEMENT OF INTRACRANIAL HYPERTENSION AND TISSUE SHIFTS

Sedation

A number of sedative medications are effective in reducing ICP. Anxiety, fear, and pain increase cerebral metabolic rate and CBF in normal volunteers (72). In confused, disoriented, or encephalopathic patients, thrashing and "bucking" the ventilator increase intrathoracic and jugular venous pressure and raise ICP. In many such patients, sedation to the point of producing a quiet and motionless state is an effective means of controlling ICP. When using the Ramsey sedation scale (Table 3.3) level 5 or 6 is desirable (see also Pharmacologic Suppression of Brain Metabolism).

A number of approaches to sedation can be used. Drugs can be administered on an as-needed basis in an attempt to minimize the amount of sedative the patient receives. Although some less agitated patients can be controlled with this approach, it carries the risk of losing control of the situation because additional drugs are not given until the patient again begins to show signs of agitation. It may be preferable in many cases to administer regularly scheduled doses or a continuous infusion along with periodic supplementation. This approach, however, limits the clinical assessment of neurological status. For this reason, some centers supplement sedation with monitoring of jugular bulb oxygen saturation, brain tissue oxygen tension, or EEG.

The utility and wisdom of periodically "awakening" patients by stopping sedation for neurological assessment are debated. Short-acting agents can be used in order to facilitate the periodic cessation of medications and allow more complete neurological assessment. In others, it may be more prudent to continue sedation and rely on a limited examination, ICP monitoring, and serial imaging studies.

TABLE 3.3. *Ramsay sedation scale*

Score	Description
1	Anxious, agitated or restless
2	Cooperative, oriented, and tranquil
3	Responds to commands only
4	Asleep, but brisk response to glabellar tap or loud auditory stimulus
5	Asleep, but sluggish response to glabellar tap or loud auditory stimulus
6	No response

Certainly, the main indicators of increasing tissue shifts, such as pupillary enlargement, are not affected much by sedation; very high doses of barbiturates make the pupils small and do not obviate their enlargement with compression of the third nerve or brainstem. On "awakening," some patients become wildly agitated and have marked rises in ICP, which may then become difficult to control. On the other hand, the approach of intermittent awakening has been reported to reduce the duration of mechanical ventilation and ICU length of stay and reduce the number of other tests to assess neurological function (73). The choice of approach should be individualized and take into account the patient's level of agitation, intracranial compliance, and disease process.

The agents most often used for sedation of patients with intracranial hypertension are the benzodiazepines, opioids, and propofol. Midazolam and lorazepam have rather different durations of action when administered intermittently (Table 3.4). When used as a prolonged continuous infusion, the effects of lorazepam clear more quickly because midazolam has long-acting metabolites that may accumulate. Although benzodiazepines are effective and easily managed sedatives, they have no analgesic properties. Therefore, the additional administration of opioid analgesics may be warranted, especially in trauma victims. A combination of morphine, fentanyl, or sufentanil with lorazepam or midazolam is frequently used. More recently, the general anesthetic propofol, 25 to 75 µg/kg per minute, has come into favor for short-term (several hours) sedation because of its very rapid onset and offset. Awakening can be expected within 15 minutes of cessation of the infusion. Its use for longer duration of sedation is less clear because propofol carries risks of hypotension, hepatic dysfunction, metabolic acidosis, excessive calories from fat and delayed offset when used for long periods (74,75). Of note, benzodiazepines, barbiturates, and propofol lowers cerebral metabolic rate, potentially adding some degree of brain protection; opiates, on the other hand do

TABLE 3.4. *Sedatives*

Class	Agent	Action	Initiation of therapy	Maintenance dose	Side effects (all produce respiratory depression)
Benzodiazepines		Anxiolysis and sedation in larger doses			
	Midazolam		2–4 mg i.v. q 5 min, increase as needed and tolerated	Infusion 2–10 mg/h	Hypotension especially with bolus Delayed clearance after infusion
	Lorazepam		2–4 mg i.v. q 15 min, increase as needed and tolerated	Infusion 2–10 mg/h	Propylene glycol toxicity
Opiates		Analgesic and sedation in larger doses			Reduced GI motility
	Fentanyl		50–100 μg i.v. q 5 min Increase as needed and tolerated	25–200 μg/h	
	Morphine		2–10 mg i.v. q 15 min Increase as needed and tolerated	1–10 mg/h	Hypotension
Propofol		Sedation		0.5–6 μg/kg/h	Hypotension Elevated trigylcerides Liver toxicity Metabolic acidosis

GI, gastrointestinal; i.v., intravenous.

not have this effect and fentanyl may increase ICP (76,77). Antipsychotic medications usually are not appropriate during the acute phase of illnesses because they often are unable to provide the degree of sedation necessary, do not suppress cerebral metabolism, and may delay recovery (78).

The use of sedatives has a number of deleterious side effects well known to all physicians. They can produce hypotension, especially in hypovolemic patients. This can be managed by avoiding oversedation, paying careful attention to maintaining euvolemia, and using vasopressors. The respiratory depressant effects of sedation can lead to hypercarbia, cerebral vasodilation, and a rise in ICP. This is prevented by careful attention to ven-

tilator settings and monitoring of end tidal CO_2 concentration. Opiates reduce gastrointestinal motility leading to intolerance of gastric feedings, constipation, and commonly ileus. These problems can be addressed in part by administering agents that promote bowel motility such as metoclopramide, erythromycin, and a stool softener combined with the periodic use of laxatives.

Pharmacologic Paralysis

In the absence of severely compromised pulmonary function and the need for completely controlled mechanical ventilation, there is little use for paralytic agents in the management of elevated ICP and brain tissue shifts. Although these agents are effective in controlling agitation and "bucking" the ventilator, these problems can be handled with appropriate doses of sedatives that do not completely obliterate the neurological examination. Paralytic agents also prevent beneficial coughing, can accumulate in liver or renal disease, and have been linked to critical illness polyneuropathy (79,80). The routine use of paralytics in head-injured patients has been associated with longer length of stay and higher incidence of pneumonia (73). In addition, a recent study has suggested that ICP control is no better with neuromuscular blocking agents than without them (81). The intermittent use of paralytic agents may be helpful when a patient must remain absolutely motionless during dangerous procedures or to eliminate muscle artifact from an EEG study that otherwise would be difficult to interpret. Of course, paralytic agents should not be administrated without sedatives.

Hyperventilation

Therapeutic hyperventilation to reduce arterial CO_2 tension and raise CSF pH (the factor that alters the diameter of cerebral vessels) (82) has played a central role in the management of intracranial hypertension. The ability of acute hyperventilation to reverse herniation syndromes is universally acknowledged. Yet, considerable controversy exists regarding the details of its clinical use. It does not need to be emphasized to those with experience in critical care, but it should be stated for completeness that hypocarbia is achieved by increasing the minute ventilation by increasing the ventilator rate or tidal volume.

Cerebrovascular Response to Hyperventilation

The cerebrovascular response to hyperventilation has been well studied in normal individuals. Acute hyperventilation produces global cerebral vasoconstriction, a decline in CBF and blood volume (83). The relationship between Pa_{CO_2} and CBF is linear over the range of Pa_{CO_2} that occurs in the clinical environment (Fig. 2.3). The reduction in cerebral blood volume, and consequently in total intracranial volume, results in a fall in ICP (84). The fall in CBF also reduces oxygen delivery (defined as CBF × arterial oxygen content), forcing the brain to increase oxygen extraction in order to continue to maintain metabolism (85). The increase in oxygen extraction is manifest as a fall in jugular venous oxygen saturation and oxygen content, and a rise in the a-vDO$_2$ (arterial venous difference in oxygen content); there is also a rise in jugular venous lactate concentration (86) that some have interpreted to represent brain ischemia, although this point remains an area of great controversy (87,88).

A more heterogeneous cerebrovascular response to hyperventilation is seen in brain-injured patients. For example, many patients with subarachnoid hemorrhage (25), and some moribund patients with severe TBI (89), entirely lose the cerebrovascular response to hyperventilation. In the majority of head-injured patients, however, global cerebrovascular CO_2 reactivity is retained (90–92), although there is considerable regional variability (93). Furthermore, the absolute reduction in ICP that might be expected for a given change in Pa_{CO_2} is somewhat unpredictable, depending as it does on the intracranial compliance and the degree of cerebrovascular reactivity. These observations raise a perennial paradox. If the ostensible purpose of therapeutic hyperventilation is to reduce ICP and thereby improve cerebral perfusion, how is it that an intervention that lowers CBF reverses the clinical signs? An extension of this concern is that hyperventilation might cause or exacerbate ischemia. The fall in jugular venous content that normally occurs with hyperventilation has been interpreted as reflecting "ischemia" (33,91). Indeed, frequent sampling of jugular venous blood following TBI has shown that oxygen desaturations below 50% are associated with worse outcomes (94). Yet, more recent positron emission tomography (PET) studies during acute hyperventilation in severe TBI have shown that regional reductions in CBF to less than 10 mL/100 g per minute were not associated with a fall in oxygen metabolism (84). Similarly, microdialysis studies have failed to demonstrate indications of energy failure in these same circumstances (95). Thus, the fall in CBF with hyperventilation does not appear to be the limiting step in cerebral oxygen metabolism, and under clinical conditions, even marked reductions in P_{aCO_2} do not produce cerebral ischemia. Little is known about regional CBF changes with hyperventilation in disease states other than trauma but the same general principles are believed to hold.

Time Course of Response to Hyperventilation

The duration of the ICP response to hyperventilation has important clinical consequences but its elaboration has been filled with misinterpretations. When arterial P_{CO_2} (P_{aCO_2}) is initially reduced, there occurs a rapid equilibration of CO_2 across the BBB, whereas hydrogen and bicarbonate ions are impeded from equilibrating. For this reason, the CSF P_{CO_2} declines, CSF pH rises, and bicarbonate concentration is unchanged initially. With continued hyperventilation, the arterial pH is gradually corrected over many hours and days, through enhanced renal excretion of bicarbonate ion. In the CSF, the choroid plexus apparently plays a role similar to the kidneys but does so by the excretion of ammonium (NH_4 which dissociates, releasing hydrogen ions). Moreover, it accomplishes the normalization of CSF pH far faster than occurs in the blood, typically over a matter of hours (96). This rapid compensation has two important clinical consequences. First, CBF, CBV, and ICP return to their preexisting levels during the first few hours of sustained hyperventilation (assuming no other interventions have taken place); the beneficial effect on ICP is lost yet a systemic hypercarbia and alkalosis have been produced. Second, once the CSF readjustment has occurred, any rise of arterial P_{CO_2} toward normal causes CSF acidosis as CO_2 freely enters the CSF. This results in cerebral vasodilation and often, a dramatic rise in ICP. From this, it has been surmised and should be emphasized that if hyperventilation has been maintained for more than 1 or 2 hours it should be withdrawn cautiously (typically by reducing the ventilator rate one or two breaths per minute at a time) with careful attention to ICP and clinical signs. We have encountered ample clinical examples to confirm this dictum, especially as it is related to head trauma and severe brain edema after stroke.

The impact of acute hyperventilation on outcome in cases of an intracranial mass is not known and designing a study to address this is daunting because of the multitude of factors that interact to raise ICP and alter outcome, not the least of which is the increase of brain edema over days. However, sustained, prophylactic hyperventilation of TBI patients appears to have a slight detrimental effect on outcome in severe head injury and cannot be recommended (97) (Chapter 12). Whether the use of a buffer to slow the acidification of the CSF pH might aid in prolonging the effects of hyperventilation has only been studied in limited populations and the results are uncertain.

In summary, hyperventilation is useful in the acute management of intracranial hypertension and the reversal of herniation syndromes, mainly as a temporizing measure while preparing for other interventions. The effective lower limit of P_{aCO_2} has not been established, but lowering it to 25 mm Hg in acute head injury does not induce ischemia and appears safe (84). Hyperventilation should be weaned cautiously in patients with poor compliance. Prophylactic hyperventilation applied without regard to the level of ICP and the clinical state should not be used.

Jugular Bulb Venous Monitoring as an Adjunct to Therapeutic Hyperventilation

Continuous measurement of jugular bulb oxygen saturation has been advocated as a means of monitoring the effects of sustained hyperventilation (98). Using this approach, the ventilator rate is increased to the desired level while assuring that an acceptable jugular venous saturation is maintained. A fall in jugular venous saturation below 50% is considered by some as a sign of excessive hyperventilation. However, the jugular venous oxygen saturation below which brain ischemia occurs cannot be stated with confidence. Patients with head injury who have frequent jugular venous desaturations from any cause below 50% have worse outcomes (99,100).

Catheters are available that provide continuous measurement of jugular bulb oxygen saturation. They are inserted in the jugular vein at the level of the thyroid cartilage and threaded cephalad until resistance is encountered. A lateral skull film is used to confirm that the tip of the catheter is at the level of the mastoid air cells. Unfortunately, the method has not been very reliable and desaturations had to be confirmed by venous blood gas analysis (101). The routine use of jugular venous monitoring cannot be strongly endorsed at this time but the information may be helpful in certain situations and it remains a useful investigative tool.

Osmotic Agents

The observation that changes in serum osmolality caused cerebral swelling and shrinkage occurred almost 100 years ago and the i.v. administration of osmotic agents has been used since the 1920s. Osmotic agents are routinely used for the treatment of intracranial hypertension and to ameliorate cerebral edema and brain tissue shifts. The sugar, mannitol, and more recently hypertonic saline have been the main modes of hypertonic treatment in the United States. Glycerol, diuretics and other agents have had periods of popularity elsewhere.

Mannitol acts by adding a very hypertonic (20% to 25%) solution to the blood (0.9% solution) producing a sudden rise in the osmolality of the ECF. In most organs mannitol is distributed freely throughout the ECF space, however, the BBB prevents it from leaving the intravascular space, thereby creating a gradient for water from the brain tissue (extracellular and intracellular compartments) to the vascular compartment. The result is shrinkage of the brain as a whole. In all other organs, an osmotic gradient is created between the ECF and the intracellular compartment, resulting in shrinkage of cells. All such gradients are short-lived because water rapidly equilibrates across cell membranes, including those of the blood vessels.

The potential for leakage of osmotic agents has led to two concerns. First, that mannitol could accumulate in damaged brain tissue and, as it disappears from the blood, reverse the osmotic gradient and cause "rebound cerebral edema." Despite one animal study to the contrary (102), there is reason to believe that the rebound phenomenon only occurs with excessive doses of mannitol, larger than used in practice. Because mannitol is not metabolized, it leaves the tissues in the same manner as it enters, by diffusing down its concentration gradient. It can be surmised that if mannitol is cleared from the blood between doses, then it should not accumulate in any brain regions. The clearance of mannitol can be determined by monitoring the osmolal gap in the blood (see the following). The second concern is that mannitol could act to shrink normal brain more than abnormal brain and worsen tissue shifts owing to a mass lesion (1). This question recently has been explored using serial magnetic resonance imaging (MRI) scans before and after a large bolus of mannitol in patients with large infarcts and midline shift. There was no demonstrable change in midline shift in the initial analysis (96). Subsequent analysis using a new technique that detects very small changes in brain volume indicated that there is indeed a reduction in the volume of normal brain with no change in the volume of the infarcted hemisphere but not to a degree that produces any measurable increase in midline shift (103).

The response to a rise in osmolality is for brain cells to shrink. Over time, however, a poorly understood osmotic compensation takes place in order to return cell sizes to normal. Over the course of 1 to 3 days the number of osmotically active particles in brain cells increases owing to a rise in intracellular potassium stores, proteins, and the formation of so-called idiogenic (unidentified) osmoles (70). This raises the intracellular osmolality and draws water inward, returning the cell size to normal despite a persistent systemic hyperosmolar state. Once this new balance is achieved, any reduction in systemic osmolality will cause water to move back into brain cells, theoretically resulting in a rebound cellular edema. This phenomenon is the most likely explanation for the so-called "rebound" edema that occurs with sustained mannitol use (104). Because of the formation of these additional intracellular osmoles once a sustained hyperosmolar state has been achieved any subsequent fall in osmolality will lead to rebound swelling. The hyperosmolar state should be corrected very slowly, over several days to a week.

Mannitol has additional effects that may contribute to its ability to lower ICP. It has been proposed that mannitol leads to a fall in cerebral blood volume through two supplementary mechanisms. One is a hemodynamic mechanism that derives from the acute intravascular volume expansion and rise in BP after mannitol, which leads to cerebral vasoconstriction and a fall in CBV (105). This theory assumes that mannitol consistently produces a significant rise in BP and that autoregulatory mechanisms are intact, assumptions that are not always valid. The second potential mechanism results from the lowered blood viscosity that follows an infusion, which raises CBF and leads to vasoconstriction and a fall in CBV (106).

Dosing and Kinetics of Osmotic Diuresis

An i.v. bolus of mannitol produces a rapid rise in ECF osmolality in most tissues (the brain excepted as discussed). The movement of water into the ECF space (which includes the intravascular compartment) quickly drives osmolality back toward its initial level and causes intravascular volume expansion. Initially, there is a fall in serum sodium concentration (since sodium content that is unchanged is diluted by the water). The

elimination half-life of mannitol is 30 to 60 minutes. Because mannitol is an osmotic diuretic it results in a very large volume of dilute urine with a subsequent rise in serum sodium concentration. The final serum sodium concentration varies considerably depending on previous mannitol doses and the i.v. fluids administered, but generally there is a rise with sustained use. For example, sodium does not change if the urine volume is replaced with free water. There is a net increase in sodium content and sodium concentration rises if it is replaced with isotonic or hypertonic sodium solutions.

Typical doses of mannitol range from 0.25 to 1.5 g/kg administered every 3 to 6 hours. When treating a patient who is deteriorating because of mass effect, doses up to 1.5 g/kg are appropriate. Further dosing is usually guided by monitoring ICP. Additional doses are generally given when the ICP exceeds 20 to 25 mm Hg. The doses and intervals should be adjusted so that ICP is maintained below that threshold. It should be kept in mind that patients can show signs of herniation with ICP below these levels, especially in the presence of temporal lobe or cerebellar lesions. When the goal of treatment is to reduce tissue shifts using ICP monitoring to guide therapy is of little use because fatal herniation following large ischemic stroke usually occurs before ICP rises. Thus, determining the appropriate dose of mannitol is difficult and must be based on serial clinical and radiographic assessments and clinical judgment.

Precautions with Mannitol

Caution is required when administering mannitol, as there are several potential complications. The potent diuretic effect may rapidly lead to hypovolemia and hypotension if urine output is not replaced. Hypotension is particularly prone to occur if high ventilator pressures are simultaneously restricting cardiac filling. Urine output should be replaced with a roughly equal volume of isotonic saline to maintain a hyperosmolar and euvolemic state. This usually can be accomplished with careful monitoring of fluid balance and serial measurements of body weight. In addition, there is excessive loss of electrolytes in the urine, primarily potassium, magnesium and phosphate. Levels of these electrolytes should be monitored closely and appropriate supplementation effected.

Mannitol use occasionally is associated with acute renal failure. The contributory factors have not been established but probably include dehydration, an exaggerated hyperosmolar state, and incomplete clearance of mannitol between doses (mannitol accumulation) (107,108). The renal failure typically manifests as a rise in creatinine, and fortunately is reversible in most cases if mannitol is discontinued.

It is frequently suggested that the use of mannitol be curtailed if serum osmolality exceeds 320 mOsm/L. Direct myocardial muscle depression and renal failure are feared. Despite frequent repetition of this tenet by authoritative sources, its validity has never been established. This, along with the concern over accumulation of mannitol in the brain with repeated dosing and "rebound edema" frequently results in the underuse of this agent. There is little indication that any of these phenomena occur outside of extreme laboratory conditions (102). Clinical deterioration is often caused by overly aggressive water replacement and a too-rapid fall in osmolality. Many neurointensivists do not rigidly adhere to these arbitrary limitations, but rather monitor mannitol clearance between doses and allow osmolality to rise above 320 mOsm/L if ICP remains uncontrolled.

Osmolal Gap and Assessing Mannitol Effect

Although routine measurement of mannitol levels is not possible in clinical work, the osmotic gap (the difference between measured and calculated osmolality) is a reasonable surrogate. The serum osmolality can be calculated by the formula:

$$([Na] \times 2) + (BUN/2.8) + (Glucose/18)$$

This is compared to the directly measured osmolality. The difference between the two is accounted for by unmeasured osmoles and is normally about 10 to 18 mOsm/L. The gap is greater in the presence of additional circulating agents (e.g., mannitol or ethanol). Determining the osmolal gap just prior to a dose of mannitol indicates whether the last dose has been completely cleared. When the osmolal gap rises over baseline (premannitol) or to excessive levels (greater than 20 mOsm/L) it is advised that either the mannitol dose should be lowered or the interval between doses should be increased. If ICP is poorly controlled despite these measures, then the use of alternating doses of mannitol and hypertonic saline should be considered.

Hypertonic Saline

There has been considerable recent interest in the use of hypertonic saline as an alternative to mannitol in the treatment of intracranial hypertension and tissue shifts. Solutions of 1.25% to 3% saline can be used as i.v. fluids to produce a sustained rise in osmolality or boluses of 23.4% saline can be used in a manner similar to mannitol (109–111). Parenthetically, 23.4% saline is used because it is routinely available in pharmacies for dilution to prepare i.v. admixtures. Hypertonic saline has no theoretical advantage over mannitol but may be less effective because, unlike mannitol, it rapidly enters the brain interstitial space and it may not reduce blood viscosity. There are numerous anecdotal reports of ICP reduction by hypertonic saline (112–115), but its ability to reduce ICP in patients has not been compared directly to mannitol. Hypertonic saline may be useful when mannitol clearance is inadequate is or there are signs of mannitol-induced renal failure.

Corticosteroids

Corticosteroids are well known to reduce cerebral edema surrounding tumors (116) and may be helpful in treating edema because of brain retraction during neurosurgery. Its routine use in the management of intracranial hypertension, however, does not appear justified. Studies in stroke (117,118), intracerebral hemorrhage (119), and head injury (120) have failed to show any benefit of steroids.

Pharmacologic Suppression of Brain Metabolism

Suppression of cerebral metabolic rate, usually accomplished with pentobarbital and now with other similar agents, has long been used as a means of controlling ICP. The rationale for this technique in the treatment of raised ICP is twofold. First, reducing metabolic rate lowers oxygen requirements and thus CBF, CBV, and ICP as discussed earlier in the section on sedation. Second, in marginally perfused regions, reducing metabolic activity may reduce oxygen requirements to the point where the limited perfusion becomes adequate to prevent cell death. Pentobarbital is not the only agent with the ability to suppress metabolism; others such as thiopental, propofol, etomidate, and benzodiazepines (lorazepam or midazolam) have been used for the same purpose.

Despite the undoubted physiologic effects, early studies in head injury demonstrated that pentobarbital was effective in lowering ICP but did not improve outcome (28,121,122). In those studies, the detrimental hypotensive effects of the barbiturates were not routinely corrected, crossover between treatment groups were common, and those who responded to treatment were analyzed separately. Because of these limitations, some neurointensivists do not consider the studies to be conclusive. The use of barbiturates in patients with edema following large hemispheric infarction also has been shown not to improve outcome (123).

A loading dose followed by a continuous infusion is required to achieve sufficient levels of pentobarbital to have a therapeutic effect. Suggested loading doses range from 5 to 36 mg/kg and suggested infusion rates range from 1 to 5 mg/kg per hour. Drug levels usually are not rapidly available and in any case,

correlate poorly with therapeutic benefit (124,125). Little data exist on guiding and monitoring this therapy, although maximal metabolic suppression is thought to occur when the EEG reaches a burst-suppression or isoelectric pattern and some units have used this as an end point. The appropriate doses for other agents have not been determined.

The question of overall efficacy aside, a rational approach would be to administer the minimum loading dose of anesthetic required to either control ICP or to achieve maximal metabolic suppression based on EEG monitoring. Once either of these goals is attained, further metabolic suppression is unlikely to be of benefit but certainly risks hypotension. Continuous EEG monitoring may be useful in determining the correct maintenance infusion rate. The duration of therapy is determined by the natural history of the condition, effectiveness of the other measures being used to control ICP, and severity of complications.

Use of metabolic suppression is associated with important complications. All of these anesthetic agents can cause significant hypotension and a net reduction in CPP. Vasopressor agents usually are required to correct drug-induced hypotension. Drugs that suppress cerebral metabolism also depress respiratory drive. It is therefore important to ensure that adequate mandatory minute ventilation is provided in order to avoid hypercarbia. Barbiturates apparently are associated with predisposition to infections and suppression of myocardial contractility. Finally, barbiturates are very lipophilic and accumulate in adipose tissue; therefore, it may take several days after discontinuation of the infusion to establish a clear idea of the patient's levels of consciousness.

Because of the difficulty in carrying out this therapy, the frequent and serious complications, and lack of established impact on outcome, barbiturates are considered a second-tier therapy for intracranial hypertension, suggested only after surgery, osmotic agents, and hyperventilation have failed (3). Use of this therapy varies widely among centers, with many having abandoned it for the treatment of intracranial hypertension. Metabolic suppression continues to be routinely used in the operating room during temporary vascular occlusion, but again, without any prospective evaluation of its impact on outcome. Hypothermia, an older nonpharmacologic approach to metabolic suppression, is gaining renewed interest.

Hypothermia

As with the pharmacologic approaches discussed previously, hypothermia reduces cerebral metabolic rate and lowers CBF, CBV, and ICP. Hypothermic metabolic suppression also may protect the brain during transient hypoperfusion, temporary vessel occlusion, or circulatory arrest during surgery.

The deep levels of hypothermia (28°C) that were used for cardiac surgery were associated with significant systemic complications, including bradycardia, hypotension, and coagulopathy (126). Subsequent studies in models of ischemic stroke and head injury suggested there was benefit with the use of moderate degrees of hypothermia (32 to 33°C) (127), even when instituted after the injury or infarct (128). When applied to patients, mild hypothermia was not found to be associated with serious systemic complications. Still, hypothermia requires intubation, mechanical ventilation, sedation, and often, use of neuromuscular blocking agents. The demand on nursing care and resources use is very high.

Despite its complexity several early trials in head injury indicated promise (129). However, they were followed by the failure to demonstrate benefit in a large National Institutes of Health–sponsored multicenter trial of early moderate hypothermia in head injury (130). Less is known about efficacy in other applications. Case series on the use of early hypothermia in patients deteriorating from large hemispheric stroke are encouraging (131–133) and controlled trials are needed. A randomized trial is currently underway to evaluate mild intraoperative hypothermia for neuroprotection during aneurysm repair based on a pilot trial that showed promise

(134) and a similar study is ongoing in severe stroke.

New techniques for lowering body temperature are being introduced. The use of cooling blankets and gastric lavage with iced solutions are cumbersome and not very effective for rapid and controlled cooling. A cooling vest that increases skin contact and speeds cooling has been introduced and intravascular devices that cool the body by circulating cold saline around a central venous catheter are now available.

SURGICAL APPROACHES TO INTRACRANIAL PRESSURE REDUCTION

Cerebrospinal Fluid Removal

Drainage of CSF from an intraventricular catheter is a rapid and effective means of lowering ICP. Drainage of just a few milliliters of CSF can dramatically reduce ICP, albeit temporarily, especially if intracranial compliance is poor. This volume required to lower ICP may seem small, but a very large (1.5 g/kg) dose of mannitol reduces whole brain volume by only 6 to 10 cc (134a). Although frequently reserved for patients with hydrocephalus, drainage of ventricular CSF can be useful in any case where there is a global increase in ICP and sufficient ventricular size to allow catheter placement. It has been recommended as the initial treatment of elevated ICP in severe head injury where feasible (3).

The catheters are typically placed in the frontal portion of the right lateral ventricle and attached simultaneously to a pressure transducer and drainage chamber. In order to obtain an accurate pressure reading the connection to the drainage chamber must be closed so that there is an airtight connection between the tip of the ventricular catheter and the transducer. Measurements are typically obtained once an hour; at other times, CSF is allowed to drain. The height of the drainage chamber is adjusted to be situated 0 to 25 cm above a reference point (usually the tragus of the ear) (Chapter 2). In this way, CSF only drains if ICP exceeds the height of the fluid column. It is also possible to keep the system closed and allow CSF to drain intermittently as the ICP surpasses a predetermined threshold, but this approach is more cumbersome and thus has greater potential for errors.

The overall utility of intraventricular catheters in patients with mass effect is unclear. In some cases drainage of CSF could shrink the ventricle and worsen tissue shifts. Upward herniation is feared in patients with posterior fossa lesions and hydrocephalus if the lateral ventricles are aggressively and rapidly decompressed. In both these situations, the height of the drainage chamber may be kept at a higher level than usual or the drainage system may be kept closed and CSF carefully drained intermittently for ICP elevations.

Evacuation of Mass Lesions

Early surgical intervention can be life saving and result in an excellent outcome in certain situations, such as the rapid removal of an acute epidural hematoma or a cerebellar hemorrhage. Surgery improves ICP control by removing sufficient mass to effectively lower ICP and it reverses tissue shifts. The mass removed may be a hematoma, tumor, or brain tissue (in extreme cases). This may be combined with craniectomy and dural augmentation.

Craniectomy

The idea of removing a segment of the cranial vault to relieve increased intracranial pressure dates back to the beginning of the last century. Hemicraniectomy, as it is currently performed, involves removal of a large bone flap on the side of the lesion with opening of the dura and dural augmentation to enlarge the cranial vault. This allows the brain to herniate out of the skull instead of compressing the brainstem and other normal structures. The craniectomy must be of sufficient size and situated low enough in the temporal bone to prevent injury to the herniating brain. The

bone flap is replaced several weeks or months later.

Hemicraniectomy has been used most effectively to treat patients with large middle cerebral artery (MCA) infarctions. Initially applied to deteriorating patients (135), subsequent case series have reported lower mortality in patients undergoing decompression prior to the onset of massive edema (136). Early hemicraniectomy also has been advocated for use in head injury, especially in those with hematoma and cerebral edema on presentation (137,138). This represents the resurrection of a practice that failed several decades ago, but under circumstances that were not comparable because it was used late in the course and without information regarding ICP and tissue shifts.

Controlled trials with careful attention to inclusion criteria and timing are required to determine if and how craniectomy should be used.

Lobectomy

Removal of injured or infarcted brain tissue, often combined with some uninjured tissue, has been used in cases in which other measures have failed to effectively reverse intracranial hypertension or tissue shifts. Lobectomy has been advocated as a useful adjuvant in the management of younger patients with relatively higher initial GCS scores who subsequently deteriorate or develop elevated intracranial pressure (139). Case series suggest that aggressive, early temporal lobectomy helps patients with posttraumatic swelling and herniation (140), but, as with hemicraniectomy, appropriate trials are required.

AN APPROACH TO TREATMENT OF MASS EFFECT AND INTRACRANIAL HYPERTENSION

The management of patients with intracranial hypertension or mass effect is influenced by many factors, including the pathophysiology and time course of the process, the severity of the insult, the presence or absence of a surgically accessible lesion, the patient's age, and overall medical condition. There is no single ideal way to combine the interventions discussed in the preceding for a given patient. However, there are some widely accepted general approaches to different clinical situations. The most common of those situations is discussed in the following.

Acute Neurological Deterioration or Clinical Signs of Herniation

This situation is often encountered at the time of initial presentation in the Emergency Department but also commonly occurs in the intensive care unit. Patients who are thought to have a structural cause for coma (GCS score less than 9) should be considered at risk for elevated ICP and tissue shifts. Initial stabilization should include rapid intubation (premedication with an ultra–short-acting anesthetic agent such as thiopental or etomidate and avoidance of neuromuscular blocking agents) hyperventilation to a $PaCO_2$ of 25 to 30 mm Hg, and administration of 1.0 to 1.5 g/kg of mannitol. Systemic hypertension should not be treated aggressively initially, whereas hypotension should be rapidly corrected. This approach is designed to empirically lower ICP and maximize CPP during stabilization and diagnostic evaluation. These measures can be instituted in a matter of minutes while preparing the patient to undergo CT scanning.

A similar approach is required for a hospitalized patient who suddenly deteriorates. The first step is to reassess the airway while considering whether there may be an enlarging or new lesion that should be treated surgically. Depending on the clinical situation, a CT scan is not always required but it should be considered. In deteriorating patients who must be transported for a CT or MRI scan, early intubation (with appropriate premedication) is advisable. Hyperventilation and mannitol should be initiated prior to CT scan in patients with signs of herniation.

Management of Sustained Intracranial Hypertension

Persistent intracranial hypertension requires further intervention. A practical treatment threshold is chosen (e.g., sustained ICP greater than 20 to 25 mm Hg for 5 to 10 minutes) and treatments are used either intermittently when ICP exceeds the determined threshold, or at regular intervals to prevent ICP from exceeding that threshold. This must occur in parallel with maintenance of sufficient BP to keep CPP greater than 50 to 70 mm Hg.

The routine patient management measures such as amelioration of fever, optimal oxygenation, and head position discussed in the preceding should be instituted. The most rapid and effective means of lowering ICP is CSF drainage in appropriately selected patients. Agitated patients should be sedated until they are calm and motionless. Mechanical ventilation should be adjusted to minimize patient discomfort and avoid hyperventilation. Often, switching a patient from a mandatory mode of ventilation (SIMV or Assist Control) to pressure support ventilation can resolve agitation and lower ICP. In patients who are being sedated, this approach should be undertaken only if respiratory drive can be followed by closely monitoring end-tidal CO_2 or arterial PCO_2.

If general measures and sedation are ineffective, the next appropriate step is osmotic treatment with mannitol. Whether it is preferable to administer mannitol on a scheduled basis or only when the ICP threshold is exceeded is not known; however, one study indicated that less mannitol was required when it was administered only as needed (141).

It is not always apparent when to institute and stop mannitol treatment. It is clear that renal failure necessitates stopping mannitol and switching to hypertonic saline. Dehydration and hypotension should be rapidly corrected with fluids and vasopressors and not considered an indication to discontinue mannitol administration. The oft-quoted maximum safe osmolality of 320 mOsm/L, however, is not well supported by data and is often surpassed. Monitoring for an increasing osmotic gap has been proposed as a means of determining if mannitol is cleared from the blood between doses, as a way of avoiding complications, but there are no published data to support this approach. Another approach is to use hypertonic (23.4%) saline when there is inadequate mannitol clearance or in the presence of complications.

If osmotic treatment is considered to have failed, then alternative "second-tier" treatments are considered, including sustained hyperventilation, anesthetic metabolic suppression, hypothermia, craniectomy, or lobectomy. No data exist to indicate whether any of these interventions is superior to another.

Management of Plateau Waves

Patients with poor intracranial compliance are subject to periodic, self-limited elevations in ICP to abnormally high levels, as discussed in Chapter 2. These "Lundburg B waves," ICP may rise 10 to 30 mm Hg either spontaneously or in response to stimulation and remain elevated for up to 1 hour. What causes this phenomenon is not known, but one theory is that transient systemic hypotension produces cerebral autoregulatory vasodilation, increasing blood volume and therefore ICP. The rise in ICP reduces CPP further, causing more vasodilation. The proponents of this theory suggest that plateau waves may be terminated by the use of peripheral vasoconstrictors to raise BP (142). Other measures have been suggested for treating plateau waves, including CSF drainage, hyperventilation, and intermittent boluses of sedatives. Of these, CSF drainage and hyperventilation appear to be the safest and most effective means of treating transient elevations in ICP.

REFERENCES

1. Frank JI. Large hemispheric infarction, deterioration, and intracranial pressure. *Neurology* 1995;45: 1286–1290.
2. Marshall LF, Barba D, Toole BM, et al. The oval pupil: clinical significance and relationship to intracranial hypertension. *J Neurosurg* 1983;58:566–568.
3. Bullock R, Chesnut RM, Clifton G, et al. Guidelines for the Management of Severe Head Injury. *J Neurotrauma* 1996;13:639–734.
4. The Brain Trauma Foundation. The American Association of Neurological Surgeons. The Joint Section on Neurotrauma and Critical Care. Use of mannitol. *J Neurotrauma* 2000;17:521–525.
5. The Brain Trauma Foundation. The American Association of Neurological Surgeons. The Joint Section on Neurotrauma and Critical Care. Critical pathway for the treatment of established intracranial hypertension. *J Neurotrauma* 2000;17:537–538.
6. The Brain Trauma Foundation. The American Association of Neurological Surgeons. The Joint Section on Neurotrauma and Critical Care. Guidelines for cerebral perfusion pressure. *J Neurotrauma* 2000;17:507–511.
7. The Brain Trauma Foundation. The American Association of Neurological Surgeons. The Joint Section on Neurotrauma and Critical Care. Recommendations for intracranial pressure monitoring technology. *J Neurotrauma* 2000;17:497–506.
8. The Brain Trauma Foundation. The American Association of Neurological Surgeons. The Joint Section on Neurotrauma and Critical Care. Intracranial pressure treatment threshold. *J Neurotrauma* 2000;17:493–495.
9. The Brain Trauma Foundation. The American Association of Neurological Surgeons. The Joint Section on Neurotrauma and Critical Care. Resuscitation of blood pressure and oxygenation. *J Neurotrauma* 2000;17: 471–478.
10. Toutant SM, Klauber MR, Marshall LF, et al. Absent or compressed basal cisterns on first CT scan: ominous predictors of outcome in severe head injury. *J Neurosurg* 1984;61:691–694.
11. Schwab S, Aschoff A, Spranger M, et al. The value of intracranial pressure monitoring in acute hemispheric stroke. *Neurology* 1996;47:393–398.
12. Marmarou A, Anderson RL, Ward JD, et al. Impact of ICP instability and hypotension on outcome in patients with severe head trauma. *J Neurosurg* 1991;75: S59–S66.
13. Clusmann H, Schaller C, Schramm J. Fixed and dilated pupils after trauma, stroke, and previous intracranial surgery: management and outcome. *J Neurol Neurosurg Psychiatry* 2001;71:175–181.
14. Qureshi AI, Geocadin RG, Suarez JI, et al. Long-term outcome after medical reversal of transtentorial herniation in patients with supratentorial mass lesions. *Crit Care Med* 2000;28:1556–1564.
15. Mindermann T, Gratzl O. Interhemispheric pressure gradients in severe head trauma in humans. *Acta Neurochir Suppl (Wien)* 1998;71:56–58.
16. Sahuquillo J, Poca MA, Arribas M, et al. Interhemispheric supratentorial intracranial pressure gradients in head-injured patients: are they clinically important? *J Neurosurg* 1999;90:16–26.
17. Mayhall CG, Archer NH, Lamb VA, et al. Ventriculostomy-related infections, a prospective study. *N Engl J Med* 1984;310:553–559.
18. Lyke KE, Obasanjo OO, Williams MA, et al. Ventriculitis complicating use of intraventricular catheters in adult neurosurgical patients. *Clin Infect Dis* 2001;33: 2028–2033.

19. Rebuck JA, Murry KR, Rhoney DH, et al. Infection related to intracranial pressure monitors in adults: analysis of risk factors and antibiotic prophylaxis. *J Neurol Neurosurg Psychiatry* 2000;69:381–384.

20. Jacobs DG, Westerband A. Antibiotic prophylaxis for intracranial pressure monitors. *J Natl Med Assoc* 1998; 90:417–423.

21. Naff NJ, Carhuapoma JR, Williams MA, et al. Treatment of intraventricular hemorrhage with urokinase: effects on 30-day survival. *Stroke* 2000;31:841–847.

22. Naff NJ, Williams MA, Rigamonti D, et al. Blood clot resolution in human cerebrospinal fluid: evidence of first-order kinetics. *Neurosurgery* 2001;49:614–619.

23. Chesnut RM, Marshall SB, Piek J, et al. Early and late systemic hypotension as a frequent and fundamental source of cerebral ischemia following severe brain injury in the Traumatic Coma Data Bank. *Acta Neurochir Suppl (Wien)* 1993;59:121–125.

24. Strandgaard S, Paulson OB. Regulation of cerebral blood flow in health and disease. *J Cardiovasc Pharmacol* 1992;19:S89–93.

25. Dernbach PD, Little JR, Jones SC, et al. Altered Cerebral Autoregulation and CO_2 reactivity after aneurysmal subarachnoid hemorrhage. *Neurosurg* 1988;22: 822–826.

26. Enevoldsen EM, Jensen FT. Autoregulation and CO_2 responses of cerebral blood flow in patients with acute severe head injury. *J Neurosurg* 1978;48:689–703.

27. Muizelaar JP, Ward JD, Marmarou A, et al. Cerebral blood flow and metabolism in severely head-injured children. Part 2: Autoregulation. *J Neurosurg* 1989;71: 72–76.

28. Eisenberg HM, Frankowski RF, Marshall LF, et al. High-dose barbiturate control of elevated intracranial pressure in patients with severe head injury. *J Neurosurg* 1988;69:15–23.

29. Narayan R, Kishore K, Pulla RS, et al. Intracranial pressure: to monitor or not to monitor? *J Neurosurg* 1982;56:650–659.

30. Unterberg AW, Kiening KL, Hartl R, et al. Multimodal monitoring in patients with head injury: evaluation of the effects of treatment on cerebral oxygenation. *J Trauma* 1997;42:S32–S37.

31. Czosnyka M, Guazzo E, Iyer V, et al. Testing of cerebral autoregulation in head injury by waveform analysis of blood flow velocity and cerebral perfusion pressure. *Acta Neurochir Suppl (Wien)* 1994;60:468–471.

32. Robertson CS, Valadka AB, Hannay HJ, et al. Prevention of secondary ischemic insults after severe head injury. *Crit Care Med* 1999;27:2086–2095.

33. Marmarou A, Anderson R, Ward J. Impact of ICP instability and hypotension on outcome in patients with severe head injury. *J Neurosurg* 1991;75:S59–S66.

34. Andrews BT, Chiles BW III, Olsen WL, et al. The effect of intracerebral hematoma location on the risk of brain-stem compression and on clinical outcome. *J Neurosurg* 1988;69:518–522.

35. Marshall LF, Marshall SB, Klauber MR, et al. The diagnosis of head injury requires a classification based on computed axial tomography. *J Neurotrauma* 1992; 9:S287–S292.

36. Diringer MN, Edwards DF, Zazulia AR. Hydrocephalus: a previously unrecognized predictor of poor outcome from supratentorial intracerebral hemorrhage. *Stroke* 1998;29:1352–1357.

37. Burney RG, Winn R. Increased cerebrospinal fluid pressure during laryngoscopy and intubation for induction of anesthesia. *Anesthesiol Analg* 1975;54: 687–690.

38. Modica PA, Tempelhoff R. Intracranial pressure during induction of anaesthesia and tracheal intubation with etomidate-induced EEG burst suppression. *Can J Anaesthesiol* 1992;39:236–241.

39. Brucia J, Rudy E. The effect of suction catheter insertion and tracheal stimulation in adults with severe brain injury. *Heart Lung* 1996;25:295–303.

40. Robinson N, Clancy M. In patients with head injury undergoing rapid sequence intubation, does pretreatment with intravenous lignocaine/lidocaine lead to an improved neurological outcome? A review of the literature. *Emerg Med J* 2001;18:453–457.

41. Frost EAM. Effect of positive end-expiratory pressure in intracranial pressure and compliance in brain-injured patients. *J Neurosurg* 1977;47:195–200.

42. Clarke JP. The effects of inverse ratio ventilation on intracranial pressure: a preliminary report. *Int Care Med* 1997;23:106–109.

43. Shapiro HM, Marshall LF. Intracranial pressure responses to PEEP in head-injured patients. *J Trauma* 1978;18:254–256.

44. Yano M, Nishiyama H, Yokota H, et al. Effect of lidocaine on ICP response to endotracheal suctioning. *Anesthesiology* 1986;64:651–653.

45. Lev R, Rosen P. Prophylactic lidocaine use preintubation: a review. *J Emerg Med* 1994;12:499–506.

46. Campbell VG. Effects of controlled hyperoxygenation and endotracheal suctioning on intracranial pressure in head-injured adults. *Appl Nurs Res* 1991;4:138–140.

47. Kerr ME, Rudy EB, Brucia J, et al. Head-injured adults: recommendations for endotracheal suctioning. *J Neurosci Nurs* 1993;25:86–91.

48. Kerr ME, Rudy EB, Weber BB, et al. Effect of short-duration hyperventilation during endotracheal suctioning on intracranial pressure in severe head-injured adults. *Nurs Res* 1997;46:195–201.

49. Feldman Z, Kanter MJ, Robertson CS, et al. Effect of head elevation on intracranial pressure, cerebral perfusion pressure, and cerebral blood flow in head-injured patients. *J Neurosurg* 1992;76:207–211.

50. Ropper AH, O'Rouke D, Kennedy SK. Head position, intracranial pressure and compliance. *Neurology* 1982; 32:1288–1291.

51. Durward QJ, Amacher AL, Del Maestro RF, et al. Cerebral and cardiovascular responses to changes in head elevation in patients with intracranial hypertension. *J Neurosurg* 1983;59:938–944.

52. Schwarz S, Georgiadis D, Aschoff A, et al. Effects of body position on intracranial pressure and cerebral perfusion in patients with large hemispheric stroke. *Stroke* 2002;33:497–501.

53. Strebel SP, Kindler C, Bissonnette B, et al. The impact of systemic vasoconstrictors on the cerebral circulation of anesthetized patients. *Anesthesiology* 1998;89: 67–72.

54. Rosner MJ, Becker DP. Origin and evolution of plateau waves. Experimental observations and a theoretical model. *J Neurosurg* 1984;60:312–324.

55. Marshall WJ, Jackson JL, Langfitt TW. Brain swelling caused by trauma and arterial hypertension. Hemodynamic aspects. *Arch Neurol* 1969;21:545–553.

56. Vandam LD, Burnap TK. Hypothermia. *N Engl J Med* 1959;261:595–603.
57. Morikawa E, Ginsberg MD, Dietrich WD, et al. The significance of brain temperature in focal cerebral ischemia: histopathologic consequences of middle cerebral artery occlusion in the rat. *J Cereb Blood Flow Metab* 1992;12:380–389.
58. Zhao W, Alonso OF, Loor JY, et al. Influence of early posttraumatic hypothermia therapy on local cerebral blood flow and glucose metabolism after fluid-percussion brain injury. *J Neurosurg* 1999;90:510–519.
59. Azzimondi G, Bassein L, Nonino F, et al. Fever in acute stroke worsens prognosis. A prospective study. *Stroke* 1995;26:2040–2043.
60. Fukuda H, Kitani M, Takahashi K. Body temperature correlates with functional outcome and the lesion size of cerebral infarction. *Acta Neurol Scand* 1999;100: 385–390.
61. Ginsberg MD, Busto R. Combating hyperthermia in acute stroke: a significant clinical concern. *Stroke* 1998;29:529–534.
62. Reith J, Jorgensen HS, Pedersen PM, et al. Body temperature in acute stroke: relation to stroke severity, infarct size, mortality, and outcome [see comments]. *Lancet* 1996;347:422–425.
63. Wang Y, Lim LL, Levi C, et al. Influence of admission body temperature on stroke mortality. *Stroke* 2000;31: 404–409.
64. Mayer SA, Commichau C, Scarmeas N, et al. Clinical trial of an air-circulating cooling blanket for fever control in neuro-ICU patients. *Neurology* 2000;56: 292–298.
65. Biestro AA, Alberti RA, Soca AE, et al. Use of indomethacin in brain-injured patients with cerebral perfusion pressure impairment: preliminary report. *J Neurosurg* 1995;83:627–630.
66. Slavik RS, Rhoney DH. Indomethacin: a review of its cerebral blood flow effects and potential use for controlling intracranial pressure in traumatic brain injury patients. *Neurol Res* 1999;21:491–499.
67. Mayberg MR, Batjer HH, Dacey R, et al. Guidelines for the management of aneurysmal subarachnoid hemorrhage. A statement for healthcare professionals from a special writing group of the Stroke Council, American Heart Association. *Stroke* 1994;25:2315–2328.
68. Broderick JP, Adams HP Jr, Barsan W, et al. Guidelines for the management of spontaneous intracerebral hemorrhage: a statement for healthcare professionals from a special writing group of the Stroke Council, American Heart Association. *Stroke* 1999; 30:905–915.
69. Diringer MN. Neuroendocrine regulation of sodium and volume following subarachnoid hemorrhage. *Clin Neuropharmacol* 1995;18:114–126.
70. McDowell ME, Wolf AV, Steer A. Osmotic volumes of distribution. Idiogenic changes in osmotic pressure associated with administration of hypertonic solutions. *Am J Physiol* 1955;180:545–558.
71. Paczynski RP, Venkatesan R, Diringer MN, et al. Effects of fluid management on edema volume and midline shift in a rat model of ischemic stroke. *Stroke* 2000;31:1702–1708.
72. Lassen NA, Christensen MS. Physiology of cerebral blood flow. *Br J Anaesthesiol* 1976;48:719–734
73. Hsiang JK, Chesnut RM, Crisp CB, et al. Early, routine paralysis for intracranial pressure control in severe head injury: is it necessary? *Crit Care Med* 1994;22: 1471–1476.
74. Cannon ML, Glazier SS, Bauman LA. Metabolic acidosis, rhabdomyolysis, and cardiovascular collapse after prolonged propofol infusion. *J Neurosurg* 2001;95: 1053–1056.
75. Perrier ND, Baerga-Varela Y, Murray MJ. Death related to propofol use in an adult patient. *Crit Care Med* 2000;28:3071–3074.
76. de Nadal M, Munar F, Poca MA, et al. Cerebral hemodynamic effects of morphine and fentanyl in patients with severe head injury: absence of correlation to cerebral autoregulation. *Anesthesiology* 2000;92:11–19.
77. Sperry RJ, Bailey PL, Reichman MV, et al. Fentanyl and sufentanil increase intracranial pressure in head trauma patients [see comments]. *Anesthesiology* 1992; 77:416–420.
78. Goldstein LB. Basic and clinical studies of pharmacologic effects on recovery from brain injury. *J Neural Transplant Plast* 1993;4:175–192.
79. Geller TJ, Kaiboriboon K, Fenton GA, et al. Vecuronium-associated axonal motor neuropathy: a variant of critical illness polyneuropathy? *Neuromuscul Disord* 2001;11:579–582.
80. Garnacho-Montero J, Madrazo-Osuna J, Garcia-Garmendia JL, et al. Critical illness polyneuropathy: risk factors and clinical consequences. A cohort study in septic patients. *Int Care Med* 2001;27:1288–1296.
81. Juul N, Morris GF, Marshall SB, et al. Neuromuscular blocking agents in neurointensive care. *Acta Neurochir Suppl* 2000;76:467–470.
82. Koehler RC, Traystman RJ. Bicarbonate ion modulation of cerebral blood flow during hypoxia and hypercapnia. *Am J Physiol* 1982;243:H33–H40.
83. Raichle ME, Plum F. Hyperventilation and cerebral blood flow. [Review]. *Stroke* 1972;3:566–575.
84. Diringer MN, Videen TO, Yundt K, et al. Regional cerebrovascular and metabolic effects of hyperventilation following severe traumatic brain injury. *J Neurosurg* 2001;96:130–138.
85. Powers WJ, Grubb RL Jr, Raichle ME. Physiological responses to focal cerebral ischemia in humans. *Ann Neurol* 1984;16:546–552.
86. Raichle ME, Posner JB, Plum F. Cerebral blood flow during and after hyperventilation. *Arch Neurol* 1970; 23:394–403.
87. Bullock R. Hyperventilation. *J Neurosurg* 2002;96: 157–159.
88. Diringer MN, Dacey RG Jr. Traumatic brain injury and hyperventilation. *J Neurosurg* 2002;96:155–156.
89. Crockard HA, Coppel DL, Morrow WF. Evaluation of hyperventilation in treatment of head injuries. *Br Med J* 1973;4:634–640.
90. Carmona Suazo JA, Maas AI, van den Brink WA, et al. CO_2 reactivity and brain oxygen pressure monitoring in severe head injury. *Crit Care Med* 2000;28:3268–3274.
91. Gopinath SP, Valadka AB, Uzura M, et al. Comparison of jugular venous oxygen saturation and brain tissue Po_2 as monitors of cerebral ischemia after head injury [see comments]. *Crit Care Med* 1999;27:2337–2345.
92. Obrist WD, Langfitt TW, Jaggi JL, et al. Cerebral blood flow and metabolism in comatose patients with acute head injury. Relationship to intracranial hypertension. *J Neurosurg* 1984;61:241–253.

93. Marion DW, Darby J, Yonas H. Acute regional cerebral blood flow changes caused by severe head injuries. *J Neurosurg* 1991;74:407–414.

94. Sheinberg M, Kanter MJ, Robertson CS, et al. Continuous monitoring of jugular venous oxygen saturation in head-injured patients [see comments]. *J Neurosurg* 1992;76:212–217.

95. Letarte PB, Puccio AM, Brown SD, et al. Effect of hypocapnia on CBF and extracellular intermediates of secondary brain injury. *Acta Neurochir Suppl (Wien)* 1999;75:45–47.

96. Lundberg N, Cronqvist S, Kjallquist A. Clinical investigations on interactions between intracranial pressure and intracranial hemodynamics. *Prog Brain Res* 1958; 30:69–75.

97. Muizelaar JP, Marmarou A, Ward JD, et al. Adverse effects of prolonged hyperventilation in patients with severe head injury: a randomized clinical trial. *J Neurosurg* 1991;75:731–739.

98. Cruz J. The first decade of continuous monitoring of jugular bulb oxyhemoglobin saturation: management strategies and clinical outcome. *Crit Care Med* 1998; 26:344–351.

99. Robertson C. Desaturation episodes after severe head injury: influence on outcome. *Acta Neurochirurg Suppl* 1993;59:98–101.

100. Sheinberg M, Kanter MJ, Robertson CS, et al. Continuous monitoring of jugular venous oxygen saturation in head-injured patients. *J Neurosurg* 1992;76: 212–217.

101. Howard L, Gopinath SP, Uzura M, et al. Evaluation of a new fiberoptic catheter for monitoring jugular venous oxygen saturation. *Neurosurgery* 1999;44: 1280–1285.

102. Kaufmann AM, Cardoso ER. Aggravation of vasogenic cerebral edema by multiple-dose mannitol. *J Neurosurg* 1992;77:584–589.

103. Manno EM, Adams RE, Derdeyn CP, et al. The effects of mannitol on cerebral edema after large hemispheric cerebral infarct. *Neurology* 1999;52:583–587.

104. Go KG. The fluid environment of the central nervous system. In: Go KG, ed. *Cerebral pathophysiology.* New York: Elsevier,1991:66–171.

105. Rosner MJ, Daughton S. Cerebral perfusion pressure management in head injury. *J Trauma* 1993;30: 933–940.

106. Muizelaar JP, Wei EP, Kontos HA, et al. Mannitol causes compensatory cerebral vasoconstriction and vasodilation in response to blood viscosity changes. *J Neurosurg* 1983;59:822–828.

107. Horgan KJ, Ottaviano YL, Watson AJ. Acute renal failure due to mannitol intoxication. *Am J Nephrol* 1989; 9:106–109.

108. Dorman HR, Sondheimer JH, Cadnapaphornchai P. Mannitol-induced acute renal failure. *Medicine (Baltimore)* 1990;69:153–159.

109. Shackford SR, Bourguignon PR, Wald SL, et al. Hypertonic saline resuscitation of patients with head injury: a prospective, randomized clinical trial. *J Trauma* 1998;44:50–58.

110. Simma B, Burger R, Falk M, et al. A prospective, randomized, and controlled study of fluid management in children with severe head injury: lactated Ringer's solution versus hypertonic saline. *Crit Care Med* 1998; 26:1265–1270.

111. Suarez JI, Qureshi AI, Bhardwaj A, et al. Treatment of refractory intracranial hypertension with 23.4% saline. *Crit Care Med* 1998;26:1118–1122.

112. Horn P, Munch E, Vajkoczy P, et al. Hypertonic saline solution for control of elevated intracranial pressure in patients with exhausted response to mannitol and barbiturates. *Neurol Res* 1999;21:758–764.

113. Khanna S, Davis D, Peterson B, et al. Use of hypertonic saline in the treatment of severe refractory posttraumatic intracranial hypertension in pediatric traumatic brain injury. *Crit Care Med* 2000;28: 1144–1151.

114. Valadka AB, Robertson CS. Should we be using hypertonic saline to treat intracranial hypertension? *Crit Care Med* 2000;28:1245–1246.

115. Walsh JC, Zhuang J, Shackford SR. A comparison of hypertonic to isotonic fluid in the resuscitation of brain injury and hemorrhagic shock. *J Surg Res* 1991;50: 284–292.

116. Hatam A, Yu ZY, Bergstrom M, et al. Effect of dexamethasone treatment on peritumoral brain edema: evaluation by computed tomography. *J Comput Assist Tomogr* 1982;6:586–592.

117. O'Brien MD. Ischemic cerebral edema. A review. *Stroke* 1979;10:623–628.

118. Shapiro HM. Intracranial hypertension therapeutic and anesthetic considerations. *Anesthesiology* 1975;43: 445–471.

119. Poungvarin N, Bhoopat W, Viriyavejakul A, et al. Effects of dexamethasone in primary supratentorial intracerebral hemorrhage. *N Engl J Med* 1987;316: 1229–1233.

120. Gudeman SK, Miller JD, Becker DP. Failure of high-dose steroid therapy to influence intracranial pressure in patients with severe head injury. *J Neurosurg* 1979; 51:301–306.

121. Schwartz ML, Tator CH, Rowed DW, et al. The University of Toronto head injury treatment study: a prospective, randomized comparison of pentobarbital and mannitol. *Can J Neurol Sci* 1984;11:434–440.

122. Ward JD, Becker DP, Miller JD, et al. Failure of prophylactic barbiturate coma in the treatment of severe head injury. *J Neurosurg* 1985;62:383–388.

123. Schwab S, Spranger M, Schwarz S, et al. Barbiturate coma in severe hemispheric stroke: useful or obsolete? *Neurology* 1997;48:1608–1613.

124. Bayliff CD, Schwartz ML, Hardy BG. Pharmacokinetics of high-dose pentobarbital in severe head trauma. *Clin Pharmacol Ther* 1985;38:457–461.

125. Heinemeyer G, Roots I, Dennhardt R. Monitoring of pentobarbital plasma levels in critical care patients suffering from increased intracranial pressure. *Ther Drug Monit* 1986;8:145–150.

126. Drake CG, Barr HWK, Coles JC, et al. The use of extracorporeal circulation and profound hypothermia in the treatment of ruptured intracranial aneurysm. *J Neurosurg* 1964;21:575–581.

127. Clifton GL, Jiang JY, Lyeth BG, et al. Marked protection by moderate hypothermia after experimental traumatic brain injury. *J Cereb Blood Flow Metab* 1991; 11:114–121.

128. Karibe H, Chen J, Zarow GJ, et al. Delayed induction of mild hypothermia to reduce infarct volume after temporary middle cerebral artery occlusion in rats. *J Neurosurg* 1994;80:112–119.

129. Marion DW, Obrist WD, Carlier PM, et al. The use of moderate therapeutic hypothermia for patients with severe head injuries: a preliminary report. *J Neurosurg* 1993;79:354–362.

130. Clifton GL, Miller ER, Choi SC, et al. Lack of effect of induction of hypothermia after acute brain injury. *N Engl J Med* 2001;344:556–563.

131. Krieger DW, De Georgia MA, Abou-Chebl A, et al. Cooling for acute ischemic brain damage (cool aid): an open pilot study of induced hypothermia in acute ischemic stroke. *Stroke* 2001;32:1847–1854.

132. Schwab S, Schwarz S, Spranger M, et al. Moderate hypothermia in the treatment of patients with severe middle cerebral artery infarction. *Stroke* 1998;29: 2461–2466.

133. Schwab S, Spranger M, Aschoff A, et al. Brain temperature monitoring and modulation in patients with severe MCA infarction. *Neurology* 1997;48:762–767.

134. Hindman BJ, Todd MM, Gelb AW, et al. Mild hypothermia as a protective therapy during intracranial aneurysm surgery: a randomized prospective pilot trial. *Neurosurgery* 1999;44:23–32.

134a. Videen TO, Zazulia AR, Manno EM, et al. Mannitol bolus preferentially shrinks non-infarcted brain in patient swith ischemic stroke. *Neurology* 2001;57: 2120–2122.

135. Delashaw JB, Broaddus WC, Kassell NF, et al. Treatment of right hemisphere cerebral infarction by hemicraniectomy. *Stroke* 1990;21:874–881.

136. Schwab S, Steiner T, Aschoff A, et al. Early hemicraniectomy in patients with complete middle cerebral artery infarction. *Stroke* 1998;29:1888–1893.

137. Coplin WM, Cullen NK, Policherla PN, et al. Safety and feasibility of craniectomy with duraplasty as the initial surgical intervention for severe traumatic brain injury. *J Trauma* 2001;50:1050–1059.

138. Meier U, Zeilinger FS, Henzka O. The use of decompressive craniectomy for the management of severe head injuries. *Acta Neurochir Suppl* 2000;76:475–478.

139. Litofsky NS, Chin LS, Tang G, et al. The use of lobectomy in the management of severe closed-head trauma. *Neurosurgery* 1994;34:628–632.

140. Nussbaum ES, Wolf AL, Sebring L, et al. Complete temporal lobectomy for surgical resuscitation of patients with transtentorial herniation secondary to unilateral hemispheric swelling. *Neurosurgery* 1991;29:62–66.

141. Marshall LF, Smith RW, Rauscher A, et al. Mannitol dose requirements in brain-injured patients. *J Neurosurg* 1978;48:169–172.

142. Rosner MJ, Rosner SD, Johnson AH. Cerebral perfusion pressure: management protocol and clinical results. *J Neurosurg* 1995;83:949–962.

143. Cottrell JE, Patel K, Turndorf H, et al. Intracranial pressure changes induced by sodium nitroprusside in patients with intracranial mass lesions. *J Neurosurg* 1978;48:329–331.

144. Turner JM, Powell D, Gibson RM, et al. Intracranial pressure changes in neurosurgical patients during hypotension induced with sodium nitroprusside or trimetaphan. *Br J Anaesthesiol* 1977;49:419–425.

4

Pulmonary Aspects of Neurological Intensive Care

Pulmonary disorders are a central feature of the practice of intensive care medicine. Furthermore, they are particularly pertinent because certain types of respiratory failure derive primarily from disorders of the nervous system. Additionally, as in other intensive care unit (ICU) settings, many patients with serious neurological conditions have coexisting pulmonary conditions such as asthma or chronic obstructive pulmonary disease (COPD); others develop complications of treatment or immobilization such as ventilator-associated pneumonia (Chapter 7) or pulmonary embolism. However, among the most interesting aspects of the interaction between the nervous and respiratory systems are the conditions summarized by the term neurogenic respiratory failure (NRF), encompassing both central and peripheral nervous causes of pulmonary distress; it is this subject which comprises the bulk of discussion in this chapter. These forms of respiratory failure derive from neuromuscular diseases (Guillain–Barré syndrome, myasthenia gravis, etc.), primary brainstem lesions, and from diseases that cause coma and secondary reduction in airway reflexes and ventilation, all of which are detailed in this volume.

Several general aspects of the subject that are necessary to the intelligent application of ventilators and endotracheal tubes in any ICU are also presented here because they are referable to all types of respiratory failure. Much of this information, particularly classic respiratory physiology which has been considered the core knowledge of respiratory intensive care, should be known to all competent neurointensivists who plan to deal with and discuss intelligently general intensive care problems.

ACUTE RESPIRATORY FAILURE

Respiratory failure may be divided into four broad classes (Table 4.1) (1). Although the first two types are the ones emphasized in most discussions of neurological critical care, the other two should be kept in mind in that there are many patients who benefit from mechanical ventilation but do not fit strictly in one of the first two categories. For example, patients in cardiogenic shock benefit from mechanical ventilation in part because they no longer need to deliver as much oxygenated blood to the diaphragm; this decrease in oxygen demand allows for the diminished cardiac output to be redistributed to other organs. Or, hyperventilation for the short-term control of increased intracranial pressure (ICP) is similar to perioperative mechanical ventilation insofar as one employs mechanical ventilation to meet a therapeutic goal that is not strictly mandated by the patient's disease.

The unifying feature of the group with failure of oxygenation is an inability to transfer sufficient oxygen from the airways into the pulmonary venous blood. In neurocritical care, most cases of primary oxygenation failure stem from pulmonary edema, pneumonia, pulmonary embolism, or severe atelectasis.

TABLE 4.1. *Classification of respiratory failure*

	Description	Conventional example	Neurological example
Type I	Oxygenation failure	Cardiogenic pulmonary edema	Neurogenic pulmonary edema
Type II	Ventilation failure	Narcotic overdose	Guillain–Barré syndrome
Type III	Perioperative	Coronary artery bypass graft	Craniectomy for tumor
Type IV	Shock	Cardiogenic shock	Acute spinal cord injury

Pulmonary Edema

Pulmonary edema in all its forms indicates an excess of extravascular lung water. Under normal circumstances, an increase in the transudation of water from the pulmonary capillaries into the interstitial space is handled by the lymphatic system, which is able to increase its flow rate severalfold in order to keep excess fluid from accumulating. The interstitial space enlarges if the rate of fluid transudation exceeds the lymphatic capacity, thereby inhibiting gas exchange by increasing the distance through which gases must diffuse in order to be transferred both to the capillary (oxygen) and from the alveolus (carbon dioxide), the capillary, and the alveolus. The lower solubility of oxygen in water also results in slower exchange, such that even under normal circumstances oxygen does not completely equilibrate between the alveolus and the capillary during the transit time of a red blood cell. As a practical matter, carbon dioxide normally equilibrates completely in less than this transit time; this is why an increase in interstitial lung water produces hypoxemia but rarely hypercarbia.

Fluid transudation further impairs gas exchange by decreasing the number of respiratory units (the parts of the lung capable of gas exchange, including the alveoli, respiratory bronchioles, and terminal bronchioles) available for ventilation. If perfusion of these alveoli continues, the blood leaving these units is still venous in its gas composition; when it mixes with blood from functioning units, the result is a mixture of blood with a low $PpvO_2$ (venous O_2); that is, a true "shunt" and a slight increase in $PpvCO_2$ (venous CO_2). The brainstem senses this hypoxemia, however, and increases minute ventilation in response; thus, the measured $PaCO_2$ is generally lower than 40 mm Hg.

The commonly recognized causes of pulmonary edema can be predicted from the Starling equation

$$Q = K\,[(P_c - P_i) - \sigma(\pi_c - \pi_i)]$$

where: Q = the net fluid flow across the capillary membrane; K = the reflection coefficient; P_c = the hydrostatic pressure within the capillary; P_i = the hydrostatic pressure in the interstitium; σ = the permeability constant; π_c = the colloid oncotic pressure in the capillary; and π_I = the colloid oncotic pressure in the interstitium. Thus, conditions that raise capillary hydrostatic pressure (e.g., elevated left atrial pressure in mitral stenosis or congestive heart failure) increase the driving force for fluid to leave the capillary and enter the interstitium. Markedly lowering the plasma oncotic pressure has the same effect but this is a rare clinical occurrence. If the permeability of the capillary to plasma proteins increases (becomes "leaky"), fluid moves out of the capillary and is difficult to return to the circulation until normal permeability is restored.

A further result of increased interstitial lung fluid flux is a decrease in lung compliance (unit change in volume per unit change in airway pressure, or $\Delta V/\Delta P$, in mL/cm H_2O, as described in the discussion of pulmonary physiology). For the spontaneously breathing patient, diminished compliance increases work of breathing. For the mechanically ventilated patient, diminished compliance increases the airway pressure required for ventilation and thereby the risk of barotrauma.

Noncardiogenic and Neurogenic Pulmonary Edema

Many patients with neurological disease have coincident cardiovascular diseases that

TABLE 4.2. *Criteria for the diagnosis of acute lung injury*

Item	Value	Score
Consolidation on chest radiograph	None	0
	One quadrant	1
	Two quadrants	2
	Three quadrants	3
	Four quadrants	4
Hypoxemia score ($Pao_2:Fio_2$ ratio)	>300	0
	255–299	1
	175–254	2
	100–174	3
	>100	4
Positive end-expiratory pressure (PEEP) score	≤5 cmH_2O	0
	6–8 cmH_2O	1
	9–11 cmH_2O	2
	12–14 cmH_2O	3
	≥15 cmH_2O	4
Final score = Divide aggregate sum by number of components used		
	0	No lung injury
	0.1–2.5	Mild–moderate lung injury
	>2.5	Severe lung injury

From Murray JF, Matthay MA, Luce JM, et al. An expanded definition of the adult respiratory distress syndrome. *Am Rev Respir Dis* 1988;138:720–723, with permission.

may produce congestive heart failure, or cardiogenic pulmonary edema, and also may have aspiration or trauma producing acute lung injury (termed noncardiogenic pulmonary edema, such as neurogenic pulmonary edema). One useful classification of acute lung injuries is listed in Table 4.2 (2). In neurocritical care practice, the intensivist is particularly alert to the development of neurogenic pulmonary edema (NPE). The conditions associated with NPE and the presumed physiology of this process are discussed in detail in Chapter 5.

Diagnosis

The suspicion of pulmonary edema arises whenever oxygenation becomes abnormal; this may manifest as tachypnea or dyspnea in patients who can make these responses, and decreased oxygen saturation or Pao_2 (or the need to increase the Fio_2 to prevent such decreases). Rales (crackles) reflect alveolar edema, and a third heart sound reflects elevated ventricular end-diastolic volume; these findings have high positive predictive values but relatively low sensitivities (3). When substantial alveolar edema occurs, the patient

may produce pink sputum. Other physical findings suggesting congestive heart failure should be sought. However, the clinical suspicion of pulmonary edema should prompt a chest radiograph, because the differential diagnosis of oxygenation difficulty is broad, and the chest film often reveals lung findings other than or in addition to pulmonary edema that require management. It also allows one to estimate the importance of cardiac dysfunction as a contributor to pulmonary edema if present. Echocardiography is a useful adjunct if cardiac dysfunction is suspected. Electrocardiography and measurement of troponin concentrations should be undertaken if there is reason to suspect myocardial damage as the cause of pulmonary edema.

Management (see also "Endotracheal Intubation," page 83)

Perhaps even more crucially than others, the patient with acute neurological disease who becomes hypoxemic requires immediate correction of this problem. Patients who have suffered head trauma or have other reasons for cerebral ischemia do not tolerate superimposed systemic hypoxia. Although recent work indicates that excessive supplemental oxygen may be deleterious to stroke patients (4), one should not fear a brief period of elevated PaO_2 during the prevention or correction of hypoxemia. Furthermore, fear of oxygen toxicity induced by prolonged inspiration of gas at an FiO_2 exceeding 0.50 to 0.60 should never be used as a reason to permit hypoxia.

Patients who are breathing spontaneously may respond to increased oxygen by nasal cannulae or face mask; if continuous positive airway pressure (CPAP) is needed to prevent respiratory units from collapsing, this can be delivered by face mask in some patients. However, many patients with acute neurological disease are unable to cooperate with this treatment. Continuous positive airway pressure masks also impair access to the patient's airway for suctioning, and may result in massive aspiration if the patient vomits without someone in the room to remove the mask immediately. Thus, most patients with critical illnesses of the nervous system who develop pulmonary edema require endotracheal intubation.

Intubation of these patients often requires some sedation, and may also require neuromuscular junction blockade (as discussed later). Sedative agents have varying effects on intracranial pressure and systemic arterial pressure. Thiopental provides good sedation and coincident decrease in intracranial pressure if the patient has stable autonomic function. We prefer the use of etomidate, which provides brief anesthesia without measurably lowering blood pressure if hypotension is present or considered likely. Should the patient already be comatose and not require sedation, intravenous (i.v.) lidocaine may blunt the increase in ICP associated with intubation and should be given shortly before the procedure. Intravenous lidocaine also should be considered if an awake intubation is planned with topical anesthesia, because the latter does not prevent ICP elevation (5).

If neuromuscular blockade is deemed necessary, one should consider the risk of hyperkalemia produced by a depolarizing agent (e.g., succinylcholine) in patients with neurological or neuromuscular disease. Succinylcholine may also increase ICP unless the patient has been pretreated with a small ("defasciculating") dose of a nondepolarizing agent. Therefore, in most circumstances, one should rely on a nondepolarizing agent (e.g., vecuronium).

In almost all circumstances, endotracheal tubes should be placed through the mouth rather than the nose. This technique helps avoid nosocomial sinusitis, which is a risk factor in the development of nosocomial pneumonia. Nasal intubation, although mechanically more stable in the long run for awake and moving patients, is more prone to local bleeding if anticoagulation or plasma exchange become necessary. Endotracheal tubes capable of continuous aspiration of subglottic secretions should be considered (see the following).

Although the usual management of cardiogenic pulmonary edema involves diuretic and vasodilator therapy to decrease the hydrostatic pressure driving edema production, this process carries substantial risk in patients with subarachnoid hemorrhage (SAH) and others in whom cerebral ischemia may be present, even if hypotension is not produced. In addition, because NPE can occur at pulmonary capillary wedge pressure (PCWP) substantially lower than those present in cardiogenic edema, attempts to further lower PCWP may produce hypotension. Thus, the initial strategy should concentrate on supplemental oxygen and either CPAP (for the spontaneously breathing patient) or positive end-expiratory pressure (PEEP) (for the mechanically ventilated patient). After initial stabilization, determination of the wedge pressure by direct measurement through a pulmonary artery catheter should be used to guide therapy. A wedge pressure of 15 to 18 mm Hg is the usual goal in this setting. At higher wedge pressures, the patient may be at risk for an additional hydrostatic contribution to edema formation. (A cardiogenic source should be sought if the pressure is elevated at the time pulmonary edema is documented.) Lower wedge pressures may be associated with hemodynamic aggravation of vasospasm in SAH patients.

Positive end-expiratory pressure and CPAP raise intrathoracic pressure and thereby decrease cardiac preload. Thus, one must be alert for their potential effects on blood pressure, particularly in dehydrated patients. In the patient who is already in a state of increased peripheral oxygen extraction (as may occur in hypoxemia), a decrease in preload that adversely affects cardiac output further lowers the oxygen content of venous blood, resulting in incomplete oxygen uptake by the blood during its passage through the lungs, and hence progressive arterial hypoxemia. It is important to transiently decrease airway pressure to determine whether this problem is present, and to increase preload by fluid administration (even in the face of pulmonary edema) if indicated.

Patients with obstructive airway disease may not allow a complete exhalation so that lung volume comes down to functional residual capacity when intubated, as the loss of elastic tissue allows the bronchioles to collapse before some of the respiratory units have emptied to the size allowed by the applied PEEP. This results in the gradual development of additional PEEP at the alveolar level that is not reflected at the pressure sensor of the ventilator during a normal respiratory cycle; this has been variously termed "dynamic hyperinflation" or "auto-PEEP." This problem also reduces preload, and may thereby produce hypotension or arterial hypoxia. Paradoxically, it is treated by increasing the level of PEEP applied at the ventilator. This maneuver keeps the bronchioles open longer during expiration, decreasing auto-PEEP and thereby improving preload.

Pneumonia

Patients with pneumonia come to the attention of the neurointensivist in one of three ways. The most common is the development of ventilator-associated pneumonia (VAP) (or other nosocomial pneumonia) in patients with any critical illnesses of the nervous system. The second is the occurrence of aspiration in patients whose acute neurological disease impairs airway control; this may also arise at the time of an emergent intubation. The third is the patient with a chronic neurological disease, such as motor neuron disease, who develops pneumonia as a reflection of progressive loss of airway control.

Prophylaxis

The intensive care unit routine should include an established protocol for the prevention of VAP. Extensive research in the past two decades confirms that most instances, as with other forms of pneumonia, result from aspiration. The measures summarized in Table 4.3 should be employed to the extent tolerated by the patient. It should be commented that this problem is also probably ubiquitous among stroke patients and some form of assessment of the safety of swallowing is highly recommended for these individuals before feeding occurs.

TABLE 4.3. *Measures for the prevention of ventilator-associated pneumonia*

Item	Comment
Head and upper body positioning to decrease risk of aspiration	Greater than 30 and preferably 45 degrees; must be balanced against concerns for cerebral perfusion
Endotracheal tube	Oral rather than nasal to decrease the risk of sinusitis; consider using a tube designed for continuous aspiration of subglottic secretions if prolonged intubation is anticipated (6)
Gastric tubes	Oral rather than nasal to decrease the risk of sinusitis
Nutrition	Institute enteral nutrition as soon as possible
Choice of gastrointestinal bleeding prophylaxis	Although sucralfate may have a slightly lower rate of associated ventilator-associated pneumonia, it is not as effective as H_2 blockers
Selective gastric decontamination	Still debated; potential improvements in pneumonia rate may be counterbalanced by the emergence of resistant microorganisms

Diagnosis

Although the diagnosis of VAP seems straightforward, studies of this condition have been difficult to perform because of disagreements about diagnostic criteria and appropriate microbiologic techniques. This diagnosis is suspected because of the presence of fever and purulent sputum. However, these findings are frequent in patients with artificial airways, and often represent tracheobronchitis rather than pneumonia. The lack of evidence that antibiotic treatment affects the natural history of patients with tracheobronchitis, coupled with the need to reduce unnecessary antibiotic usage to reduce both costs and the selective pressure driving antibiotic resistance, suggests that antibiotics not be instituted for this problem alone.

Conversely, recent studies establish that early and microbiologically correct treatment of pneumonia improves outcome (7). Thus, the strategy that appears to be optimal is one that correctly identifies patients with pneumonia, covers the important microorganisms for that patient group, and allows early tailoring or termination of therapy as appropriate.

Most neurocritical care patients are too ill for routine chest films. Portable films usually suffice, but evanescent infiltrates often are noted. If these infiltrates are coupled with fever and purulent sputum, clinicians often begin presumptive treatment for pneumonia, which continues for days or weeks, even when the infiltrates are absent on the next film. Therefore, a strategy that terminates antibiotic therapy if the chest radiograph clears rapidly is most appropriate. Although chest computed tomography (CT) scanning is more precise than plain radiography for the diagnosis of pneumonia, its utility for this purpose remains to be determined.

A protocol such as that presented in Table 4.4 is useful to address all of these concerns.

Pulmonary Embolism

Patients with critical illness of the nervous system seem particularly predisposed to develop deep venous thrombosis (DVT) and pulmonary embolism. Most such patients are immobilized by a neurological deficit, coma, hemiparesis, or spinal instability. Some have underlying disorders, which include hypercoagulability; others have contraindications to anticoagulation for the prophylaxis of pulmonary embolism. A few have cardiac or pulmonary problems predisposing them to right-to-left shunting. Venous thrombosis may lead to systemic as well as pulmonary embolism in this group.

The optimal prophylactic regimen in these patients is under constant discussion. For patients without a contraindication to anticoagulation, a combination of pharmacologic and mechanical therapies is probably optimal. Although the use of low molecular weight heparins for this purpose has steadily increased since their approval, enthusiasm for their use must be tempered by the recognition that the lack of a readily available technique for measurement of their effects may result in excessive anticoagulation in some patients. Many neurointensivists favor weight-adjusted-dose subcutaneous unfractionated heparin, or simply give unfractionated heparin subcutaneously every 8 to 12 hours, depending on the patient's habitus. The multiplicity of opinions regarding anticoagulation in various clinical settings is beyond the scope of this text; therefore, the reader should consult recent guideline statements such as that of the American College of Chest Physicians (available at *http://www.chestnet.org/health.science.policy/ quick.reference.guides/antithrombotic/6th_an tithrom_qrg.pdf*).

The diagnosis of uncomplicated DVT requires a high index of suspicion. Physical findings such as lower extremity edema, a palpable venous cord, or Homan's sign may suggest the diagnosis but are frequently absent. Upper extremity venous thromboses are increasingly recognized, especially in patients with central venous catheters or immobilized or paretic extremities. If the involved vein has been used for venous access, one should consider the possibility of septic thrombophlebitis. Otherwise, systemic signs of inflamma-

TABLE 4.4. *Protocol for the diagnosis and management of ventilator-associated pneumonia (VAP)*

1. Suspect VAP in patients mechanically ventilated for ≥48 hours if
   a. the chest radiograph or chest CT shows a new or progressive *and* persistent infiltrate
      AND
   b. at least one of the following is present:
      1. Fever (temperature >38°C)
      2. Leukopenia (<4,000 white blood cell [WBC]/cm^3) or leukocytosis (≥12,000 WBC/cm^3)
      3. Altered mental status in patients ≥70 years
         AND
   c. at least one of the following:
      1. New onset of purulent sputum
      2. New onset or worsening of cough, dyspnea, or tachypnea
      3. Rales or bronchial breath sounds
      4. Worsening gas exchange
2. In patients suspected of having VAP by these criteria, calculate the clinical pulmonary infection score for day 1 (CPIS-1) (8):

	0 Points	1 Point	2 Points
Temperature (°C)	36.5–38.4	38.5–38.9	≤36 or ≥39
WBC count	4–11 K	<4 K or >11 K plus one additional point for >50% bands	
Secretions	None	Nonpurulent	Purulent
Pao$_2$/Fio$_2$ ratio	>240 (no points if Pao$_2$/Fio$_2$ ratio abnormal for another reason, such as the acute respiratory distress syndrome)		<240 and no other etiology
Radiographic abnormalities	None	Diffuse or patchy	Localized

3. Obtain blood cultures and sputum for quantitative culture (QC) according to the preferred local technique (e.g., endotracheal aspirate mixed with diluted acetylcysteine, or protected brush bronchoscopy, or bronchoalveolar lavage).
4. Initiate appropriate antibiotic therapy for 3 days, based on the organisms and susceptibilities of the intensive care unit. Because initial adequate antibiotic coverage is an important determinant of outcome, this choice should be adequately broad (e.g., consider two agents active against *Pseudomonas aeruginosa*) at this point, and narrowed on day 3.
5. On day 3, calculate CPIS-3:

	0 Points	1 Point	2 Points
Temperature (°C)	36.5–38.4	38.5–38.9	≤36 or ≥39
WBC count	4–11 K	<4 K or >11 K plus one additional point for >50% bands	
Secretions	None	Nonpurulent	Purulent
Pao$_2$/Fio$_2$ ratio	>240 (no points if Pao$_2$/Fio$_2$ ratio abnormal for another reason, such as the acute respiratory distress syndrome)		<240 and no other etiology
Radiographic abnormalities	None	Diffuse or patchy	Localized
Progression of infiltrate	No		Yes (and no other etiology)

   a. If QC yields <10^5 cfu/mL *and* CPIS-3 ≤ 4, discontinue antibiotics (9).
   b. If QC yields >10^5 cfu/mL *and/or* CPIS-3 > 4, continue antibiotics; adjust choice of antibiotics according to culture and sensitivity results.
6. On day 6, assess need for prolonged antibiotic therapy. Unless indicated by a slow clinical response, discontinue antibiotics on day 7.

Protocol developed by the ventilator-associated pneumonia medical management team of the University of Virginia (courtesy of Thomas P. Bleck, M.D.).

tion usually are lacking. Although DVT is sometimes detected in the course of a search for the etiology of a fever, neither venous thrombosis nor pulmonary embolism are likely to cause substantial fever; hence, the search for a source of fever should not end with the discovery of a clot (10).

The commonly employed tests for lower extremity DVT include ultrasound examination and impedance plethysmography. In the upper extremity, the evaluation often is limited to ultrasound. These techniques are reliable for the diagnosis of thrombosis in the extremities and the central veins of the chest; however, useful techniques for the diagnosis of pelvic thrombi are lacking. We have taken the position that screening for venous thrombosis should be undertaken before the application of "air boots" unless the patient has been ambulatory in the day or two before the neurological disability.

Measurement of the serum concentration of fibrin degradation products by newer sensitive techniques is a useful adjunct to the diagnosis of DVT or pulmonary embolism. However, patients with trauma or recent surgery have elevated levels of these products, which may then be difficult to distinguish from thrombosis. Thus, for many patients in neurocritical care units, this test has good specificity but poor predictive value (11).

The suspicion of pulmonary embolism in neurocritical care practice is typically raised by the abrupt development of tachypnea and difficulty with oxygenation. The main alternative consideration is airway plugging. Classic findings for embolism such as hemoptysis, chest pain, or a pleural friction rub are rarely present. The commonest electrocardiographic change owing to pulmonary embolism is sinus tachycardia; however, more suggestive findings include acute right axis deviation, a new right bundle branch block, or the development of an $S_1Q_3T_3$ pattern. With emboli of sufficient size and number, the pulmonary artery (PA) pressure becomes elevated; this can be detected as a change in the pressure recorded from a PA catheter, or from an echocardiographic estimate of PA pres-

sure. The diagnosis is typically confirmed with a radiographic study. Ventilation-perfusion scanning was the traditional test for this purpose, but is being rapidly supplanted by spiral CT scanning. Pulmonary angiography is infrequently necessary for the detection of large thrombi, but may still be required to diagnose smaller clots and it offers a potential avenue for thrombolytic treatment if the embolism is found to be very sizable.

Therapy for DVT and pulmonary embolism is often limited in neurocritical care practice by the risks of systemic anticoagulation. If no contraindications exist, one may choose either unfractionated heparin by infusion or intermittent injections of low molecular weight heparin. Although the latter option has become more common, the risks of excessive anticoagulation in patients with acute nervous system disease, the attendant difficulty of measuring the effect of low molecular weight heparin and the lack of an agent to reverse its effects often argue in favor of unfractionated heparin therapy that we still use. Weight-based nomograms for heparin dosing are available; in general, however, one should initially begin with a heparin dose that is slightly below that predicted. If the patient's risk of hemorrhage is low, one may choose to administer a 5,000 U initial dose of heparin. From our own experience we emphasize that it is imperative to stop the heparin infusion if a PTT above the measurable limit found (100 or 120 s in most laboratories), and to resume at a lower rate when the test value has returned to a measurable range. Treatment with enoxaparin or other low molecular weight heparins is easier to manage, but its effects are more difficult to measure and it is more difficult to reverse if hemorrhagic complications ensue.

Therapeutic anticoagulation carries substantial bleeding risks in patients who have recently suffered CNS hemorrhages or have had recent intracranial or spinal trauma or surgical procedures. Data to quantitate these risks are lacking; however, many avoid systemic anticoagulation for the first 3 days after an ictus. Should patients develop DVT or pulmonary embolism during this period, or have another contraindication to anticoagulation (e.g., active peptic ulcer disease), the best option may be placement of an inferior vena cava filter. Such patients should still be anticoagulated when possible (12).

The duration of anticoagulation depends on many factors, but typically is continued for 6 months. Warfarin therapy is substituted after the patient is on a therapeutic heparin regimen and no surgical procedures (e.g., tracheostomy) are anticipated. When warfarin is instituted, the older practice of giving large doses of warfarin for the first few days of therapy should be discouraged, because the measurement of prothrombin time is highly dependent on factor VII levels. The international normalized ratio thus calculated may suggest that the patient has been adequately anticoagulated when only the shortest half-life vitamin K–dependent factors actually have been reduced. Furthermore, concentrations of the anticoagulant proteins C and S fall before that of factor II, which may leave the patient in a relatively procoagulant state at the time heparin is discontinued.

Patients with pulmonary emboli hemodynamically significant enough to cause hypotension may require volume resuscitation and vasopressor therapy. Those not rapidly responsive to these measures should be considered for either thrombolytic therapy or thrombectomy; however, most patients in neurocritical care units have relative contraindications to both of these procedures. If such a patient is dying from hemodynamically significant pulmonary embolism, one may still wish to consider these options.

Severe Atelectasis and Mucus Airway Obstruction

Some degree of atelectasis is ubiquitous among patients receiving mechanical ventilation, but large areas of atelectasis, or collapse of segments or entire lobes, often produces substantial difficulties with oxygenation. This often results from mucous plugging of the airways, a problem to which neurocritical care patients seem commonly predisposed. Per-

haps this reflects autonomic dysfunction, although the precise etiology is unknown. Although the pulmonary circulation normally responds to this problem by decreasing local perfusion (hypoxic vasoconstriction), many patients with critical diseases of the nervous system seem particularly predisposed to this problem, resulting in more severe hypoxemia than one expects.

Attempts to treat atelectasis in patients receiving mechanical ventilation often include increasing the FiO_2, as well as enhancing the tidal volume and the PEEP in an attempt to ventilate the collapsed regions. Delivering a higher concentration of oxygen is useful as long as the other portions of the lung are normal, and the extent of pulmonary arteriovenous shunting is not too great. Indeed, one can assess the relative proportion of shunting versus ventilation–perfusion mismatching by observing the degree of correction of hypoxemia with 100% inspired oxygen, only the latter being corrected by this maneuver. Some shunting is to be expected with airway plugging and atelectasis, but early on the majority of the difficulty relates to mismatching. Increasing the inspired oxygen fraction should be instituted immediately in order to avoid systemic hypoxemia while measures are instituted to correct the underlying problem. However, increasing the tidal volume only overdistends the other areas of the lung, and by itself does not improve oxygenation. Increasing the PEEP may recruit areas of microatelectasis and usually thereby improve oxygenation, but will not reinflate larger regions of collapse that are lost to reexpansion once their surfactant coating has been reabsorbed.

Physical measures such as suctioning, postural drainage, and external percussion sometimes are effective in relieving the obstruction producing atelectasis, but some patients require bronchoscopic suctioning and lavage. Patients with reactive airway disease may benefit from inhaled β-agonist treatments to relieve obstruction in smaller airways. Occasional patients with substantial secretion volumes also may benefit from either inhaled or systemic anticholinergic agents, but one must be wary of producing secretions that become too tenacious to clear. Once the obstruction is relieved, maintaining the patient on higher PEEP levels to increase functional residual capacity may help to prevent this problem. Although some have suggested that ventilation with very high tidal volumes (e.g., 20 mL/kg) may help to prevent this condition (and speed weaning) in patients with normal lungs, this should be considered unproved at present. We prefer to ventilate most of these patients with sufficient pressure support to achieve tidal volumes of 7 to 8 mL/kg if they are able to trigger the ventilator, or a similar tidal volume in a controlled volume mode if they are unable to do so.

Neurogenic Ventilatory Failure

Patients with neurogenic ventilatory failure comprise one of the most important and interesting groups in neurocritical care practice. The major causes of this problem are summarized in Table 4.5 and a more detailed account of diaphragmatic failure owing to neuromuscular conditions is discussed in more detail elsewhere in this volume, particularly the one on Guillain–Barré syndrome (Chapter 18). The conditions included in the table do not represent a complete list, but are intended to provide examples of each of the types of neurogenic ventilatory failure (13).

Regardless of the etiology, patients respond to reduced ventilation in one of two characteristic ways, depending on the ability of the brainstem to sense and respond to pH, and the ability of the effector mechanisms to operate, extending from the medulla to the cervical spinal motor neurons, motor nerves, and diaphragmatic neuromuscular junction. It should be noted that extracellular pH drives this response; the Pa_{CO_2} is not an independent driver but rather exerts its influence through the pH. Local (brainstem) or systemic acidosis should trigger an increase in minute ventilation, whereas alkalosis does the opposite. If the effector mechanisms fail completely, the patient becomes apneic. The remainder of this discussion assumes that brainstem commands

are able to affect the respiratory musculature. If the brainstem is unable to sense or respond to a fall in pH, the patient's minute ventilation is not increased appropriately, and CO_2 retention occurs; however, the actual Pa_{CO_2} must be interpreted in terms of the patient's overall acid–base balance.

If the brainstem is functioning normally but the effectors are impaired, the patient's response depends in part on the rate of progression of weakness. Abrupt failure of the peripheral mechanisms, as in neuromuscular junction blockade, produces a progressive rise in Pa_{CO_2} (and a concomitant fall in pH). Rapidly progressive disorders such as Guillain–Barré polyneuropathy or myasthenic crisis produce weakness that increases over hours or days. In this setting, the initial fall in tidal volume initially elicits a compensatory increase in that efferent signal in an attempt to restore the tidal volume to normal. However, as the weakness progresses, inadequate lung expansion causes a degree of atelectasis, which by itself usually is not sufficient to cause hypoxemia. This atelectasis appears to be sensed by afferents from the lung as inadequate stretch, however, which is translated into a signal requesting an increase in minute ventilation. At about the same time, the ventilatory system loses the ability to increase the tidal volume further, and as a consequence all requests for increasing minute ventilation can only be met by increasing respiratory rate. The exact points during the progressive fall in muscle strength that the relative contributions of atelectasis (producing the inadequate stretch signal) and the need for a higher respiratory rate (to insure CO_2 excretion) are exerting greater influence over the brainstem control mechanisms are unclear, and probably vary among patients. However, the consequence is an increase in respiratory rate that typically overshoots the rate required to compensate for the fall in tidal volume; this increases the minute ventilation above that needed for the amount of CO_2 produced and thus results in a slight respiratory alkalosis. The clinician caring for such a patient must not let the finding of a Pa_{CO_2} under 40 mm Hg

TABLE 4.5. *Major causes of neurogenic ventilatory failure*

Type	Anatomic class	Representative entities	Clinical manifestations
Type IIa	Central failure to respond to falling pH (inadequate respiratory rate and inadequate tidal volume)	Medullary infarction or other lesion disrupting the nucleus of the solitary tract	Apnea, if complete; CO_2 retention if incomplete
		Narcotic overdose or other intoxication	Absent or inadequate response to falling pH and Pa_{O_2}
Type IIb	Disconnection of medullary efferents from lower motor neurons	Cervical spine injury or other lesion between lower medulla and C4 producing diaphragmatic paralysis	Apnea, if pathways are completely disrupted; tachypnea with inadequate tidal volume and consequent rise in Pa_{CO_2} if incomplete; attempted use of accessory muscles
		Cervical spine injury or other lesion between C4 and T6 producing paralysis of parasternal intercostal muscles	Paradoxical respiration; use of accessory muscles; rise in Pa_{CO_2}
Type IIc	Disorders of lower motor neurons in spinal cord	Amyotrophic lateral sclerosis and other motor neuron diseases	Slowly progressive weakness resulting in CO_2 retention and compensatory metabolic alkalosis
		Tetanus	Acute or subacute spasticity of musculature causing acute respiratory acidosis; superimposed airway obstruction
Type IId	Disorders of peripheral nerve	Acute inflammatory polyradiculoneuropathy (Guillain–Barré syndrome)	Progressive fall in tidal volume with compensatory rise in respiratory rate (often overcompensate early in the disease)
		Chronic inflammatory polyneuropathy Diphtheric neuropathy Porphyric neuropathy	Ventilatory failure is uncommon
		Tick paralysis	*Dermacentor* tick produces neuropathy
		Ciguatera Saxitoxin (and other nerve toxins) Thallium intoxication Acute hyperkalemic paralysis Heavy metals producing peripheral neuropathy	Arsenic
		Critical illness polyneuropathy Motor neuropathy of critical illness	
Type IIe	Disorders of the neuromuscular junction	Myasthenia gravis	Similar respiratory problems to acute inflammatory polyradiculoneuropathy
		Botulism	Associated autonomic disturbances are often prominent from the outset
		Organophosphate intoxication Hypermagnesemia	Carbamate insecticides and nerve agents
		Tick paralysis	*Ixodes* tick toxin produces neuromuscular junction dysfunction
		Snake bites Prolonged effect of drugs producing therapeutic neuromuscular junction blockade	Pancuronium
Type IIf	Disorders of respiratory muscles	Rhabdomyolysis Polymyositis/dermatomyositis Acid maltase deficiency Carnitine palmityl-transferase deficiency Necrotizing myopathy of critical illness Thick filament myopathy Depolarization failure Nemaline rod myopathy Acute hypokalemic paralysis Acute hypophosphatemic paralysis Stonefish myotoxin poisoning Barium poisoning Trichinosis	

produce a false sense of security. One must interpret the $Paco_2$ in the context of the respiratory rate and the vital capacity, also recognizing that weakness of the cranial musculature may impair the patient's ability to form a tight seal around the spirometer mouthpiece and hence make the vital capacity artifactually low.

Eventually, progressive weakness results in a further decline in the tidal volume, for which the patient is unable to compensate with further elevations in respiratory rate; as the minute ventilation falls, the $Paco_2$ increases, with a concomitant fall in pH. Such patients usually require mechanical ventilation, although one can opt to permit hypercapnia in the patient who maintains good airway control and intact consciousness. On rare occasions, we have allowed such patients to reach $Paco_2$ values in the 90- to 100-mm Hg range while waiting for the effect of therapy (e.g., i.v. immunoglobulin therapy for myasthenic crisis) (14). However, such patients must be managed in an intensive care unit where any decompensation will be discovered and managed immediately.

Weakness of the cranial musculature is a frequent, although not invariable, accompaniment of this decline in ventilatory strength. As a consequence, endotracheal intubation may be required for airway control (to prevent aspiration and facilitate suctioning) before the patient requires mechanical ventilation. When the time comes to intubate the patient, recall that the extra work of breathing imposed by the endotracheal tube often forces the patient to depend on mechanical ventilation as well. Because the resistance imposed by the tube is directly proportional to its length but proportional to the inverse fourth power of its radius, one should place the largest diameter tube that comfortably fits the patient's larynx. If neuromuscular junction blockade is required to intubate a patient with neuromuscular respiratory failure, the action of the agent used likely lasts much longer than the duration to which one is accustomed. Although the initial sedation and neuromuscular junction blockade are active, the patient requires mechanical

ventilation with a fixed rate. When these medications have worn off, the patient may or may not need mechanical ventilation. Five cm H_2O of CPAP is often useful to prevent atelectasis in this group of patients, but one must observe the patient carefully for signs of fatigue because CPAP slightly increases work of breathing, in addition to the increase imposed by the endotracheal tube.

Patients who require mechanical ventilation because of respiratory muscle weakness but who maintain airway protection may be candidates for noninvasive mechanical ventilation. In general, patients with rapidly progressive neurogenic respiratory failure (e.g., acute inflammatory polyradiculoneuropathy) do not tolerate noninvasive ventilation well and are usually better candidates for endotracheal intubation. Conversely, patients with slowly progressive neuromuscular diseases who need short-term mechanical ventilation (e.g., during treatment of an intercurrent illness) occasionally do very well with noninvasive ventilation by mask. Such patients must always have someone in attendance in case their tightly fitting mask should become filled with vomitus. Although some patients also may be managed with negative pressure ventilators (e.g., cuirass ventilators), these devices are more commonly used for long-term home ventilation.

Once the patient with neurogenic ventilatory failure is committed to positive pressure mechanical ventilation via an endotracheal tube, five basic principles must be kept in mind. First, if the patient has developed ventilatory failure over several days or weeks, renal compensation for the respiratory acidosis has produced a high serum bicarbonate concentration. One should not attempt to correct the elevated $Paco_2$ immediately, because this produces a severe systemic alkalosis. Rather, one should achieve and maintain a minute ventilation that results in a pH near 7.50; this triggers renal loss of bicarbonate and other bases, eventually bringing the serum bicarbonate back to the normal range. Because the minute ventilation necessary to do this is often quite low, one usually selects a reasonable tidal volume (e.g., 6 to 8 mL/kg) at a low rate; lower tidal volumes may promote atelectasis.

Second, there is no clear value to "resting" patients by using full ventilatory support, even at night, with the exception of selected patients with chronic obstructive lung disease. One should make maximal use of the patient's own respiratory capabilities in order to prevent muscle deconditioning to the extent possible. Pressure support ventilation is usually the most easily tolerated ventilator mode for these patients, because it supplies a high gas flow rate at the start of the breath. The optimal level of pressure support is generally that producing a tidal volume in the 6- to 8-mL/kg range, a respiratory rate below 20/min, and no signs of distress (diaphoresis, tachycardia, nasal flaring, and use of accessory muscles of respiration). However, there is no evidence to prove that one mode of ventilation leads to faster weaning than another; if the patient seems more comfortable when a volume mode of ventilation is employed, one should consider using that mode.

Third, at a time when weaning seems feasible, it is useful to "challenge" the patient once or twice daily to ensure that weaning from mechanical ventilation proceeds as quickly as possible. One can either decrease the level of pressure support, or introduce periods (e.g., 1 hour at a time) of CPAP in place of mechanical ventilatory support. The patient should be prepared for these changes by careful explanation and reassurance. If the patient requires sedation to tolerate the ventilator, this should also be reduced or discontinued daily to insure that changes in the patient's tolerance or accumulation of medication have not produced too deep a level of sedation.

Fourth, one should be cognizant of changes in oxygenation and ventilatory mechanics. The origin of most problems with oxygenation is discussed in the preceding. A fall in tidal volume in a patient on pressure support ventilation, or an increase in peak or mean airway pressure in a patient on a volume ventilatory mode, indicate a fall in pulmonary compliance that must be investigated. Some of the common causes include pulmonary edema, pneumonia, and mucus plugging, which produces large areas of atelectasis. One must always be alert, most of all, for the possible development of a pneumothorax.

Fifth, most patients with neurogenic respiratory failure are quite cognizant of their situation, including their potential discomfort from the endotracheal tube. Some patients tolerate the tube without difficulty, but most are troubled by it. Local measures for pain control are useful sometimes, but systemic narcotics and sedatives are necessary more commonly. The development of the percutaneous technique has lowered the threshold for tracheostomy in these patients, and we typically offer it to patients in whom weaning from mechanical ventilation is expected to be prolonged. Weaning usually is hastened by tracheostomy, in part because of decrease in dead space and airway resistance as well as better clearance of airway secretions. Several devices are now available to allow the patient with a tracheostomy to speak, a major advantage in conditions in which weakness prevents the patient from using a letter board or otherwise communicating by hand.

THE PHYSIOLOGY OF RESPIRATORY FUNCTION

In order to grasp the changes effected by pulmonary diseases and neuromuscular respiratory failure and the reasoning behind various uses of artificial ventilation, it is necessary to introduce a number of physiologic concepts (e.g., dead space and compliance) and the formulas that are used to express them. As mentioned, acquisition of this knowledge allows the neurointensivist to think intelligently about ventilators and their settings and discuss more sophisticated concepts of pulmonary care in any ICU setting.

The respiratory function of the lung can be divided into two separate but interrelated components: *ventilation,* or the bulk movement of gas in and out of the lung to achieve the excretion of carbon dioxide, and *oxygenation,* or the delivery of oxygen-containing gas to the alveolar space and its diffusion into the blood. The first is more of an issue in the mechanical ventilatory failure of neuromuscular diseases that weaken the diaphragm and the latter, in the airway disease of pneumonia and its extension to adult respiratory distress syndrome.

Ventilation

Predicting Ventilatory Requirements: Dead Space

In the steady state, carbon dioxide is produced as a byproduct of metabolism and excreted by the lungs. Regardless of the absolute Pa_{CO_2} level, in order to keep that level constant it is necessary to excrete exactly the same amount of carbon dioxide as is produced by the body in a given period of time. Excretion is achieved by exhaling gas that contains more carbon dioxide than was inhaled. For practical purposes, room air and oxygen mixtures used in the ICU contain no carbon dioxide. A portion of the inhaled tidal volume is delivered to the functioning alveolar space, where carbon dioxide diffuses passively from the blood across the alveolar capillary membrane and into the air space. Diffusion is driven by a CO_2 tension gradient across the membrane and continues until the P_{CO_2}, in alveolar capillary blood has decreased to a tension equal to that which has built up in the alveoli. Because CO_2 diffuses readily, time is not a limiting factor, and it is assumed that equilibration occurs virtually immediately. Therefore, the P_{CO_2} in blood leaving the lungs should be equal to P_{CO_2} in the alveolar gas that is exhaled.

A portion of the inhaled tidal volume goes to parts of the respiratory system that are not perfused and therefore do not take part in gas exchange. This wasted ventilation, referred to as *dead space,* is made up first of those fixed anatomic parts of the respiratory system that are normally ventilated but not perfused, namely, the conducting airways *(anatomic dead space)* and an additional *physiologic dead space* composed of the conducting airways plus alveolar units that are normally not perfused and those that cannot be recruited because of a pathologic process. The normal anatomic dead space is approximately 1 mL/lb of lean body weight and can be measured by Fowler's method, a nitrogen concentration technique. Physiologic dead space, usually expressed as the ratio of dead space to tidal volume, V_D/V_T, is calculated from the Bohr equation.

$$\frac{V_D}{V_T} = \frac{Pa_{CO_2} - PE_{CO_2}}{Pa_{CO_2}}$$

Physiologic dead space is that portion of an inhaled tidal volume that does not participate in gas exchange and is therefore of greater clinical significance than the anatomic dead space. It should be recognized that the normal V_D/V_T is approximately 0.3, or restated, that a third of pulmonary volume is not used in gas exchange. PE_{CO_2} signifies the end tidal concentration of CO_2.

If V is the minute ventilation (in liters per minute) delivered to a patient and V_D/V_T is the fraction of that ventilation that does not participate in gas exchange, $(1 - V_D/V_T) \times V$ is the amount of remaining alveolar ventilation, termed V_A. Recalling that the PPV_{CO_2} (i.e., after blood has passed the alveolus) equals the PA_{CO_2}, one assumes that the Pa_{CO_2} closely approximates the PA_{CO_2}. From the gas laws, the ratio of CO_2 volume (V_{CO_2}) to total volume of alveolar gas (V_A) equals the ratio of CO_2 tension to tension of the total gas. Thus,

$$\frac{Pa_{CO_2}}{760} = \frac{V_{CO_2}}{V_A}$$

Therefore, during each minute,

$$\frac{Pa_{CO_2}}{760} = \frac{V_{CO_2}}{V_A}$$

which is the volume of CO_2 excreted per minute divided by the alveolar minute ventilation. Substituting for VA yields the equation:

$$V_{CO_2} = \frac{Pa_{CO_2}}{760} \times (1 - V_D/V_T) \times V$$

In the steady state, CO_2 excretion must equal CO_2 production for the Pa_{CO_2} to remain constant. The point of these calculations is that, assuming a normal V_D/V_T of 0.3 and CO_2 production equal to 3 mL/min per kg, *a minute ventilation of approximately 80 mL/kg/min is necessary to maintain a P_{CO_2} of 40 mm Hg and a minute ventilation of about 100 mL/kg per minute to maintain P_{CO_2} at 30 mm Hg.*

Additionally, when estimating minute ventilation requirements for a patient on a mechanical ventilator, the difference between tidal volume set on the ventilator and tidal volume delivered to the patient should be kept in mind. During inspiration, some of the tidal volume displaced by the ventilator is compressed in the ventilator and tubing and is not delivered to the airway. Depending on the characteristics of the ventilator, the compression volume may be an important factor, particularly when peak inspiratory pressure is high and tidal volume low.

Lung Compliance and the Work of Breathing

These subjects relate to the distensibility of the lung and the effort required to expand the chest wall. They come in to play mainly when high pressures are required to deliver a given tidal volume by mechanical ventilation. The bulk movement of air in and out of the lung is achieved by rhythmic changes in lung volume. The lung is a distensible organ, and like any such elastic structure, its volume is a function of the distending pressure across its surface. The lungs, being contained within the airtight system made up of the muscular thoracic cage and diaphragm, have a distending pressure, or transmural pressure (P_{TM}), equal to the difference between airway pressure (P_{AIR}, representing the pressure within the lung) and the intrapleural pressure (P_{PL}). The lungs expand as positive transmural pressure is applied to the pulmonary system. This is normally achieved in spontaneous ventilation by the diaphragmatic pull that creates negative intrapleural pressure while airway pressure remains atmospheric, or artificially by applying positive pressure to the airway with

a mechanical ventilator. The amount of expansion or change in volume for a given increase in pressure is referred to as the compliance of the lung system, expressed as the ratio

$$\text{Compliance} = \frac{\Delta V}{\Delta P}$$

Where there is no gas flow in the pulmonary system, the major determinant of compliance is the elasticity of the lung. When elastic tissue in the lung is destroyed, as in emphysema, the lungs become "floppy" and compliance increases; that is, relatively little pressure is required to increase the volume of the lung. However, at the end of inspiration, relatively little elastic recoil is available to help achieve exhalation. Conversely, an increase of the inelastic substances in the lung decreases compliance. Lungs stiffened by alveolar edema or infected fluid or fibrosis from chronic lung disease require higher pressure to achieve a given degree of inflation; that is, they have low compliance.

Figure 4.1 is a classic pressure–volume curve of lung expansion and contraction. With pressure plotted on the abscissa and volume on the ordinate, the slope of the curve repre-

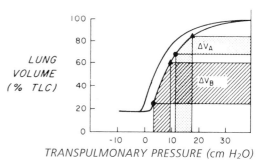

TRANSPULMONARY PRESSURE (cm H₂O)

FIG. 4.1. The classic pressure–volume curve of the lung, relating transpulmonary pressure (P_{TM}) to lung volume, which is expressed as percent of total lung capacity. A given increase in lung volume, ΔV, depends on the slope of the curve where pressure is added. The more compliant the lung, the steeper the slope, and the greater increase in lung volume is achieved ($\Delta V_B > \Delta V_A$). (Adapted from DC Sabiston Jr, ed. *Davis-Christopher: textbook of surgery,* 11th ed. Philadelphia: Saunders, 1977:2026, with permission.)

sents the compliance of the lung. Initially, as pressure is increased, volume in the lung increases only slowly. This initially flat portion of the curve reflects low compliance. Greater increases in volume are seen as pressure is increased further. The curve becomes steeper as lung compliance increases. The lung becomes overdistended and difficult to inflate at high lung volume. This is seen in the final flat portion of the curve, where lung compliance again decreases. In the spontaneously breathing patient, the airway and alveolar pressures are atmospheric, or a reference point of zero. Therefore, P_{TM} is numerically equivalent to P_{PL}. In the mechanically ventilated patient, P_{PL} may still remain slightly negative; therefore, P_{TM} may be slightly larger than the airway pressure measured at the ventilator.

Compliance is an important measure of lung elasticity but can be affected by numerous other factors. Imagine, for example, a normal, healthy patient anesthetized, paralyzed, and placed on a mechanical ventilator. A tidal volume of 1,000 mL is delivered through an endotracheal tube. The peak pressure measured in the airway might be expected to be in the range of 15 to 20 cm H_2O. It is possible to reach much higher pressures if the tidal volume is delivered rapidly; that is, if high peak flow rates are used. In this case, high peak pressures might be reached because resistance in the airways becomes an increasingly important factor. When compliance is considered in this dynamic situation using pressures measured during periods of high gas flow, the resulting value is called the *dynamic compliance*. To eliminate the effect of airway resistance on the pressure required to generate a given lung volume, measurements are made at a time when there is no gas flow. If a 1-L syringe is attached to the endotracheal tube and small increments of volume are administered, allowing equilibration of airway pressure after each aliquot, the airway pressure at the end of inflation will be a function of the lung's elasticity only. Measured under conditions of no flow, this value is termed *static compliance*. In practice, static compliance is cumbersome and difficult to measure.

However, a surrogate method can be used that diminishes the influence of high flow rate on airway pressure. A brief "inspiratory hold" setting is used on the ventilator and the exhalation port is occluded for a period of 2 to 3 seconds at the moment the ventilator has finished delivering a prescribed tidal volume; during this time the peak airway pressure settles briefly to a plateau level. When this plateau pressure is used in the calculation, the resulting value is known as the *effective compliance*. In normal subjects these three measures of compliance are similar. With a disease state or a high inspiratory flow rate, the values become more disparate. In the clinical setting, effective compliance is a reasonably reliable value.

Work is obviously performed in moving the lungs and chest wall. This work is proportional to the product of pressure, volume, and respiratory rate. It is easy to appreciate that any change that increases the pressure necessary to generate a given lung volume increases the work of breathing. For a given amount of minute ventilation (tidal volume × rate), the less compliant the lungs, the greater pressures are required to inflate the lung and therefore the greater the work of breathing. Conversely, for a given lung compliance, as the amount of minute ventilation increases, the work of breathing increases. It follows that high carbon dioxide production, which causes an increase in minute ventilation, or an increase in the ratio of dead space to tidal volume, both increase the *work of breathing*.

Mechanical Ventilation

The inception of mechanical ventilation virtually defined the era of intensive care. As discussed in the Introduction to this book, the polio epidemics of the 1940s and 1950s led to technical innovations that were the progenitors of the modern volume cycled ventilator. Mechanical ventilation is indicated in a patient who is unable to meet his or her own ventilatory demands or, alternatively, it may be used to induce hypocapnia in the patient with an intracranial mass lesion.

The ability to meet ventilatory demands and maintain $Paco_2$ within a normal range by spontaneous ventilation requires an intact medullary control system, adequate neuromuscular function to move the diaphragm and accessory respiratory muscles, and V_D/V_T, Vco_2, and pulmonary compliance within normal limits. For example, the otherwise healthy patient who has received large doses of narcotics that suppress medullary activity may require mechanical ventilation solely to maintain normal $Paco_2$. Or, the patient with normal medullary function and healthy lungs may require mechanical ventilation because neuromuscular disease has weakened the diaphragm (advanced cases of Guillain–Barré syndrome, myasthenia gravis, or a cervical spinal cord lesion). A patient with normal medullary and neuromuscular function may require mechanical assistance when pulmonary pathology either increases the dead space (V_D/V_T), resulting in the retention of carbon dioxide, or decreases in pulmonary compliance, thereby increasing the work of breathing. The work of breathing may then increase to the point that even an otherwise normal patient cannot meet the demands for gas excretion. Except for the rare case of malignant hyperthermia, it is unlikely that an increase in CO_2 production alone will create the indication for mechanical ventilation; however, fever, for example, which greatly raises CO_2 production, certainly exacerbates any other underlying conditions.

The decision to institute mechanical ventilation is based on the patient's clinical appearance, including presence of dyspnea, severity of the underlying pulmonary or neuromuscular lesion, age, and $Paco_2$. Other physiologic parameters that do not themselves constitute indications for ventilation but have been found in various clinical studies to correlate with the need for it include *vital capacity less than 15 to 20 mL/kg, inspiratory force less than −30 cm H_2O, V_D/V_T greater than 0.6, spontaneous minute ventilation greater than 10 L/min, and inability to achieve a spontaneous minute ventilation of 20 L/min on command.* Conversely, the ability of the patient to exceed these measurements usually correlates with the ability to wean mechanical ventilation.

The goal of mechanical ventilation in these patients is to maintain the $Paco_2$ near what is normal for the patient while minimizing the impact of the positive intrathoracic pressure on cardiac output (see the following). This requires maintenance of adequate intravascular volume, occasionally the use of vasopressors or inotropic drugs, and an attempt to keep positive airway pressure to the necessary minimum. This is best done by titrating the ventilator settings, similar to any drug, to meet the patient's needs. The intermittent mandatory ventilation (IMV) rate is kept at the lowest possible that produces adequate $Paco_2$ and pH without taxing the patient by forcing him to carry too high a proportion of the minute ventilation. When the ventilator is managed in this fashion, weaning conceptually begins as soon as ventilatory assistance begins. After the IMV has been reduced to rates as low as one per minute or one every few minutes, a trial of spontaneous ventilation with CPAP may be undertaken. In the patient recovering from serious respiratory failure of some weeks' duration, the trial period may be on the order of 24 to 48 hours. The patient recovering from a recent drug overdose may require a trial of only 1 or 2 hours. The endotracheal tube is removed when the patient is successfully weaned from the respirator and no other indication is present for intubation.

The ventilator is also an established tool in the therapy of patients with intracranial mass lesions. Acutely lowering the $Paco_2$ produces an abrupt rise in the pH of brain's extracellular fluid (ECF), as discussed in Chapter 2. This occurs because CO_2 equilibrates rapidly across the blood–brain barrier (BBB), lowering the concentration of carbonic acid (H_2CO_3) in brain ECF. The concentration of bicarbonate, which does not cross the BBB, does not immediately change; therefore, the pH of brain ECF rises with acute hypocapnia regardless of what happens to arterial bicarbonate concentration (Fig. 4.2). Within hours, the bicarbonate concentration begins to decrease, and by 30 hours the pH is back to nor-

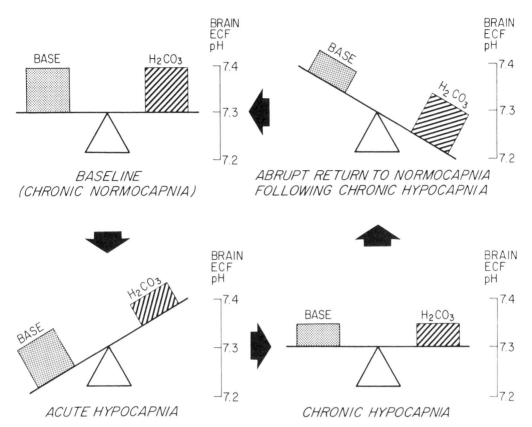

FIG. 4.2. Brain extracellular fluid pH changes with alterations in Paco$_2$. Base represents bicarbonate concentration. H$_2$CO$_3$, carbonic acid concentration, is determined by Paco$_2$, which rapidly equilibrates across the blood–brain barrier. Acute hypocapnia produces local alkalosis and vasoconstriction. With time, pH returns to normal, even though Paco$_2$ remains low. An abrupt return to normal Paco$_2$ in the presence of low bicarbonate concentration lowers the pH, producing vasodilatation.

mal (15). The ability of acute hyperventilation to reduce ICP is presumably because of vasoconstriction and reduction of cerebral blood volume secondary to increased pH. Therefore, the beneficial effect of hyperventilation should be short-lived.

Experimental verification of this has been found by Muizelaar and colleagues, who demonstrated that rabbit pial arterioles constricted 13% when Paco$_2$ was acutely reduced from 38 to 25 mm Hg (16). Vasoconstriction decreased by about 3% every 4 hours during hyperventilation. After 20 hours of hyperventilation to 25 mm Hg, vessel diameter was slightly greater than baseline at 38 mm Hg. After 52 hours of hypocapnia, the vessel di-

ameter had returned to 105% of baseline. When Paco$_2$ was acutely restored to 38 mm Hg, vessel diameter increased to 122% of baseline. Blood and cerebrospinal fluid bicarbonate were reduced throughout the period of hyperventilation, presumably contributing to the vasodilation observed whenever Paco$_2$ was returned to baseline.

In cats with experimental fluid-percussion cerebral injury, prolonged hyperventilation has been associated with indications of mild brain ischemia and increased brain lactate production. Intravenous tromethamine (THAM), a buffering agent, along with hyperventilation, reduced brain lactate, and edema (17). However, in an influential prospective study of head-injured patients, there was no difference in outcome 1 year after injury among patients treated with prolonged hyperventilation ($Paco_2$ = 25 mm Hg); hyperventilation plus i.v. THAM; and control ($Paco_2$ = 35 mm Hg) (18). At 3 to 6 months postinjury, among patients with motor scores of 4 to 5, the hyperventilation-only group had poorer outcome than both control and hyperventilation plus THAM. (Biochemical data indicated that hyperventilation could not sustain alkalinization in the CSF, although THAM could.) The authors concluded that "prophylactic hyperventilation is deleterious in head injured patients with motor scores of 4 to 5. When sustained hyperventilation becomes necessary for intracranial pressure control, its deleterious effect may be overcome by the addition of THAM." This feature of ICP control is still controversial and has not been adopted into standard practice; it must be viewed in the context of an individual situation as discussed more extensively in Chapter 3.

When using hyperventilation in the treatment of raised ICP, several points should be kept in mind. First, not all patients benefit from the same degree of hyperventilation, particularly from profound hyperventilation to $Paco_2$ of 25 mm Hg or lower. Vasoconstriction tends to reduce ICP but at some point may jeopardize adequate perfusion. Also, increasing levels of hyperventilation generally are associated with higher levels of mean airway pressure, which may tend to raise ICP. We have observed several patients whose ICP increased when $Paco_2$ was reduced from 30 to 25 mm Hg. Second, the longer a patient is hyperventilated, and certainly after 24 hours, the greater the reduction in bicarbonate is. At this point, any increase in $Paco_2$, inadvertent or owing to fever or other causes, even to levels below the patient's previous normal level, may produce a decrease in brain pH and corresponding increase in ICP. For this reason, hyperventilated patients with intracranial mass lesions should be very slowly returned to their normal $Paco_2$ over 24 to 48 hours by a gradual increase in the ventilator rate. Third,

consideration should be given to using acute hyperventilation as a short-term therapy only, whereas other measures are taken to control ICP. If $Paco_2$ can be maintained at normal levels and the ICP otherwise controlled, acute hyperventilation to 30 mm Hg could then be used if a sudden increase in ICP should occur. Abrupt hyperventilation from 40 to 30 mm Hg is associated with less increased mean airway pressure than would be required to take the patient from 30 to 20 mm Hg (Chapter 3).

Ideally, hyperventilation is titrated to a desired endpoint of ICP control as measured directly by an intracranial monitor. Initial ventilator settings in the acute situation and subsequent ventilator changes may be guided by the end-tidal CO_2 monitor. In the absence of clinically important lung damage, $Paco_2$ in head-injured patients is accurately reflected by the end-tidal CO_2 measurement, a technique that we favor if hyperventilation is to be used for more than 1 or 2 days (19).

Although autoregulation is a sensitive mechanism that appears to be altered with even slight head injury, the response of cerebral blood flow (CBF) to $Paco_2$ tends to be maintained except in severe head injury. Loss of carbon dioxide reactivity is considered a grave prognostic sign. Furthermore, carbon dioxide reactivity can be reduced or eliminated during pharmacologically induced hypotension (20).

Complications of Positive Airway Pressure

The application of positive pressure to the airway, whether by continuous positive airway pressure (CPAP) or by the standard volume cycled mechanical ventilation, affects many organ systems in the body. Among other effects, antidiuretic hormone production is stimulated (6), renal blood flow is decreased and redistributed so that medullary perfusion increases, and urine output falls (21,22). In the lung, there is a net increase in water content (23).

However, the most clinically significant problems related to positive pressure generally fall into three categories: barotrauma of the lung (e.g., pneumothorax), hemodynamic disturbances, and increases in ICP. In each case, the magnitude of the problem is a function of the increase in the applied intrathoracic–intrapleural pressure, which in turn is determined by mean airway pressure and by lung compliance. Although there is no clinically practical method of measuring the change in intrapleural pressure produced by an increase in mean airway pressure, one can at least make some qualitative predictions based on an assessment of the patient's lung and chest wall compliance. *Most often this problem presents itself in the opposing needs to raise airway pressure in order to expand a diseased and noncompliant lung for the purpose of delivering more oxygen, and the desire to keep these ventilator pressures low in order to minimize the effects on cardiac output and blood pressure.*

The application of a given amount of positive airway pressure increases lung volume by an amount that depends on the compliance of the lung. The more compliant the lung, the greater is the increase in lung volume. However, this increase in lung volume will not be as great as predicted from an idealized pressure–volume curve of the excised lung, because the patient's lungs are contained within the chest cavity, which is itself a distensible, compliant structure. An increase in lung volume increases the intrapleural pressure within the chest cavity, the magnitude of which is determined by the chest wall compliance. The intrapleural pressure increases more as the chest wall compliance decreases. However, the increase in pressure is not as great as predicted from the compliance curve of the isolated chest wall, because as the pleural pressure increases, the distending pressure across the lung ($P_{AIR} - P_{PL}$) also decreases, thereby reducing the increase in lung volume initially predicted from the isolated lung pressure–volume curve. Somewhere between these two extremes of the isolated lung and isolated chest wall lies an equilibrium that reflects the clinical circumstance. The patient with compliant lung and noncompliant chest wall has the greatest increase in pleural pressure for a given increase in airway pressure. This might

occur in a barrel-chested, emphysematous patient, for instance. However, the patient with noncompliant lungs and compliant chest wall has the least increase in intrapleural pressure. Other things being equal, the young, previously healthy trauma victim with "shock lung" and flail chest should tolerate the hemodynamic and intracranial side effects of a given increase in airway pressure better than the former patient.

Alterations in intrapleural pressure have a profound effect on other pressures measurements in the thorax, particularly atrial and pulmonary artery measurements. In clinical work, mechanical ventilation has the effect of reducing cardiac filling pressures and blood pressure, both of which are detrimental in most neurological processes, and can be disastrous in instances of raised intracranial pressure. The central venous pressure or right atrial pressure is usually measured relative to the ambient atmospheric pressure. For purposes of hemodynamic assessment, cardiac chamber compliance is assumed to be constant, and pressure is used as a measure of volume. In fact, it is the transmural pressure, for example, in the right atrium (central venous pressure − P_{PL}), that is the distending pressure that best represents the pressure–volume relationship in the thorax. During spontaneous respiration, mean intrapleural pressure is approximately −2 to −5 cm H_2O, so the central venous pressure is a reasonable approximation of the right atrial transmural pressure. However, this relationship becomes unreliable once a patient is placed on positive airway pressure for the following reasons. If a patient is mechanically ventilated and pleural pressure increase by 10 cm H_2O and if one assumes that right atrial compliance and volume remain unchanged, the central venous pressure should increase by 10 cm H_2O. In other words, the hemodynamic status characterized by a central venous pressure of 5 cm H_2O, off the ventilator, is now characterized by a central venous pressure of 15 cm H_2O while on the ventilator. In practice, intrapleural pressure is not measured, so the clinician would have no way of demonstrating that the new central venous pressure of 15 cm H_2O reflected no change in hemodynamic status. Once a patient is placed on a ventilator, new standards of normal are established, and the absolute numbers cannot be predicted. The patient's clinical status must be evaluated, and cardiac output, urine output, and other measures of adequate perfusion must be obtained to determine the atrial pressures necessary to maintain adequate hemodynamic performance in a given patient. With ventilation held constant, changes in central venous pressure are as reliable as in the spontaneously breathing patient.

Because of these unpredictable influences on cardiovascular pressure measurements, some have suggested temporarily removing the patient from the ventilator while "true" pressure measurements are taken. There are several problems with this reasoning. First, positive airway pressure may profoundly affect the hemodynamic status of a patient, so that documenting adequate central venous pressure off the ventilator may be of little use if patients suffer serious depression of cardiac output as soon as they have returned to the ventilator. Second, it is not always possible to predict how long a period off the ventilator is necessary before cardiac pressures reach a new equilibrium. Finally, these rapid shifts in atrial pressure and cardiac output may be detrimental not only to the patient's hemodynamic status but also to potential intracranial lesions as well. Given these limitations, the practice in our units has been to make all pressure measurements at end expiration, thereby eliminating some of the artifacts introduced by mechanical ventilation at high tidal volume. This is best performed by taking measurements from a calibrated screen or calibrated recording paper. In the end, however, the adequacy of cardiac filling pressure is determined by the patient's clinical response rather than by any absolute normal value.

Hemodynamic Effects

As stated, as mean airway pressure is increased, cardiac output decreases. This ob-

servation was made more than 50 years ago (24), and even then the change in cardiac output was recognized to be related to a decrease in right ventricular transmural pressure. Increased pleural pressure impedes venous return to the heart, decreasing right ventricular preload and thereby decreasing cardiac output. The expected response to mechanical ventilation, therefore, is a decreased cardiac output and blood pressure, which is indeed, commonly observed. *The changes are more pronounced when hypovolemia is present and may be prevented if transmural filling pressures are maintained with intravascular volume expansion* (25,26). In most cases, positive pressure ventilation produces an increase in central venous pressure, whereas the transmural right atrial pressure decreases. Depressed myocardial function also has been suggested as a cause of decreased cardiac output and blood pressure with positive pressure ventilation (27). This notion has been based on the observation that cardiac output is not restored to baseline values even after calculated left atrial transmural filling pressures are restored to normal. This hypothesis assumes that cardiac compliance remains constant, so that restoration of transmural filling pressures implies restoration of baseline chamber volumes as well. More recent studies measuring end-diastolic and end-systolic volume have demonstrated that cardiac output may be restored to normal when end-diastolic volume is returned to normal with volume expansion (28). Transmural end-diastolic pressures at this point were higher, indicating a decrease in ventricular compliance as mean airway pressure was increased.

It should be further pointed out that pulmonary vascular resistance is influenced by lung volume, being minimal at functional residual capacity. As mean airway pressure increases, pulmonary vascular resistance increases. A sudden increase in right ventricular afterload may strain the right ventricle to the point that cardiac output is compromised. The intraventricular septum is displaced to the left as the right ventricle dilates, decreasing left ventricular compliance and left ventricular stroke volume (29–31).

There are several ways to minimize the deleterious effects of decreased cardiac output and blood pressure during mechanical ventilation. As emphasized, the mean airway pressure should be kept at the minimum necessary, for example by using PEEP only when required to keep the FiO_2 within safe limits and by using IMV. The IMV is titrated to the patient's ventilatory needs, keeping the number of mechanical breaths to a minimum and allowing the patient to breathe spontaneously, thereby creating intermittent, negative intrapleural pressure, which further reduces mean airway pressure. Another approach is vigorous intravascular volume expansion to restore transmural filling pressures to baseline. Whether such volume expansion, either with crystalloid or colloid, is detrimental to patients with intracranial lesions is unknown. Alternatively, inotropic drugs may be administered. Dopamine is useful in restoring cardiac output as well as increasing urinary output and sodium excretion (32). The role of rapid, "jet" or high-frequency ventilation that uses frequent small volume breaths and minimizes the pressure required to deliver a given minute volume has yet to be established in neurological intensive care.

Effects of Positive Pressure Ventilation on Intracranial Pressure

Intracranial pressure may increase when positive airway pressure is applied; however, the more important effect is likely to be an alteration in cerebral perfusion pressure, produced by changes in systemic blood pressure (Chapters 2 and 3). Regardless of the effect on right atrial transmural pressure, the central venous pressure increases during positive pressure ventilation. As discussed, depending on the patient's lung and chest wall compliance, some of the mean airway pressure increase is transmitted to the pleural space, raising the central venous pressure. Through venous backflow pressure from the thorax to the jugular veins (ignoring the valves that limit

transmission of pressure) and from pressure transmitted more directly to the spinal foramina and adjacent CSF, this produces an increase in cerebral venous pressure that may raise the ICP. The greater the *intracranial compliance,* the better tolerated is this intracranial volume challenge. Patients with decreased intracranial compliance are likely to show substantial increases in ICP as cerebral venous pressure is increased during positive pressure ventilation. For example, Apuzzo and colleagues studied the effects of PEEP in 25 patients with severe head injury (33). Intracranial pressure increased significantly in 12 patients, all of whom had decreased compliance measured by the volume pressure response. No significant increase in ICP occurred in patients with normal volume pressure response. Cerebral perfusion pressure dropped below 60 mm Hg in six of the 12 patients with increased ICP. Aidinis and coworkers (34) studied the intracranial responses to PEEP in experimental cats. They found that PEEP tended to reduce cerebral perfusion pressure and produce electroencephalographic abnormalities in cats with normal lungs. In another group of cats, oleic acid embolization to the lungs produced a respiratory distress syndrome characterized by pulmonary edema and decreased lung compliance. These cats suffered less reduction in cerebral perfusion pressure and electroencephalographic abnormalities. *This is consistent with our observation that decreased lung compliance results in less transmission of mean airway pressure to the pleural space and less increase in ICP.* A similar ability of decreased lung compliance to blunt the effect of positive airway pressure on ICP was described by Huseby and colleagues (35). In a later study, they showed that PEEP increased ICP to a lesser extent in animals with preexisting intracranial hypertension (36). They postulated a "waterfall effect." When ICP is elevated, pressure in cortical veins must increase to a slightly higher level to prevent collapse and cessation of blood flow. However, Huseby and coworkers postulated that bridging veins connecting cortical veins to the superior sagittal sinus do, in fact, collapse, preventing pressure changes in the sagittal sinus from affecting cortical veins. Therefore, increased venous pressure produced by increased positive airway pressure is seen in the rigid sagittal sinus but not in the cortical veins. Furthermore, in regard to this waterfall effect, *elevation of the patient's head should obviate most of the impact of raised intrathoracic pressure on ICP because the added pressure then must exceed the pressure of the column of CSF in the spine and the venous blood column in order to have an impact on intracerebral pressure.*

Occasionally, the application of positive airway pressure produces an increase in ICP that exceeds the increase in central venous pressure, as discussed in Chapter 3. In this case, the increase in cerebral venous pressure alone could not account for raised ICP. This situation probably results from an increase in cerebral edema produced by ischemia resulting from decreased cerebral perfusion pressure.

Results in human studies have been variable. Investigating 12 head-injured patients, Shapiro and Marshall found that six patients increased their ICP by 10 mm Hg or more with the application of 4 to 8 cm H_2O of PEEP (37). Burchiel and colleagues studied 18 patients, 16 with severe head injury. Eleven patients with normal intracranial compliance as measured by the volume–pressure response (VPR) had no change in ICP when airway pressure was increased with PEEP (38). Decreased intracranial compliance and normal lung compliance were associated with increases in ICP when PEEP was applied. Two patients with decreased lung and brain compliance showed no change in ICP. Other investigators have found use of PEEP to be a safe technique in patients with severe head injury and associated lung injury (39,40). In clinical practice, the maintenance of adequate oxygenation is of paramount importance; therefore, use of PEEP is often necessary in severely head-injured patients.

In a given patient, the intracranial response to a given application of positive airway pressure cannot be predicted. The patient with increased lung compliance and decreased chest wall compliance experiences the greatest increase in intrapleural and therefore cerebral venous pressure. Should this patient leave decreased intracranial compliance, then the ICP is likely to increase as a result of positive airway pressure. In clinical practice, it is important to note not only the response of ICP but, more important, the change in cerebral perfusion pressure. Just as application of positive pressure depresses systemic arterial pressure, its sudden removal may cause an abrupt increase in blood pressure and occasionally a sudden increase in ICP (15,41). This is another reason to avoid repeatedly removing a patient from a ventilator to make hemodynamic pressure measurements and should also be kept in mind when performing such procedures as endotracheal suctioning and servicing respiratory equipment.

Conventional ventilation raises airway pressure in a rhythmic fashion, producing peak pressure at inspiration substantially greater than the mean airway pressure. High-frequency ventilation (HFV), also termed jet ventilation, allows ventilation to be achieved at nearly constant airway pressures, comparable with the mean airway pressure required with conventional ventilation. For a general discussion of HFV, still relevant although published in 1989, readers are referred to symposia on HFV summarized in the *British Journal of Anaesthesia* (42). Theoretically, avoiding these peaks in the airway pressure and the corresponding peaks in ICP should be advantageous.

In a randomized prospective trial of conventional mechanical ventilation and HFV among a general population of surgical intensive care unit patients at risk for developing acute respiratory failure, Hurst and coworkers (43) found that patients on HFV were maintained at a lower level of continuous positive airway and mean airway pressures, but there was no significant difference in outcome. In another study by the same group, patients with head injury and acute respiratory failure were managed initially with conventional mechanical ventilation. They were then switched to high-frequency percussive ventilation (HFPV), 240 to 480 cycles per minute. "Satisfactory oxygenation was obtained at approximately half the level of continuous positive airway pressure and peak inspiratory pressure as that on conventional ventilation. HFPV resulted in a statistically significant decrease in ICP in patients when ICP remained greater than 15 mm Hg in spite of optimum medical management." However, several studies have compared HFV with conventional ventilation and found no important difference in CBF, cerebral perfusion pressure (CPP), or ICP (44–49). At least one case report demonstrates a reduction in ICP in a 12-year-old boy with severe head injury when HFV was substituted for conventional ventilation. At the present time, there is no consistent, convincing evidence that HFV improves outcome after severe head injury compared with conventional ventilation but it appears that its application is at least safe in circumstances of raised ICP (50).

Oxygenation and Shunt

Oxygenation is the process by which oxygen is presented to the alveolar space, where it diffuses into blood across the alveolar capillary membrane. The oxygen tension in the alveolus (PA_{O_2}) is calculated from the somewhat cumbersome alveolar gas equation:

$$PA_{O_2} = (P_B - P_{H_2O}) \times FI_{O_2} - \frac{1}{R} (PA_{CO_2})$$

P_{H_2O} is the vapor pressure of water, which equals 47 mm Hg at body temperature. Because complete humidification of inspired gases is assumed, this value must be subtracted from the total gas tension, which equals barometric pressure, P_B. The value ($P_B - P_{H_2O}$) represents the tension of the inspired gas mixture and is multiplied by FI_{O_2} (the fraction of the inspired mixture that is oxygen) to give the oxygen tension of the inspired mixture. This represents the P_{O_2} of inspired gas in the trachea and conducting airways. In the alveolar space, oxygen is taken up and

carbon dioxide excreted in a ratio that depends on the nutrients metabolized by the patient. The respiratory quotient, R, is the ratio of CO_2 production to O_2 consumption and, on a normal diet, equals 0.8. The reciprocal of the respiratory quotient multiplied by the alveolar CO_2 tension, which is assumed to be equal to the arterial CO_2 tension, represents the drop in oxygen tension from the conducting airways to the alveolar space. From this equation it is clear that, except at high altitude, the major determinant of alveolar P_{O_2} is the inspired oxygen concentration. If ventilation and perfusion were ideally matched, Pa_{O_2} would always equal PA_{O_2}. This, of course, is not the case. Pa_{O_2} is always less than PA_{O_2}, and the difference between the two is determined by what is commonly called the *shunt fraction*.

The P_{O_2} of mixed venous blood in a normal patient is approximately 40 mm Hg, which corresponds to 75% saturation of hemoglobin. This blood is presented to the alveolar space, where, assuming an adequate supply of oxygen to the alveoli, oxygen diffuses across the membrane and fully saturates hemoglobin. Approximately 2% to 5% of the normal right ventricular cardiac output is shunted past the alveolar space through the bronchial, pleural, and thebesian veins directly into the left-sided circulation. This addition of desaturated blood from the right heart into the left-sided circulation lowers the systemic arterial oxygen tension slightly. An atrial or ventricular septal defect could produce a similar right-to-left shunt. Although a true anatomic shunt of desaturated blood from the right heart into the left-sided circulation produces hypoxia, the term *shunt* is applied to any lesion in the cardiopulmonary system that produces a lower systemic arterial oxygen tension than is present or predicted in the pulmonary venous system.

When applied to primary respiratory lesions, the term *shunt* really refers to an "as-if" shunt. For example, when pneumonia produces collapsed or fluid-filled alveoli that are still perfused, desaturated venous blood passes through these portions of the lung without increasing its oxygen content. This desaturated blood mixes in the pulmonary veins and lowers the oxygen content of pulmonary venous blood below that which would be predicted if there were no pathology in the lung. This represents the extreme example of shunt, namely, perfusion of an area that is not ventilated. A similar but less severe lesion is created when ventilation (V) is low relative to perfusion (Q). When venous blood is presented to the alveoli, oxygen diffuses into it. The drop in alveolar PAO_2 is linearly related to the amount of oxygen crossing the alveolar membrane. The increase in blood PaO_2 follows the sigmoid-shaped hemoglobin dissociation curve. If a sufficient quantity of oxygen is not present in the alveolus or, conversely, if too much blood is presented to the alveolus, the equilibrium may be met while hemoglobin is still on the steep portion of the dissociation curve (i.e., not fully saturated). When this blood mixes with fully saturated blood from other alveolar units better matched for V/Q, the resulting PaO_2 is lower than predicted. The magnitude of shunting of desaturated blood past unventilated or underventilated alveoli is a measure of the severity of the pulmonary lesion. It is described in terms of the magnitude of a true anatomic shunt that would produce the same degree of hypoxemia. The shunt fraction, Q_S/Q_T, is the ratio of blood flow shunted past alveoli to total blood flow. It is often estimated by $AaDO_2$, the alveolar arterial oxygen tension difference, commonly referred to as the gradient.

A shunt may result from gross pulmonary pathology such as pneumonia or pulmonary edema or from more subtle forms of V/Q abnormalities or atelectasis. In any event, the common denominator in these lesions is decreased functional residual capacity, and therapy usually includes positive airway pressure.

Functional Residual Capacity, Closing Volume, and Positive End-Expiratory Pressure

The resting intrapleural pressure in normal subjects is −3 to −5 cm H_2O (atmospheric pressure equals zero). This negative intrapleural pressure at rest is the result of an equilibrium between two opposing forces, namely, the tendency of the chest wall to expand and that of the lung to collapse. Depending on the compliance of the lung, that negative intrapleural pressure will result in a certain lung volume. That volume is known as the functional residual capacity (FRC) and equals the volume contained in the lung at the end of exhalation during normal tidal breathing. The FRC represents the volume of gas in the lungs with which each new tidal volume mixes. The FRC is also important in determining the extent of airway closure at rest. For any lung, there is a certain critical volume known as the closing volume (CV) below which airway closure begins to develop and shunting of blood in the lungs may occur.

In the spontaneously breathing patient, baseline airway pressure is atmospheric: it is defined here as zero. Positive pressure may be applied to the airway in such a way as to increase the baseline above zero, thereby raising the resting lung volume at the end of exhalation, that is, the FRC. Closing volume is that lung volume at which small airways (less than 1 mm) begin to close. Small airway closure impairs ventilation to lung units that remain perfused, thereby increasing shunt, and may lead to atelectasis and worsening of the shunt. Because CV is the volume of gas that must remain in the lung to keep the airway open, CV may be thought of as a measure of the tendency of small airways to collapse. As airways lose their ability to support themselves, collapse becomes more likely, and greater lung volumes are required to maintain airway patency. In particular, conditions such as aging or emphysema, which decrease the amount of elastic supporting tissue in the airway, result in an increased CV. Figure 4.3 demonstrates the inevitable, slow increase in CV with aging. By the seventh decade of life, CV typically exceeds FRC in the standing position. In the course of normal breathing, there are intermittent periods of small airway closure, which disrupt normal ventilation–perfusion patterns. This is presumably an important contributing factor in the pro-

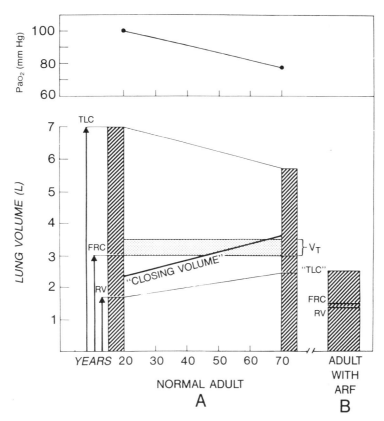

FIG. 4.3. Changes in PaO2 and lung volumes with age in normal adults in the supine position (*A*) and atypical values for functional residual capacity (*FRC*) and vital capacity (*B*) in an adult patient with acute respiratory failure (*ARF*). *RV*, residual volume; *TLC*, total lung capacity. The *shaded horizontal band* represents normal tidal breathing range (*V$_T$*). Vital capacity (TLC – RV) falls progressively with age. Closing volume increases linearly with age and in the supine position exceeds FRC at age 44 years. Note the progressive fall in normal PaO2 with age. (Reprinted from Pontoppidan H, Geffin B, Lowenstein E. Acute respiratory failure in the adult (first of three parts). *N Engl J Med* 1972;287: 690–698, with permission from the Massachusetts Medical Society.)

gressive decline in normal PaO2 with age. The normal FRC is about 15% to 20% lower in the supine than in the standing position. Figure 4.3 demonstrates that the CV exceeds FRC in the supine position in the fifth decade. If pulmonary pathology is present, a further decrease in FRC occurs, increasing the shunt.

Figure 4.1, showing the pressure–volume curve of the lung, demonstrates the expected response to an increase in the baseline airway pressure. If the resting P_{PL} equals –3 cm H_2O and P_{AIR} equals zero, P_{TM} equals 3. On a pressure curve, this corresponds to resting lung volume (FRC) between 20% and 25% of total lung capacity. When 12 cm H_2O positive pressure is applied to the airway at the end of exhalation, P_{AIR} becomes 12. P_{PL} also increases. If P_{PL} increases to 3 cm H_2O, P_{TM} equals 9 cm H_2O. This corresponds to a lung volume of 60% of total lung capacity, a substantial increase in FRC represented by ΔV_B in Figure 4.1. The same increase in P_{TM} produces a much smaller increase in lung volume, ΔV_A, as the slope of the pressure–volume curve decreases. In the normal patient, after an initial steep portion, the slope of the pressure–volume curve decreases as P_{TM} increases. Most pulmonary pathology produces an overall decreased slope of the pressure–volume curve. The increase in FRC with PEEP depends on the compliance of the lung, which is in turn influenced by disease states as well as the position on the pressure–volume curve at the time PEEP is applied. The purpose of PEEP is to raise the FRC and improve the shunt, allowing the use of lower inspired oxygen concentrations to achieve the same PaO_2.

Positive end-expiratory pressure increases the FRC and improves intrapulmonary shunting. This is owing to recruitment of previously perfused but underventilated or collapsed alveolar units, which are now supplied with oxygen and take part in gas exchange. The effects of positive pressure in the lung are not uniform, however, and this may contribute to mismatch of ventilation and perfusion. The focal areas of pathology in the lung that are responsible for the increase in shunt are the areas in which alveolar expansion is most needed. These areas are likely to be less compliant than surrounding normal tissue and therefore are distended less with positive airway pressure. As greater amounts of positive airway pressure are applied, the collapsed alveoli begin to reexpand, but normal alveoli, being more compliant, expand even more. At some point, overdistension of normal alveoli may occur, producing an excess of ventilation relative to perfusion (i.e., an increase in V_D/V_T). In addition, cardiac output and blood pressure fall as mean airway pressure increases with increments of PEEP. The appropriate level of PEEP in patients with pulmonary pathology is a tradeoff between improvement in shunt on the one hand and worsening hemodynamics and dead space on the other. This is variously described as optimal PEEP, maximal reduction of intrapulmonary shunt without significant decrease of cardiac function (51,52), or as best PEEP, "the end expiratory pressure resulting in maximum oxygen transport (cardiac output times arterial oxygen content) and the lowest dead space fraction" (53). The ideal PEEP (best PEEP) is based on the reasoning that the deleterious effect of PEEP, namely, overdistension, decreases compliance, whereas the desired effect of PEEP, recruitment of atelectatic alveoli, increases FRC and compliance. Suter and colleagues (53) reasoned that the level of PEEP that produced maximum compliance in the pulmonary system should provide optimal lung function. They demonstrated that, in fact, this level of PEEP coincided with the point of maximum oxygen transport and lowest V_D/V_T.

Atelectasis

The pattern of normal breathing includes an occasional hyperinflation or sigh. If normal minute ventilation is maintained only with normal tidal volumes (5 to 8 mL/kg), normal $PaCO_2$ are maintained; however, there is a progressive decrease in compliance and increase in shunt (54–56). This is produced by progressive, diffuse, miliary atelectasis, and is prevented with an occasional deep breath (15 to 20 mL/kg). In the totally mechanically ventilated patient, tidal volumes of 12 to 15 mL/kg prevents this progressive atelectasis. Atelectasis is exacerbated by retention of pulmonary secretions. The normal mechanism for clearing these secretions is a vigorous cough. The patient with progressive neuromuscular disease is at great risk of developing atelectasis because of lack of sighing and decreased ability to cough. For this reason, the vital capacity and inspiratory force are followed closely in these patients. The relevance of respiratory measurements and atelectasis are discussed later in the book and they relate to Guillain–Barré syndrome (Chapter 18) and myasthenia gravis (Chapter 19).

Vital capacity (VC) is perhaps the most important measurement that can be made in a cooperative patient. To generate an adequate vital capacity, a patient must have sufficient strength for the given compliance of the lung. Because peak expiratory flow rate is dependent on lung volume, the ability to cough depends on the ability of a patient to achieve a substantial total lung volume, which is to say a substantial vital capacity. In addition, to counteract the inevitable progressive microatelectasis that occurs with monotonous breathing at low tidal volume (8), the patient must be able to take an occasional large tidal volume. A low vital capacity suggests inability to take such a sigh.

Inspiratory force (IF) is the negative airway pressure generated when an inspiratory effort is made in the presence of an airway obstruction. Strictly speaking, this is not a measurement of force but of pressure. It is usually performed as a maximum inspiratory force maneuver after full exhalation and corresponds to the maximum negative intrapleural pressure. This pressure then generates a certain volume. Performed at the end of maximum exhalation (i.e., at residual volume), the maximum inspiratory force is the negative pressure that generates the vital capacity. In general, pressure times compliance equals volume, which in this case should approximate the vital capacity.

When caring for patients with progressive neuromuscular disease such as myasthenia gravis or Guillain–Barré syndrome, the practice, as discussed in subsequent chapters, is to serially follow the vital capacity. When the vital capacity falls below 10 to 12 mL/kg, the patient is intubated and placed on IMV at a tidal volume of 12 to 14 mL/kg at a rate of 3 to 6 breaths/min, with 5 to 10 cm H_2O CPAP (see pages 289–291). Without such intervention, the early pulmonary lesion in such patients is often hypoxia, not hypercarbia.

AIRWAY MANAGEMENT

Skillful management of the airway is a crucial part of therapy in a substantial proportion of patients in any intensive care setting. Airway problems may present as an acute life-threatening emergency or as part of the long-term management of a chronically ill patient. The solution to such problems is often an artificial airway device, commonly an endotracheal tube. For this reason the discussion of airway management focuses on use of the endotracheal tube. Although the endotracheal tube is often relied on, it is rarely the unique solution, and the indication for intubation is rarely absolute. In the emergency situation, for instance, the skilled physician using only

two hands and minimal, if any, equipment can usually manage the patient equally well. In chronic airway management, the tracheostomy replaces the endotracheal tube. Regardless of the devices used, the basic skills and principles underlying acute and chronic airway management are the same.

Indications

Using endotracheal intubation as the prime example of an airway intervention, one can separate airway management problems into five categories. These somewhat arbitrary divisions may be thought of as the indications for endotracheal intubation.

Airway Maintenance

Maintenance of a patent airway is obviously crucial in the care of any patient. Total airway obstruction is a rapidly lethal condition. With the respiratory system deprived of its oxygen supply, the body's continuing metabolic demand draws on oxygen stores present at the time of obstruction. These stores primarily consist of oxygen trapped in the lung in the gas phase, and the blood oxygen content. The duration of total airway obstruction that a patient will tolerate before becoming profoundly hypoxic, therefore, is a function of oxygen consumption (body metabolic rate), blood volume and hemoglobin concentration, and lung volume (usually functional residual capacity) and the inspired oxygen concentration (FiO_2) before obstruction. When acute airway obstruction is experimentally produced in anesthetized animals during normal tidal breathing of room air, PaO_2 goes from 92 to 40 mm Hg after 1 minute, to 10 mm Hg after 3 minutes, and to 4 mm Hg after 5 minutes (34). Arterial carbon dioxide tension ($PaCO_2$) increases somewhat, but the major pathologic lesion is clearly hypoxia and the priority in therapy is to oxygenate the patient. This implies immediate reestablishment of an airway and application of high concentrations of oxygen. The pathology of partial airway obstruction is similar, but the pace is slower.

The most common cause of airway obstruction in the neurological intensive care unit is posterior displacement of oropharyngeal soft-tissue structures in patients who are not fully awake or those with oropharyngeal weakness from neuromuscular disease. Awake patients with intact innervation and musculature of the oropharynx maintain sufficient tone to ensure a patent airway. In states of depressed consciousness or neuromuscular dysfunction, the tongue may become flaccid and fall back against the posterior pharyngeal wall, occluding the airway. Airway obstruction may also occur with direct trauma (e.g., in motor vehicle accidents) or after endotracheal extubation or occasionally even after brief-duration intubation. In the latter case, obstruction is usually at the level of the larynx.

The responses of the body to airway obstruction, hypoxia, and hypercarbia stimulate ventilation. The patient tries vigorously to inhale, with increasing efforts of the diaphragm and accessory muscles, producing substantial negative intrapleural pressure. This is manifested clinically as tensing of the accessory muscles of the neck, intercostal and supraclavicular retractions, and descent of the larynx (the "tracheal tug"). In the normal situation, descent of the diaphragm displaces abdominal structures and the abdomen protrudes. Negative intrapleural pressure expands the lungs and thoracic cage. With the airway obstructed, diaphragmatic descent still causes abdominal protrusion, but the chest wall retracts, producing a rocking respiratory pattern. If the obstruction is complete, no movement of air is detected either by listening or feeling with the hand for the warmth or humidity of exhaled air. If obstruction is partial, the flow of air past a relatively small lumen is likely to be noisy. The sound may resemble snoring or the higher-pitched squeal termed stridor. As a rule, noisy breathing is a sign of obstruction until proven otherwise.

One should consider the differential diagnosis in the immediate treatment of upper airway obstruction. Stridor, usually a high-pitched squeal but occasionally a musical wheezing sound, is produced by flow through a narrowed lumen at any level in the respiratory system. For this reason, upper airway obstruction may be difficult to distinguish from lower obstruction such as bronchospasm or asthma. Intercostal retractions and tracheal tugging are a direct result of substantial negative intrapleural pressures. Airway obstruction increases the resistance between the alveolar space and the ambient environment, requiring a much greater pressure gradient to maintain the same flow. Increased negative intrapleural pressures are also necessary when lungs become noncompliant from parenchymal lung disease with no change in airway resistance. The labored breathing of pulmonary edema, acute respiratory failure, and airway obstruction may appear clinically similar at first.

Emergency management of the compromised airway is aimed at relieving functional soft-tissue obstruction. For the most part, the obstructing soft tissues attach to the mandible. Sufficient elevation of the mandible occasionally is achieved by merely extending the head. Most often, the jaw itself must be elevated. This is accomplished by first opening the mouth to prevent the lower teeth from locking behind the upper teeth and then grasping the vertical ramus of the mandible and lifting it in an axis perpendicular to the plane of the face. When performed correctly, the lower teeth protrude beyond the upper teeth. When the chin is grasped and tipped back to extend the head, the protruding lower teeth may lock into the upper teeth, helping to keep the tongue off the posterior pharyngeal wall. If the lower teeth do not protrude beyond the upper teeth, any tilting back of the jaw to extend the head runs the risk of locking the jaw in a posterior position, forcing the tongue back onto the posterior pharyngeal wall and obstructing the airway. Alternatively, the patient may be rolled onto the side in a "swimmer's position," allowing the tongue to fall laterally and away from the pharyngeal wall.

Artificial devices such as the oropharyngeal or nasal airways may be used. These devices are based on the same principle, namely, placement of a tubular structure between the back of the tongue and the posterior pharyngeal wall. The comatose patient with depressed pharyngeal reflexes is likely to tolerate an oropharyngeal airway. The obtunded but not yet comatose patient may respond to the oral airway with gagging, making the nasal airway better suited to this situation.

Stridor after extubation may result from glottic or subglottic edema. The patient should be kept in a sitting position and oxygen given in a cool, humidified mist. Some try racemic epinephrine, 0.5 mL of a 1:200 solution in 2.5 mL of saline, through a face mask nebulizer every 4 hours for six doses. The benefit of steroids or diuretics in this condition is unknown, and they are generally not used.

Unless the lesion producing upper airway obstruction is obviously self-limited and likely to persist for a brief period during which skilled airway management is available, the only practical treatment is an endotracheal airway device, usually an endotracheal tube, or occasionally a tracheostomy.

Airway Protection

With a patent airway established, it becomes important to ensure that the airway is protected from aspiration of foreign substances such as pharyngeal secretions or regurgitated gastric contents. As with airway obstruction, the patient with depressed mental status or neuromuscular compromise of the larynx is at risk. In the comatose patient, passive regurgitation rather than actual vomiting of gastric contents is likely to occur. In these patients, there probably are no clinical signs of inability to protect the airway until aspiration pneumonitis or pneumonia develops. However, in awake patients with conditions such as myasthenia gravis or Guillain–Barré syndrome, paroxysms of coughing or nasal regurgitation, particularly when swallowing liquids, suggest that the patient is unable to protect the airway.

Because this lesion is unlikely to be short-lived, a cuffed endotracheal or tracheostomy tube is the practical solution. For brief periods of time, such as while preparing to intubate a patient with sudden loss of consciousness from cardiac arrest, the airway may be protected from aspiration of regurgitated gastric contents with cricoid pressure. The technique, often termed the Sellick maneuver (57), is illustrated in Figure 4.4 (58). With the head and neck extended, the cricoid cartilage (the only circumferential tracheal cartilage) is pressed firmly against the cervical vertebrae, thereby occluding the esophagus. In Figure 4.4, with the thumb and first two fingers pressing down on the cricoid, a latex balloon filled with barium to a pressure of 100 cm H_2O is occluded. This maneuver is not effective and is not recommended in the case of active vomiting, during which high intragastric pressures are generated.

Application of Positive Pressure

Whether the intent is to apply a constant low level of positive pressure (CPAP), intermittent bursts of substantial positive pressure [intermittent positive pressure breathing (IPPB) or mechanical ventilation], or combinations of both, efficient application of pressure to the respiratory system requires an airtight mechanical connection between the airway and respiratory equipment. This can be achieved with a tight-fitting face mask applied by someone skilled in its use. In the obtunded patient, this technique is likely to produce gastric dilatation, particularly when airway pressures exceed 20 cm H_2O, at which point the competence of the cricopharyngeus cannot be relied on and air is likely to be forced into the esophagus and stomach. The awake or semialert patient is likely to fight efforts at artificial ventilation. In any event, except for brief periods of time, the tight-fitting face mask is cumbersome, uncomfortable, and unreliable. The safe, practi-

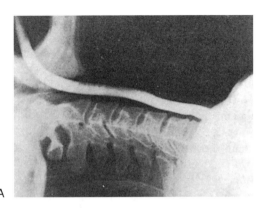
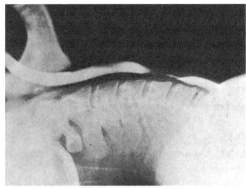

A

B

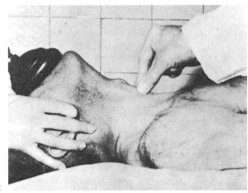

C

FIG. 4.4. A: Lateral x-ray film of neck showing a latex tube, distended with contrast medium to a pressure of 100 cm H_2O, lying within the lumen of the pharynx and esophagus of an anesthetized, paralyzed patient. **B:** Extension of the neck and application of pressure on the cricoid cartilage obliterates the esophageal lumen at the level of the fifth cervical vertebra. **C:** Application of cricoid pressure. (From Sellick BA. Cricoid pressure to control regurgitation of stomach contents during induction of anaesthesia. *Lancet* 1961;2:404–406, with permission.)

cal solution is again an endotracheal or tracheostomy tube.

Oxygen Administration

Commonly used oxygen face masks and nasal prongs are necessarily limited in their ability to deliver high concentrations of oxygen. With maximum effort, a normal subject is easily able to achieve peak inspiratory flow rate of several hundred liters per minute. During normal tidal breathing, peak flow rates on the order of 40 to 50 L/min are not unusual. The flow of oxygen to a face mask is commonly on the order of 5 to 10 L/min. Consequently, as soon as the patient's inspiratory flow rate exceeds the rate of oxygen flow to the mask, room air is entrained and the oxygen concentration drops. The inspired oxygen fraction, FiO_2, increases if the patient's intermittent high demand can be met with an adequate flow of oxygen. Rather than continuously administer the excessively high flow rate needed to match the peak inspiratory flow rate, a reservoir bag may be attached to the face mask. The patient can draw on this supply of oxygen during inspiration and the decrease in FiO_2 is lessened. Between inspirations, the continuous flow of oxygen to the face mask refills the reservoir bag. These masks are generally not tight-fitting and, in fact, are usually vented to allow unobstructed exhalation. This means that some degree of room air entrainment is inevitable.

Under the best of circumstances, FiO_2 between 50% and 60% may be expected from such an arrangement, but varying degrees of room air entrainment make this technique unpredictable. For the same reasons discussed in the preceding, a tight-fitting mask is impractical except in the short term, and again the endotracheal or tracheostomy tube is indicated. The patient may now be reliably connected to an oxygen delivery system using either a high continuous flow of humidified, enriched oxygen, a reservoir bag, or a combination of both.

Tracheal Access

Occasionally a patient may require repeated instrumentation of the trachea. A severely obtunded or weakened patient with pneumonia, copious secretions, and inability to cough may benefit from frequent endotracheal suctioning or even bronchoscopy with lavage for diagnostic or therapeutic purposes. An endotracheal tube may be indicated if personnel skilled in blind endotracheal suctioning are not regularly available or if that technique proves difficult in a particular patient. It is important to note that deep endotracheal suctioning is effective in removing secretions only from large airways. It cannot compare with the ability of a normal cough to clear secretions from distal airways. A forceful cough depends on the ability to create high airway pressure and flow rate. Because peak expiratory flow rate is dependent on lung volume, the patient must be able to achieve a reasonable vital capacity. The ability to create high airway pressure requires not only an adequate muscular effort, but also the ability to narrow the glottic opening, creating high resistance. The endotracheal tube holds the glottis open and thereby substantially decreases the patient's ability to cough effectively.

Endotracheal Intubation

The technique of endotracheal intubation is a motor skill that is not well taught on the printed page. It is best learned under the tutelage of an experienced practitioner in a controlled environment such as the operating room. This section deals with some of the practical aspects of intubation and management of tracheal tubes once the decision to intubate has been made, based on the five broad indications discussed in the preceding.

Oral Versus Nasal Intubation

The choice between oral and nasal intubation is determined by the clinical situation, because each route offers distinct advantages and disadvantages. As a rule, oral intubation is the technique of choice in an emergency when immediate control of the airway is sought. Laryngoscopy followed by oral intubation is almost always faster than nasal techniques and requires the least interruption of resuscitative efforts.

Placed under direct vision, the orotracheal tube may be carefully and reliably placed in the trachea to prevent mainstem intubation. This is a relatively common and entirely preventable complication of endotracheal intubation. The average distance between vocal cords and carina is approximately 10 cm in the adult. When placing an endotracheal tube, the cuff must be placed entirely below the vocal cords to achieve a satisfactory pressure-tight seal. However, the tip of the endotracheal tube must be kept above the carina to assure equal ventilation of both lungs. If the tip is less than 2 cm above the carina, a streaming effect may direct a disproportionate amount of ventilation to one lung. With the tip below the carina, virtually all the ventilation is directed to one lung as the cuff occludes the opposite mainstem bronchus. Oxygen in the obstructed lung is rapidly absorbed and atelectasis soon develops. A substantial shunt is produced as perfusion to the obstructed lung persists while gas exchange is prevented. The distance from the top of the cuff to the tip of the tube is commonly about 5 cm. Because the tip must be at least 2 cm above the carina, proper placement of the endotracheal tube is achieved when the top of the cuff is passed 1 to 3 cm beyond the vocal cords. An additional advantage to placement of the endotracheal tube under direct vision is the ability to estimate the largest size endotracheal tube that the larynx will safely accommodate. In adults, the maximum orotracheal tube size is limited by the size of the glottic opening. An 8-mm tube may be placed easily in most women, an

8.5- to 9-mm tube in most men. A tube is too large for a patient if, with the cuff deflated, airway pressure of 10 to 15 cm H_2O can be applied without detecting an air leak. The size of nasotracheal tubes is limited not by the glottic opening but by the nasal passage, which is smaller. If the size of the endotracheal tube is an important factor in the care of the patient (for instance, if fiberoptic bronchoscopy is contemplated), oral intubation is likely to be the route of choice.

Oral intubation may not be well suited to some patients. Laryngoscopy is a particularly stressful procedure, which may not be well tolerated by patients with heart disease or the potential for raised ICP. Tachycardia and hypertension are commonly seen in well-sedated patients. With adequate monitoring available, evidence of cardiac strain and increased PCWP may be seen in the absence of hypertension and tachycardia. As well as being quite uncomfortable for the awake patient, laryngoscopy is technically difficult to perform in this setting. Even after oral intubation is satisfactorily achieved (e.g., under brief anesthesia), the awake patient generally finds the oral tube more uncomfortable than the nasal tube. It is difficult to give adequate mouth care to orally intubated patients, and gagging is a more common problem. The oral tube is less stable than the nasal, because it is firmly held at only one point, namely, where it is taped to the face. As the tube warms to body temperature it becomes more pliable, and with the proximal end taped to the face, the distal end migrates out of the larynx. With the cuff herniating above the cords, an adequate pressure-tight seal cannot be achieved. Occasionally, the orotracheal tube is itself a source of complete airway obstruction. An agitated, semiconscious, or seizing patient may bite down on the tube, occluding the lumen. For this reason, a bite block should be placed between the teeth of an orally intubated patient. Oropharyngeal airways are often used for this purpose, but it is important to note that the curved body of the airway is generally pliable and will not prevent occlusion of the endotracheal tube. Only the short (1/2- to 3/4-inch) horizontal portion of the airway near the flange is made of firm material and serves as an adequate bite block.

Nasotracheal tubes may be passed blindly without much difficulty in most patients. For this reason, it is the technique of choice when even brief periods of anesthesia or muscle relaxation are relatively contraindicated, such as in patients with a full stomach or compromised airway, or when it is not clear that oral intubation can be rapidly and reliably achieved. With adequate topical anesthesia, blind nasal intubation is reasonably well tolerated by most patients and seems to be less hemodynamically stressful than laryngoscopy. Held in place by the bony structures of the nasal passage, the nasal tube tends to be stable, which makes gagging less of a problem as well.

The nasal tube presents some problems of its own. As discussed, a smaller tube is required when the nasal route is selected. Epistaxis is common but can be reduced with 4% cocaine sprayed or applied with pledgets to the nasal passage before intubation. Any coagulopathy is a relative contraindication to nasal intubation, because bleeding may be profuse. Nasal intubation should be avoided in the presence of pharyngeal abscess or hematoma, because these structures may be ruptured by the tube. A mild edematous reaction to the nasotracheal tube may occlude the eustachian tube and sinus passages, producing serous otitis or sinusitis that persists for the duration of intubation, resolves after extubation, and is rarely of clinical significance. The issue of nasal intubation in the presence of basilar skull or facial fracture is controversial. The fear is that bony fragments may be dislodged during intubation, causing further brain damage, or that prolonged nasal intubation would make infection, particularly meningitis, more likely.

Problems in Endotracheal Tube Management

Patients in a neurological intensive care unit (neuro-ICU) present a number of specific problems in airway management, particularly relating to intubation. Laryngoscopy and intubation elicit a substantial hemodynamic response, which may be taxing to the patient with ischemic heart disease. The results may be catastrophic in a patient with an intracranial mass lesion, as discussed in Chapter 3. Whether or not intracranial hypertension is present before laryngoscopy, if the intracranial compliance is decreased, the patient may be unable to withstand a marked increase in blood pressure without raising the ICP to dangerous levels during instrumentation of the airway. Large doses of sodium thiopental (3 to 5 mg/kg) or similar drugs help to blunt the ICP response to intubation but should be used only when there is reasonable confidence that the endotracheal tube can be placed rapidly. Cricoid pressure should be applied to help prevent aspiration of regurgitated gastric contents. Intravenous lidocaine just before laryngoscopy also helps to blunt the ICP response (59). Figure 4.5 demonstrates the effect of lidocaine, 1.5 mg/kg, administered intravenously and intratracheally to patients undergoing elective craniotomy for brain tumor.

Occasionally a patient with a recently ruptured intracranial aneurysm requires intubation, usually for airway maintenance or protection. In this situation, control of blood pressure is crucial to avoid rebleeding. One alternative is to intubate under general anesthesia in the operating room, but this is often impractical. These patients may be intubated in the neuro-ICU under close blood pressure monitoring, preferably with an indwelling arterial catheter and continuous readout of blood pressure. Vasodilator drugs are administered as a slow, continuous i.v. drip, and the dose is titrated to reduce the blood pressure in anticipation of a hypertensive response to intubation. Our practice is to lower the mean blood pressure approximately 20% to 25% before intubation, but other factors such as vasospasm, cardiovascular disease, or the likelihood of intracranial hypertension influence this decision. The patient may be intubated awake under heavy sedation or after a sleep dose of thiopental or methohexital.

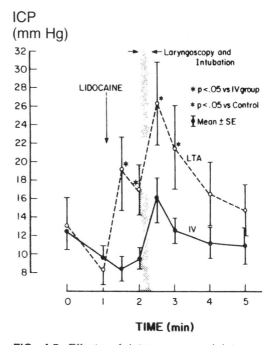

FIG. 4.5. Effects of intravenous and intratracheal lidocaine on intracranial pressure (*ICP*) during laryngoscopy and intubation in patients with brain tumor. Intravenous (*IV*) administration was more effective than laryngotracheal (*LTA*). (From Hamill JF, Bedford RF, Weaver DC, et al. Lidocaine before endotracheal intubation: intravenous or laryngotracheal? *Anesthesiology* 1981;55:578–581, with permission.)

A patient with normal gastrointestinal function who has taken no food or drink in the previous 8 hours may be considered to have an empty stomach. Trauma, pain, surgery, and many drugs, especially analgesics and tranquilizers, delay gastric emptying. In any of these situations, the patient is assumed to have a full stomach. If intubation is necessary, steps must be taken to reduce the likelihood of aspiration. There are two options: The patient is intubated awake, relying on the laryngeal and pharyngeal reflexes to protect the airway, or the patient is given a sleep dose of a rapid-acting hypnotic (sodium thiopental or methohexital) and immediately laryngoscoped and orally intubated, while cricoid pressure is applied to prevent regurgitation during the brief period between onset of hypnosis and inflation of the cuff in the trachea. Rapid-sequence oral intubation, often accompanied by short-acting muscle relaxants, should be attempted only by personnel skilled in the technique. Because most patients intubated in the neuro-ICU require an airway device for a number of days, a nasal tube is often preferable. For this reason, after rapid-sequence oral intubation, the patient may be kept asleep with incremental doses of a short-acting barbiturate while a nasotracheal tube is passed into the pharynx, laryngoscopy is performed, and the tip of the nasal tube is grasped with the end of a Magill forceps, with care taken to avoid touching the cuff. With cricoid pressure applied, an assistant deflates the orotracheal tube cuff and removes the oral tube. The nasal tube is immediately advanced and placed into the trachea using the Magill forceps. The immediate change to a nasal tube is only performed when rapid-sequence laryngoscopy and oral intubation have been achieved easily.

A patient with cervical spine fracture demands particularly careful airway management. If intubation is necessary, care must be taken to avoid dislocating the fracture. Rapid-sequence intubation and the use of hypnotics or muscle relaxants are inappropriate. Awake nasal intubation with topical anesthesia and minimal sedation is usually successful. The flexible fiberoptic laryngoscope is particularly useful in this situation. The flexible device may be inserted to the tip of the nasal tube, which is then manipulated under guidance into the trachea. A rigid, malleable fiberoptic laryngoscope is also available for oral intubation.

Once the endotracheal tube has been secured, a number of common problems may arise. One of the most rapidly lethal complications is obstruction of the endotracheal tube by mucous plugs, blood clot, or rarely, herniation of the cuff around the tip of the tube. In the ventilated patient, this is heralded by the sudden onset of high airway pressures. In any event, other signs of airway obstruction are usually present such as intercostal retractions and vigorous inspiratory efforts without movement of air. The patient should be re-moved from the ventilator immediately, and manual ventilation with a self-inflating bag (Ambu bag or equivalent) attempted. This maneuver rules out mechanical problems with the ventilator or ventilator tubing and gives one an immediate feel for the airway, to help differentiate bronchospasm from mechanical obstruction. If obstruction is suspected, the endotracheal tube cuff is deflated. This solves the problem in the rare event of herniation, but in any event provides another potential channel for air exchange. The suction catheter is now passed down the endotracheal tube to ascertain the level of obstruction. If the obstruction seems to be within the tube and manipulation fails to relieve a kink, the tube is immediately removed and, if possible, replaced with another. These maneuvers are performed in rapid succession with every attempt made to oxygenate the patient.

The appearance of hypoxia in an intubated patient should always raise the question of mainstem intubation. The angulation of the right mainstem bronchus from the carina is shallower than the left, making right mainstem intubation more common. Diffuse atelectasis and shunting result. The tip of the endotracheal tube should be positioned at least 2 cm above the carina, and the position of the tube should be documented with reference to fixed landmarks, such as marking on the endotracheal tube relative to fixed points on the patient's anatomy. At the time of intubation, careful placement under direct vision is the best assurance of adequate tube position. Breath sounds should be equal over both lung fields (assuming they were equal before intubation), but this is an unreliable sign because, even after mainstem intubation, transmission of breath sounds to the contralateral side may confuse the picture. If the tube is well positioned, rapid inflation and deflation of the cuff may be detected by palpating the trachea just below the cricoid cartilage. The most reliable confirmation of tube position is obtained with a chest film. This is useful only if the position of the tube with reference to landmarks on the tube and the patient are noted at the time the film is taken. Notes on tube placement (e.g., "proximal end of tube 4 cm from nose") should be recorded along with other pertinent respiratory data and be available at the patient's bedside. It is also useful to record the volume of air injected into the cuff and the resulting pressure required to achieve a seal. By keeping cuff pressures within a reasonable range (less than 20 cm H_2O), the risk of tracheal damage is lessened. A progressive increase in the cuff volume required to achieve a seal may be an early sign of tracheomalacia.

One of the most common endotracheal tube malfunctions is the "leaking cuff." If detected promptly, this should be nothing more than a minor annoyance. If the leak is substantial and not detected, the patient may be inadequately ventilated or become hypoxic from lack of PEEP. The cause is rarely a ruptured cuff, so the patient can almost always be spared the trauma and risks of reintubation. Often the cause is migration of the endotracheal tube cephalad, bringing the cuff into the glottis where it is difficult to achieve a seal. This often presents as a sudden marked increase in cuff volume and pressure required to achieve a seal. Repositioning of the tube obviously solves the problem. If a leak persists with the tube in proper position and if air introduced into the cuff cannot be withdrawn back into the syringe, there is a leak in the system. These leaks are often caused by a crack in the valve where the syringe is inserted. This is diagnosed and remedied by pinching or clamping the pilot tubing immediately after injecting air into the cuff. If neither of these maneuvers has eliminated the leak, the problem may well be a ruptured cuff; however, immediate reintubation may not be absolutely necessary. It may be to the patient's advantage to wait for a clinical problem to stabilize, for experienced personnel to be available, or to avoid reintubation altogether if for some reason the initial intubation was difficult. A moistened pharyngeal pack may be placed deep in the pharynx, impacted on the glottis, and a pressure-tight seal obtained. It is important to have a functioning nasogastric tube in place to decompress any leaking gas

that might otherwise produce gastric dilatation. The nasogastric tube is also useful in obtunded patients intubated through the nasal route, in whom small amounts of gas leaking around the cuff may be directed toward the stomach when the tongue rests against the posterior pharynx.

Tracheostomy

With the development of high-volume, low-pressure endotracheal tube cuffs, the risk of tracheal stenosis from long-term oral or nasal intubation has markedly decreased. The controversy over when tracheostomy is indicated in the patient with a need for long-term airway support centers around the side effects of either device. The indications and timing of tracheostomy in patients with Guillain–Barré (Chapter 18) and myasthenia (Chapter 19) are discussed in later sections of this book. Prolonged oral or nasal intubation creates the risk of laryngeal damage, which may result in airway obstruction or diminished ability to phonate. Tracheal stenosis at the stoma may occur after tracheostomy. These are both relatively rare complications.

A review by Lanza and colleagues (59) of 52 previously healthy head-injured patients with Glasgow Coma Scale scores of 12 or less who required intubation or tracheostomy within 24 hours of hospitalization had an early complication rate for intubation of 61%, and for tracheostomy, 20%. Increasing duration of intubation was the most significant predictor of airway complication. Of the 52 patients, ten had documented sinusitis. All ten had simultaneous nasotracheal tube and nasogastric tube for an average of 8.4 days before the diagnosis of sinusitis was established and seven had maxillofacial injuries. These authors noted that "tracheostomy in head injured patients is associated with less morbidity and mortality than in chronically ill patients; it should be performed early if protracted airway support is necessary." In another study, 44 head-injured patients were admitted to an inpatient rehabilitation service; ten had only endotracheal intubation; 32 had endotracheal intubation (mean duration, 6 days) followed by tracheostomy; and two had immediate tracheostomy (60). Eleven patients had airway complications, all in the endotracheal tube followed by the tracheostomy group. Five had documented stenosis or granuloma above the tracheostomy stoma; four weaned successfully from mechanical ventilation but failed decannulation, suggesting airway pathology; and two were reintubated for recurrent pneumonia. Airway injury, especially at the arytenoid level, is exacerbated by coughing, head movement, and posturing in the head-injured patient (61).

The decision to perform tracheostomy is often influenced by other factors. Awake patients generally find a tracheostomy more comfortable than oral or nasal tubes. Once the stoma has matured (7 to 10 days after tracheostomy), the tracheostomy tube may be replaced easily should it become accidentally dislodged. This is an important feature to the patient who requires chronic airway management, because adequate care can be given without the need for immediate availability of highly skilled personnel. The tracheostomy can be well cared for outside the hospital setting.

Percutaneous tracheostomy has become the procedure of choice in many neuro-ICUs. With this technique, the trachea is entered with a needle, through which a wire is placed; an introducer is then placed over the wire. Bronchoscopy is often used to conform correct placement of the wire. This introducer is then used to dilate the space between tracheal rings and also carries the tracheostomy tube into position. The entire procedure is performed in the patient's bed.

The awake patient with a cuffed tube is unable to phonate. Several specially modified tracheostomy tubes (e.g., the Pitt Speaking Tube, National Catheter Co, Argyle, NY, U.S.A.) is available that restores at least partial ability to vocalize. In these "talking trachs," a short length of tubing is incorporated in the tracheostomy tube, which channels an external source of gas (usually oxygen at a flow rate of 5 to 15 L/min) to a point just above the cuff. The gas flows through the larynx, producing audible speech.

With an endotracheal tube in place, it is generally impossible to evaluate a patient's ability to maintain or protect the natural airway without a clinical trial of extubation. Tracheostomy, however, permits such evaluation without seriously jeopardizing the airway. Airway protection may be assessed with a methylene blue test. Several drops of methylene blue are added to water or custard, which the patient swallows while the tracheostomy cuff is deflated. A suction catheter is passed into the trachea through the tube. Any sign of blue coloring in the catheter indicates the patient is unable to protect the airway.

Patency of the airway is tested by deflating the cuff and occluding the lumen of the tube for a brief clinical trial.

The acceptable duration of translaryngeal endotracheal intubation is controversial. In a study of general trauma patients, there was no difference in airway complications after either early or late tracheostomy (after up to 2 weeks of translaryngeal intubation) (41). Head-injured patients with posturing had the highest airway complication rate in both groups. In contrast, another study found an increased risk of airway damage after 7 days, increasing sharply after 10 days of translaryngeal intubation (62) Because most head-injured patients with a Glasgow Coma Scale score of less than 8 are likely to require tracheostomy (63), there is strong support for early tracheostomy, within 3 to 4 days, in these patients. An endotracheal tube or tracheostomy tube is left in place as long as any of the five original indications for intubation exists. When that is no longer the case, the patient is extubated.

Equipment and personnel should be assembled to treat postextubation stridor (airway obstruction) or to reintubate if necessary. Preoxygenation with FiO_2 of 0.9 or more is a useful safety measure; it provides a reservoir of alveolar oxygen that supports passive oxygenation for up to several minutes if there is a mishap. The patient is asked to cough, take a deep breath and then exhale or cough again as the tube is being withdrawn. A face mask that delivers approximately FiO_2 of 0.4 with humidified air is applied immediately after withdrawal of the tube. After prolonged intubation, or if deflating the cuff does not provide adequate airflow around the tube, we sometimes, as mentioned, find useful aerosolized racemic epinephrine through a face mask immediately after extubation.

SUMMARY

Respiratory complications a play central role in the morbidity and mortality of patients in a neuro-ICU. Care of these patients begins with proper assessment and management of the airway. Problems in airway maintenance, potentially rapidly lethal, constitute a medical emergency. Other airway problems tend to be slower-paced but may produce serious complications (e.g., aspiration pneumonia).

Positive airway pressure (CPAP, IMV, PEEP) is used to prevent and treat pulmonary complications and to treat raised ICP. The loss of the normal sighing mechanism, either through altered mental status or depressed neuromuscular function, predisposes the patient to atelectasis or pneumonia. Early intubation, CPAP, and low-rate IMV along with vigorous chest physical therapy may help prevent pulmonary complications in susceptible patients. Should complications develop, the basic principles underlying management of respiratory failure apply; however, the neurological patient may be particularly vulnerable to certain side effects of therapy. Techniques of intubation, fluid management, and the effect of positive airway pressure on ICP require careful attention in these patients.

Some basic concepts in respiratory physiology such as ventilatory requirements, V_D/V_T, compliance, gradient, and shunt have been presented. Familiarity with these concepts helps in understanding the etiology and consequences of pulmonary pathology in neurological patients. In addition, these principles may be applied in the rapid assessment of a patient's pulmonary status. Knowing the gradient, V_D/V_T, and compliance, the clinician can estimate the severity of the pulmonary pathology and help direct therapy. The gradient is estimated by comparing the PaO_2 observed to that predicted on the basis of the inspired oxygen concentration: V_D/V_T is estimated by comparing the $PaCO_2$ observed to that predicted on the basis of the measured minute ventilation. Compliance is estimated from the measured tidal volume and airway pressure, either directly in the ventilated patient or, when there are gross disturbances, estimated in the spontaneously breathing patient based on intercostal retractions and other signs. The high gradient suggests the need for oxygen and end-expiratory pressure. Increased dead space and poor compliance increase the work of breathing and may create the need for mechanical ventilation. Severe head injury may be complicated by "shock lung," aspiration, or associated chest injuries or fat embolism. These lesions may then become the limiting factor in determining outcome. Finally, an indirect neural mechanism may cause vascular disruption in the lung and neurogenic pulmonary edema, a subject discussed in detail in Chapter 5.

REFERENCES

1. Wood LDH, Schmidt GA, Hall JB. Principles of critical care of respiratory failure. In: Murray JFNJ, Mason RJ, Boushey HA, eds. *Textbook of respiratory medicine.* Philadelphia: Saunders, 2000:2377–2411.
2. Murray JF, Matthay MA, Luce JM, et al. An expanded definition of the adult respiratory distress syndrome. *Am Rev Respir Dis* 1988;138:720–723.
3. Connors AF Jr, McCaffree DR, Gray BA. Evaluation of right-heart catheterization in the critically ill patient without acute myocardial infarction. *N Engl J Med* 1983;308:263–267.
4. Ronning OM, Guldvog B. Should stroke victims routinely receive supplemental oxygen? A quasi-randomized controlled trial. *Stroke* 1999;30:2033–2037.
5. Donegan MF, Bedford RF. Intravenously administered lidocaine prevents intracranial hypertension during endotracheal suctioning. *Anesthesiology* 1980;52:516–518.
6. Kollef MH, Skubas NJ, Sundt TM. A randomized clinical trial of continuous aspiration of subglottic secretions in cardiac surgery patients. *Chest* 1999;116:1339–1346.
7. Kollef MH, Sherman G, Ward S, et al. Inadequate antimicrobial treatment of infections: a risk factor for hospital mortality among critically ill patients. *Chest* 1999; 115:462–474.
8. Pugin J, Auckenthaler R, Mili N, et al. Diagnosis of ventilator-associated pneumonia by bacteriologic analysis of bronchoscopic and nonbronchoscopic "blind" bronchoalveolar lavage fluid. *Am Rev Respir Dis* 1991;143:1121–1129.
9. Singh N, Rogers P, Atwood CW, et al. Short-course em-

piric antibiotic therapy for patients with pulmonary infiltrates in the intensive care unit. A proposed solution for indiscriminate antibiotic prescription. *Am J Respir Crit Care Med* 2000;162:505–511.

10. Kazmers A, Groehn H, Meeker C. Do patients with acute deep vein thrombosis have fever? *Am Surg* 2000; 66:598–601.

11. Lee AY, Hirsh J. Diagnosis and treatment of venous thromboembolism. *Annu Rev Med* 2002;53:15–33.

12. Swann KW, Black PM, Baker MF. Management of symptomatic deep venous thrombosis and pulmonary embolism on a neurosurgical service. *J Neurosurg* 1986;64:563–567.

13. Bennett DA, Bleck TP. Diagnosis and treatment of neuromuscular causes of acute respiratory failure. *Clin Neuropharmacol* 1988;11:303–347.

14. Juel VC, Bleck TP. Neuromuscular disorders in critical care. In: Shoemaker WC, ed. *Textbook of critical care.* Philadephia: Saunders, 2000:1186–1894.

15. Christensen MS. Acid–base changes in cerebrospinal fluid and blood, and blood volume changes following prolonged hyperventilation in man. *Br J Anaesthesiol* 1974;46:348–357.

16. Muizelaar JP, van der Poel HG, Li Z, et al. Pial arteriolar vessel diameter and CO_2 reactivity during prolonged hyperventilation in the rabbit. *J Neurosurg* 1988;69: 923–927.

17. Yoshida K, Marmarou A. Effects of tromethamine and hyperventilation on brain injury in the cat. *J Neurosurg* 1991;74:87–96.

18. Muizelaar JP, Marmarou A, Ward JD, et al. Adverse effects of prolonged hyperventilation in patients with severe head injury: a randomized clinical trial. *J Neurosurg* 1991;75:731–739.

19. Mackersie RC, Karagianes TG. Use of end-tidal carbon dioxide tension for monitoring induced hypocapnia in head-injured patients. *Crit Care Med* 1990;18:764–765.

20. Artru AA, Colley PS. Cerebral blood flow responses to hypocapnia during hypotension. *Stroke* 1984;15: 878–883.

21. Drury DR, Henry JP, Goodman J. The effects of continuous positive pressure breathing on kidney function. *J Clin Invest* 1947;26:945–951.

22. Hall SV, Johnson EE, Hedley-Whyte J. Renal hemodynamics and function with continuous positive-pressure ventilation in dogs. *Anesthesiology* 1974;41:452–461.

23. Sladen A, Laver MB, Pontoppidan H. Pulmonary complications and water retention in prolonged mechanical ventilation. *N Engl J Med* 1968;279:448–453.

24. Cournand A, Motley HL, Werko L, et al. Physiological studies of the effects of intermittent positive pressure breathing on cardiac output in man. *Am J Physiol* 1948: 152–174.

25. Morgan BC, Crawford EW, Guntheroth WG. The hemodynamic effects of change in blood volume during intermittent positive-pressure ventilation. *Anesthesiology* 1969;30:297–305.

26. Qvist J, Pontoppidan H, Wilson R, et al. Hemodynamic response to mechanical ventilation with PEEP: the effect of hypervolemia. *Anesthesiology* 1975;42:45–55.

27. Cassidy SS, Robertson CH, Pierce AK, et al. Cardiovascular effects of positive end-expiratory pressure in dogs. *J Appl Physiol* 1978;44:743–750.

28. Prewitt RM, Oppenheimer L, Sutherland JB, et al. Effect of positive end-expiratory pressure on left ventric-

ular mechanics in patients with hypoxemic respiratory failure. *Anesthesiology* 1981;55:409–415.

29. Bemis CE, Serur JR, Brockenhagen D, et al. Influences of right ventricular filling pressure on left ventricular pressure and dimension. *Circ Res* 1974;34:498–504.

30. Stool EW, Mullins CB, Leshin SJ, et al. Dimensional changes of the left ventricle during acute pulmonary arterial hypertension in dogs. *Am J Cardiol* 1974;33: 868–875.

31. Taylor RR, Covel IW, Sonnenblick EH, et al. Dependence of ventricular distensibility on filling of the opposite ventricle. *Ana J Physiol* 1967;213:711–718.

32. Hemmer M, Suter PM. Treatment of cardiac and renal effects of PEEP with dopamine in patients with acute respiratory failure. *Anesthesiology* 1979;50:399–403

33. Apuzzo MLJ, Weiss MH, Petersons V, et al. Effect of positive end expiratory pressure ventilation on intracranial pressure in man. *J Neurosurg* 1977;46:227–232.

34. Aidinis SJ, Lafferty J, Shapiro HM. Intracranial responses to PEEP. *Anesthesiology* 1976;45: 275–286.

35. Huseby JS, Pavlin EG, et al. Effects of positive end-expiratory pressure on intracranial pressure in dogs. *J Appl Physiol* 1978;44:25–27.

36. Huseby JS, Luce JM, Cary JM. Effects of positive end-expiratory pressure on intracranial pressure in dogs with intracranial hypertension. *J Neurosurg* 1981;55:704–707.

37. Shapiro HM, Marshall LF. Intracranial pressure responses to PEEP in head-injured patients. *J Trauma* 1978;18:254–256.

38. Burchiel KJ, Steege TD, Wyler AR. Intracranial pressure changes in brain-injured patients requiring positive end-expiratory pressure ventilation. *Neurosurgery* 1981;8:443–449.

39. Cooper KR, Boswell PA, Choi SC. Safe use of PEEP in patients with severe head injury. *J Neurosurg* 1985;63: 552–555.

40. Frost EAM. Effects of positive end-expiratory pressure on intracranial pressure and compliance in brain-injured patients. *J Neurosurg* 1977;47:195–200.

41. Papo I, Caruselli G. The effects on intracranial pressure of stopping controlled ventilation in patients with head injury. *Neurochirurgia* 1978;21:157–163.

42. Sykes MK. High frequency ventilation. *Br J Anaesthesiol* 1989;62:475–477.

43. Hurst JM, Branson RD, Davis K, et al. Comparison of conventional mechanical ventilation and high-frequency ventilation. *Ann Surg* 1990;211:486–491.

44. Auffant RA, Shuptrine JR, Gal TJ. Effects of HFV vs IPPV on cerebral perfusion pressure and cardiopulmonary function. *Anesthesiology* 1982;57:A88.

45. Babinski MF, Albin M, Smith RB. Effect of high frequency ventilation on ICP (abstract). *Crit Care Med* 1981;9:159.

46. Grasberger RC, Spatz EL, Mortara RW. Effect of high-frequency ventilation versus conventional mechanical ventilation on ICP in head-injured dogs. *J Neurosurg* 1984;60:1214–1218.

47. O'Donnell JM, Thompson DR, Layton TR. The effect of high-frequency jet ventilation on intracranial pressure in patients with closed head injuries. *J Trauma* 1984; 24:73–75.

48. Raju TNK, Braverman B, Nadkarny V. Intracranial pressure and cardiac output remains stable during high frequency oscillation. *Crit Care Med* 1983;11:856–858.

49. Toutant SM, Todd MM, Drummond JC, et al. Cerebral

blood flow during high-frequency ventilation in cats. *Crit Care Med* 1983;11:712–715.

50. Schragl E, Pfisterer W, Reinprecht A, et al. Behavior of cerebral blood flow velocity in conventional ventilation and superimposed high frequency jet ventilation. *Anasthesiol Intensivmed Notfallmed Schmerzther* 1995;30: 283–289.

51. Civetta JM, Barnes TA, Smith LO. "Optimal PEEP" and intermittent mandatory ventilation in the treatment of acute respiratory failure. *Respir Care* 1975;20:551–557.

52. Kirby RR, Downs JB, Civetta JM, et al. High level positive end-expiratory pressure (PEEP) in acute respiratory insufficiency. *Chest* 1975;67:156–163.

53. Suter PM, Fairley HB, Isenberg MD. Optimum end-expiratory airway pressure in patients with acute pulmonary failure. *N Engl J Med* 1975;292:284–289.

54. Bendixen HH, Hedley-Whyte J, Laver MB. Impaired oxygenation in surgical patients during general anesthesia with controlled ventilation. A concept of atelectasis. *N Engl J Med* 1963;269:991–996.

55. Ferris BG, Pollard DS. Effect of deep and quiet breathing on pulmonary compliance in man. *J Clin Invest* 1960;39:143–149.

56. Mead J, Collier C. Relation of volume history of lungs to respiratory mechanics in anesthetized dogs. *J Appl Physiol* 1959;14:669–678.

57. Sellick BA. Cricoid pressure to control regurgitation of stomach contents during induction of anesthesia. *Lancet* 1961;2:404–406.

58. Hamill JF, Bedford RF, Weaver DC, et al. Lidocaine before endotracheal intubation: Intravenous or laryngotracheal. *Anesthesiology* 1981;55:578–581.

59. Lanza DC, Parnes SM, Koltai PJ, et al. Early complications of airway management in head injured patients. *Laryngoscope* 1990;100:958–961.

60. Klingbiel GEG. Airway problems in patients with traumatic brain injury. *Arch Phys Med Rehabil* 1988;69: 493–495.

61. Dunham CM, LaMonica C. Prolonged tracheal intubation in trauma patients. *J Trauma.* 1984;24:120–124.

62. Whited RE. Prospective study of laryngotracheal sequelae in long-term intubation. *Laryngoscope* 1984;94: 364–377.

63. Lanza DC, Koltai PJ, Parnes SM. Predictive value of the Glasgow Coma Scale for tracheotomy in head injured patients. *Ann Otol Rhinol Laryngol* 1990;99:38–41.

5

Cardiovascular Aspects of Neurological Intensive Care

A number of interesting cardiovascular problems arise in relation to acute cerebral lesions. Although infrequent, they are unique to this setting and expose the mechanisms by which the brain participates in the control of the heart and vasculature. In addition, more mundane acute cardiovascular issues are frequent in the neurological intensive care unit (neuro-ICU); they include coronary ischemia, cardiac arrhythmias, and congestive failure that are seen in all general critical care settings. Management of these latter conditions in the neurocritical care setting must take into account the potential neurological complications of hypotension and hypertension, and the neurointensivist must establish strategies and priorities in their management.

ACUTE CORONARY ISCHEMIA

Atherosclerotic vascular disease causes a broad overlap between neurological and cardiac illnesses. Myocardial infarction (MI) is common in the stroke population, probably accounting for the most common causes of death in the weeks and months following stroke. Surgical and neurovascular interventional procedures also stress underlying coronary disease, which is why cardiac complications are frequently encountered in the neuro-ICU.

The diagnosis of acute coronary ischemia can be difficult in neurocritical care patients, as the classic complaint of chest pain may be masked by coma, intubation, and sedation. In patients with cardiac risk factors (including

mainly ischemic and hemorrhagic strokes), surveillance should be heightened and routine screening with electrocardiogram (ECG) and serum markers should be part of the neuro-ICU protocol. Cardiac monitoring generally includes continuous ECG and invasive or noninvasive blood pressure monitoring. Twelve lead ECGs and serum markers such as troponin levels should be monitored after surgical or interventional procedures requiring general anesthesia. It is reasonable to "rule out MI" with ECG and serum for troponin level at admission to the neuro-ICU. Patients with risks for further myocardial injury, such as those with ECG changes, should have repeated screening for myocardial injury after major procedures such as craniotomy.

Treatment of acute coronary ischemia with nitrates, β-blockers, calcium antagonists, and analgesics usually can be undertaken without particular complication in neurological disease. Difficulty arises when the blood pressure falls as a result of treatment and reduces cerebral perfusion. As detailed in Chapter 2, cerebral perfusion pressure (CPP) is defined as the difference between the mean arterial pressure (MAP) and the intracranial pressure (ICP). The CPP is usually well maintained through cerebrovascular autoregulation, but it can be compromised in the setting of recent acute stroke or vasospasm following subarachnoid hemorrhage (SAH). Although traditional clinical prioritization in coronary ischemic syndromes calls for preserving the myocardium, the neurointensivist must balance risks in order to preserve brain viability. Lower levels of medication may be most appropriate in this set of patients. Doses can be titrated upward to just begin to lower MAP, rather than the more standard lowering of MAP by 20% or more. In the authors' experience, it is usually possible to treat the coronary ischemia adequately without marked reductions in blood pressure.

Heparin and aspirin are standard treatments in the acute coronary syndromes, both unstable angina and MI. The use of these agents may pose additional risks in patients with recent craniotomy, intracerebral hemorrhage, and perhaps in cerebral infarction. Heparin usually can be used with low risk following ischemic stroke. Most clinicians are reluctant to use systemic anticoagulation with heparin within the first several days after a craniotomy. Antiplatelet drugs also may pose special risks in cases of acute hemorrhage, trauma, or acute craniotomy, although there are little data that quantify the actual risk, and decisions need to be made based on individual circumstances. Furthermore, thrombolytic therapy for acute MI is generally not an option in this patient population because of the increased risk of cerebral hemorrhage.

CARDIAC ARRHYTHMIAS

Arrhythmias occur in the neuro-ICU in patients with known cardiac disease as well as in those without apparent cardiac risk factors. Again, many neurocritical care patients have cardiac disease, and some of these disturbances are attributable to coronary artery insufficiency, whereas others have conduction disturbances that result from the neurological illness. In addition, a fair number of patients manifest atrial arrhythmias (mainly atrial fibrillation) while under observation in the first few days after stroke. The implication of this finding is generally held to be that there was a similar previous arrhythmia that created the substrate for the (embolic) stroke, but it may be that some rhythm disturbances arise as a result of infarction of brain areas that modulate cardiac conduction (see Tachyarrhythmias).

Animal models of cardiac changes in relation to acute brain injury have demonstrated some cerebral localization of these effects (1). Acute focal injuries to brain tissue, ischemic stroke, hemorrhage, and trauma lead to cardiac effects, as well as electrical activation of brain tissue as seen in epilepsy. Tachycardia and pressor responses are more common after stimulation of the right insular cortex and stimulation of the left vagus, which innervates the atrioventricular node and cardiac conduction system. Bradycardia seems to be more common after stimulation of the left insular cortex or the right vagus nerve, which innervates the sinoatrial node (2). Tachycardias are most commonly seen with seizure and epilepsy, although bradycardias and sinus arrest have been reported (3).

It should be emphasized also that certain neuromuscular diseases affect cardiac muscle and conduction pathways as a primary manifestation of the neurological disease, leading to cardiac dysfunction in a more direct fashion (Table 5.1) (4).

TABLE 5.1. *Neuromuscular diseases involving myocardium and cardiac conduction*

Neuromuscular disease	*Common cardiac abnormality*
Kearns–Sayre syndrome	Conduction block
Friedreich ataxia	Hypertrophic cardiomyopathy; subaortic stenosis
	Hypokinetic-dilated left ventricle; abnormal electrocardiogram
Charcot–Marie–Tooth disease	Conduction block
Myotonic dystrophy	Conduction defects; tachyarrhythmias ± cardiomyopathy
Fascioscapulohumeral dystrophy	Arrhythmia or conduction block
Limb girdle dystrophy	A-V conduction block; dilated cardiomyopathy
Multicore myopathy	Septal defects; conduction block; cardiomyopathy
Polymyositis	Arrhythmias; inflammatory cardiomyopathy

Bradycardias

Excepting the effects of β-adrenergic blocking drugs, a heart rate below 60 beats per minute (BPM) is usually the result of sinus node dysfunction or an atrioventricular conduction disturbance. Very acute cerebral diseases can also produce a vasovagal response that is pronounced enough to cause the heart rate to drop and blood pressure to fall to the point of causing syncope. Closed head injury is one setting that leads to bradycardia and conduction block, likely through a vagal mechanism (5). Whether similar mechanisms pertain in SAH and epilepsy is not known, although similar bradycardia is seen. Vagal influences inhibit sinus nodal activity but a sympathetic discharge of medullary origin probably accounts for the concurrent vasodepressor effect. When the vasodepressor component is prominent, even cardiac pacing may not eliminate hypotension but vasopressor drugs may reverse it. Atropine can be helpful in the reversing the bradycardic component in acute setting but, in extreme and protracted cases, external pacing may be necessary for short periods of time.

Some patients have similar responses after carotid angioplasty and stenting procedures (6). Stimulation of the carotid sinus by the angioplasty balloon can lead to profound bradycardia, including complete heart block. Pacing may be required for a brief period, although pretreatment with an anticholinergic usually is adequate. The stenting procedure may cause a more sustained stimulation of the carotid sinus, in which case hypotension and bradycardia may persist for 24 to 48 hours. Some of these patients require vasopressor therapy to maintain adequate perfusion (7). The vasovagal response is obviated during and after carotid endarterectomy by regional blockade of the carotid sinus, but other problems arise in the postoperative period, mainly hypertension.

Finally, bradycardia in a neuro-ICU raises concern as a possible indication of increased intracranial pressure. The Cushing reflex (bradycardia, hypertension, and respiratory depression) (Chapter 2) results from acutely increased intracranial pressure and diminished cerebral perfusion. Animal models demonstrate increases in circulating catecholamines as the probable cause of hypertension, possibly as a compensatory effect to increase cerebral perfusion (8,9). The bradycardia appears to be the result of pressure that is transmitted to mechanically sensitive centers in the floor of the fourth ventricle. However, it should be pointed out that in clinical circumstances tachycardia is as often observed as bradycardia with episodes of ICP elevation.

Tachycardias

Supraventricular tachycardias are common in all critical care settings. Sinus tachycardia is defined here as a heart rate exceeding 100 BPM, and usually represents a physiologic response to pain, stress, hypotension, congestive heart failure, or excessive catecholamine drive. It is generally not treated as a primary dysrhythmia, but rather the precipitating conditions are sought and corrected.

Paroxysmal supraventricular tachycardias (PSVT) related to a reentry or similar mechanism at the atrioventricular node are also common. Treatment with vagal stimulation maneuvers, especially carotid sinus massage, are useful. Low doses of verapamil, 2.5 to 10 mg, by intravenous (i.v.) injection or of adenosine, 6 to 12 mg, also can be used to "break" the tachycardia. Adenosine has a very short half-life, and in our experience is quite effective in this setting. β-Blockade reduces the risk of recurrent episodes of PSVT but there are a number of alternative approaches.

Atrial fibrillation with a rapid ventricular response is also very common in relation to neurological disease, particularly in older age groups. In the neuro-ICU, pain, infections, intravascular volume overload, and neurological injuries such as SAH are the most common precipitants. The rapid ventricular response is usually the most urgent issue, because the high rate may precipitate coronary ischemia or compromise cardiac function. Short-acting β-adrenergic blockers such as labetalol and esmolol can be used by i.v. bolus or continuous infusion. Diltiazem also is quite effective as an infusion that can be titrated to achieve rate control and is the approach we have preferred. The major limitation of β-blockade and calcium channel antagonists in the neurological patients relates to the induced hypotension that often accompanies doses adequate to slow rate. There is also some concern that certain calcium antagonists may increase intracranial pressure; however, the clinical effects have been minor in our experience. When hypotension must be avoided in order to maintain tenuous cerebral perfusion (e.g., soon after an ischemic stroke), treatment with digoxin may be preferable. The effects of digoxin, of course, are slower, requiring several hours, and may not always be effective, but the lack of associated hypotension makes it valuable in care of the neurological patient.

Ventricular tachycardias are less frequent than are atrial ones in the neuro-ICU, but their implications and potential for severe hypotension underscores their importance. Isolated premature ventricular contractions (PVCs) are seen commonly in many monitored patients, and rarely require treatment. The use of dopamine as a vasopressor agent may be associated with more frequent PVCs and at some point the ventricular irritability mandates the use of alternate agents. The Lown classification (Table 5.2) has long been used to grade ventricular ectopy in terms of potential morbidity and risk of cardiac sudden death. Although much more sophisticated information can now be gathered by electrophysiologic studies, this classification still provides a simple and useful guide (10,11). Low-grade ectopy (grades I and II), usually are benign; treatment usually is considered in grade III and IV arrhythmias.

Ventricular flutter and fibrillation are most commonly seen in patients with underlying ischemic heart disease. Prolonged Q-T intervals are a risk for ventricular ectopy. This circumstance arises with hypokalemia and in relation to some medications, including phenothiazines and tricyclic antidepressants. The ventricular tachycardias are emergent problems for which management protocols are essential.

A specific type of ventricular tachycardia, torsade de pointes, is also related to Q-T prolongation and deserves special mention because it has been reported in relation to acute neurological injuries such as SAH and cranial trauma (12,13). Repletion of potassium and magnesium is critical and low-dose β-blockade may be helpful. Careful monitoring and support are essential until the arrhythmia ceases and the Q-T interval shortens.

HYPERTENSIVE CRISIS

Markedly elevated blood pressure can be a reflection of accelerated hypertension. When it is associated with evidence of end-organ damage, the term malignant hypertension is applied and urgent intervention is necessary. Papilledema, retinal hemorrhages, and hematuria are indicative of malignant hypertension, and this clinical syndrome overlaps with hypertensive encephalopathy when cerebral features appear. The latter include headache, confusion, visual disturbances (cortical blindness and its variants), seizures, obtundation, and coma, and are usually associated with diastolic blood pressures of 130 mm Hg or greater. Most but not all affected patients have papilledema and retinal vascular changes. Cerebral hyperperfusion and pathologic changes of fibrinoid necrosis and microvascular thrombosis are felt to underlie the encephalopathy. Similar changes are seen in eclamp-

TABLE 5.2. *Lown's grading of cardiac arrhythmias*

Grades	Frequency and forms of premature ventricular contractions (PVCs)
I	Isolated PVCs, <30/h
II	Frequent PVCs, >1/min or >30/h
III	Multifocal PVCs
IV	Repetitive multiform PVCs Couplets Salvos

Adapted from Lown B, et al. Monitoring for serious arrhythmias and high risk of sudden death. *Circulation* 1975;52:189–198.

sia as well, although the precise mechanisms are not known in either circumstance. It has become apparent that changes in the appearance of the posterior cerebral white matter on magnetic resonance imaging and computed tomography scans are highly characteristic of hypertensive encephalopathy.

Hypertensive crisis represents a neurological emergency. Cerebral perfusion may be markedly increased initially, but the CPP can be quickly compromised as MAP drops. Monitoring of the intracranial pressure may be optimal, although in practice it is not always practical to monitor ICP, and therapy to lower ICP is often empiric. As a general guide, awake patients usually have an ICP less than 30 mm Hg, and the MAP can be lowered to approximately 100 mm Hg without compromising CPP. Intracranial pressure in patients in coma is uncertain, and lowering MAP significantly is most safely done after placement of an ICP monitoring device.

Treatment is optimally undertaken with central venous access and continuous blood pressure monitoring in the intensive care unit. The optimal pharmacologic agent should provide rapid, predictable control of blood pressure. Commonly used drugs are listed in Table 5.3. Intravenous bolus injection of labetalol can provide control in many cases and we usually resort to it first. Doses of 10 to 40 mg every 10 minutes can be used. Intravenous enalaprilat at 0.625 to 1.25 mg i.v. can be used, as well as sublingual captopril, 6.25 to 12.5 mg. Sublingual nifedipine has been associated with precipitous and profound drops in MAP, and other agents offer better control.

Hydralazine, 10 to 40 mg i.v. every 4 to 6 hours also can be useful, but associated tachycardias can be seen. Nitroprusside remains the most rapidly effective and widely available agent for the control of profound hypertension, and can be used as a continuous infusion at 0.3 to 10 µg/kg per minute. The vasodilatory effect has the potential to exacerbate elevated ICP, but this is uncommon in practice and the effectiveness of the drug argues for its use in emergent situations. More conventional agents can be initiated for more prolonged effect once control is achieved.

Accelerated hypertension with systolic pressure more than 200 mm Hg is commonly seen in the acute presentation of patients with stroke, intracerebral hemorrhage, trauma, and mass lesions. Although many of these issues are covered in more detail in other chapters, a similar approach is usually appropriate. Cautious lowering of blood pressure is reasonable, with efforts to avoid compromising cerebral perfusion.

NEUROGENIC CARDIAC ABNORMALITIES

The influence of the nervous system on the heart has been known for some time, but careful study of this relationship has been undertaken only in recent decades. Early reports of electrocardiographic changes in association with acute neurological disease focused on T wave and Q-T interval changes. Byer and colleagues reported on five patients (four with strokes and one with hypertensive encephalopathy) with large upright T waves and long Q-T intervals (14). In 1953, Levine described a pa-

TABLE 5.3. Drugs used for acute treatment of hypertension

Drugs	Mode of administration	Class of action
Labetalol	10–40 mg i.v. q 10 min	β-adrenergic blockade[a]
Esmolol	1 mg/kg i.v. bolus, then 150–300 µg/kg/min i.v. infusion	β-adrenergic blockade[b]
Enalaprilat	0.625–1.25 i.v. q 6 h, maximum 5.0 i.v. q 6 h	ACE inhibitor
Nitroprusside	0.3–10 µg/kg/min i.v. infusion	Direct vascular dilator
Hydralazine	5–10 mg i.v. q 10 min (maximum of 50 mg)	Direct vascular dilator[c]

[a]Has both selective α-1 and nonselective β-adrenergic receptor-blocking actions.
[b]Maintenance dose titrated to heart rate or goal blood pressure.
[c]Causes reflex tachycardia; avoid in patients with coronary artery disease.
ACE, angiotensin converting enzyme; i.v., intravenous.

tient with SAH whose ECG showed an apparent MI (15). The heart was said to be normal at autopsy. Levine thought that the abnormalities were caused by vagal stimulation and referred to Fulton's work, which suggested that area 13 in the orbitofrontal cortex was the major cortical representation of the vagus nerve. This was based on stimulation studies in which bradycardia could be elicited with stimulation of Brodmann area (13,17). It was Burch and colleagues who drew attention to peaked T waves, long Q-T intervals, and U waves as manifestations of central nervous system disease, primarily but not exclusively in SAH patients (18). It is from their article that the popular term cerebral T waves probably arose.

Cropp and Manning (19) later reported on a series of 15 patients with SAH with electrocardiographic changes. Four of these patients died, and each was said to have a normal heart at autopsy. The authors postulated that the electrocardiographic changes resulted from autonomic nervous system abnormalities arising from area 13 in the orbitofrontal cortex. Hugenholtz reported on six patients with various neurological events with associated Q-T prolongation, deeply inverted and widened T waves, and prominent U waves (20). Electrolyte determinations were normal, and an abnormality in hypothalamic influence on cardiac repolarization was postulated. No consistent electrolyte abnormalities were noted and pathologic studies failed to reveal consistent myocardial lesions.

Sympathetic influences on cardiac activity include an extensive noradrenergic innervation of the myocardium, with the highest density of nerve terminals situated in the cardiac base. The rapid appearance and disappearance of certain of the ECG changes support the concept that the effects are mediated by neurogenic and humoral factors. Although elevated systemic levels of catecholamines are seen in some patients with ECG changes in the context of acute neurological processes, normal levels may also occur frequently. A direct effect of the local sympathetic innervation on the myocardium and conduction system have been proposed as the mechanism (21).

The cardiac enzymes that are used as markers of myocardial cellular injury are frequently elevated in the setting of acute neurological events, particularly, SAH (22). Troponin levels are more sensitive markers than CK of this disturbance, and are quite commonly elevated. Pathologic studies suggest that the cellular injury involves myofibrillar degeneration, or a histopathologic entity called "contraction band necrosis." It is possible that failure to recognize myocardial lesions in many of the older studies was a result of insensitivity of observation techniques. Clearly, gross examination of the heart fails to reveal the vast majority of lesions now known to be present in such hearts. Even light microscopy may sometimes be too insensitive, in that electron microscopy shows widespread lesions when light microscopic examination is unimpressive or equivocal. The myofibrillar necrosis noted in the more recent studies is identical histologically to the cardiac lesion of catecholamine infusion, stress plus or minus steroids, nervous system stimulation in animals, and reperfusion of transiently ischemic cardiac muscle. Furthermore, it is identical to the so-called catecholamine cardiomyopathy described in human beings with pheochromocytoma (23).

However, the rapid appearance and disappearance of these electrocardiographic changes with perturbations of the nervous system suggest that these effects, even in humans, are caused by neural rather than humoral factors. For example, Hammer and colleagues (24) reported on a patient who had the sudden appearance and disappearance of electrocardiographic abnormalities during resection of a basilar artery aneurysm. The effects appeared and disappeared too rapidly to be attributed to any humoral abnormality. A similar phenomenon was reported by Cropp and Manning (19); intraoperative recordings showed evidence of rapidly reversible arrhythmias during surgical treatment of a cerebral aneurysm. Although they may be imitated and perhaps even exacerbated by excessively high circulating catecholamines, these electrocardiographic abnormalities can occur without elevations of systemic catecholamines, presumably by release of norepinephrine directly into cardiac muscle by sympathetic nerve terminals. In the human, one cannot separate the effect of systemic elevations of catecholamines caused by "stress" and that of local cardiac catecholamines caused by specific release from cardiac nerves. The two are presumably additive with regard to the production of cardiac lesions. Systemic catecholamines may be elevated when measured in patients with neurologically induced electrocardiographic changes but also may be normal (25).

The diagnosis of neurologically related cardiac effects is facilitated by the common association with SAH or other major intracranial events such as severe cerebral trauma or massive cerebral hemorrhage. Minor changes may be attributable to ischemic stroke at times; however, more often ECG changes are a separate and primary problem related to coronary artery disease. Abrupt elevations in ICP also are thought to lead to excessive sympathetic discharge. At times in this setting, the ECG changes are diffuse, suggesting subendocardial injury, rather than patterns typical coronary arterial insufficiency.

Generally speaking, the clinical cardiac effects include at least three features (Fig. 5.1) (26). Dysrhythmias ranging from asystole to both atrial and ventricular tachycardias are

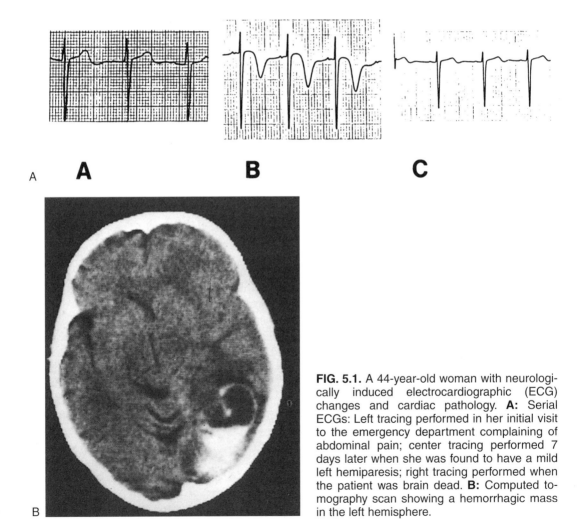

A

B

C

A

B

FIG. 5.1. A 44-year-old woman with neurologically induced electrocardiographic (ECG) changes and cardiac pathology. **A:** Serial ECGs: Left tracing performed in her initial visit to the emergency department complaining of abdominal pain; center tracing performed 7 days later when she was found to have a mild left hemiparesis; right tracing performed when the patient was brain dead. **B:** Computed tomography scan showing a hemorrhagic mass in the left hemisphere.

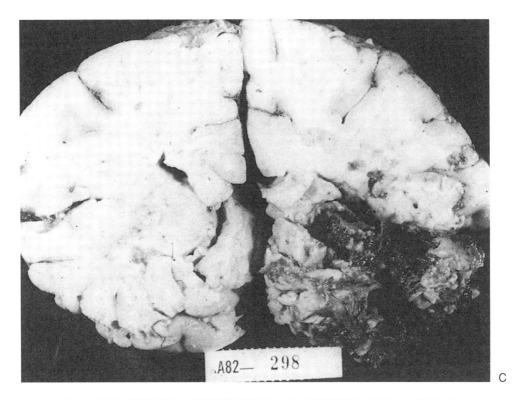

.A82— 298

C

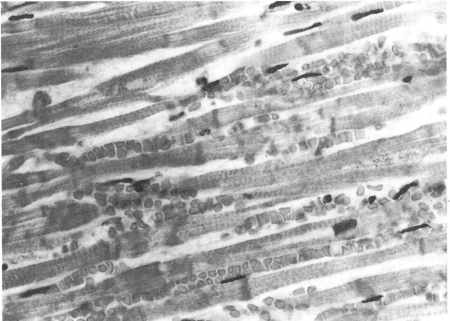

D

FIG. 5.1. *(Continued)* **C:** Gross brain pathology showing hemorrhage into a metastatic tumor. **D:** Microscopic cardiac pathology showing contraction bands with hemorrhage.

Continued on next page

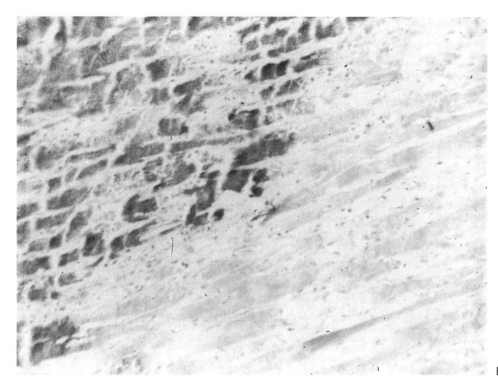

FIG. 5.1. *(Continued)* **E:** Microscopic cardiac pathology showing intensive calcification of the lesion.

seen. Effects on repolarization may lead to ECG changes with or without other cardiac effects. Cellular injury may be associated with incidental elevation of serum markers such as troponin, or may lead to profound contractility dysfunction. Some patients rapidly develop hypotension and left ventricular failure with diffuse hypocontractility, and resemble stunned myocardium. The ventricular function usually recovers over several days despite an initial need for inotropic support. In the case of SAH, alterations in the morphology of the ECG as well as conduction disturbances such as sinus arrest and ventricular tachycardia are clearly the secondary effect of brain injury (27,28). Although patients with SAH require cardiac monitoring and support, the underlying neurological disorder must be addressed and managed effectively (Chapter 15). Surgical and interventional procedures directed at the aneurysm may need to proceed expeditiously despite ongoing cardiac events (29). No specific therapy has been

demonstrated to be useful in minimizing neurogenic cardiac injury. β-Blockade has been advocated, but supportive therapies and time usually lead to resolution of cardiac dysfunction (29).

NEUROGENIC PULMONARY EDEMA

The mechanisms underlying neurogenic pulmonary edema (NPE) are still uncertain despite 40 years of physiologic research in animals and clinical observations. Neurogenic pulmonary edema has been described in multiple clinical settings (Table 5.4). In SAH, a surge of catecholamine at the time of the aneurysmal rupture has been postulated to result in transient myocardial dysfunction, perhaps because of abrupt systemic hypertension and a marked increase in left ventricular afterload. The excessive catecholamine response is in part a fragment of the Cushing response but probably has an alternative more direct mechanism, perhaps originating in the

TABLE 5.4. *Conditions associated with neurogenic pulmonary edema*

Commonly associated	Rarely associated
Subarachnoid hemorrhage	Brainstem infections
Status epilepticus	Medullary tumors
Severe head trauma	Multiple sclerosis
Intracerebral hemorrhage	Spinal cord infarction
	Increased intracranial hemorrhage from other causes

hypothalamus. In a minority of cases, there has been evidence of global left ventricular dysfunction, suggesting that this mechanism at least contributes to the development of what is essentially a cryptic neurogenically induced cardiogenic pulmonary edema (30). Some of these patients have had documented elevations of pulmonary capillary wedge pressure, corroborating this element of the process. Another small group develop pulmonary edema as a consequence of cardiac ischemia in this setting because of preexisting coronary artery disease (but this is not the usual cause of elevations in creatine kinase or troponin concentrations; see further on). However, the majority of patients developing pulmonary edema soon after aneurysmal rupture have neither echocardiographic nor pulmonary arterial catheter-based evidence of such left ventricular dysfunction. Measurements of extravascular lung water confirm that pulmonary edema is present even though abnormalities of neither hydrostatic nor colloid oncotic pressure are detectable.

The most favored mechanism for NPE implicates pulmonary venous sphincters, which are under neural control. Several lines of experimental evidence suggest the presence of these sphincters and their importance in the development of NPE but direct evidence of their role in patients has proved somewhat elusive. For example, studies of the rodent pulmonary circulation immediately after head injury implicate the existence of neurogenically innervated pulmonary conductance vessels (Fig. 5.2) (31).

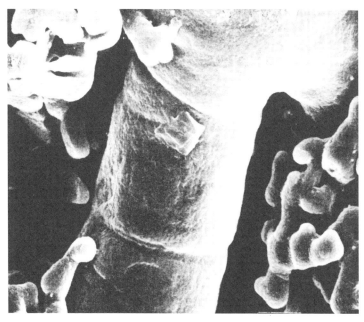

FIG. 5.2. Cast of rat pulmonary venule showing indentations corresponding to sphincters. (From Nakamura J, Zhang SW, Ishikawa N. Role of pulmonary innervation in canine in situ lung-perfusion preparation: a new model of neurogenic pulmonary oedema. *Clin Exp Pharmacol Physiol* 1987;14:535–542, with permission.)

Pulmonary venous hypertension, presumably because of contraction of these sphincters, appears to be necessary for the development of NPE (32). Studies in dogs in which one lung has undergone removal and vascular reanastomosis (leaving the lung denervated and without lymphatic drainage) have shown that a stimulus producing NPE resulted in edema only in the lung with intact innervation (33). The replanted lung, which should have been more prone to edema formation because the lymphatics were interrupted, and which was exposed to the same arterial and venous hydrostatic forces, did not become edematous. The integrity of the cardiopulmonary innervation appeared necessary for edema development in another dog model of NPE (34).

Another aspect of NPE requiring further explanation is the unanticipated high protein content of the fluid. Several experimental studies suggest the presence of a pulmonary capillary leak in NPE because the protein concentration of the fluid recovered from the lung or its lymphatic drainage is quite high. This escape of protein from the circulation into the interstitium and alveoli usually reflects fracture of the junctions between capillary endothelial cells. However, a study in humans employing bronchoalveolar lavage to obtain specimens showed that about half the patients in NPE had a normal alveolar protein concentration, whereas the concentration was elevated in the remainder (35). Thus, it appears likely that NPE has more than one mechanism; in some a true neurogenic leak and in others, perhaps a cardiogenic mechanism predicated on brief myocardial pump failure—or perhaps both are operative.

ANATOMIC STRUCTURES IMPLICATED IN NEUROGENIC PULMONARY EDEMA

Centers in the medullary reticular formation in the region of the nuclei reticularis gigantocellularis and reticularis parvicellularis mediate the hypertension and pulmonary edema seen with the Cushing response (36). Under normal circumstances, these centers are inhibited by neurons in the nucleus solitarius, a medullary nucleus to which afferents from arterial baroreceptors and chemoreceptors project through the vagus and glossopharyngeal nerves. Thus, bilateral lesions in the nucleus solitarius will produce systemic hypertension and pulmonary edema identical to that caused by the Cushing response (37). Both of these forms of pulmonary edema and hypertension are prevented by cervical spinal cord transection or sympathetic blockade with either ganglion blockade, α-adrenergic receptor blockage, or surgical sympathectomy.

Part of the caudal hypothalamus produces a similar form of systemic hypertension and pulmonary edema that is prevented by sympathetic blockade. This center is under tonic inhibition from a nucleus in the lateral preoptic region because lesions there produce hypertension and NPE, a phenomenon that is prevented by prior lesions in the caudal hypothalamus (38).

Some balance exists between the sympathetic and parasympathetic limbs of the autonomic nervous system, because bilateral vagotomy, bilateral lesions in the dorsal motor nuclei of the vagus, or parasympatholytic drugs such as atropine enhance the pulmonary edema associated with volume overloading (39).

Pulmonary Innervation

The pulmonary vessels have both a sympathetic and parasympathetic nerve supply. The parasympathetic fibers arise from the trunk of the vagus nerve. Their stimulation results in some pulmonary vasodilation and a drop in capillary hydrostatic pressure. It is not clear how important this innervation is in the normal physiologic functioning of the pulmonary vessels (40). The sympathetic supply probably arises from several contiguous thoracic levels and, through the sympathetic ganglia, innervate the pulmonary vascular bed to a high degree. There is pharmacologic evidence that α-receptor–mediated innervation causes vasoconstriction, whereas β-receptor innervation causes vasodilation. Furthermore, there is evidence that the α-receptor–mediated sympathetic activity has a greater effect on the venous site of the pulmonary circulation. Thus, sympathetic nerve stimulation can cause a rise in capillary pressure and pulmonary artery pressure without an associated rise in systemic blood pressure and left atrial pressures (41).

PHYSIOLOGIC MECHANISMS OF NEUROGENIC PULMONARY EDEMA

Because α-receptor–mediated sympathetic fibers are widely distributed throughout the vessels of the body, it is evident that a non-specific "sympathetic storm" could result in systemic hypertension as well as pulmonary venoconstriction with a rise in capillary hydrostatic pressure and consequent pulmonary edema.

Sympathetic nerve stimulation leads to an increase in pulmonary capillary permeability to protein, possibly because sympathetic nerve fibers innervate contractile elements in the endothelial cells. Thus, sympathetic activity may lead to physical opening of the tight junctions in the capillary, allowing protein flux; however, this mechanism can be demonstrated only in restricted experimental circumstances (42). Systemic release of catecholamines does not appear to result in increased pulmonary permeability in an experimental model (43). Inhibition of nitric oxide synthesis in the medulla appears to block the increase in capillary permeability in NPE (44).

Sympathetic stimulation also may cause lymphatic constriction. This could lead to alveolar pulmonary edema with only a small shift of fluid from the capillaries to the interstitial tissue space. Thus, a number of regions in the brainstem and hypothalamus are associated with the development of systemic hypertension and pulmonary edema. All share increased sympathetic activity. The mechanisms of neurogenic pulmonary edema are not necessarily exclusive. Furthermore, it is likely that milder subclinical forms of this syndrome commonly occur, whereas fulminate NPE is quite rare.

ACKNOWLEDGMENT

The authors thank Dr. Martin Samuels for use of material from his chapter in the third edition.

REFERENCES

1. Evans DE, et al. Cardiac arrhythmias resulting from experimental head injury. *J Neurosurg* 1976;45:609–616.
2. Keller C, Williams A. Cardiac dysrhythmias associated with central nervous system dysfunction. *J Neurosci Nurs* 1993;25:349–355.
3. Kiok MC, et al. Sinus arrest in epilepsy. *Neurology* 1986;36:115–116.
4. Anan R, et al. Cardiac involvement in mitochondrial diseases. A study on 17 patients with documented mitochondrial DNA defects. *Circulation* 1995;91:955–961.
5. Wirth R, Fenster PE, Marcus FI. Transient heart block associated with head trauma. *J Trauma* 1988;28:262–264.
6. Dangas G, et al. Postprocedural hypotension after carotid artery stent placement: predictors and short- and long-term clinical outcomes. *Radiology* 2000;215:677–683.
7. Qureshi AI, et al. Postoperative hypotension after carotid angioplasty and stenting: report of three cases. *Neurosurgery* 1999;44:1320–1323; discussion 1324.
8. Beiner JM, Olgivy CS, DuBois AB. Cerebral blood flow changes in response to elevated intracranial pressure in rabbits and bluefish: a comparative study. *Comp Biochem Physiol A Physiol* 1997;116:245–252.
9. Ogilvy CS, DuBois AB. Effect of increased intracranial pressure on blood pressure, heart rate, respiration and catecholamine levels in neonatal and adult rabbits. *Biol Neonate* 1987;52:327–336.
10. Lown B, Wolf M. Approaches to sudden death from coronary heart disease. *Circulation* 1971;44:130–142.
11. Lown B, et al. Monitoring for serious arrhythmias and high risk of sudden death. *Circulation* 1975;52:189–198.
12. Di Pasquale G, et al. Torsade de pointes and ventricular flutter-fibrillation following spontaneous cerebral subarachnoid hemorrhage. *Int J Cardiol* 1988;18:163–172.
13. Rotem M, et al. Life-threatening torsade de pointes arrhythmia associated with head injury. *Neurosurgery* 1988;23:89–92.
14. Byer E, Ashman R, Toth LA. Electrocardiogram with large upright T wave and long Q-T intervals. *Am Heart J* 1947;1947:796–801.
15. Levine HD. Non-specificity of the electrocardiogram associated with coronary heart disease. *Am J Med* 1953;15:344–350.
16. Drislane FW, et al. Myocardial contraction band lesions in patients with fatal asthma: possible neurocardiologic mechanisms. *Am Rev Respir Dis* 1987;135:498–501.
17. Fulton JF. *Functional localization in the frontal lobes.* London: Oxford University Press, 1949.
18. Burch GE, Myers R, Abildskov JA. A new electrocardiographic pattern observed in cerebrovascular accidents. *Circulation* 1954;9:719–726.
19. Cropp CF, Manning GW. Electrocardiographic change simulating myocardial ischemia and infarction associ-

ated with spontaneous intracranial hemorrhage. *Circulation* 1960;22:24–27.

20. Hugenholtz PG. Electrocardiographic abnormalities in cerebral disorders: report of six cases and review of the literature. *Am Heart J* 1962;63:451–461.

21. Zarof JG, et al. Regional myocardial perfusion after experimental subarachnoid hemorrhage. *Stroke* 2000;31: 1136–1143.

22. Connor RC. Myocardial damage secondary to brain lesions. *Am Heart J* 1969;78:145–148.

23. Rona G. Catecholamine cardiotoxicity. *J Mol Cell Cardiol* 1985;17:291–306.

24. Hammer WJ, Luessenhop AJ, Weintraub AM. Observations on the electrocardiographic changes associated with subarachnoid hemorrhage with special reference to their genesis. *Am J Med* 1975;59:427–433.

25. Grad A, Kiauta T, Osredkar J. Effect of elevated plasma norepinephrine on electrocardiographic changes in subarachnoid hemorrhage. *Stroke* 1991;22:746–749.

26. Di Pasquale G, et al. Cardiologic complications of subarachnoid hemorrhage. *J Neurosurg Sci* 1998;42:33–36.

27. Andreoli A, et al. Subarachnoid hemorrhage: frequency and severity of cardiac arrhythmias. A survey of 70 cases studied in the acute phase. *Stroke* 1987;18: 558–564.

28. Marion DW, Segal R, Thompson ME. Subarachnoid hemorrhage and the heart. *Neurosurgery* 1986;18: 101–106.

29. Syverud G. Electrocardiographic changes and intracranial pathology. *Aana J* 1991;59:229–232.

30. Mayer SA, et al. Cardiac injury associated with neurogenic pulmonary edema following subarachnoid hemorrhage. *Neurology* 1994;44:815–820.

31. Schraufnagel DE, Patel KR. Sphincters in pulmonary veins. An anatomic study in rats. *Am Rev Respir Dis* 1990;141:721–726.

32. Maron MB. Pulmonary vasoconstriction in a canine model of neurogenic pulmonary edema. *J Appl Physiol* 1990;68:912–918.

33. Grauer SE, et al. Effect of autotransplantation of a lung on development of neurogenic pulmonary edema. *Surg Forum* 1978;29:199–201.

34. Nakamura J, Zhang SW, Ishikawa N. Role of pulmonary innervation in canine in situ lung-perfusion preparation: a new model of neurogenic pulmonary oedema. *Clin Exp Pharmacol Physiol* 1987;14:535–542.

35. Smith WS, Matthay MA. Evidence for a hydrostatic mechanism in human neurogenic pulmonary edema. *Chest* 1997;111:1326–1333.

36. Dampney RA, Kumada M, Reis DJ. Central neural mechanisms of the cerebral ischemic response. Characterization, effect of brainstem and cranial nerve transections, and simulation by electrical stimulation of restricted regions of medulla oblongata in rabbit. *Circ Res* 1979;45:48–62.

37. Doba N, Reis DJ. Role of central and peripheral adrenergic mechanisms in neurogenic hypertension produced by brainstem lesions in rat. *Circ Res* 1974;34:293–301.

38. Maire FW, Patton HD. Neural structures involved in the genesis of preoptic pulmonary edema, gastric erosions and behavioral changes. *Am J Physiol* 1956;184:345–350.

39. Luisada AA, Sarnoff SJ. Paroxysmal pulmonary edema consequent to stimulation of cardiovascular receptors: pharmacologic experiments. *Am Heart J* 1946;13: 293–307.

40. Nandiwada PA, Hyman AL, Kadowitz PJ. Pulmonary vasodilator responses to vagal stimulation and acetylcholine in the cat. *Circ Res* 1983;53:86–95.

41. Maron MB, Dawson CA. Pulmonary venoconstriction caused by elevated cerebrospinal fluid pressure in the dog. *J Appl Physiol* 1980;49:73–78.

42. Rosell S. Neuronal control of microvessels. *Annu Rev Physiol* 1980;42:359–371.

43. Shibamoto T, et al. No effects of large doses of catecholamines on vascular permeability in isolated blood-perfused dog lungs. *Acta Physiol Scand* 1995;155: 127–135.

44. Hamdy O, et al. Role of central nervous system nitric oxide in the development of neurogenic pulmonary edema in rats. *Crit Care Med* 2001;29:1222–1228.

6

Fluid and Metabolic Derangements

Metabolic derangements are frequent in patients with severe central and peripheral neurological illnesses. These alterations may occur as part of the critical illness itself or as sequelae of a number of treatments for acute neurological problems. Many of these disorders are not clinically obvious until they become severe. For these reasons, monitoring of metabolic parameters and strategies to maintain fluid and electrolyte balance have become a routine parts of intensive care unit (ICU) protocols, and neurological illnesses are no exception.

PHYSIOLOGY OF SODIUM AND WATER BALANCE

Water comprises approximately 50% to 60% of the human body weight and is distributed in extracellular fluid (ECF) and intracellular fluid (ICF) compartments. About 55% to 75% of body water is intracellular, and the remaining 25% to 45% is extracellular, divided between the intravascular plasma fraction and interstitial spaces.

The particle, or solute, concentration in fluid is referred to as osmolality, and is expressed in milliosmoles per kilogram (mOsmol/kg) of fluid. Water tends to be freely permeable across cell membranes, resulting in an equilibration between the ICF and ECF osmolalities. However, the solutes in ECF and ICF are vastly different based on differential membrane permeabilities and active transport mechanisms. The major ECF particles are Na and the associated anions, Cl and HCO_3, whereas the ICF contains predominantly K and organic anions. Sodium is largely restricted to the ECF, therefore, it is the dominant contributor to tonicity. Its concentration also reflects ECF volume and can be used as a surrogate measure of that volume. The concentration of the intracellular particles (K and associated anions) are held fairly constant, for which reason changes in the osmolality of the ICF are most often a reflection of changes in ICF water, usually driven by an equilibration with ECF osmolality. Brain cells apparently lose or generate effective osmoles to defend against major fluid shifts in some situations. The added "idiogenic osmoles" alluded to in Chapter 3 in relation to brain swelling are most prone to arise in chronic circumstances of hyponatremia, hypernatremia, and hyperglycemia. This osmotic adaptation occurs slowly and requires the synthesis or transport of solutes.

Water Balance

Normal plasma osmolality is maintained between 275 and 290 mOsmol/kg. Homeostatic mechanisms sense a 1% to 2% change in tonicity and drive the maintenance of water balance as long as water intake exceeds the minimal physiological requirements. Water intake is normally stimulated by thirst, resulting from either hypertonicity or hypovolemia. Osmoreceptors in the anterolateral hypothalamus are sensitive to a rise in tonicity, the thirst threshold being approximately 295 mOsmol/kg. Freely permeable osmoles such as urea or glucose have little effect on the thirst threshold (1).

Water intake normally exceeds physiological needs and water balance; therefore, it is tightly maintained by renal water excretion and largely controlled by arginine vasopressin (AVP) and antidiuretic hormone (ADH). As is well known, AVP is synthesized in the hypothalamus and secreted by the posterior pituitary. Binding of AVP to receptors in the renal collecting tubules stimulates water reabsorption. Other factors facilitate AVP release, including hypovolemia, pain, nausea, stress, hypoglycemia, and various drugs.

Sodium Balance

Sodium (Na) intake is generally in excess of the physiological sodium requirements. Excessive dietary intake of Na increases ECF volume, leading to a renal response of enhanced sodium excretion.

The renin–angiotensin–aldosterone system and sympathetic activity promote Na retention, whereas a natriuretic system fosters Na excretion. Baroreceptors that sense decreased intravascular volume and reduced blood pressure are the main stimuli for the release of renin. Other receptors monitor Na concentration in the nephron and modulate renin release. Renin leads to production of angiotensin II, via angiotensinogen and angiotensin, resulting in aldosterone release from the adrenal medulla. Angiotensin II stimulates thirst, aldosterone leads to Na resorption, and renal sympathetic activity also promotes Na retention (2). The factors favoring Na retention are countered by a natriuretic system that is less well understood. Atrial natriuretic factor (ANF), released from the heart in response to increased cardiac filling pressures, inhibits Na resorption (3,4). Atrial natriuretic factor is found in brain also, mainly in perihypothalamic regions, and it (as well as other central factors) appears to be involved in Na homeostasis (5).

CLINICAL DERANGEMENTS OF WATER AND SODIUM BALANCE IN THE NEUROLOGICAL INTENSIVE CARE UNIT

Disorders occur in various combinations of volume status and sodium concentration (Table 6.1) because water and sodium are independently regulated. This is the case as well when therapies such as hyperosmolar treatment create or exacerbate these disorders.

Hyponatremia

Hyponatremia is the result of excess ECF water in relation to Na. This circumstance occurs in relation to excess total body sodium in congestive heart failure. In contrast, normal Na with excess free water result from inappropriate ADH, and with decreased Na, in salt-wasting syndromes (natriuresis). The clinical distinction among these three states depends on an understanding of the time course, volume status, and associated medical conditions (Fig. 6.1). In the neurocritical care setting, a steady-state of water balance is rarely allowed since intravenous fluids and interventions are common. It may be difficult to determine if the disorder would lead to decreased volume without intervention. Slowly evolving perturbations can be significant yet clinically silent; for example, chronic hyponatremia often reaches levels of 110 to 115

TABLE 6.1. *Characteristics of commonly seen fluid and electrolyte disturbances in neurocritical patients*

	Vascular volume	Serum sodium	Urine sodium	Urine osmolality
Diabetes insipidus	↓	↑	↔	↓
SIADH	↔↑	↓	↔↑	↑
Cerebral salt wasting	↓	↓	↑	↔↑

SIADH, syndrome of inappropriate antidiuretic hormone.

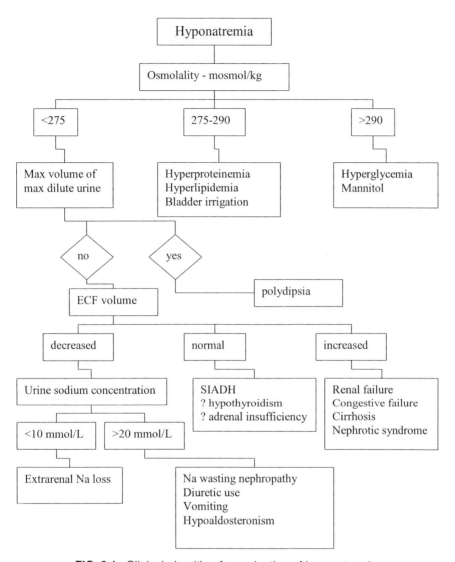

FIG. 6.1. Clinical algorithm for evaluation of hyponatremia.

mEq/L without symptoms. Lower levels, or acute reductions of Na below 125 mEq/L, generally are associated with somnolence, confusion, or seizures. Moreover, seizures resulting from this degree of hyponatremia are refractory to anticonvulsants.

Hypernatremia

Hypernatremia usually results from water loss, or occasionally from sodium excess (Fig. 6.2). Mild hypernatremia (serum Na less than 160 mEq/L) is frequent and usually well tolerated in the neurocritical care setting. Profound hypertonic states with Na greater than 160 can be associated with confusion, lethargy, and seizure, and excessive mortality is associated with serum Na greater than 180 mEq/L.

Mild hypernatremia in the neurological intensive care unit (neuro-ICU) is most frequently related to the administration of normal saline solution, which contains 154

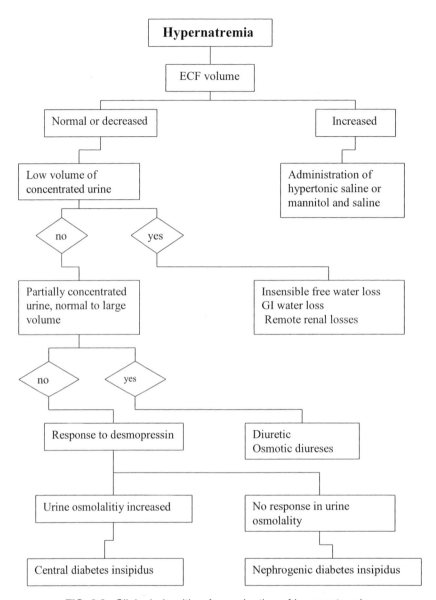

FIG. 6.2. Clinical algorithm for evaluation of hypernatremia.

mEq/L of Na, tending to drive serum sodium upward. The use of osmotic diuretics such as mannitol exaggerate this, especially if normal saline is used to replace the lost volume. Excessive sweating, diarrhea, and increased losses from mechanical ventilation also can contribute to mild hypernatremia.

Severe hypernatremia is most often the result of an osmotic diuresis without adequate volume replacement. Diabetes insipidus (DI) is another common occurrence in the neuro-ICU. Inadequate AVP leads to excessive loss of free water (decreased renal reabsorption) and the classical sign of large volumes of dilute urine (specific gravity less than 1.005). Without rapid recognition and intervention, profound volume contraction and hypernatremia result.

DIABETES INSIPIDUS

Diabetes insipidus justifies additional comment because of its special relationship to diseases of the brain. A central form of diabetes insipidus is known in relation to focal brain lesions in the region of the pituitary fossa and optic chiasm. (Tumors such as germinomas, epidermoids, and metastatic lesions are the most common causes.) Transient partial or more profound DI frequently is seen in patients following exploration or resection of pituitary tumors or after varying degrees of head injury, often severe in cases with section of the pituitary stalk. A pronounced type can be expected after resection of a craniopharyngioma. A more diffuse process, such as basilar meningitis, also may lead to some degree of DI. Rarely, it complicates the Guillain–Barré syndrome (Chapter 18). Brain death is associated with profound DI, reflecting the loss of pituitary and hypothalamic functions, but as commented on in Chapter 9, sometimes the typical features are not evident at the time the clinical criteria for brain death are first documented.

It should be emphasized that the large output of dilute urine that characterizes DI also may be the result of an appropriate postoperative diuresis of large volumes of previously administered intravenous fluids. The osmotic diuresis related to mannitol administration and hyperglycemia can appear excessive, but all these states are differentiated from DI by the presence of isoosmotic or hyperosmotic urine. As a practical matter, the contribution of mannitol to the total serum osmolarity can be estimated by calculating the difference between measured osmolarity and the contribution of normal serum constituents ($2 \times Na + gluc/18 + BUN/3$, as discussed in Chapter 3).

The diagnosis of DI also requires an abnormal and excessive water loss relative to sodium that is reflected by an increasing serum sodium concentration. Treatment of DI can be initiated with the replacement of water losses by oral or preferably intravenous routes; needless to say, this requires assiduous recording of urinary volume and is aided by regular weighing. Fluid replacement alone is not sufficient when the urine output approaches 300 to 500 mL/hour. Although the intranasal administration of 10 to 20 µg desmopressin acetate (DDAVP) is useful in some settings, profound DI in the neuro-ICU is best treated by the intravenous administration of 1 to 5 µg desmopressin acetate. This controls urine output for 12 to 24 hours, during which time intravascular volume and serum sodium can be further corrected by intravenous fluid replacement.

SYNDROME OF INAPPROPRIATE ANTIDIURETIC HORMONE

The syndrome of inappropriate antidiuretic hormone (SIADH) represents a primary disruption in the regulation of water, with intact sodium and volume regulation (6). The water retention that is characteristic of SIADH leads to mildly increased ECF volume, triggering increased sodium excretion and an inappropriately concentrated urine. The intravascular volume remains mildly increased and leads to sodium loss and hyponatremia. The diagnostic criteria include hypoosmotic *hyponatremia* (the main clinical marker and the feature that most often leads to its recognition) with urine that is excessively concentrated relative to serum. Renal and thyroid disease must be excluded as causes of hyponatremia, as well as transient nonosmotic stimuli of ADH release such as pain, nausea, hypotension, or hypovolemia. The list of drugs that have been associated with SIADH at one time or another is long and includes carbamazepine, opiates, many oral hypoglycemic agents, phenothiazine, tricyclics, and the selective serotonin reuptake inhibitors (7).

The syndrome of inappropriate antidiuretic hormone arises in a wide variety of medical conditions (8). Pulmonary processes and systemic malignancies are common in general medical practice. The more salient neurological disorders include central processes such as stroke, brain tumor, encephalitis, brain abscess, and trauma, as well as peripheral processes, mainly the Guillian–Barré syndrome. Some individuals (but especially those with one of the mentioned underlying causes) have a proclivity to display the syndrome when they are receiving positive pressure ventilation. The increase in intrathoracic pressure apparently causes aortic baroreceptors and other volume sensing receptors to behave as if there were hypotension. Elderly patients in general seem most susceptible to SIADH.

Mild hyponatremia related to SIADH is often subacute or chronic and little treatment is necessary. Restriction of fluid intake to an amount less than urinary output (while attempting to maintain normal sodium intake) gradually corrects the hyponatremia in most cases. In cases of moderate and minimally symptomatic hyponatremia (Na 110 to 118 mEq/L and drowsiness) a favored approach is to induce a furosemide diuresis, which causes excretion of dilute urine, and replacement of urinary volume with 0.9% saline solution. More profound and symptomatic hyponatremia requires more rapid intervention, particularly if there are seizures that can be attributed to the electrolyte disorder. In these cases, the correction of sodium can be initiated more rapidly by repeated doses of intravenous hypertonic 3% saline, 50 to 100 cc, with monitoring of electrolytes every 1 to 2 hours, until the serum sodium reaches 125 mEq/L. Further correction should be accomplished more slowly for reasons discussed in the following. Restriction of fluid intake then can be used to maintain the increase in serum sodium. The total sodium load required to reach a given level of serum sodium may be calculated by multiplying the volume of distribution in the extracellular water, assumed to be 60% of body weight, by the desired change in serum sodium [Na infused in mmols = body weight in kilograms $\times$ 0.6 $\times$ (target serum sodium − current serum sodium)].

Despite some controversy, a reasonably firm relationship has been established between the overly rapid correction of profound hyponatremia and the evolution of central pontine myelinolysis (CPM) (9). Overcorrection or other hyperosmolar conditions also may play a role in CPM. Most clinicians attempt to correct serum sodium concentrations slowly (not faster than 1 mEq/L per hour) and avoid raising the sodium concentration above approximately 135 mEq/L.

HYPONATREMIA IN SUBARACHNOID HEMORRHAGE

This problem arises frequently and is comparable to the hyponatremia that sometimes occurs after head injury, the condition in which "cerebral salt wasting" (CSW) was first identified. (10). In CSW, hyponatremia is the result of renal sodium loss, which causes hypovolemia, the opposite of the circumstance in SIADH. The frequency and better-elaborated physiology of SIADH have led many to consider SIADH to be the most common mechanism of hyponatremia in patients with neurological disease (11). Although not as well understood, the syndrome of cerebral salt wasting clearly occurs in subarachnoid hemorrhge (SAH) (12,13). As a consequence, in the past fluid restriction often was imposed on patients following SAH; when sodium and water loss were responsible, this led to even further hypovolemia and frequent ischemic injury from vasospasm (14).

The mechanisms that have now been proposed to explain cerebral salt wasting include a disruption of neural input to the kidney and (more likely in the authors' opinion) the elaboration or release by the brain of a central circulating natriuretic factor, presumably ANF (15,16).

It is likely that some combination of both salt wasting and inappropriate ADH exists in some patients (17,18). The clinical presentation is one of hyponatremia that arises 3 to 7 days after the hemorrhage. The degree of hyponatremia can be profound, and vigorous treatment with both sodium replacement and volume is necessary. Fluid restriction is not used as the primary treatment, because volume must be maintained in patients at risk for vasospasm following SAH. Oral replacement can usually be increased to 2 g of salt three or four times per day. More intensive replacement may require hypertonic 3% saline at rates of 10 to 50 cc per hour. Sodium homeostasis usually recovers within 2 to 3 weeks, and salt replacement can be discontinued. The clinical course often parallels that of the vasospasm of SAH.

HYPERGLYCEMIA

Hyperglycemia is another frequent issue in the neuro-ICU, particularly in patients with diabetes and in the context of corticosteroids use. Many factors, including stress, glucocorticoid administration, sepsis, possibly the use of phenytoin, and interruption of diabetic medications lead to elevated serum glucose. There is considerable animal and some human research data (the latter admittedly ambiguous) to suggest that hyperglycemia is potentially harmful to the injured brain, and control of serum glucoses probably deserves more emphasis than has been given typically in neurocritical care (19). The control of serum glucose is best achieved by attending to all contributing factors. Nutritional support always should be initiated a soon as possible, and specific dietary modifications can facilitate control. The frequency with which serum glucose should be monitored has not been established, but finger stick measurements can be used easily. Insulin administration by sliding scale has not been reliable in controlling serum glucose in extreme conditions, making insulin by continuous infusion preferable in the intensive care setting. Routine protocols allow insulin drip infusions to be managed safely, and serum glucoses can be maintained in the 120 to 180 mg/dL range (20).

CALCIUM AND MAGNESIUM

Both calcium and magnesium circulate as free divalent cations or as protein-bound ions. The physiologically active free ionized fraction of calcium is carefully controlled by parathyroid hormone (PTH) and vitamin D. Parathyroid hormone stimulates the release of calcium from bone and its reabsorption in the kidney and absorption from gut. Release of PTH is inhibited by hypercalcemia and hypermagne-

semia. Vitamin D, either dietary or synthesized, favors calcium release from bone and intestinal absorption. Magnesium is regulated primarily by renal excretion. Excessive magnesium loss occurs in hypercalcemia, ECF expansion, phosphate depletion, acidosis, and diuresis. The main implications of low serum levels of calcium and magnesium are the proclivity to muscle twitching and seizures. Routine monitoring beyond determinations on admission is probably not necessary unless there has been malnutrition or renal disease.

POTASSIUM

As is well known, the serum potassium is strictly controlled, largely by the kidney. Additional influence is exerted by aldosterone, which promotes potassium excretion. Acid–base status influences potassium concentration, via shifts across cell membranes, in exchange for hydrogen ions. Acidosis is associated with shifts of potassium out of the intracellular compartment. In the neuro-ICU, potassium regulation usually has most impact on cardiac issues, and both hypokalemia and hyperkalemia must be avoided.

REFERENCES

1. Abraham WT, Schrier RW. Body fluid volume regulation in health and disease. *Adv Intern Med* 1994;39:23–47.
2. DiBona GF. Neural regulation of renal tubular sodium reabsorption and renin secretion. *Fed Proc* 1985;44: 2816–2822.
3. Lang RE, Unger T, Ganten D. Atrial natriuretic peptide: a new factor in blood pressure control. *J Hypertens* 1987;5:255–271.
4. Needleman P, Greenwald JE. Atriopeptin: a cardiac hormone intimately involved in fluid, electrolyte, and blood-pressure homeostasis. *N Engl J Med* 1986;314:828–834.
5. Hamlyn JM, et al., Purification and characterization of digitalislike factors from human plasma. *Hypertension* 1987;10:171–177.
6. Miller M. Syndromes of excess antidiuretic hormone release. *Crit Care Clin* 2001;17:11–23.
7. Kirby D, Ames D. Hyponatraemia and selective serotonin re-uptake inhibitors in elderly patients. *Int J Geriatr Psychiatry* 2001;16:484–493.
8. Schrier RW. Pathogenesis of sodium and water retention in high-output and low-output cardiac failure, nephrotic syndrome, cirrhosis, and pregnancy (1). *N Engl J Med* 1988;319:1065–1072.
9. Laureno R, Karp BI. Myelinolysis after correction of hyponatremia. *Ann Intern Med* 1997;126:57–62.
10. Peters JP, et al., A salt-wasting syndrome associated with cerebral disease. *Trans Assoc Am Phys* 1950;63:57–64.

11. Schwartz WB, et al., A syndrome of renal sodium loss and hyponatremia probably resulting from inappropriate antidiuretic hormone secretion. *Am J Med* 1957;13: 529–542.
12. Harrigan MR. Cerebral salt wasting syndrome. *Crit Care Clin* 2001;17:125–138.
13. Nelson PB, et al. Hyponatremia in intracranial disease: perhaps not the syndrome of inappropriate secretion of antidiuretic hormone (SIADH). *J Neurosurg* 1981;55: 938–941.
14. Wijdicks EF, et al. Hyponatremia and cerebral infarction in patients with ruptured intracranial aneurysms: is fluid restriction harmful? *Ann Neurol* 1985;17: 137–140.
15. Nakao K. et al. Atrial natriuretic polypeptide in brain—implication of central cardiovascular control. *Klin Wochenschr* 1987;65:103–108.
16. Samson WK. Atrial natriuretic factor and the central nervous system. *Endocrinol Metab Clin North Am* 1987;16:145–161.
17. Palme BF. Hyponatraemia in a neurosurgical patient: syndrome of inappropriate antidiuretic hormone secretion versus cerebral salt wasting. *Nephrol Dial Transplant* 2000;15:262–268.
18. Wijdicks EF, et al., Atrial natriuretic factor and salt wasting after aneurysmal subarachnoid hemorrhage. *Stroke* 1991;22:1519–1524.
19. Cherian L, et al. Hyperglycemia increases neurological damage and behavioral deficits from post-traumatic secondary ischemic insults. *J Neurotrauma* 1998;15: 307–321.
20. Brown G, Dodek P. Intravenous insulin nomogram improves blood glucose control in the critically ill. *Crit Care Med* 2001;29:1714–1719.

7

Fever and Infections in the Neurological Intensive Care Unit

Fever and infection are major concerns in the daily practice of neurocritical care. Recognition of the importance of fever and its implications in neurocritical care patients in particular has surged in recent years because of increased awareness of the potential detrimental effects of elevated temperature on acute brain injury. In experimental models of cerebral ischemia and traumatic brain injury (TBI), even 1 to 2 degrees of hyperthermia appears to have deleterious effects on outcome (1–3). The relevance of these findings in humans is underscored by the association of fever with poor functional outcome after ischemic stroke (4,5), intracerebral hemorrhage (ICH) (6), and aneurysmal subarachnoid hemorrhage (SAH) (7). Brain temperature elevations also have been associated with elevated intracranial pressure after SAH and TBI (8). These recent insights suggest that fever in patients with acute brain injury should be prevented whenever possible, and aggressively treated when it does occur (9).

PHYSIOLOGY OF THERMOREGULATION

Body temperature is normally tightly regulated at approximately 37.0°C (98.0°F). The term fever is generally used in clinical practice (as well as in this chapter) when body temperatures exceed 38.3°C (101.0°F). Strictly speaking, however, the term fever specifically denotes temperature elevation resulting from an increased temperature set point. Set point elevation results from local hypothalamic prostaglandin E synthesis, which is stimulated by circulating systemic inflammatory (pyrogens) such as tumor necrosis factor or interferon 1β (10). The mediators often but not always originate from a tissue infection such as pneumonia, meningitis, or bacteremia; conditions associated with the systemic inflammatory response syndrome (SIRS), drug allergy, deep vein thrombosis, and a variety of other processes also can lead to cytokine elevation and fever (10). Vasoconstriction and shivering are the body's principal means of generating heat when body temperature is lower than the hypothalamic set point. An example of this process occurs during the "chill phase" of a fever; despite having an elevated and rising body temperature, the patient feels cold and shivers because his temperature is below the set point (11).

By contrast, the term hyperthermia (or hyperpyrexia) refers to clinical conditions in which body temperature exceeds the hypothalamic set point (11). This scenario occurs when either an external or internal source of heat production overwhelms the normal heat-dissipating mechanisms of the body (vasodilation and sweating). The best example of hyperthermia from an external source is heat stroke; prolonged exercise and neuroleptic malignant syndrome are examples of hyperthermia resulting from endogenous heat production. Distinguishing between fever and hyperthermia may have important implications for treatment. Antipyretic nonsteroidal antiinflammatory agents are effective for fever, but not hyperthermia. External cooling, by contrast, can result in shivering when used to treat fever, but not hyperthermia.

CENTRAL FEVER

Although regularly encountered and routinely diagnosed by exclusion in clinical practice, "central fever" remains a highly controversial entity, which may relate in part to difficulty in establishing the diagnosis with certainty. Many experts advocate complete avoidance of the term central fever (12). Regardless, refractory high fever (greater than 42°C) in the immediate aftermath of massive supratentorial or brainstem hemorrhage is well described, and these unusual but remarkable cases support the notion that acute brain injury can cause fever in the absence of systemic inflammation or infection (13–15). The highest such fevers we have observed have occurred in the preterminal phase of massive anterior cerebral artery aneurysm rupture, where core temperatures of 106°F were exceeded.

A more liberal definition of central fever might be any temperature elevation that occurs after brain injury for which no other explanation exists despite an exhaustive diagnostic evaluation. Unexplained fever of this type occurs in approximately 15% of hospitalized stroke patients, and these fevers develop earlier than infection-related fevers (16). In a study of 367 neurological intensive care unit (neuro-ICU) patients, 28% of fevers were unexplained, and external ventricular drainage (EVD) for intraventricular hemorrhage (IVH) was associated with fevers of this type (17). This observation and others (6,7) support the notion that IVH can cause *de novo* central fever in humans, or at least disrupt normal thermoregulation and exacerbate temperature elevations resulting from conventional pyrogenic stimuli. The mechanism by which IVH may alter hypothalamic function remains speculative. In fact, it is unclear whether central fever primarily reflects fever (set point elevation) or hyperthermia (via

sympathetically mediated vasoconstriction and anhidrosis) per se. Direct hemotoxic damage to thermoregulatory centers in the preoptic region, interference with tonic inhibitory inputs from the lower midbrain that ordinarily suppress thermogenesis, and stimulation of prostaglandin production leading to temperature set point elevation all have been invoked (18).

INCIDENCE OF FEVER AND INFECTION IN NEUROLOGICAL INTENSIVE CARE UNIT PATIENTS

Prospective clinical epidemiologic studies indicate that fever eventually develops in 25% to 50% of neuro-ICU patients. Kilpatrick and colleagues (19) identified at least one febrile episode in 47% of 428 consecutively admitted neurosurgical ICU patients. In this study, fever was associated with increased ICU stays and cranial (as opposed to spinal) procedures. Commichau and colleagues (17) identified fever in 23% of 387 neuro-ICU patients. Fifty-two percent of fevers were explained by an infection, which is similar to the frequency of infection among febrile medical ICU patients (20), and the predominant source of infection was the lung (82%), which parallels the experience of stroke patients in general (21,22). By contrast, a more diverse spectrum of nosocomial infections occur in febrile medical ICU patients (20). Coma and mechanical ventilation increased the risk of infectious fever in neuro-ICU patients, which likely reflects the high frequency of ventilator-associated pneumonia associated with these risk factors (17). Among specific diagnoses, SAH was the only condition associated with an increased risk of infectious or unexplained fever after controlling for other predictors, suggesting a generalized disturbance of thermoregulation in these patients (17).

Dettenkofer and coworkers (23) calculated the frequency of nosocomial infections in 545 neurosurgical ICU patients using Centers for Disease Control criteria and found an overall incidence of 20.7 per 100 patients, which is well within the range of published data from

TABLE 7.1. *Site-specific incidence rates for nosocomial infections in neurosurgical intensive care unit patients*

	Incidence per 100 patients	Incidence density per 1,000 days (procedure)
Pneumonia	9.0	15.1 (ventilator days)
Urinary tract infection	7.3	8.5 (urinary catheters)
Bloodstream infection	1.0	0.9 (central line days)
Meningitis	1.1	NC
Brain abscess/ventriculitis	0.7	NC
Other[a]	1.7	NC
TOTAL	20.7	NC

NC, not calculated.
[a]Most often wound infection, bronchitis, local intravenous cellulitis, and diarrhea.
Data from Dettenkofer M, Ebner W, Hans F-J, et al. Nosocomial infections in a neurosurgery intensive care unit. *Acta Neurochir* 1999;141:1303–1308.

medical ICUs. Pneumonia was the most common site of infection (Table 7.1), and *E. coli, Enterococci,* and *S. aureus* were the most common pathogens identified by culture.

EVALUATION OF THE FEBRILE NEUROLOGICAL INTENSIVE CARE UNIT PATIENT

The initial task for the neurointensivist when evaluating fever is to identify its cause.

Although infection is always the main concern, a large number of noninfectious causes of fever must also be considered, particularly drug-induced ones (Table 7.2). In addition to performing the traditional initial evaluation for infectious fever in hospitalized patients (chest radiograph, urinalysis, and blood, sputum, and urine cultures), the clinician should obtain a recent history from the nursing staff and patient or family, perform a careful physical examination, and review the patient's cur-

TABLE 7.2. *Noninfectious causes of fever in neurocritical care patients*

Condition	Key to diagnosis
Common	
Blood product reaction	Recent transfusion
Cocaine intoxication	Toxicology screen
Central fever	Exclusion
Deep vein thrombosis	Lower extremity Doppler
Drug fever	Rash, eosinophilia, transaminitis
Gout or pseudogout	Joint tenderness and erythema
Postsurgical local tissue injury	Erythema and tenderness with negative cultures
Pulmonary embolism with infarction	Hypoxemia on room air, chest computed tomography (CT) angiogram
Retroperitoneal hemorrhage	Hematocrit, abdominal/pelvic CT scan
Sterile chemical meningitis	Meningismus
Systemic inflammatory response syndrome	Leukocytosis, tachycardia, tachypnea
Uncommon	
Adrenal insufficiency	History, serum electrolytes
Bowel ischemia	Abdominal tenderness and rigidity
Neuroleptic malignant syndrome	Muscle turgor and rigidity
Malignancy (lymphoma, leukemia)	Complete blood cell count, chest/abdomen CT scan
Malignant hyperthermia	Anesthetic exposure
Myocardial infarction	Electrocardiogram
Pancreatitis	Serum amylase
Pericarditis	Pericardial rub, electrocardiogram
Thyrotoxic crisis	Thyroid function tests

rent medications (24). Most causes of noninfectious fever are identified by taking the extra time for these often-neglected "fundamentals" of hospital practice. In doing so, the astute clinician may preclude a potentially serious medical complication, such as pulmonary embolism, or at the very least protect the patient from unnecessary empiric antibiotic therapy.

Noninfectious Causes of Fever

Some causes of noninfectious fever in neuro-ICU patients deserve special comment. A truncal maculopapular rash, eosinophilia, mild transaminates, or relative bradycardia may be clues to the presence of a *drug fever*. Phenytoin and β-lactamase antibiotics (penicillins and cephalosporins) are the most common culprits; the diagnosis is confirmed by improvement after stopping the offending agent (25). The aromatic anticonvulsants (phenytoin, carbamazepine, phenobarbital) are almost as common in neurological practice. Both, of course, may be associated with a rash. *Deep vein thrombosis* occurs in 9% of neuro-ICU patients, and should be excluded with lower extremity Duplex ultrasonography or plethysmography (26). The systemic *inflammatory response syndrome* may be invoked when fever is associated with tachypnea, tachycardia, or leukocytosis in the absence of a infection; subtle consumption coagulopathy (d-dimer elevation, hypofibrinogenemia, prothrombin time elevation) corroborates its presence (27).

Another often unsuspected cause of fever is the *neuroleptic malignant syndrome,* a rare, idiosyncratic reaction to treatment with a dopamine receptor blockers (e.g., haloperidol, Thorazine, and rarely, L-dopa and other drugs) (28). It is characterized by generalized muscle rigidity with rhabdomyolysis, fever, altered mental status, dysautonomia, elevated creatine kinase levels, and leukocytosis. In some cases the rigidity is mild and the fever is not easily recognized as part of the syndrome. Treatment includes discontinuation of the offending agent, surface cooling, dantrolene [1 to 10 mg/kg per day intravenously (i.v.) given every 4 to 6 hours], and/or bromocriptine (2.5 to 5 mg every 8 hours).

Subarachnoid hemorrhage, IVH, and posterior fossa surgery can lead to a *sterile inflammatory meningitis* that is characterized by a progressive increase in CSF white blood cell counts and hypoglycorrhachia. The inflammation is caused by red blood cell breakdown and reabsorption, and is associated with the intrathecal production of proinflammatory cytokines such as tumor necrosis factor, IL-1, and IL-6 (29). In addition to fever, worsening headaches and meningismus are typical, and in some cases mental status changes may occur; these signs usually respond to treatment with dexamethasone. Finally, brief low-grade temperature elevations are common after surgery of any type, and in most cases are not associated with atelectasis and infection. *Postoperative fever* of this type results from local tissue inflammation and injury at the site of surgery. Although atelectasis is often invoked, no correlation exists between the presence or severity of atelectasis and postoperative fever (30). The temperature elevation is typically low grade, and resolves spontaneously within 72 hours. Nonetheless, chest physical therapy is a reasonable treatment for all febrile patients, especially in the absence of an obvious cause.

Diagnostic Studies

The incidence of nosocomial infection rises substantially after the third hospital day. Within the hospital, patients in ICUs have the highest risk for nosocomial infection because of the high intensity of invasive drains and monitors as well as their relative immobility. The most common hospital-acquired infections include urinary tract infections (especially in patients with Foley catheters), pulmonary infections (particularly in mechanically ventilated patients), vascular–catheter related bloodstream infections, antibiotic-associated *Clostridium difficile* colitis, and wound infections. Less common are infected decubitus ulcers, nosocomial sinusitis related to nasotracheal intubation, and acalculous cholecystitis. Beyond obtaining a chest radiograph and urinalysis and culturing blood, sputum, and urine, additional tests and directed cultures should be prompted by findings on examination. White blood cell count and erythrocyte sedimentation rate elevation reflect the presence of systemic inflammation, which may or may not be caused by infection. The Foley catheter should be changed if infection is suspected, and all indwelling central venous catheters should be removed and cultured. The presence of diarrhea should prompt testing for *C. difficile* toxin. Lumbar puncture should be performed in patients who have recently undergone craniotomy or placement of a ventricular drain, or in patients with a traumatic CSF fistula to rule out meningitis. After spinal surgery, osteomyelitis may be an occult source of fever and is difficult to detect. The sedimentation rate is elevated and magnetic resonance imaging (MRI) shows signal change in the spinal marrow and often in the adjacent disc space, quite unlike the pattern in neoplastic invasion. In specific circumstances, computed tomographic (CT) scans of the sinuses, chest, abdomen, or pelvis may be helpful to rule out sinusitis, empyema, acalculous cholecystitis, bowel ischemia, or other conditions, but these ancillary tests should be guided by the physical examination.

NOSOCOMIAL INFECTIONS

The epidemiology, pathogenesis, and pathophysiology of nosocomial infections have become increasingly well understood over the past 30 years. Although effective means of decreasing the risk of acquiring many of these infections are now available, nosocomial infections contribute significantly to morbidity and mortality, and still cannot be entirely prevented (31). The principles of prevention can best be understood by considering the pathogenetic, anatomic, and microbiologic features involved in the acquisition of infection. In many cases, nosocomial infection arises as the direct result of violation of a local host defense. The organisms that cause infection in each site are usually found at the mucosal or skin surface at which the local defenses have been breached. In many cases, an indwelling tube or catheter provides intraluminal fluid through which organisms can be infused. Acquired infections can be caused by either endogenous organisms that were part of the patient's own flora, or exogenous organisms transmitted within the hospital.

The acquisition of nosocomial infection is increasingly recognized as a complex phenomenon with many stages, often including a change in surface flora; change in characteristics of mucosal surfaces or bacterial strains leading to enhanced adherence; interactions between adherence to tissue and foreign bodies; ability to grow (or survive) on foreign bodies or altered sites; modification of local host defenses; and alteration of flora by antibiotics. The aspect of these changes most visible to the clinician, because it is reflected in changing bacteriologic reports from clinical isolates and therefore may affect therapy, is the change in the patient's flora after admission to the hospital. For example, the pharyngeal flora often begin to include increasing numbers of enteric Gram-negative bacilli, and fecal and skin flora also can become altered to include more resistant hospital-associated strains (31). Many of these changes in colonizing flora result from the direct transfer of organisms through the hands of hospital personnel.

Patients with acute TBI, at least theoretically, have defects in the cellular arm of the immune system that further increase the risk of nosocomial infection. Wolach and associates (32) found significant deficiencies in neutrophil superoxide release, immunoglobulin production, and T-cell function in 14 comatose TBI patients studied within 72 hours of injury. The use of corticosteroids to treat cerebral edema related to ICH, TBI, and cerebral infarction is ineffective, further increases the risk of infection, and should be avoided (33).

Respiratory Infection

Epidemiology

Pneumonia is by far the most common nosocomial infection among critically ill neurological patients. Approximately half of all nosocomial pneumonias are associated with mechanical ventilation, a condition known as ventilator-associated pneumonia (VAP) (34). The rate of pneumonia increased 5- to 20-fold in intubated patients, and increases with the duration of mechanical ventilation (34). The crude risk of developing VAP is about 1% to 3% per day in intubated patients (35).

Berrouane and coworkers (36) studied the incidence of pneumonia in 569 neurosurgical ICU patients over a period of 1 year. Pneumonia developed in 22%, and the risk was highest in mechanically ventilated and comatose TBI patients. The risk of pneumonia was greatest during the first 3 days in the ICU, with a second smaller peak at days 5 and 6. The incidence rate of nosocomial pneumonia among TBI patients in this study (34.2 per 1,000 ventilation days) is among the highest reported in any ICU population.

Pathogenesis and Prevention

Although nosocomial pneumonia can result from bacteremia or direct inoculation via an endotracheal tube or bronchoscope, aspiration of bacteria from the oropharynx or stomach is by far the most common route of infection. Obviously, neurological patients with an impaired swallowing mechanism and cough reflex are at particularly high risk for aspira-

tion. Most of this aspiration results from subclinical "microaspiration" and is not associated with major aspiration events after vomiting or eating. Aspiration of acidic gastric contents may lead promptly to widespread pulmonary infiltrates, which result in large part from the combined effects of physical obstruction by food particles and the chemical effect of an acute acid burn (37). Although some of these patients subsequently become infected, many do not, and the role of prophylactic antibiotics in preventing subsequent infection is not clear (38). Although histamine blockers and proton pump inhibitors can result in gastric colonization with bacteria and potentially increase aspiration risk, their benefits in patients who are mechanically ventilated, coagulopathic, or have a history of peptic ulcer disease probably outweighs this risk (39).

Most pneumonias that develop early during hospitalization are caused by highly penicillin-sensitive flora, including the *pneumococcal* and *streptococcal* species, and various penicillin-sensitive microaerophilic and anaerobic species (Table 7.3) (34,40). This rule may be violated in some situations, such as in epidemics of influenza, which may predispose to staphylococcal pneumonia, or among certain groups of patients, such as alcoholics, who have an increased incidence of Gram-negative pneumonia. Neurological in-

TABLE 7.3. *Empiric treatment of nosocomial pneumonia*

Risk factors	Usual pathogens	Antibiotics
None (early infection)	S. pneumoniae H. influenzae Nonpseudomonal Gram-negative bacilli[a] S. aureus	Ceftriaxone or ampicillin/sulbactam
Long intensive care unit stay or prior antibiotics (late infection)	Nonpseudomonal Gram-negative bacilli P. aeruginosa	Ceftazidime, piperacillin, aztreonam, merapenem, ciprofloxacin, tobramycin[b]
Gross aspiration	Pathogens with no risk factors plus anaerobes	Treat as for no risk factors plus clindamycin or metronidazole

[a]*Klebsiella* sp, *Enterobacter* sp, *Proteus* sp, *Serratia marcescens*, *Escherichia coli*.
[b]Combine any two of these agents.
Modified from Niederman MS. An approach to empiric therapy of nosocomial pneumonia. *Med Clin North Am* 1993;78:1123–1141.

tensive care unit patients appear to have an increased frequency of Gram-negative early nosocomial pneumonia as well: In one study, *Haemophilus* species accounted for 23% of early-onset pneumonias, and other Gram-negative bacilli for an additional 19% (36).

Pneumonia that develops after day 3 in the ICU is caused by a Gram-negative organism in over 50% of cases (Table 7.3) (34,36). Conversion of the normal oropharyngeal flora to enteric Gram-negative bacilli is particularly accelerated in patients with advanced critical illness and in those treated with antibiotics (41–43). Wound infection around a tracheostomy site presents a special risk, because organisms from the wound can find direct access to the lower respiratory tract around the outside of the tube; in these cases, the risk of acquiring subsequent pneumonia may be quite high (44). Outbreaks of *Legionella pneumophila,* which causes a particularly virulent necrotizing pneumonia, have been associated with contamination of humidifiers, nebulizers, tracheostomy tubes, and tap water (34).

Prevention of nosocomial pneumonia rests on three approaches. First, upright positioning, frequent oral suctioning, and chest physical therapy can minimize the flow and collection of upper respiratory secretions into the lower respiratory tract. Second, when delivering respiratory care, hand washing, meticulous local care, and attention to standard protocols of change and cleaning of tubing and nebulizer reservoirs can decrease the risk of introducing additional microbial populations. Finally, the type and placement of tubes that traverse the upper airway should be considered. Continuous aspiration of subglottic secretions that collect above the endotracheal cuff can reduce the risk of VAP (45). Placement of feeding and endotracheal tubes via the oral as opposed to nasal route may reduce the flow of organisms from the nasopharynx into the lower respiratory tract, and also reduce the risk of sinusitis. Prophylactic antibiotics do not prevent VAP, and only pave the way for the development of more resistant infections in the future (42).

Diagnosis

Clinical criteria for the diagnosis of nosocomial pneumonia include fever, leukocytosis, purulent sputum, and a persistent infiltrate on chest radiograph. However, the specificity of these findings has been reported to be 30% or lower, and in many cases the diagnosis can be difficult to establish with certainty. In some cases, a chest CT scan can be helpful for differentiating infiltrate from a pleural effusion or pulmonary infarction or edema. Although tracheal aspirate cultures are often used to identify the causative agent, these specimens are often contaminated by oropharyngeal and upper airway flora and can be misleading. The gold standard for establishing the diagnosis requires quantitative cultures of deep specimens obtained by bronchoalveolar lavage or bronchoscopic-protected brush specimens (34). Given the widespread use of broad-spectrum empiric antibiotic treatment, the utility of invasive diagnostic testing of this type in routine clinical practice remains controversial.

Treatment

Empiric antibiotic therapy, using combinations of antibiotics, is often prescribed initially because of the polymicrobial and sometimes cryptic nature of nosocomial pneumonia (34). The indiscriminate use of empiric treatment is not recommended given the potential for antibiotic-associated drug fever, drug side effects, and later infection with resistant organisms. Initial therapy should be broad enough to cover the potential pathogens, taking into account length of hospitalization, local bacterial sensitivity patterns, and concurrent treatment with steroids (Table 7.3) (46). In general, early infections (less than 3 days) require coverage for *S. aureus, H. influenzae, S. pneumoniae,* and nonpseudomonal Gram-negative rods, whereas patients with late infections require double coverage for resistant *Pseudomonas* or *Acinetobacter,* and treatment with vancomycin for methicillin-resistant *S. aureus.* Treatment can be modified, if necessary, after the results of cultures and sensitivities become available. Treatment should not be changed simply because of a change in the microbiology of tracheal secretions after treatment has been begun, because new organisms almost inevitably appear as secondary colonizers. However, treatment should be altered if there is a clear deterioration in the clinical status, usually in the form of increasing secretions or purulence, fever, leukocytosis, or decline in respiratory status with a new infiltrate. The duration of treatment with an effective agent should range from 7 to 14 days depending on the circumstances.

Urinary Tract Infection

Pathogenesis and Prevention

Most nosocomial urinary tract infections (UTIs) appear after chronic, indwelling bladder catheterization (47). The initial insertion of the Foley catheter poses two risks: Organisms may be directly inserted into the bladder or catheterization may create a transient bacteremia, particularly if the urine is already infected. Initial catheterization results infrequently in significant bacteriuria (in approximately 1% to 2% of ambulatory patients), but this may reach 5% in hospitalized patients (47).

If the catheter is left in place, bacteriuria often develops despite meticulous care. The longer the catheter is left in place, the more frequently this occurs. Even if the catheter is maintained as an absolutely closed system, the rate of development of significant bacteriuria inevitably seems to be about 3% to 5% per day. After 10 days, nearly 50% of all catheterized patients have acquired significant bacteriuria (48). This rate is slightly higher in women than men. Although the extent to which any single violation of this system modifies this rate of development is not known, repeated breaks in the catheter tubing are associated with an increased tendency to develop infection (48). Other errors in handling, such as elevation of the drainage bag, also add to the risk.

Organisms often are introduced around the outside of the catheter, in the thin rim of fluid between it and the urethral mucosa. There is a strong correlation between meatal colonization and subsequent bladder infection with these organisms (49). These organisms are found in the fecal flora as well.

There is no effective means for preventing nosocomial UTI other than removing the Foley catheter as soon as possible. Initial attempts to maintain physical cleanliness by cleaning, washing, or applying antibacterial agents to the periurethral do not substantially reduce the incidence of infection, despite universal recommendations for their use (50). Antibacterial materials incorporated into the catheter, prophylactic antibiotic administration, and local irrigation of the bladder with antibiotic-containing solutions and lubricants also have been unsuccessful (47).

Diagnosis and Treatment

Because asymptomatic bacterial colonization is extremely common, treatment generally should be reserved for patients with pyuria (greater than 10 cells/mm^3) and fever or leukocytosis. Uncomplicated UTI diagnosed early in the ICU stay can be treated with trimethoprim/sulfamethoxazole 160/800 mg or ciprofloxacin 100 mg twice a day for 3 to 7 days. Nosocomial UTIs are usually caused by E. coli and Proteus mirabilis, but in patients previously treated with antibiotics, resistant Pseudomonas aeruginosa, Serratia marcescens, and Enterobacter spp. may be involved. Treatment should be guided on the results of previously obtained culture and sensitivity results when available. Options for the empiric treatment of uncomplicated cases are shown in Table 7.4. To avoid problems with bioabsorption, therapy for nosocomial UTI always should be given intravenously for a total of 7 to 10 days.

TABLE 7.4. Empiric treatment of nosocomial urinary tract infection

Agent	Intravenous dose
Gentamicin	1–1.5 mg/kg q8h
Ceftriaxone	1–2 q12–24h
Ciprofloxacin	0.2–0.4 g q12h

Catheter-related UTIs present a special problem because antibiotics may not eradicate an organism if the catheter is left in place. Treatment also may be associated with the development of a secondary resistant infection. Changing the catheter prior to treatment may reduce the rate of secondary infection and improve the initial response to treatment because organisms on the catheter surface may be embedded in a mucoid film that makes them relatively resistant to antibiotics (51).

Bloodstream Infection

Epidemiology

The incidence of central venous catheter (CVC)–related bloodstream infection (BSI) in the ICU is 5.3 per 1,000 catheter days (52). Infection can double the LOS, and 12% to 25% of cases are fatal (53). Each episode is estimated to add $25,000 to the cost of care (53).

Pathogenesis and Prevention

Bacteremia can result from infection anywhere in the body, but is most often associated with infection arising from an intravenous or intraarterial catheter. Infection may or may not be associated with suppurative infection or phlebitis at the site. Most serious BSIs are associated with CVC-related sepsis. The organisms most frequently involved in catheter-related BSI include *S. epidermis* (37%), *S. aureus* (13%), *Enterococcus* (13%), *Klebsiella-Enterobacter* (11%), *Candida* spp. (8%), and *Serratia* (5%) (54,55).

Routine replacement of CVCs every 3 days did not prevent BSI in a prospective study of 160 patients (56). Among those who did undergo routine catheter replacement, exchange over a guidewire was associated with an increased risk of infection. A recent consensus statement found that although subclavian CVCs have a slightly lower risk of infection than femoral or internal jugular lines, this risk is offset by an increased risk of mechanical complications such as pneumothorax. Accordingly, the site of insertion primarily should be dictated by clinical circumstances (i.e., presence of a hard collar or need for central venous pressure monitoring) and operator expertise. Measures that can minimize the risk of catheter-related BSI include: (a) the use of strict aseptic technique during insertion, including use of a gown, mask, and chlorhexidine (rather than povidone) to prepare the site; (b) vigilant surveillance for local site infection; and (c) the use of antibiotic-impregnated catheters for ICU patients with expected line placement of more than 4 days.

Diagnosis

The diagnosis of catheter-related BSI is suggested by unexplained fever in any patient who has had an intravascular catheter in place for more than 48 hours. Two sets of blood cultures should be obtained via the catheter and a distant venipuncture site, and the catheter should be removed if purulence, erythema, or sepsis syndrome is present. The diagnosis is confirmed by positive blood and catheter tip cultures in the appropriate clinical setting. Semiquantitative culture techniques are available that may help distinguish the bacteriologic results obtained in catheter sepsis from those resulting from simple contamination at the time of removal.

Treatment

Ceftazidime 2 g every 8 hours and vancomycin 1 g every 12 hours is the preferred regimen for empiric coverage. In cases of septic shock, double coverage with an agent with antipseudomonal activity (Table 7.3) should be considered. Further treatment is dictated by the results of blood cultures. Activated protein C (drotrecogin alfa) 200 µg/kg per hour infused over 96 hours reduces mortality in patients with sepsis-induced organ dysfunction (hypotension, oliguria, acute respiratory distress syndrome, acidosis, or thrombocytopenia) (57).

Nosocomial Gastrointestinal Infection

Pathogenesis and Prevention

Nosocomial gastroenteritis is usually manifested by diarrhea, but the appearance of diarrhea does not imply an infectious cause. *Clostridium difficile* is most often implicated. The presenting features of *C. difficile* colitis can be subtle, with only a subtle change in the liquidity of stools and fever; more severe cases are associated with leukocytosis and abdominal tenderness. Treatment with antibiotics is the main risk factor for *C. difficile* colitis, but some cases may result from patient-to-patient transfer. In a survey, second- and third-generation cephalosporins were a more important risk factor than exposure to clindamycin (58).

Diagnosis and Treatment

Assay for the *C. difficile* cytotoxin may be positive in only 30% to 60% of cases confirmed by colonoscopy, which reveals mucosal inflammatory changes and pseudomembra-

nous lesions. Accordingly, empiric treatment despite negative toxin studies is often indicated. Treatment should begin with metronidazole 500 mg orally (p.o.) every 6 hours for 10 days; vancomycin 250 mg p.o. every 6 hours is reserved for resistant infections.

Ventriculostomy-Related Infections

Epidemiology

This problem is particularly relevant to neuro-ICU practice and much has been learned recently regarding its prevention and treatment. The incidence of ventriculostomy-related meningitis or ventriculitis is approximately 8% (59). Although studies are conflicting, the risk of infection seems to increase with time during the first 10 days of catheterization, and remains stable thereafter (Fig. 7.1) (60–62). Compared to external–ventricu-

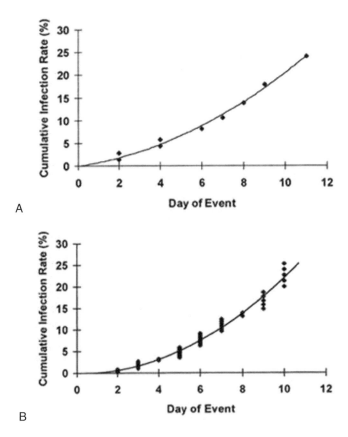

A

B

FIG. 7.1. Survival analysis graphs of external ventricular drainage–related infection risk. They depict the relationship between the cumulative infection rate, corrected for censoring and the time at which events occur. Under the assumption of constant risk, the relationship is a straight line through the origin, with the slope equal to the hazard rate. Both graphs show clear departures from linearity, with the risk of infection increasing with duration the first 10 days of catheterization. **A:** From Kanter RK, Weiner LB, Patti AM, et al. Infectious complications and duration of intracranial pressure monitoring. *Crit Care Med* 1985;13:837–839, with permission. **B:** From Holloway KL, Barnes T, Choi S, et al. Ventriculostomy infections. *J Neurosurg* 1996;85:419–424, with permission.

lar drains, nonfluid coupled (mainly fiberoptic) parenchymal intracranial pressure monitors have an extremely low incidence of infection (approximately 1% at 5 days).

Pathogenesis and Prevention

Infection results from either spread of skin flora along the catheter tract to the subarachnoid or intraventricular space, or via direct inoculation when the system is flushed or irrigated with a contaminated syringe. Other risk factors for EVD-related ventricular meningitis include intraventricular or subarachnoid hemorrhage, cranial fracture with cerebrospinal fluid leak, craniotomy, systemic infection, and catheter irrigation (59). Prophylactic catheter exchange does not appear to modify the risk of developing EVD-related infection (59). Gram-positive cocci consistent with skin flora *(S. epidermidis, P. acnes, S. aureus)* comprise the majority of isolates on CSF culture. Gram-negative ventriculitis is more likely to occur with prophylactic antibiotic treatment with a penicillin and is more virulent (63). Despite this, most neurointensivists administer prophylactic antibiotics with Gram-positive activity such as oxacillin 1 to 2 g every 6 hours to patients who have a ventricular drain. In 1972, Wyler and Kelly reported that prophylactic antibiotic administration decreased the drain infection rate from 27% to 9% (64), and in a more recent clinical trial of 228 such patients, Poon and coworkers (65) found that ampicillin-sulbactam significantly reduced the frequency of CSF infection (from 11% to 3%). Most other negative studies that have examined this question in the past were substantially underpowered (59). In a small but well-conducted randomized trial, attempts to reduce the infection rate by changing the ventricular catheter at 5-day intervals was found to be of no benefit (66). In fact, the infection rate for the group with regular exchanges was 7.8% compared to 3.8% in the group with a catheter in place for an average of 11 days.

Diagnosis

The diagnosis is based on the presence of systemic signs of infection (fever and leukocytosis) or deterioration in level of consciousness, in conjunction with positive CSF cultures and increased CSF white blood cell counts and reduced glucose levels from baseline. Establishing the diagnosis can be challenging, because in some cases a sterile meningitis resulting in similar inflammatory CSF changes can occur, and occasionally CSF cultures are negative because of partial treatment with antibiotics. Elevated CSF lactate levels may be helpful for differentiating bacterial infection from sterile inflammation, but we have not used this test (67).

Treatment

Ceftazidime 2 g every 8 hours and vancomycin 1 g every 12 hours is the preferred regimen for empiric coverage. The infected catheter should be removed, and the patient should be treated with serial lumbar punctures or a spinal drain for persistent hydrocephalus if indicated. It is the current consensus that treatment should be given for a minimum of 14 days.

Neurosurgical Wound Infections

Epidemiology

Most ostensibly clean neurosurgical procedures have a relatively low risk of infection, with an overall rate in most institutions of 3% to 5% (68,69), but this risk is related to the specific procedure (70). For this reason, an overall "clean-wound infection rate" cannot be used to compare hospitals, surgeons, or the same unit over time, unless the surgical-specific procedures (and perhaps even the severity of illness) are taken into account.

Pathogenesis and Prevention

When wound infection occurs following a clean operation, infection is usually caused by contamination with organisms that colonize the skin or nares of the patient or hospital personnel. Procedures that traverse more contaminated sites, or are less easy to decontaminate (e.g., sinus or oropharyngeal mucosa), present a higher risk of infection. Contamination may occur either at the time of the operation, when the wound is open, or in the early postoperative period. The potential for postoperative bacterial seeding is higher when the wound remains open or has a direct conduit from the skin to the subcutaneum, such as with subdural drains (3,53). Traumatic injury represents quite another issue altogether, because entry of organisms from skin or foreign bodies into the subarachnoid space and fractures that cross the middle or external ear, sinuses, nose, or oropharyngeal cavity may directly cause contamination before treatment.

Rigorous surgical aseptic technique is probably the most effective means of preventing intraoperative infections. Epidemics of virulent Gram-negative wound infection can result from contamination of a particular piece of equipment (i.e., a drill) or from a single health care worker (71).

In addition to maintaining aseptic technique, the available evidence suggests that perioperative antibiotics (one or two doses given at the end of the procedure and within 24 hours thereafter) can further reduce the risk of wound infection following clean neurosurgical procedures. Zhang and associates (72) found that the risk of postoperative meningitis fell from 7.2% to 1.8% after instituting a policy of perioperative ceftriaxone administration. Although evidence from properly designed prospective clinical trials is lacking, reviews of the existing literature agree that antibiotics probably exert a protective effect for clean, nonimplant procedures, for which a first- or second-generation cephalosporin is most appropriate (73,74). A review of one institution's experience over 10 years concluded that long-term antibiotic therapy in the neuro-ICU offered no advantage to perioperative prophylaxis (75).

Contaminated or dirty wounds almost certainly benefit from antibiotic therapy. Early administration of antibiotics in this setting, especially when upper airway flora have entered the subarachnoid space, should be considered early treatment for infection rather than prophylaxis, and should be directed at organisms expected to be found in that site.

Whether prophylactic antibiotics can prevent meningitis in patients with traumatic CSF fistulae is unknown. Short-term treatment during or immediately after the acute event has some logic and support, as noted, but even so remains controversial (76). Long-term treatment, intended to decrease the risk of seeding with *pneumococcus* (by far the most common invader in adults) has its advocates, but no documented success and has too many potential drawbacks to make this a sound or certain recommendation (77). A rational approach is to withhold antibiotics and monitor patients closely for early signs of meningitis, and institute empiric antibiotic therapy should this complication arise (73).

Diagnosis

Gram stain and culture should always be obtained from any draining wound. If any central nervous system or meningeal signs are present, or if the infected focus is contiguous with the subarachnoid space even without such signs, CSF also should be obtained for gram stain and culture. Contrast MRI and CT scans may be helpful to document the presence of associated subdural empyema or cortical abscess drainage that may require drainage. Direct surgical exploration usually is necessary if the diagnosis remains in question. Lumbar puncture alone has a low diagnostic yield for diagnosing clinically symptomatic postoperative wound infection (78).

Treatment

When selecting antibiotics, one must consider the wide range of organisms that may infect the postoperative wound. Gram-negative meningitis represents a particularly difficult problem, because many antibiotics penetrate poorly into the subarachnoid space. This is especially true for first- and second-generation cephalosporins and for all of the aminoglycosides (79). Many of the newer third-generation cephalosporins often treat these infections, but they may be less effective against Gram-positive organisms. Whether determination of CSF drug levels is helpful is still controversial. If the illness is critical or worsening in the face of conventional therapy, direct intrathecal administration may be required simply to deliver adequate antibiotics to the area of infection. In most cases, the administration of intrathecal antibiotics via a lumbar catheter or EVD is heroic, and data regarding the optimal dosing of this type of intervention is lacking.

SYSTEMATIC INFECTION CONTROL

Means for control of specific infections have been mentioned, but these should form part of a much larger program of infection control that plays an important part in the quality assessment programs of the hospital. Such a preventive program should be established in each hospital and unit. Its components begin with issues as individual as hand washing, which is thought by some to be the most effective single measure to control nosocomial infections (80). For patients colonized or infected with methicillin-resistant *Staphylococcus aureus,* vancomycin-resistant *Enterococcus faecalis,* or *C. difficile,* contact isolation can provide increased protection against the cross-contamination of other patients by health care workers (81). Finally, hospital-wide efforts to monitor and control infections should be applied to individual units by infectious disease and nursing epidemiology specialists (82).

TREATMENT OF FEVER

Despite increasing recognition of the importance of treating fever in patients with stroke or other forms of acute brain injury (9), effective methods for combating fever in critically ill neurological patients are lacking to date. In most neuro-ICUs, fever is initially treated with acetaminophen, and patients with refractory temperature elevations are treated with water-circulating cooling blankets (83,84). Although acetaminophen is well established as an antipyretic in children (85), its efficacy in critically ill adult patients has never been carefully evaluated. Few controlled studies have evaluated the efficacy of external cooling for lowering body temperature in humans. Three experimental studies have shown that the combination of evaporative and convection cooling, with water sprays or sponging and forced airflow, is more effective than conduction cooling or either method alone for reducing temperature in patients with hyperthermia induced by exercise and heat exposure (86–88).

Water-circulating cooling blankets, a form of conductive cooling, are the most commonly used treatment for acetaminophen-refractory fever in critically ill adults. However, there are little data confirming their efficacy. O'Donnell and associates (84) found no difference in the mean cooling rate between patients treated with or without water-circulating cooling blankets in an observational study of medical ICU patients. In a clinical trial comparing an air-circulating cooling blanket to acetaminophen for fever control in neuro-ICU patients, Mayer and associates (89) found a 30% rate of treatment failure (sustained fever) with both interventions, and no difference between the treatments. These finding suggests that more robust interventions are needed to maintain normothermia in neurological patients at risk for fever-related secondary brain damage. Novel external and endovascular cooling devices are currently in development that may improve our ability to combat fever in patients at risk for temperature-related brain injury (90,91). If normothermia can be effectively maintained in these patients, it then remains to be seen if this can improve functional outcome.

REFERENCES

1. Baena RC, Busto R, Dietrich WD, et al. Hyperthermia delayed by 24 hours aggravates neuronal damage in rat hippocampus following global ischemia. *Neurology* 1997;48:768–773.

2. Kim Y, Busto R, Dietrich WD, et al. Delayed postischemic hyperthermia in awake rats worsens the histopathologic outcome of transient forebrain ischemia. *Stroke* 1996;27:2274–2281.

3. Dietrich WD, Alonso O, Halley M, et al. Delayed posttraumatic brain hyperthermia worsens outcome after fluid percussion brain injury: a light and electron microscopic study in rats. *Neurosurgery* 1996;38:533–541.

4. Hajat C, Hajat S, Sharma P. Effects of post-stroke pyrexia on stroke outcome. A meta-analysis of studies on patients. *Stroke* 2000;31:410–414.

5. Wang Y, Lim LL-Y, Levi C, et al. Influence of admission body temperature on stroke mortality. *Stroke* 2000;31:404–409.

6. Schwarz S, Häfner K, Aschoff A, et al. Incidence and prognostic of fever following intracerebral hemorrhage. *Neurology* 2000;54:354–361.

7. Oliveira-Filho J, Ezzeddine MA, Segal AZ, et al. Fever in subarachnoid hemorrhage: relationship to vasospasm and outcome. *Neurology* 200;56:1299–1304.

8. Rossi S, Roncati Zanier E, Mauri I, et al. Brain temperature, body core temperature, and intracranial pressure in acute cerebral damage. *J Neurol Neurosurg Psychiatry* 2001;71:448–454.

9. Ginsberg MD, Busto R. Combating hyperthermia in acute stroke: a significant clinical concern. *Stroke* 1998;29:529–534.

10. Holtzclaw BJ. The febrile response in critical care: state of the science. *Heart Lung* 1992;21:482–501.

11. Guyton AG. Body temperature, temperature regulation and fever. In: Guyton AG, ed. *Textbook of medical physiology,* 8th ed. Philadelphia: Saunders, 1991:797–808.

12. Wijdicks EFM. Management of nosocomial infections. In: *The clinical practice of critical care neurology.* Philadelphia: Lipincott–Raven, 1997:386–398.

13. Chin RL. High temperature with cerebral hemorrhage. *Ann Emerg Med* 1999;34:411.

14. Kitanaka C, Inoh Y, Toyoda T, et al. Malignant brain stem hyperthermia caused by brain stem hemorrhage. *Stroke* 1994;25:518–520.

15. Erickson TC. Neurogenic hyperthermia (a clinical syndrome and its treatment). *Brain* 1939;62:172–190.

16. Georgilis K, Plomaritoglou A, Dafni U, et al. Aetiology of fever in patients with acute stroke. *J Int Med* 1999; 246:203–209.

17. Commichau C, Scarmeas N, Mayer SA. Risk factors for fever in the neurologic intensive care unit. *Neurology* 2003;60:837–841.

18. Shibata M. Hyperthermia in brain hemorrhage. *Med Hypoth* 1998;50:185–190.

19. Kilpatrick MM, Lowry DW, Firlik AD, et al. Hyperthermia in the neurosurgical intensive care unit. *Neurosurgery* 2000;47:850–856.

20. Circiumaru B, Baldock G, Cohen J. A prospective study of fever in the intensive care unit. *Int Care Med* 1999; 25:668–673.

21. Georgilis K, Plomaritoglou A, Dafni U, et al. Aetiology of fever in patients with acute stroke. *J Int Med* 1999; 246:203–209.

22. Przelomski MM, Roth RM, Gleckman RA, et al. Fever in the wake of stroke. *Neurology* 1986;36:427–429.

23. Dettenkofer M, Ebner W, Hans F-J, et al. Nosocomial infections in a neurosurgery intensive care unit. *Acta Neurochir* 1999;141:1303–1308.

24. O'Grady NP, Barie PS, Bartlett J, et al. Practice parameters for evaluating new fever in critically ill adult patients. *Crit Care Med* 1998;26:392–408.

25 Mackowiak PA, Lemaistre CF. Drug fever: a critical appraisal of conventional concepts. *Ann Int Med* 1987; 106:728–733.

26. Frank JI, Mirabelli J, Goldenberg F, et al. Pre-symptomatic detection and treatment of deep vein thrombosis in neurocritical care patients. *Neurology* 1997;48: A411–A412.

27. Yoshimoto Y, Tanaka Y, Hoya K. Acute systemic inflammatory response syndrome in subarachnoid hemorrhage. *Stroke* 2001;32:1989–1993.

28. Susman VL. Clinical management of neuroleptic malignant syndrome. *Psychiatric Quarterly* 2001;72: 325–336.

29. Gruber A, Rossler K, Graninger W, et al. Ventricular cerebrospinal fluid and serum concentrations of sTNFR-I, IL-1ra, and IL-6 after aneurysmal subarachnoid hemorrhage. *J Neurosurg Anesthesiol* 2000;12: 297–306.

30. Roberts J, Barnes W, Pennock M, et al. Diagnostic accuracy of fever as a measure of postoperative pulmonary complications. *Heart Lung* 1988;17:166–169.

31. Wenzel RP. *Prevention and control of nosocomial infections.* Baltimore: Williams & Wilkins, 1987.

32. Wolach B, Sazbon L, Gavrieli R, et al. Early immunological defects in comatose patients after acute brain injury. *J Neurosurg* 2001;94:706–711.

33. Poungvarin N, Bhoopat W, Viriyavejakul A, et al. Effects of dexamethasone in primary supratentorial intracerebral hemorrhage. *N Engl J Med* 1987;316: 1229–1233.

34. Craven DE, Steger KA. Ventilator-associated bacterial pneumonia: challenges in diagnosis, treatment, and prevention. *New Horizons* 1998;6:S30–S43.

35. George DL. Epidemiology of nosocomial ventilator-associated pneumonia. *Infect Control Hosp Epidemiol* 1993;14:163–169.

36. Berrouane Y, Daudenthun I, Riegel B, et al. Early onset pneumonia in neurosurgical intensive acre unit patients. *J Hosp Infect* 1998;40:275–280.

37. du Moulin GC, Paterson DG, Hedley-White J, et al. Aspiration of gastric bacteria in antacid-treated patients: a frequent cause of postoperative colonization of the airway. *Lancet* 1982;i:242–245.

38. Bartlett JG, Gorbach SL. The triple threat of aspiration pneumonia. *Chest* 1975;68:560–566.

39. Murray HW. Antimicrobial therapy in pulmonary aspiration. *Am J Med* 1979;66:188–190.

40. Bartlett JG, Gorbach SL, Finegold SM. The bacteriology of aspiration pneumonia. *Am J Med* 1974;56: 202–207.

41. Valenti WM, Trudell RG, Bentley DW. Factors predisposing to oropharyngeal colonization with gram-negative bacilli in the aged. *N Engl J Med* 1978;298: 1108–1111.

42. Tillotson JR, Finland M. Bacterial colonization and clinical superinfection of the respiratory tract complicating antibiotic treatment of pneumonia. *J Infect Dis* 1969;119:597–624.

43. Meduri GU, Mauldin GL, Wunderink RG, et al. Causes of fever and pulmonary densities in patients with clinical manifestations of ventilator-associated pneumonia. *Chest* 1994;106:221–235.

44. Stauffer JL, Olson DE, Petty TL. Complications and

consequences of endotracheal intubation and tracheotomy: a prospective study of 150 critically ill adult patients. *Am J Med* 1981;70:65–76.

45. Valles J, Artigas A, Rello J, et al. Continuous aspiration of subglottic secretions in the prevention of ventilator associated pneumonia. *Ann Int Med* 1995;122:179–186.

46. Niederman MS. An approach to empiric therapy of nosocomial pneumonia. *Med Clin North Am* 1993;78: 1123–1141.

47. Kunin CM. *Detection, prevention and management of urinary tract infections,* 4th ed. Philadelphia: Lea & Febiger, 1987.

48. Garibaldi RA, Burke JP, Dickman ML. Factors predisposing to bacteriuria during indwelling urinary catheterization. *N Engl J Med* 1974;291:215–219.

49. Garibaldi RA, Burke JP, Britt MR, et al. Meatal colonization and catheter-associated bacteriuria. *N Engl J Med* 1980;303:316–318.

50. Burke JP, Garibaldi RA, Britt MR, et al. Prevention of catheter-associated urinary tract infections: efficacy of daily meatal care regimens. *Am J Med* 1981;70:655–658.

51. Nickel JC, Ruseska I, Wright JB, et al. Tobramycin resistance of *Pseudomonas aeruginosa* cells growing as a biofilm on urinary catheter material. *Antimicrob Agents Chemother* 1985; 27:619–624.

52. Centers for Disease Control and Prevention. National Nosocomial Infections Surveillance (NNIS) System report, data summary from October 1986–April 1998, issued June 1998. *Am J Infect Control* 1998;26:522–533.

53. Heiselman D. Nosocomial bloodstream infections in the critically ill. *JAMA* 1994;272:1819–1820.

54. Centers for Disease Control and Prevention. National Nosocomial Infections Surveillance (NNIS) System report, data summary from January 1990–May 1999, issued June 1999. *Am J Infect Control* 1999;27:520–532.

55. Hampton AA, Sheretz RJ Vascular-access infections in hospitalized patients. *Surg Clin North Am* 1988;68: 57–71.

56. Cobb DK, High KP, Sawyer RG, et al. A controlled trial of scheduled replacement of central venous and pulmonary-artery catheters. *N Engl J Med* 1992;327: 1062–1068.

57. Bernard GR, Vincent JL, Laterre PF, et al. Efficacy and safety of recombinant human activated protein C for severe sepsis. *N Engl J Med* 2001;344:699–709.

58. McFarland LV, Mulligan ME, Kwok RY, et al. Nosocomial acquisition of *Clostridium difficile* infection. *N Engl J Med* 1989;320:204–210.

59. Lozier AP, Sciacca RR, Romagnoli MF, et al. Ventriculostomy-related infections: a critical review of the literature. *Neurosurgery* 2002;51:170–182.

60. Holloway KL, Barnes T, Choi S, et al. Ventriculostomy infections. *J Neurosurg* 1996;85:419–424.

61. Kanter RK, Weiner LB, Patti AM, et al. Infectious complications and duration of intracranial pressure monitoring. *Crit Care Med* 1985;13:837–839.

62. Mayhall CG, Archer NH, Lamb VA, et al. Ventriculostomy-related infections. *N Engl J Med* 1984;310: 553–559.

63. Alleyne CH, Hassan M, Zabramski JM. The efficacy and cost of prophylactic and periprocedural antibiotics in patients with external ventricular drains. *Neurosurgery* 2000;47:1124–1129.

64. Wyler AR, Kelly WA. Use of antibiotics with external ventriculostomies. *J Neurosurg* 1972;37:185–187.

65. Poon WS, Ng S, Wai S. CSF antibiotic prophylaxis for neurosurgical patients with ventriculostomy: a randomised study. *Acta Neurochir Suppl* 1998;71:146–148.

66. Wong GkC, Poon WS, Wai S, et al. Failure of regular external ventricular drain exchange to reduce cerebrospinal fluid infection: results of a randomised controlled trial. *J Neurol Neurosurg Psychiat* 2002;73: 759–761.

67. Leib SL, Boscacci R, Gratzl O, et al. Predictive value of cerebrospinal fluid (CSF) lactate level versus CSF/blood glucose ratio for the diagnosis of bacterial meningitis following neurosurgery. *Clin Infect Dis* 1999;29: 69–74.

68. Balch RE. Wound infections complicating neurosurgical procedures. *J Neurosurg* 1967;26:41–45.

69. Wright RI. A survey of possible etiologic agents in postoperative craniotomy infection. *J Neurosurg* 1966;25: 125–132.

70. Tenney JH, Vlahov D, Salcman M, et al. Wide variation in the risk of wound infection following clean neurosurgery. Implications for perioperative antibiotic prophylaxis. *Am J Infect Control* 1985;62:243–247.

71. Trick WE, Kioski CM, Howard KM, et al. Outbreak of *Pseudomonas aeruginosa* ventriculitis among patients in a neurosurgical intensive care unit. *Infect Control Hosp Epidemiol* 2000;21:204–208.

72. Zhang JZ, Wang S, Li JS, et al. The perioperative use of ceftriaxone as infection prophylaxis in neurosurgery. *Clin Neurol Neurosurg* 1995;97:285–289.

73. Brown EM. Antimicrobial prophylaxis in neurosurgery. *J Antimicrob Chemother* 1993;31(suppl B):49–63.

74. Shapiro M. Prophylaxis in otolaryngologic surgery and neurosurgery: a critical review. *Rev Infect Dis* 1991;13 (suppl 10):S858-S868.

75. Santilli F, Narciso N, Bifano D, et al. Antibiotic prophylaxis in elective neurosurgery: epidemiological study. *Minerva Chirurg* 1994;49:829–836.

76. Mincy JE. Post traumatic cerebrospinal fluid fistula of the frontal fossa. *J Trauma* 1966;6:618–622.

77. Hand W, Sanford JP. Post traumatic bacterial meningitis. *Ann Intern Med* 1970;72:869–874.

78. Adelson-Mitty J, Fink MP, Lisbon A. The value of lumbar puncture in the evaluation of critically ill, non-immunocompromised, surgical patients: a retrospective analysis of 70 cases. *Int Care Med* 1997;23:749–752.

79. Swartz MN. Intraventricular use of aminoglycosides in the treatment of gram-negative bacillary meningitis: conflicting views. *J Infect Dis* 1981;143:293–296.

80. Steere AC, Mallison GE. Handwashing practices for the prevention of nosocomial infections. *Ann Intern Med* 1975;83:683–690.

81. Lynch P, Jackson MM, Cummings MJ, et al. Rethinking the role of isolation practices in the prevention of nosocomial infections. *Ann Intern Med* 1987;107:243–246.

82. Haley RW, Culver DH, White JW. The efficacy of infection surveillance and control programs in preventing nosocomial infections in U.S. hospitals. *Am J Epidemiol* 1985;121:182–204.

83. Isaacs SN, Axelrod PI, Lorber B. Antipyretic orders in a university hospital. *Am J Med* 1990;88:31–35.

84. O'Donnell J, Axelrod P, Fisher C, et al. Use and effectiveness of hypothermia blankets for febrile patients in the intensive care unit. *Clin Infect Dis* 1997;24:1208–1213.

85. Ameer B, Greenblatt DJ. Acetaminophen. *Ann Int Med* 1977;87:202–209.

86. Wyndham CH, Strydom NB, Cooke HM, et al. Methods of cooling subjects with hyperpyrexia. *J Appl Physiol* 1959;14:771–776.

87. Weiner JS, Khogali M. A physiologic body-cooling unit for treatment of heat stroke. *Lancet* 1980;1: 507–508.

88. Kielblock AJ, Van Rensberg JP, Franz RM. Body cooling as a method for reducing hyperthermia. *S Afr Med J* 1986;69:378–380.

89. Mayer SA, Commichau C, Scarmeas N, et al. Clinical trial of an air-circulating cooling blanket for fever control in critically ill neurological patients. *Neurology* 2001;56:292–298.

90. Mayer SA, Kowalski RG, Ostapkovitch N, et al. Normalization of body temperature in febrile neuro-ICU patients with the Arctic Sun Temperature Management System. *Neurology* 2002;58(Suppl 3):A93.

91. DeGeorgia M, Abou-Chebl, Devlin T, Jauss M, et al. Endovascular cooling for patients with acute ischemic stroke. *Neurology* 2002;58(Suppl 3):A506.

8

Electrophysiologic Monitoring in the Neurological Intensive Care Unit

Monitoring neurological functioning is of paramount importance in the neurological intensive care unit (neuro-ICU). However, even when performed conscientiously, serial neurological examinations are discontinuous, may miss important changes in the patient's condition, and can vary according to the expertise of the examiner. Neurophysiologic monitoring with electroencephalography (EEG) and evoked potential (EP) are the primary tools available to the neurointensivist for objective evaluation of the functional status of the brain. In addition to supplementing the neurological examination as a measure of physiologic activity, EEG and EP can also provide unique diagnostic information related to specific brain wave patterns (e.g., burst-suppression, spindles, abnormal alpha, attenuation, seizures, and diurnal cycling on EEG studies) or anatomic function (e.g., evidence of brainstem damage on EP studies).

There are four primary applications for neurophysiologic monitoring in the neuro-ICU: (a) the detection of seizure activity and epileptic foci; (b) monitoring of neurological status (e.g., early detection of neurological deterioration owing to ischemia); (c) prognostication; and (d) evaluation of the effects of sedation and therapeutic interventions (1–8). In this rapidly evolving field, computer technology is being developed that can allow neurophysiologic monitoring to be fully integrated with other data collected in the neuro-ICU, such as cerebral perfusion pressure (CPP), intracranial pressure (ICP), and brain tissue oxygen tension. Multimodal monitoring of this type allows the neurointensivist to optimize physiologic variables that are directly under our control, such as CPP and P_{CO_2}, and provide insights into how different physiologic derangements affect neurological function.

A single or even repeated electrophysiologic study may suffer from the same problems as does the neurological examination: It is a discrete, brief sample of data that may not reflect the patient's overall condition. Many comatose patients, for example, show cycling of EEG patterns over the course of the day; these diurnal patterns cannot be detected by performing discrete electrophysiologic examinations. Seizures are usually brief and paroxysmal, and can be missed easily when EEGs are performed intermittently. For these reasons, monitoring of central nervous system (CNS) integrity or function in the neuro-ICU is best accomplished with continuous monitoring. Technologic advances have now made possible the collection, storage, analysis, and transmission of large amounts of continuous EEG and EP data (3). The ultimate goal of such monitoring is to enable the clinician to predict impending CNS injury at a time when intervention is still possible. For example, by the time temporal lobe herniation has reached the stage of third cranial nerve compression and pupillary dilation, a common clinical signpost, some irreparable damage probably has occurred already. In the case of cerebral vasospasm, hours can intervene between the onset of ischemia and the detection of clinical deficits on examination. Nonconvulsive status epilepticus (NCSE), left untreated, can exacerbate neuronal injury and become increasingly refractory to treatment. These instances easily come to mind as examples in which continuous EEG (cEEG) monitoring might dramatically influence management in the neuro-ICU. Similarly, the reliable, objective data provided by EP studies can be useful sources of information about the level of functioning of specific CNS structures. This is especially true because short-latency somatosensory and brainstem auditory EPs are closely tied to anatomic structures, and are resistant to alterations by anything other than structural pathology. For example, brainstem auditory evoked potentials (BAEPs) and other subcortical EPs are essentially unchanged by high-dose barbiturate therapy sufficient to render the EEG isoelectric and clinical function virtually absent.

ELECTROENCEPHALOGRAPHY

Background

As recently as ten years ago, EEG monitoring in most neuro-ICUs was performed intermittently with paper recordings. The use of digital cEEG monitoring initially was limited to dedicated epilepsy monitoring units, where the emphasis was on seizure classification and quantification, identification of interictal epileptiform discharges, and the presurgical evaluation of candidates for epilepsy surgery (9). Continuous electroencephalography monitoring has become increasingly accepted as a neuro-ICU monitoring technique with the advent of modern computer technology, which makes post hoc filtering, remontaging, adjusting of the sensitivity, and off-site read-

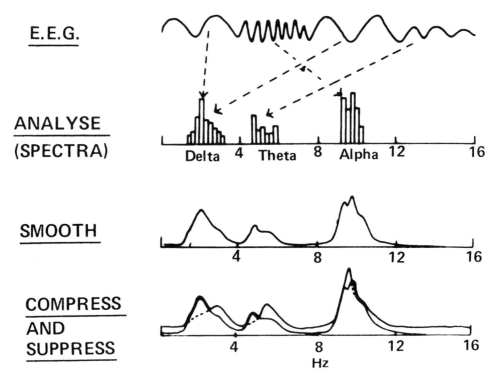

FIG. 8.1. Steps in generation of a compressed spectral array from segments of raw electroencephalographic (*E.E.G.*) data. (From Bickford RG. Newer methods of recording and analyzing EEGs. In: Klass DW, Daly DD, eds. *Current practice of clinical electroencephalography.* New York: Raven Press, 1979:451–480, with permission.)

ing possible (10). Common indications for cEEG in the neurocritical care setting include the detection of nonconvulsive status epilepticus (NCSE), monitoring for cerebral ischemia and other causes of neurological deterioration, prognostication, and titration of sedation (best exemplified by titration of pentobarbital to attain burst suppression).

Computer processing of cEEG data also has the potential to reveal subtle changes over long periods of time that may not be evident when reviewing the raw EEG. Electroencephalography data collected over long periods of time can be transformed into power spectra by fast Fourier transformation (FFT), creating quantitative EEG (qEEG) parameters (Fig. 8.1). These can be displayed graphically as compressed spectral arrays (CSAs) (Fig. 8.2), and may reveal subtle changes in the EEG earlier than other monitoring techniques. With the advent of powerful microprocessors, data processing of this type can be performed in real time at the patient's bedside. However, qEEG parameters of this type can be contaminated by artifact, and should not be

attempted without proper training in electroencephalography and access to the raw EEG, to avoid the inclusion of signals related to artifact.

Technical Considerations

The practical challenges of cEEG recording in the neuro-ICU are substantial. The major hurdle is not owing to the complexity of the equipment or computer technology, but that of maintaining a low-impedance, low-noise connection between patient and machine. This challenge alone mandates special training of nursing staff and frequent daily visits by the EEG technician. In addition, there are multiple generators of electrical noise and artifact in the ICU, which can be unusually perplexing. Ventilators produce both mechanical and electric rhythmic artifacts. Nursing procedures such as chest physical therapy are another source of activity that can be in the frequency range of normal or pathologic brain electrical activity. Completely disconnected electrodes occasionally

METHOD OF ANALYSIS AND DISPLAY

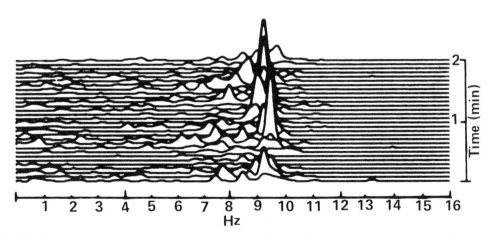

FIG. 8.2. Compressed spectral array of a normal adult, showing a large peak corresponding to the alpha rhythm. (From Bickford RG. Newer methods of recording and analyzing EEGs. In: Klass DW, Daly DD, eds. *Current practice of clinical electroencephalography.* New York: Raven Press, 1979:451–480, with permission.)

may record activity that looks similar to a comatose patient with moderate to severe diffuse slowing and attenuation. Finally, sedating medications that can affect the EEG are routinely used in the neuro-ICU setting. For these reasons, the technologist, clinical neurophysiologist, ICU nurse, and neurointensivist must work closely together to ensure that the EEG accurately reflects cerebral activity. Team training and continuing education for clinicians are crucial to the success of any neuro-ICU cEEG monitoring program (5). For cEEG, valid interpretation is often only possible when either the ICU staff makes notes in the EEG record, or when a continuous video recording is combined with the EEG recording. Digital video has been shown to be particularly helpful for identifying subtle ictal phenomena (e.g., facial twitching or rhythmic eye movements) and EEG abnormalities related to artifact (12).

Specific Applications of Continuous Electroencephalographic Monitoring in the Neurological Intensive Care Unit

Detection of Seizure Activity

Indications

Patients in coma often experience nonconvulsive seizures that have few or no clinical manifestations. Continuous electroencephalographic monitoring is essential for the detection and prompt treatment of these events, which may contribute to the patient's depressed level of consciousness or cause additional brain damage. Nonconvulsive seizures and nonconvulsive status epilepticus (NCSE) are common in all types of acute brain injury, and are not restricted to patients with epilepsy or those with a clinical diagnosis of seizures. In unselected neuro-ICU patients, cEEG monitoring reveals nonconvulsive seizures in up to 34%, and up to 75% of these cases have NCSE (13). Even after excluding patients with any clinical suspicion of seizures, cEEG detects NCSE in 5% to 10% of comatose medical intensive care unit (14), traumatic brain injury (TBI) (15), or subarachnoid hem-

orrhage (SAH) patients (16). Similarly, cEEG detects nonconvulsive seizures in up to 27% of patients with altered level of consciousness from any cause (17), in 36% of patients after the termination of generalized convulsive SE (18), in 22% of severe TBI patients (15), and in up to 23% of patients with intracerebral hemorrhage (19,20). It is important to diagnose NCSE in these patients, because the excessive metabolic demand of ictal activity may increase ICP and further compromise brain tissue at risk for ischemic or excitotoxic injury (8). The prognosis of NCSE in the ICU setting is poor: The overall mortality rate is 30% to 50% (16,21–23), and medically refractory NCSE after severe TBI and SAH has been associated with 100% mortality (16,17). The challenge for the neurointensivist remains in demonstrating that the aggressive, early termination of NCSE in these patients can result in better outcomes.

In the absence of cEEG monitoring, appropriate treatment for patients with NCSE without overt clinical symptoms of seizures often is delayed. This may have a deleterious impact on outcome because delayed anticonvulsant therapy for SE has been associated with poor outcome (23,24) and an increased likelihood of refractory SE (25,26). Patients on continuous intravenous antiepileptic drugs (cIV-AEDs) for the treatment of refractory SE always should be monitored with cEEG, because subclinical seizures may occur in up to half of patients during treatment, and up to 26% after the initial discontinuation of therapy (27). Although the outcome of NCSE is often poor, termination of ongoing electrographic seizure activity can result in recovery of consciousness and clinical improvement (25), and there remains little doubt that nonconvulsive seizures can directly injure the brain and cause enduring neurological impairment (28,29). In years past, "seizures, coma, and death" was an all-too-common course of events for victims of acute, severe brain injury. The advent of cEEG monitoring raises the possibility that untreated NCSE played a major role in prolonging coma and exacerbating brain injury in many of these cases.

Challenges of Electroencephalography Interpretation in Status Epilepticus

The accurate identification of electrographic seizures in comatose, severely brain injured patients presents special challenges for the electroencephalographer and neurointensivist (Table 8.1). Classic ictal patterns (Fig. 8.3) showing paroxysmal high-voltage spike and sharp-wave discharges (gleaned from epilepsy patients with otherwise normal brain function) may not be evident in the seizing patient with diffuse brain injury and profound EEG background suppression. Instead, more subtle discharges—such as paroxysmal waxing-and-waning focal slow wave activity or periodic lateralized epileptiform discharges (PLEDs)—may represent ictal activity in the comatose patient (Fig. 8.4) (30,31). In patients with known staus epilepticus, these EEG findings may be considered as part of an ictal/interictal continuum because they do not meet formal seizure criteria, and because their exact nature and significance remain poorly understood. Some have used serial EEG data (31,32), focal increased blood flow on single photon-emission computed tomography (SPECT) (33), and increased metabolism on fluorodeoxyglucose positron emission tomography (PET) scanning (34) to argue that PLEDs and other subtle EEG findings following SE can be ictal. Others regard PLEDs as a purely nonictal phenomenon. Further work in this controversial area is badly needed.

TABLE 8.1. *Criteria for electrographic seizures*

Repetitive spikes exceeding three per second
Repetitive spikes less than three per second, if changes after antiepileptic drug administration
Rhythmic waves with incrementing onset or decrementing offset, and postdischarge slowing or attenuation

---

From Jordan KG. Continuous EEG monitoring in the neuroscience intensive care unit and emergency department. *J Clin Neurophysiol* 1999;16:14–39, with permission.

Seizure Detection Software

Specialized EEG signal processing software can be used for screening large cEEG datasets for possible electrographic seizure activity, thus improving the efficiency of cEEG analysis. However, technical challenges remain. The data reduction techniques used in most cEEG CSA displays make recognition of spikes and sharp waves impossible, burst suppression almost impossible, and electrographic seizure activity difficult. Specific patterns related to the rhythmicity of electrographic seizure activity (35) or accompanying muscle artifact (36) may be helpful indicators. Tasker and associates (37) described continuous monitoring using the cerebral function analyzing monitor (CFAM) and found that paroxysmal events were clearly seen, although the sensitivity of this system for detecting partial seizures was limited. Another approach to solving the problem of seizure detection has been developed by Gotman, who published an algorithm for selecting parameters extracted from the digital EEG to identify ictal activity (38). Although the false-positive rate was quite high, the sensitivity was good, and few real ictal events are missed. Vespa and coworkers (15) have developed automated seizure detection software based on multichannel, digitized real-time FFT (2 seconds per epoch, 2 minutes average) and trends of total EEG power with some success.

Existing automated seizure detection software that has been developed for use in epilepsy monitoring units has largely been "trained" on seizures obtained from healthy, neurologically intact patients with seizure disorders. However, these seizures differ from those of comatose brain-injured patients, in whom ictal activity is often less organized, slower in maximum frequency, of longer duration, and without a clear on- and off-set. In order to use seizure detection programs in the neuro-ICU, new software needs to be developed that can more accurately identify potentially ictal patterns in patients with brain injury.

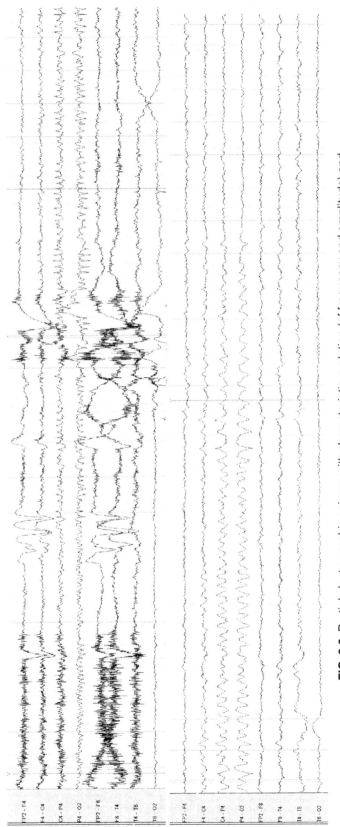

FIG. 8.3. Partial electrographic seizure with characteristic evolution (of frequency and amplitude) and offset. **Top panel:** The probable onset of the seizure is in the right parietal-occipital region (P4-O2 leads); prominent muscle artifact is seen in the other leads. It evolves into a run of high-frequency spike wave activity in the C4-P4 and P4-O2 leads. **Bottom panel:** The seizure evolves into slower frequency sharp wave activity. (Figure provided courtesy of Dr. Bryan Young.)

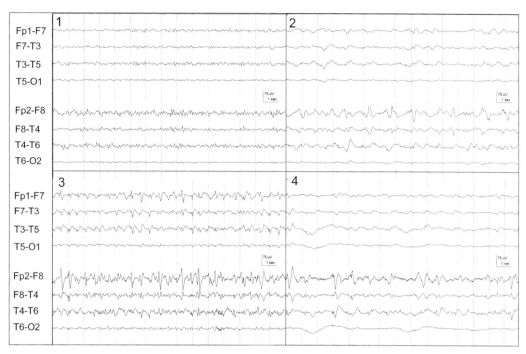

FIG. 8.4. Evolution of electroencephalographic findings in a 55-year-old woman with nonconvulsive status epilepticus after subarachnoid hemorrhage (selected montage of temporal electrodes only). **Panel 1:** Day 5 after subarachnoid hemorrhage: Mild to moderate diffuse background slowing, higher voltages on the right owing to skull defect from craniotomy, no epileptiform discharges. **Panel 2:** Day 5 (2 hours after panel 1): Broadly distributed right hemispheric periodic lateralized epileptiform discharges with underlying semirhythmic delta, diffuse background slowing, and left hemisphere attenuation. **Panel 3:** Day 5 (4 hours after panel 2): Bilateral seizure activity, right greater than left. **Panel 4:** Day 6 (24 hours after panel 3): Similar pattern to electroencephalograph in panel 2. (From Dennis LJ, Claassen J, Hirsch LJ, et al. Nonconvulsive status epilepticus after subarachnoid hemorrhage. *Neurosurgery* 2002;51;1136–1144, with permission.)

Neurological Monitoring

Electroencephalographic Signal Processing

The sensitivity of the EEG to changes in CBF and pharmacologic agents suggests that monitoring cEEG might bridge the gap between serial neurological examinations in the neuro-ICU setting, particularly in comatose patients. The primary challenge is to convert the complex EEG signal into a more "user-friendly" summary format that can be interpreted by nonelectroencephalographers in real time. The computer analysis technique most commonly used to accomplish this is transformation of the EEG into CSA. Compressed spectral array based on FFT of

the EEG signal can be plotted as total power or overall amplitude, frequency activity totals (e.g., total or percent alpha power), spectral edge frequencies (e.g., the frequency below which 75% of the EEG record resides), and frequency ratios (e.g., alpha-delta ratio, ADR) (39–42). Other EEG data reduction display formats include the CFAM, the pEEG monitor, EEG density modulation, automated analysis of segmented EEG (AAS-EEG), and the bispectral index (BIS) monitor (6,43,44). Despite great promise, the utility of these compressed cEEG parameters for neurological monitoring in the neuro-ICU setting has yet to be demonstrated.

Cerebral Ischemia

Cerebral ischemia results in EEG changes because cortical layers 3 and 5, which are particularly sensitive to oxygen deficits, contribute most to the generation of electrical dipoles detected by EEG (8). It has long been known that infarction may result in polymorphic delta, loss of fast activity and sleep spindles, and focal attenuation (45,46). These EEG findings have been shown to reflect abnormal cerebral blood flow (CBF) and metabolism (cerebral metabolic rate of oxygen) as demonstrated by PET and Xenon-CT-CBF imaging (47,48). Electroencephalography is very sensitive for ischemia, and usually begins to change at the time reversible neuronal dysfunction occurs (CBF 25 to 30 mL/100 g per minute) (46), a level at which therapeutic interventions might be instituted to prevent permanent brain damage. On the reverse side, EEG is also very sensitive for recovery and may demonstrate recovery of brain function from reperfusion earlier than the clinical examination (8).

Intracranial Pressure

Relatively little work has explored the relationship between EEG patterns and ICP. In one study of 16 patients, Munari and Calbucci (49) found no single EEG pattern that correlated with mean ICP values. However, when the ICP was stable and without pressure waves, the EEG contained regular high-voltage slow waves, whereas an alternating EEG was seen in those patients with Lundberg B waves. Other human studies have also shown a poor correlation between ICP levels and EEG activity (50). It appears likely that EEG activity is not reliably influnced by increased ICP until very high levels are reached and CPP and CBF is compromised. In monkeys, Langfitt and associates (51) found that a gradual rise in ICP produced by an intracranial balloon produced no EEG changes until near levels approaching mean systemic arterial pressure were reached.

Intraoperative Monitoring

The relationship between EEG and ischemia was first applied in the early 1970s to intraoperative monitoring during carotid endarterectomy (52,53). Detailed studies of EEG parameters during carotid clamping show three patterns corresponding to increasingly severe changes in CBF. At the first level, conventional EEG traces remain unchanged to visual inspection, but computer analysis shows a 5% to 15% drop in amplitude without changes in peak or median power frequencies (52,53). This EEG pattern presumably corresponds to a minor drop in CBF. At the second level, the EEG shows marked slowing and an increase in amplitude. At the third and most critical level of ischemia, the EEG shows a marked loss of amplitude (greater than 50%) and further slowing of the dominant frequencies. This has been considered to be a significant change and an indication for a temporary bypass shunt if the clamp is to be maintained for more than a few minutes. Though the usefulness of EEG monitoring for carotid surgery is well established, the most sensitive parameters to monitor have not been clearly determined. However, it is established that computerized qEEG is more sensitive to change than routine visual analysis (54), and that the ADR is highly sensitive to the effects of ischemic stroke (55). Future innovations to improve the sensitivity and specificity of intraoperative monitoring may include automatied multiparameter EEG analysis using sophisticated methods such as wavelet analysis, fuzzy logic, and neural networks (56).

The techniques of interventional radiology also have spurred efforts to improve neurological monitoring, and have provided a rich source of information applicable to the neuro-ICU (Fig. 8.4). Hacke and coworkers (57) originally proposed that cEEG monitoring might be useful during angiographically guided balloon test occlusion (BTO) of the carotid artery. Several investigators have described EEG CSA slowing in response to BTO, which presumably reflects critical perfusion failure and CBF reduction (58,59). The endovascular treatment of arteriovenous malformations (AVMs) has provided another opportunity for monitoring CNS function under highly controlled conditions. In one study, focal EEG slowing during preembolization superselective amytal testing was been shown in some series to predict subsequent neurological events (60). More recently, interventional neuroradiologists have described the use of intraarterial catheter tip EEG electrodes for the detection of seizure foci related to AVMs and deep brain structures not detected by conventional EEG (61,62).

Neurological Intensive Care Unit Monitoring for Delayed Ischemia After Subarachnoid Hemorrhage

The EEG changes observed during iatrogenic CBF changes in the operating room and angiography suite suggest that cEEG might be helpful in monitoring cortical function in the ICU. This application is best exemplified by SAH patients at risk for developing cerebral vasospasm (Fig. 8.5) (63–65). Several studies have attempted to identify specific EEG parameters that correlate with the development of delayed cerebral ischemia after SAH, with varying results. Labar and colleagues (64) found that the trend analysis of total power (1 to 30 Hz) correlated with the development of delayed ischemia. Vespa and coworkers (63) identified the variability of relative alpha (6 to 14 Hz/1 to 20 Hz) as a predictor of vasospasm. Claassen and associates (65) found in a systematic analysis of 20 derived cEEG parameters that the poststimulation ADR (PSADR, 8 to 13 Hz/1 to 4 Hz) had the best sensitivity and specificity for delayed ischemia. Surprisingly, all of these studies found that focal ischemia sometimes resulted in global or bilateral changes in the EEG, and two found clear evidence that EEG changes can precede clinical deterioration by several days (63,64). Claassen and associates (65) studied poor-grade SAH patients (Hunt-Hess grade 4 or 5), in whom delayed ischemia and infarction is often not detectable by the clinical examination. They found that both a one-

time 50% reduction or a prolonged greater than 10% decrease in PSADR from baseline were equally sensitive and specific (70% to 80%) for detecting delayed ischemia. Rivierez and coworkers (66) did not monitor EEG continuously, but obtained EEGs on days 1 and 5 after SAH in 151 patients. They found that a normal EEG correctly predicted a vasospasm-free course in 73%, but did not determine whether the EEG added value after considering clinical grade. Certain abnormal EEG patterns, especially one showing broad, repetitive slow waves, termed "axial bursts," predicted clinical or angiographic evidence of vasospasm 97% of the time. Although cEEG monitoring for delayed ischemia is a promising application, additional research is needed to develop online real-time cEEG parameters continuously displayed in the neuro-ICU.

One drawback of quantitative EEG interpretation is that absolute values have to be interpreted cautiously because of intersubject differences. For this reason, cEEG is likely to be most useful for trending cerebral activity after a baseline assessment can be obtained. Within-subject state changes, variations in physiologic parameters (e.g., cerebral perfusion pressure), medications (i.e., sedatives), and artifacts can heavily influence qEEG parameters (67). For this reason, most studies have found that relative qEEG parameters are more useful than absolute parameters (63,65). These studies also have found that the best data are obtained when artifact-free clips of EEG are obtained following physical stimulation.

Other Neurological Intensive Care Unit Continuous Electroencephalography Monitoring Applications

A variety of additional applications for cEEG monitoring in the neuro-ICU setting have been explored. Suzuki and colleagues (68) studied patients with stenotic arterial lesions that were subjected to hypertensive and hypotensive stress while monitoring EEG frequency in the neuro-ICU. Two thirds (12 of 18) showed deterioration of the EEG after in-

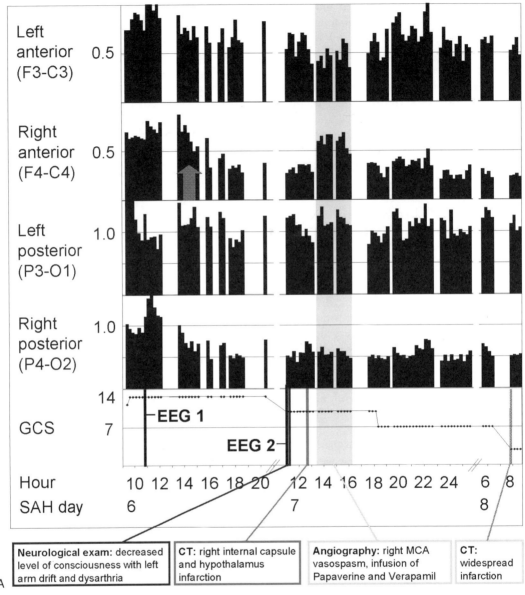

FIG. 8.5. Continuous electroencephalograph [*EEG* (cEEG)]–derived alpha-delta ratio (ADR) calcu-lated every 15 minutes in a 57-year-old woman admitted for acute subarachnoid hemorrhage (*SAH*) (admission Hunt-Hess grade 4) from a right posterior communicating aneurysm **(Panel A).** The aneurysm was clipped on SAH day 2; no infarcts were seen on postoperative computed tomography (*CT*) (Fig. 8.3). She had a Glasgow Coma Scale (*GCS*) of 14 postoperatively. CEEG monitoring was performed from SAH day 3 to 8. The ADR progressively decreased after day 6, particularly in the right anterior region *(arrow)*, to settle into a steady trough level later that night, reflecting loss of fast frequencies and slowing over the right hemisphere in the raw cEEG (Fig. 8.4). On SAH day 6 tran-scranial Doppler flow velocity in the right middle cerebral artery (*MCA*) was marginally elevated (144 cm/sec), but the patient remained clinically stable with hypertensive hypervolemic therapy (systolic blood pressure greater than 180 mm Hg).

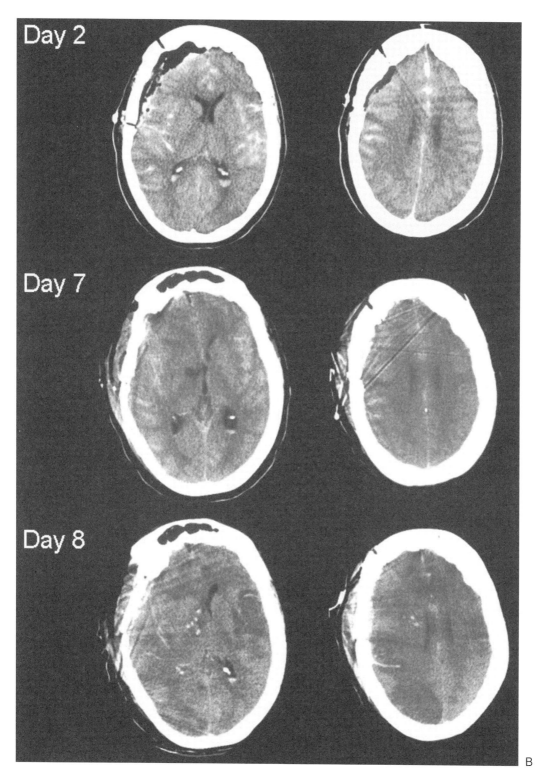

Day 2

Day 7

Day 8

B

FIG. 8.5. *Continued.* On day 7, the GCS dropped from 14 to 12 and a CT scan showed a possible right internal capsule and hypothalamic infarction **(Panel B).** Angiography demonstrated severe distal right MCA and left vertebral artery spasm owing to the marked tortuosity of the parent vessels. A decision was made not to perform angioplasty, but instead to infuse verapamil and papaverine. This resulted in a marked, but transient increase of the right anterior ADR *(vertical bar).* Later that day, the patient further deteriorated clinically to a GCS of 7, with a new left hemiparesis, and died on SAH day 9 from widespread infarction caused by vasospasm.

duced hypotension, and six of 11 patients showed an increase in EEG frequencies with induced hypertension. These data were considered helpful in deciding whether to place a bypass graft. Jordan and colleagues (69) described 21 stroke patients studied with cEEG and xenon-enhanced computed tomography (CT) CBF. A group with low CBF and focal slowing and a preserved background EEG improved significantly with hypervolemic therapy. Matousek and coworkers (70) correlated EEG slowing, using both CSA processing and a qualitative visual EEG assessment scale, with level of consciousness scores in comatose patients. The degree of correlation between the coma scores and EEG was highest ($R = 0.68$) when multiple rather than single CSA-derived EEG parameters were analyzed. Gilbert and associates (71) tested whether the EEG-derived bispectral index (BIS), an empiric index of EEG scaled from 0 to 100, correlated with neurological status in 31 awake, unsedated critically ill adults in a medical ICU. The BIS significantly correlated with a variety of neurological scores, and was more strongly correlated than other conventional CSA parameters. However, the degree of correlation was not great: In a multivariate analysis, the combination of BIS and relative theta power accounted for only 38% of the variability of Glasgow Coma Scale scores.

Prognostication

The Electroencephalograph and Coma

A number of studies have reported associations between EEG findings and outcome in comatose patients. The EEG allows insight into thalamocortical function in comatose patients that is inaccessible clinically. In the past, EEGs were predominantly used to diagnose electrocerebral silence for the diagnosis of brain death. Most of these studies did not systematically categorize EEG findings, and very few have analyzed EEG findings in conjunction with other potential predictors of poor outcome. For this reason, the independent predictive power of EEG findings re-

TABLE 8.2. *Electroencephalographic classification system for prognosis in coma*

Delta/theta >50% of record (not theta coma)
  Reactivity
  No reactivity
Triphasic waves
Burst-suppression
  With epileptiform activity
  Without epileptiform activity
Alpha/theta/spindle coma (unreactive)
Epileptiform activity (not in burst-suppression pattern)
  Generalized
  Focal or multifocal
Suppression
  Amplitude 10–20 µV
  <10 µV

From Young GB, McLachlan RS, Kreeft JH, et al. An electroencephalographic classification for coma. *Can J Neurol Sci* 1997;24:320–325, with permission.

mains unknown. In one study of unselected comatose patients, unreactive delta was associated with poor outcome (death or vegetative state) in 95%, compared to 30% of those with reactivity (72). Prognostic categorization schemes have been proposed on the basis of routine EEGs in the ICU (Table 8.2) (73,74). Poor prognostic findings in these classification schemes include invariant unreactive, monotonous alpha or theta activity ("alpha-theta" coma), burst-suppression patterns, loss of reactivity to external stimuli, and periodic bursts of epileptiform discharges (Fig. 8.6) (73–76). These grading scales have not been evaluated using cEEG, in which diurnal variability, state changes, and trends over time may add additional prognostic value.

Epileptiform Activity and Prognosis

As cEEG has become more readily available in the management of ICU patients, comatose patients with highly epileptiform EEGs are increasingly being identified, with findings ranging from nonconvulsive seizure activity, periodic epileptiform discharges, and stimulus-responsive potentially ictal discharges (SRPIDS) (77). Although PLEDS and recurrent ictal discharges are predictive of poor outcome after SE (78), the prognostic significance of these findings in patients

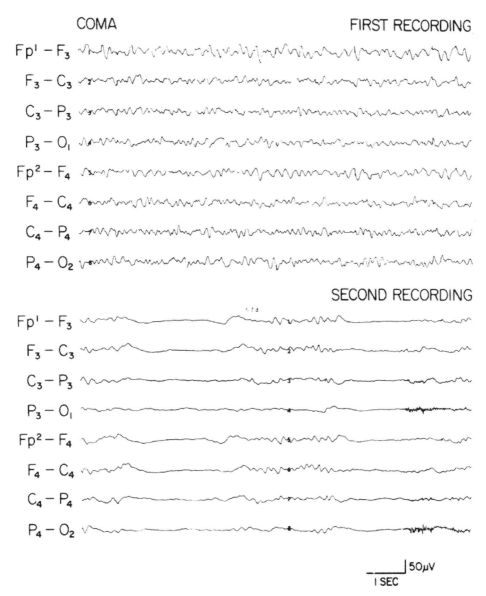

FIG. 8.6. Evolution of electroencephalogram in a comatose patient following cardiac arrest to a burst-suppression pattern (second recording), which is indicative of an extremely poor prognosis. (Figure provided courtesy of Dr. Bryan Young.)

without obvious clinical seizures remains unknown. In one study of patients with highly epileptiform EEG patterns, a scale incorporating disease etiology, age, neurological examination, and EEG findings was shown to correlate highly with mortality and functional outcome in unselected neuro-ICU patients; however, EEG findings were the weakest contributor to this score (79).

Sleep and Diurnal Variation

Although the presence of normal sleep patterns—particularly rapid eye movement sleep—in comatose patients implies a favorable prognosis (80,81), spontaneous diurnal alterations of the EEG appear to be even more important. Variation of EEG activity (cycling) in comatose patients who otherwise appear to be in a constant level of coma, has been observed for approximately 25 years (82–85). A good prognosis has been reported when the EEG pattern is variable; Bricolo and coworkers (84) and Bergamasco and associates (82) found that a monophasic (invariant) EEG carries a worse prognosis than an alternating (cycling) EEG. Similarly, Karnaze and colleagues (86) studied 24 comatose patients with cEEG CSA and found that spontaneously alternating patterns were significantly associated with survival in head-injured and anoxic patients. They felt that the EEG analysis was as useful as the Glasgow Coma Scale or neurological examination for predicting outcome, and occasionally added additional prognostic information.

Other Continuous Electroencephalogram Patterns

Other phenomena detectable with cEEG monitoring also may have prognostic significance. Rae-Grant (87) has described episodic low-amplitude events—brief periods of spontaneous EEG background attenuation—which appear to be correlated with poor prognosis. Schwartz and Scott (88) have noted abnormal, stimulus-related slow-wave arousal responses in the EEG of comatose patients, but their prognostic significance remains unclear. Guerit and associates (89) found that the presence of event-related potentials in response to auditory stimuli—a cortical orienting response that can occur in the absence of consciouness—implies a good prognosis in comatose neuro-ICU patients. Similarly, Alster and colleagues (90) found that reactivity to auditory stimuli (change in EEG frequency or the appearnace of sharp waves or k-complexes) was the single best physiologic predictor of recovery. Compressed spectral array can also assess the distribution of dominant EEG frequencies better than conventional

studies, and these features may have prognostic value. For instance, Bricolo and coworkers (72) found worse outcomes among comatose patients who had significant interhemispheric amplitude asymmetries on CSA.

Alpha-Theta, and Spindle Coma

Recently, metaanalyses of "alpha-theta" and "spindle" coma have been published (91–93). These EEG patterns, which have been recognized for many years, are characterized by a monotonous and invarying patterns, often with a frontal predominance. The overall rate of poor outcome (dead or vegetative) for alpha-theta coma is 75%, and for spindle coma is 25% (91,93). In both conditions, prognosis depends primarily on the cause of coma (with hypoxic–ischemic injury carrying the worst outlook and trauma or intoxication the best) and the presence or absence of EEG reactivity to noxious stimuli.

Hypoxic–Ischemic Coma

Burst-supression, profound waveform attenuation, and loss of reactivity to external stimuli are well-established markers of poor outcome in patients with hypoxic–ischemic coma, whereas the presence of a normal posterior dominant rhythm with normal reactivity implies a good prognosis (81). In a study of 60 hypoxic–ischemic coma patients who underwent comprehensive clinical, electrophysiologic, and biochemical testing, 80% remained in a vegetative state or died after one year. When viewed individually, EEG was not particularly helpful: Clinical examination correctly predicted outcome in 58% of patients, somatosensory EPs in 59%, and EEG in 41% (94). In a multivariate analysis which analyzed EEG and EP findings, Bassetti and associates found that a GCS score less than 8 at 48 hours with abnormal or absent early cortical somatosensory EPs was the best predictor of poor outcome (positive predictive value 97%, 95% confidence interval 86% to 99%). These findings are reinforced by the results of a metaanalysis by Zandbergen and colleagues

(95), who found that the bilateral absence of cortical somatosensory EPs was the best predictor of death or a vegetative outcome (positive predictive value 100%, 95% confidence interval 98% to 100%). The only EEG finding with 100% specificity for no possiblility of recovery of consciousness is that of complete generalized suppression (less than 10 µV) beyond 24 hours after the arrest (81).

Traumatic Coma

Even after years of study, the utility of EEG for determining prognosis after severe TBI remains controversial. Most evidence suggests that EEG can supplement but not replace the clinical examination. Bricolo and associates (96) combined clinical and EEG examinations to predict outcome in 1,600 patients in coma after traumatic head injury, and found that spontaneous EEG cycling and physiologic sleep implied a good prognosis. Among 500 patients with clinical evidence of impairment of the upper midbrain, the mortality was 93% if the EEG was slow and monotonous, 46% if it showed cycling, and only 28% if it contained evidence of physiologic rhythms of sleep. Of 666 patients with only cortical signs, the respective mortality rates were 63%, 40%, and 9%. Valente and associates (97) also found that the presence of normal sleep patterns on EEG was the best predictor of recovery from coma. Hakkinen and coworkers (98) studied cEEG in 20 severe TBI patients. The CSA was graded into five levels, using criteria including the presence of isoelectric segments, variability, number of peaks in the power spectra, and reactivity. They found that the combination of CSA and Glasgow Coma Scale scores improved the ability to predict outcome over that of either variable alone. Steudel and Kruger (99) performed serial EEGs during the first week after head injury in 50 TBI patients in an attempt to predict survival. An increase or decrease in the absolute and percentage power in the alpha range correctly predicted survival or death in 80% of patients. Theilen and associates (100) derived an electroencephalogram

silence ratio (ESR) from cEEG data in 32 TBI patients. After careful exclusion of artifacts, the ESR was superior to EPs for predicting outcome at 6 months, although the authors did not indicate if the ESR added to clinical predictors.

Others have found the value of EEG in determining prognosis to be limited. Rae-Grant and coworkers (101) studied 69 comatose patients, and found that EEGs performed during the first week did not add to the predictive value of the Glasgow Coma Scale score on day 7 after the injury. Kane and colleagues (102) were unable to demonstrate any relationship between EEG interhemispheric coherence (a statistical measure of cross-correlation in the frequency domain) and outcome or the severity of diffuse axonal injury.

Future Directions

The prognostic value of cEEG in neurocritical care patients will have to be confirmed in large prospective studies of specific disease entities, including SAH, TBI, and hypoxic–ischemic encephalopathy. Serial EEGs, continuous raw and automated "trending," testing of reactivity, and the inclusion of multiple variables hold promise for an improved role in the prognostic determination in these patients.

Monitoring Sedation and Response to Interventions

Response to Therapeutic Interventions

Continuous electroencephalography provides a measure of global cerebral function, and hence may be used to monitor the effects of therapeutic interventions in the neuro-ICU. Huang and coworkers (103) evaluated the usefulness of cEEG monitoring in 38 patients with intracerebral hemorrhage given 50 g of intravenous mannitol. After mannitol infusion, visual analysis of the EEG showed improvement in 58%, no change in 34%, and worsening in 8%. Compressed spectral array showed that mannitol resulted in increased alpha and decreased delta power in the ipsilateral hemisphere, which was maximal at 30 minutes and persisted for up to 2 hours. These investigators found a similar effect after infusion of 50 mL of 20% albumin solution, but not with furosemide administration (104). The authors concluded that cEEG may be useful for monitoring the effects of antiedema treatments in stroke patients. Confirmation of these findings is needed.

Titration of Sedation

The BIS index is a processed cEEG parameter that was developed as a tool for intraoperative and ICU neurological monitoring. BIS scores, which range from range 0 (no cerebral activity) to 100 (normal cerebral function), have been reported to correlate with standard clinical sedation and coma scores in some studies (105,106) but not others (107), casting doubt on its validity as a measure of consciousness level. Bispectral index readings can be influenced by artifact such as body temperature and muscle activity (106), which may explain the weak correlation with clinical sedation scores that some have found. High intrapatient variability of BIS scores in comatose patients suggests that its use may be limited to trending cortical function in normal subjects. In a study of mechanically ventilated pediatric patients, Berkenbosch and associates (105) found that BIS scores of 50 to 70 corresponded with an optimal clinical level of sedation. A nonrandomized retrospective study found that titration of intraoperative sedation to BIS levels of 40 to 50 was associated with improved blood pressure stability, and less residual sedation and respiratory depression postoperatively (108). Another open-label pilot study found that an alfentanil bolus (15 g/kg) blunted increases in blood pressure, heart rate, and BIS activity that occurred during tracheal suctioning, suggesting a possible role in monitoring the adequacy of analgesia during procedures (109).

EVOKED POTENTIALS

Background

Evoked potentials can be used to follow the level of functioning of the central nervous system (CNS) in comatose patients (110,111). Clinical use of BAEPs and somatosensory evoked potentials (SEPs) stems from the close relationship between the EP waveforms and specific anatomic structures. This specificity allows localization of conduction defects to within a centimeter or so (BAEPs) or a few centimeters (SEPs). In addition, EPs are essentially unaffected by intravenous sedatives, or even general anesthesia or high-dose barbiturate therapy (112,113). These factors of anatomic specificity and physiologic and metabolic immutability are the basis of clinical utility of EPs. Thus, they provide a reliable look at "physiologic anatomy." However, abnormalities demonstrated by these tests are etiologically nonspecific and must be carefully integrated into the clinical situation by a physician familiar with the clinical use of the tests.

Somatosensory evoked potentials shows special promise in the neurocritical care because components generated supratentorially in the thalamus and primary sensory cortex can be identified and followed over time. Shifts in intracranial structures leading to herniation syndromes can be reflected in abnormalities in this test, whereas BAEPs are generated entirely at or below the lower midbrain and are less likely to be affected in the early stages of herniation.

Auditory and somatosensory stimuli cause small electric signals to be produced by neural structures along the corresponding sensory pathways (114). These EPs are generally much smaller than ongoing spontaneous cortical electrical activity, and are not apparent in ordinary EEG recordings; they are detected with the use of averaging techniques. Evoked potential studies involve short-, middle-, and long-latency components. The short-latency components reflect the activity of deep structures up to the cortex (i.e., brainstem and thalamocortical connections), whereas the middle- and long-latency componenets allow the exploration of cortical structures. The analysis of short-latency EPs includes their presence or absence, as well as measurement of the latency and amplitude of the characteristic waveforms. The auditory central conduction time (CCT), defined as the interpeak latency between waves I and V, allows one to get information at the pontomesencephalic level, whereas the somatosensory CCT, defined as the N13 to N20 latency (Fig. 8.7), evaluates the cervicocortical tracts.

Brainstem Auditory Evoked Potentials

Recording from earlobe and scalp vertex after a brief click stimulus, a series of five sub-μV waveforms can be recorded from a single channel in the first 7 msec after the stimulus. These are generated in brainstem auditory structures as follows: I wave, cochlear nerve; II wave, proximal cochlear nerve and vestibular nucleus; III wave, pontine auditory relays (superior olivary complex); IV through V waves, mesencephalic auditory pathways (lateral lemniscus and inferior colliculus).

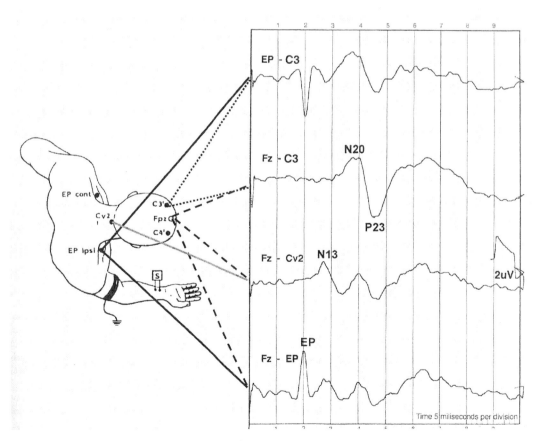

FIG. 8.7. Somatosensory evoked potential (*EP*). (From Rothstein T. The role of evoked potentials in anoxic-ischemic coma and severe brain trauma. *J Clin Neurophysiol* 2000;17:486–497, with permission.)

Absence of BAEP waves II through V despite a normal wave I indicates a significant lack of function in brainstem auditory tracts. The metabolic and physiologic immutability of BAEPs provides a safety margin for use of the test in comatose patients. For example, in a case of barbiturate overdose sufficient to produce a clinical appearance of brain death and an almost isoelectric ("flat") EEG, BAEPs were essentially unchanged, indicating preserved brainstem function (112). Similarly, high doses of anesthetic agents do not significantly alter BAEP components (113).

If wave I is absent, no inferences can be made as to the localization of the interruption of the auditory signal, because the integrity of the peripheral apparatus in any individual patient often is not known. For example, a traumatic transverse fracture of the temporal bone might have damaged the cochlea, or in a case where the clinical history is poor, the patient might have had preexisting deafness in the only ear available for BAEP testing. Wave I absence also may result from cochlear infarction, which results from occlusion of the anterior inferior cerebellar and internal auditory arteries.

Somatosensory Evoked Potentials

Electrical stimulation of large nerves (e.g., median or posterior tibial) in the upper limbs elicits a set of waveforms that are generated in the brachial plexus, upper cervical cord, dorsal column nuclei, thalamic nuclei (presumably mostly ventroposterolateral), and primary sensory cortex. Four-channel recording is required to measure SEPs, as opposed to single-channel recording for BAEPs. In the case of median nerve SEPs, electrodes are placed on the wrist, Erb's point, neck, and head (Fig. 8.7). Components of SEP testing include the Erb point potential, recorded as the afferent volley traverses the brachial plexus; the N13 wave, which reflects postsynaptic central gray activity in the cervical cord; the P14 and N18 waves, which reflect caudal brainstem function at the medial lemniscus and nucleus cuneatus; and the N20,

which corresponds to activation of the primary cortical somatyosensory receiving area (114).

Event-related potentials (ERPs), also referred to as "cognitive EPs," are a newer form of EP testing that is felt to reflect very high-level cortical functioning. It is based on the administration of occasional different stimuli within a repetitive standard stimulation (the so-called "oddball" paradigm), which allows one to record long-latency components that differ from those elicited by the standard stimulation. These ERPs are felt to reflect internal cognitive processing, rather than the activity of specific sensory structures, and therefore may be related to consciousness. The use of ERPs in the evaluation of vegetative and minimally conscious states is promising, but investigational (115).

Evoked Potential Studies in the General Evaluation of Coma

Apart from the use of SEPs to "rule in" hopelessness in patients with hypoxic–ischemic coma (95), the role of EPs in determining prognosis in the general evaluation of coma is limited. The most important reason for this is the lack of large datasets allowing for electrophysiologic-outcome correlations to be made with a high degree of precision. In addition, in general prognosis tends to depend more on the cause than the depth or anatomic basis of coma (116). In one of the larger studies relating SEP findings to prognosis, Zentner and colleagues (117) studied 213 patients between 1 and 3 days after the onset of traumatic or nontraumatic coma. Although normal SEPs generally corresponded with a favorable outcome and absent N20 responses with a poor outcome (dead or vegetative), there were frequent exceptions that prevented firm conclusions to be drawn. Smaller studies that have reported a 100% frequency of poor outcome in coma patients lacking cortical N20 or P22 responses bilaterally studied either insufficient numbers to allow firm conclusions to be drawn, or evaluated outcome at an early timepoint (less than 3 months)

(118–132). A systematic review of 324 reported patients with bilaterally absent EP cortical responses (Table 8.3) indicates an overall frequency of recovery of 5%, with most cases occurring in children or adults with traumatic coma. The prognosis is even more favorable if the N20 to P22 is unilaterally absent (113,117). Brainstem auditory evoked potentials are of considerably less utility than SEPs in determining prognosis in coma, because patients with severe hemispheric damage sparing the brainstem may have a poor outcome despite normal BAEPs (118,133).

Some investigators have reported a high degree of accuracy in coma prognostication using coma assessment profiles that combine clinical or radiographic findings with EP data; these studies require independent replication before their use can be widely adopted (134–137). The ability of normal or improving EP findings to predict a good recovery generally has been found to be unreliable, owing in large part to the fact that many other variables related to critical illness can impact on outcome besides the extent of neurological damage (118). However, there is evidence that improvement on EP studies implies a favorable outlook. In a study of 24 comatose patients from various causes, Hume and associates (138) found that central conduction times corresponding to the lower medullary level (N19) normalized during the first month in all patients who made a good recovery.

Traumatic Coma

The bilateral absence of N20 responses on SEP testing is the most consistently reported poor prognostic finding in TBI patients. However, recovery of consciousness can occur: Of 85 reported TBI patients with absent N20 responses who were followed for at least 2 months, 5 (6%) recovered consciousness (119,122,124,128,129,132). Although several investigators have reported uniformly poor outcomes in TBI patients with clinical evidence of brainstem injury and abnormal BAEPs 3 days or more after injury, sufficient experience to permit broad generalization of these findings is lacking (138–141). Claassen and coworkers (132) studied 31 severe TBI patients, and found that in many cases, elec-

TABLE 8.3. *Outcome of coma in patients with bilaterally absent N20/P22 responses on somatosensory evoked potentials (SEPs) testing*

Authors (ref)	Age	Etiology	Total studied (N)	Absent N20/P22 (N)	Outcome (N)			SEP timing
					Died	PVS	Disabled	
Anderson et al. (119)	A	T	23	8	2	4	2	<5 days
Biniek et al. (120)	A/C	G	4	4	3	1	0	Not stated
Brunko et al. (121)	A	H	50	30	30	0	0	<8 hours
Cant et al. (122)	A	T	40	7	6	0	1	<4 days
Claassen et al. (132)	A	T	31	8	8	NA	0	<7 days
De Meirleir (123)	C	G	33	13	4	0	9	1 week
de Weerd et al. (124)	A	T	18	8	6	2	0	<1 week
Facco et al. (125)	A	T	49	19	19	NA	0	<4 days
Frank et al. (126)	C	G	5	5	0	5	0	<1 day
Goldie et al. (118)	A	G	65	41	35	6	0	<3 weeks
Goodwin et al. (127)	A/C	G	41	27	23	4	0	<3 days
Judson et al. (128)	A	T	100	30	27	2	1	<5 days
Lindsay et al. (129)	A	T	101	24	22	1	1	<13 days
Taylor et al. (130)	C	G	37	19	15	3	1	Not stated
Walser et al. (131)	A	G	63	23	22	1	0	<3 weeks
Zenter et al. (117)	A/C	G	213	58	44	12	2	<3 days
TOTAL			873	324	266 (82%)	41 (13%)	17 (5%)	

A, adults; C, children; G, general causes; H, hypoxia–ischemia; NA, not applicable; PVS, persistent vegetative state; T, trauma.

trophysiologic recovery preceded clinical recovery by days to weeks. Graded SEP abnormalities also have been correlated with the extent of neurological disability at 1 year (142), but it is unlear whether such predictions are accurate enough to be clinically useful.

Hypoxic–Ischemic Coma

As mentioned, a metaanalysis comparing the value of clinical, EEG, and SEP examinations predicting death or vegetative survival found absence of the N20 response within the first week to be highly specific for poor outcome, with no reported cases of recovery given this finding. The estimated pooled positive likelihood ratio of a false-positive result in this situation (recovery despite blateral absence of the N20 response) was 0% to 2.0%; 33% of patients exhibited this abnormality (95).

Brainstem Stroke

Stern and associates (143) studied 35 patients with recent pontomesencephalic infarction and noted that abnormal BAEPs correlated with an unstable clinical course and a poor prognosis (141).

Subarachnoid Hemorrhage

Symon and associates (144) used central conduction times to follow comatose SAH patients and noted a close correlation with CBF values. The correlation with prognosis was more problematic. Of ten patients with normal SEPs and BAEPs on at least one side, five remained in a vegetative state and five experienced functional recovery. Of 11 patients with absent N20 responses, five died, five remained vegetative, and one remained conscious but disabled. BAEP findings did not appear to add further prognostic value.

Evoked Potentials in Brain Death

Evoked potential studies are not sufficiently reliable to be used as a confirmatory test for establishing the diagnosis of brain death (118,145–149). For example, Goldie and associates (118) found that only 27 of 35 brain-dead patients (77%) had no identifiable BAEP waveforms, including wave I, even though in nine, external auditory canal (EAC) needle electrodes were used. Of 29 patients who underwent SEP testing, 69% showed preservation of the P/N13 waves, though none had cortical N20 responses. These findings support the postulate that the P/N13 wave originates in structures caudal to the pons (i.e., the lower medulla), and is probably explained by the collateral blood supply to this region from extracranial sources.

Continuous Evoked Potentials Monitoring

The data cited in the preceding largely used individual studies at discrete points in the course of the patients ICU stay. More recently, advances in computer technology have made more continuous monitoring possible, although relatively few reports have documented its use, perhaps owing to the technical complexity of continuous EP monitoring. Miskiel and Ozdamar (150) described a system for rapid collection and analysis of BAEP data. Digital filtering of the signal was performed and the peaks were analyzed using the first derivative of waveform. Several criteria were applied to these data to detect and name peaks. These included slope and zero crossing. The computer was able to accurately identify peaks when compared with human visual inspection. The added advantage was the computer's ability to trend interpeak latencies, amplitude ratios, and others extracted features. Bertrand and coworkers (151) also described a system for rapid acquisition and trending of BAEP data. In TBI patients, two patterns of change in the BAEP were seen: simultaneous gradual deterioration of peaks I, III, and IV or rapid loss of peaks III and IV. Hypothermia and the combination of lidocaine and thiopental produced changes that were similar to the first pattern, which could have been confused with "preterminal" changes. Pfurtscheller and associates (152) recorded EEG and EP data simultaneously in the neuro-ICU and described examples in which ICP elevations resulted in loss of fast activity on CSA without changes in BAEPs or SEPs. Finally, Hilz and colleagues (153) described a computer-based system for monitoring EEG and EP data continuously. In addition to two channels of EEG displayed as spectra, the BAEP, SEP N14, and SEP N20 waveforms were displayed in a compressed array. Central conduction time also was calculated and displayed.

Little recent work has been conducted in this area. This may reflect the fact that given the robustness of EP subcortical signals to all but profound structural injury, continuous EP monitoring offers relatively little in the way of advance warning of impending neurological inury, with most abnormalities developing in the context of simultaneous clinical deterioration.

ACKNOWLEDGMENTS

The authors gratefully acknowledge Jan Claassen and Keith Chiappa, who contributed material to this chapter, Bryan Young, for providing figures and advice, and Lawrence Hirsch, for critical review of the manuscript.

REFERENCES

1. Vespa PM, Nenov V, Nuwer MR. Continuous EEG monitoring in the intensive care unit: early findings and clinical efficacy. *J Clin Neurophysiol* 1999;16: 1–13.
2. Langford RM. Clinical applications of cerebral monitoring. *Comp Meth Prog Biomed* 1996;51:29–33.
3. Scheuer ML. Continuous EEG monitoring in the intensive care unit. *Epilepsia* 2002;43 (suppl 3);114–127.
4. Kay J. Continuous EEG monitoring in the intensive care unit. *Can J Neurol Sci* 1998;25:S12–S15.
5. Procaccio F, Polo A, Lanteri P, et al. Electrophysiologic monitoring in neurointensive care. *Curr Op Crit Care* 2001;7:74–80.
6. Newton DEF. Electrophysiologic monitoring of general intensive care patients. *Int Care Med* 1999;25: 350–352.
7. Claassen J, Mayer SA. Continuous electroencephalographic monitoring in neurocritical care. *Curr Neurol Neurosci Rep* 2002;2:534–540.
8. Jordan KG. Continuous EEG monitoring in the neuroscience intensive care unit and emergency department. *J Clin Neurophysiol* 1999;16:14–39.
9. Legatt AD, Ebersole JS. Options for long-term monitoring. In: Engel J, Pedley TA, eds. *Epilepsy: a comprehensive textbook.* Philadelphia: Lippincott–Raven, 1997:1002–1010.
10. Scheuer ML. Portable remote wireless EEG review using a cellular CDMA network. *Epilepsia* 2001;42: 27–28 [abstract].
11. Lopes da Silva F. EEG analysis: theory and practice. In: Niedermayer E, Lopes da Silva F, eds. *Electroencephalography* Baltimore: Williams & Wilkins, 1999: 1135–1163.
12. Cascino GD, Clinical indications and diagnostic yield of video-electroencephalographic monitoring in patients with seizures and spells. *Mayo Clin Proc* 2002; 77:1111–1120.
13. Jordan KG. Nonconvulsive seizures (NCS) and nonconvulsive status epilepticus (NCSE) detected by continuous EEG monitoring in the neuro ICU. *Neurology* 1992;42:180 [abstract].
14. Towne AR, Waterhouse EJ, Boggs JG, et al. Prevalence of nonconvulsive status epilepticus in comatose patients. *Neurology* 2000;54:340–345.
15. Vespa PM, Nuwer MR, Nenov V, et al. Increased incidence and impact of nonconvulsive and convulsive seizures after traumatic brain injury as detected by continuous electroencephalographic monitoring. *J Neurosurg* 1999;91:750–760.
16. Dennis LJ, Claassen J, Hirsch LJ, et al. Nonconvulsive status epilepticus after subarachnoid hemorrhage. *Neurosurgery* 2002;51;1136–1144.
17. Privitera M, Hoffman M, Moore JL, et al. EEG detection of nontonic-clonic status epilepticus in patients with altered consciousness. *Epilepsy Res* 1994;18: 155–166.
18. DeLorenzo RJ, Waterhouse EJ, Towne AR, et al. Persistent nonconvulsive status epilepticus after the control of convulsive status epilepticus. *Epilepsia* 1998; 39:833–840.
19. Vespa PM, Nuwer MR, O'Phelan KH, et al. Nonconvulsive seizures after intracerebral hemorrhage: influence of seizures on delayed neurological deterioration. *Stroke* 2002;33:343 [abstract].
20. Choi H, Claassen J, Mayer SA, et al. Continuous EEG monitoring of patients with intracranial hemorrhage. *J Clin Neurophysiol* 2002;43:39 [abstract].
21. Krumholz A, Sung GY, Fisher RS, et al. Complex partial status epilepticus accompanied by serious morbidity and mortality. *Neurology* 1995;45:1499–1504.
22. Litt B, Wityk RJ, Hertz SH, et al. Nonconvulsive status epilepticus in the critically ill elderly. *Epilepsia* 1998;39:1194–1202.
23. Young GB, Jordan KG, Doig GS. An assessment of nonconvulsive seizures in the intensive care unit using continuous EEG monitoring: an investigation of variables associated with mortality. *Neurology* 1996;47: 83–89.
24. Waterhouse EJ, Garnett LK, Towne AR, et al. Prospective population-based study of intermittent and continuous convulsive status epilepticus in Richmond, Virginia. *Epilepsia* 1999;40:752–758.
25. Claassen J, Hirsch LJ, Mayer SA. Critical care management of refractory status epilepticus. In: Vincent JL, ed. *Yearbook of intensive care and emergency medicine.* Berlin: Springer, 2002:754–764.
26. Lowenstein DH, Alldredge BK. Status epilepticus at

an urban public hospital in the 1980s. *Neurology* 1993; 43:483–488.

27. Claassen J, Hirsch LJ, Emerson RG, et al. Continuous EEG monitoring and midazolam infusion for refractory nonconvulsive status epilepticus. *Neurology* 2001;57:1036–1042.

28. Young GB, Jordan KG. Do nonconvulsive seizures damage the brain? Yes. *Arch Neurol* 1998;55:117–119.

29. Hosford DA. Animal models of nonconvulsive status epilepticus. *J Clin Neurophysiol* 1999;16:306–313.

30. Treiman DM. Electroclinical features of status epilepticus. *J Clin Neurophysiol* 1995;12:343–362.

31. Garzon E, Fernandes RM, Sakamoto AC. Serial EEG during human status epilepticus: evidence for PLED as an ictal pattern. *Neurology* 2001;57:1175–1183.

32. Treiman DM, Walton NY, Kendrick C. A progressive sequence of electroencephalographic changes during generalized convulsive status epilepticus. *Epilepsy Res* 1990;5:49–60.

33. Assal F, Papazyan JP, Slosman DO, et al. SPECT in periodic lateralized epileptiform discharges (PLEDs): a form of partial status epilepticus? *Seizure* 2001;10: 260–265.

34. Handforth A, Cheng JT, Mandelkern MA, et al. Markedly increased mesiotemporal lobe metabolism in a case with PLEDs: further evidence that PLEDs are a manifestation of partial status epilepticus. *Epilepsia* 1994;35:876–881.

35. Talwar D, Torres F. Continuous electrophysiologic monitoring of cerebral function in the pediatric intensive care unit. *Pediatr Neurol* 1988;4:137–147.

36. Prior P. Electroencephalography in cerebral monitoring: coma, cerebral ischemia and epilepsy. In: Stalbert E, Young RR, eds. *Clinical neurophysiology.* London: Butterworths, 1981:347–383.

37. Tasker RC, Boyd SG, Harden A, et al. The cerebral function analyzing monitor in paediatric medical intensive care: applications and limitations. *Int Care Med* 1990; 16:60–68.

38. Gotman J. Automatic seizure detection: improvements and evaluation. *Electroencephalogr Clin Neurophysiol* 1990;76:317–324.

39. Suzuki A, Mori N, Hadeishi H, et al. Computerized monitoring system in neurosurgical intensive care. *J Neurosci Meth* 1988;26:133–139.

40. Bricolo A, Faccioli F, Grosslercher JC, et al. Electrophysiologic monitoring in the intensive care unit. *Electroencephalogr Clin Neurophysiol* 1987;39(suppl): 255–263.

41. Chiappa KH, Ropper AH. Long-term electrophysiologic monitoring of patients in the neurology intensive care unit. *Semin Neurol* 1984;4:469–479.

42. Agarwal A, Gotman J, Flanagan D, et al. Automated EEG analysis during long-term monitoring in the ICU. *Electroencephalogr Clin Neurophys* 1998;107:44–58.

43. Flemming RA, Smith NT. Density modulation: a technique for display of three variable data in patient monitoring. *Anesthesiology* 1979;50:543–546.

44. Maynard DE, Jenkinson JL. The cerebral function analysing monitor. *Anesthesia* 1984;39:678–690.

45. Astrup J, Siesjo BK, Symon L. Thresholds in cerebral ischemia: the ischemic penumbra. *Stroke* 1981;12: 723–725.

46. Cohn HR, Raines RG, Mulder DW, et al. Cerebral vascular lesions: electroencephalographic and neuropathologic correlations. *Arch Neurol* 1948;60: 163–181.

47. Nagata K, Tagawa K, Hiroi S, et al. Electroencephalographic correlates of blood flow and oxygen metabolism provided by positron emission tomography in patients with cerebral infarction. *Electroencephalogr Clin Neurophysiol* 1989;72:16–30.

48. Tolonen U, Sulg IA. Comparison of quantitative EEG parameters from four different analysis techniques in evaluation of relationships between EEG and CBF in brain infarction. *Electroencephalogr Clin Neurophysiol* 1981;51:177–185.

49. Munari C, Calbucci F. Correlations between intracranial pressure and EEG during coma and sleep. *Electroencephalogr Clin Neurophysiol* 1981;51:170–176.

50. Chiappa KH, Ropper AIL. Long-term electrophysiologic monitoring of patients in the neurology intensive care unit. *Semin Neurol* 1984;4:469–479.

51. Langfitt TW, Tannanbaum HM, Kassell NF, et al. Acute intracranial hypertension, cerebral blood flow, and the EEG. *Electroencephalogr Clin Neurophysiol* 1966;20:139–148.

52. Sundt TM Jr, Sharbrough FW, Anderson RE, et al. Cerebral blood flow measurements and electroencephalograms during carotid endarterectomy. *J Neurosurg* 1974;41:310–320.

53. Sharbrough FW, Messick JM Jr, Sundt TM Jr. Correlation of continuous electroencephalograms with cerebral blood flow measurements during carotid endarterectomy. *Stroke* 1973;4:674–683.

54. Ahn SS, Jordan SE, Nuwer MR, et al. Computed electroencephalographic topographic brain mapping. A new and accurate monitor of cerebral circulation and function for patients having carotid endarterectomy. *J Vasc Surg* 1988;8:247–254.

55. Nuwer MR, Jordan SE, Alm SS. Evaluation of stroke using EEG frequency analysis and topographic mapping. *Neurology* 1987;37:1153–1159.

56. Nahm W, Stockmanns G, Petersen J, et al. Concept for an intelligent anesthesia EEG monitor. *Med Inform Internet Med* 1999;24:1–9.

57. Hacke W, Zeumer H, Ringelstein EB. EEG controlled occlusion of the internal carotid artery during angiography. *Neuroradiology* 1981;22:19–22.

58. Morioka T, Matsushima T, Fujii K, et al. Balloon test occlusion of the internal carotid artery with monitoring of compressed spectral arrays (CSAs) of electroencephalogram. *Acta Neurochir* 1989;101:29–34.

59. Herkes GK, Morgan M, Grinnell V, et al. EEG monitoring during angiographic balloon test carotid occlusion: experience in sixteen cases. *Clin Exp Neurol* 1993;30:98–103.

60. Paiva T, Campos J, Baeta E, et al. EEG monitoring during endovascular embolization of cerebral arteriovenous malformations. *Electroencephalogr Clin Neurophysiol* 1995;95:3–13.

61. Nakase H, Ohnishi H, Touho H, et al. An intra-arterial electrode for intracranial electro-encephalogram recoedings. *Acta Neurochir* 1995;136:103–105.

62. Stoeter P, Dieterle L, Meyer A, et al. Intracranial electroencephalographic and evoked-potential recording from intravascular guide wires. *AJNR* 1995;16: 214–217.

63. Vespa PM, Nuwer MR, Juhasz C, et al. Early detection of vasospasm after acute subarachnoid hemorrhage us-

ing continuous EEG ICU monitoring. *Electroencephalogr Clin Neurophysiol* 1997;103:607–615.

64. Labar DR, Fisch BJ, Pedley TA, et al. Quantitative EEG monitoring for patients with subarachnoid hemorrhage. *Electroencephalogr Clin Neurophysiol* 1991; 78:325–332.

65. Claassen J, Hirsch LJ, Kreiter KT, et al. Quantitative continuous EEG analysis for detection of delayed cerebral ischemia in poor grade subarachnoid hemorrhage patients. *J Clin Neurophys* 2002;43:45(abstract).

66. Rivierez M, Landau-Ferey J, Grob R, et al. Value of electroencephalogram in prediction and diagnosis of vasospasm after intracranial aneurysm rupture. *Acta Neurochir* 1991;110:17–23.

67. Adams DC, Heyer EJ, Emerson RG, et al. The reliability of quantitative electroencephalography as an indicator of cerebral ischemia. *Anesthesiol Analg* 1995;81:80–83.

68. Suzuki A, Yoshioka K, Yasui N. Clinical application of EEG topography in cerebral ischemia: detection of functional reversibility and hemodynamics. *Brain Topogr* 1990;3:167–174.

69. Jordan K. Correlative xenon-enhanced CT cerebral blood flow (XeCTCBF) and EEG to functionally stratify acute cerebral infarction. *Neurology* 1991;41(suppl 1):336.

70. Matousek M, Takeuchi E, Starmark JE, et al. Quantitative EEG analysis as a supplement to the clinical coma scale RLS-85. *Acta Anesthesiol Scand* 1996;40: 824–831.

71. Gilbert TT, Wagner MR, Halukurike V, et al. Use of bispectral electroencephalogram monitoring to assess neurological status in unsedated, critically ill patients. *Crit Care Med* 2001;29:1996–2000.

72. Bricolo A, Turazzi S, Faccioli F, et al. Clinical application of compressed spectral array in long-term EEG monitoring of comatose patients. *Electroencephalogr Clin Neurophysiol* 1978;45:211–225.

73. Synek VM. EEG abnormality grades and subdivisions of prognostic importance in traumatic and anoxic coma in adults. *Clin Electroencephalogr* 1988;19:160–166.

74. Young GB, McLachlan RS, Kreeft JH, et al. An electroencephalographic classification for coma. *Can J Neurol Sci* 1997;24:320–325.

75. Celesia GG. EEG and coma: is there a prognostic role for EEG? *Clin Neurophysiol* 1999;110:203–204.

76. Young GB, Kreeft JH, McLachan RS, et al. EEG and clinical association with mortality in comatose patients in a general intensive care unit. *J Clin Neurophysiol* 1999;16:354–360.

77. Hirsch LJ, Claassen J, Emerson RG. Beware the SR-PIDS: stimulus-responsive pseudo-ictal discharges, a common and important EEG pattern in critically ill patients. *Epilepsia* 2002;43(suppl 7):283–284[abstract].

78. Jaitly R, Sgro JA, Towne AR, et al. Prognostic value of EEG monitoring after status epilepticus: a prospective adult study. *J Clin Neurophysiol* 1997;14:326–334.

79. Hirsch LJ, Claassen J, Mayer SA, et al. Systematic design of a prognostic scale for ICU patients with highly epileptiform EEGs. *Epilepsia* 2001;42:256[abstract].

80. Alexandre A, Rubini L, Nertempi P, et al. Sleep alterations during post-traumatic coma as a possible predicator of cognitive defects. *Acta Neurochir* 1979;28 (suppl):188–192.

81. Young GB. The EEG in coma. *J Clin Neurophysiol* 2000;17:473–485.

82. Bergamasco B, Bergamini L, Doriguzzi T. Clinical value of the sleep electroencephalographic patterns in post-traumatic coma. *Acta Neurol Scand* 1968;44: 495–511.

83. Bricolo A, Gentilomo A, Rosadini G, et al. Long-lasting post-traumatic unconsciousness. *Acta Neurol Scand* 1968;44:512–532.

84. Bricolo A, Turella G, Ore GD, et al. A proposal for the EEG evaluation of acute traumatic coma in neurosurgical practice. *Electroencephalogr Clin Neurophysiol* 1973;34:789.

85. Passouant P, Cadilhac J, Delange M, et al. Differential electrical stages and cyclic organisation of posttraumatic comas; polygraphic recording of long duration. *Electroencephalogr Clin Neurophysiol* 1965;18:720.

86. Karnaze DS, Marshall LF, Bickford RG. EEG monitoring of clinical coma: spectral array. *Neurology* 1982;32:289–292.

87. Rae-Grant AD, Strapple C, Barbour PJ. Episodic low-amplitude events: an under-recognized phenomenon in clinical electroencephalography. *J Clin Neurophysiol* 1991;8:203–211.

88. Schwartz MS, Scott DF. Pathologic stimulus-related slow wave arousal responses in the EEG. *Acta Neurol Scand* 1978;57:300–304.

89. Guerit JM, Verougstraete D, de Tourtchaninoff M, et al. ERPs obtained with the auditory oddball paradigm in coma and altered states of consciousness: clinical relationships, prognostic value, and origin of components. *Clin Neurophysiol* 1999;110:1260–1269.

90. Alster J, Pratt H, Feinsod M. Density spectral array, evoked potentials, and temperature rhythms in the evaluation and prognosis of the comatose patient. *Brain Injury* 1993;7:191–208

91. Kaplan PW, Genoud D, Ho TW, et al. Etiology, neurological correlations, and prognosis in alpha coma. *Clin Neurophysiol* 1999;110:205–213.

92. Berkhoff M, Donati F, Bassetti C. Postanoxic alpha (theta) coma: a reappraisal of its prognostic significance. *Clin Neurophysiol* 2000;111:297–304.

93. Kaplan PW, Genoud D, Ho TW, et al. Clinical correlates and prognosis in early spindle coma. *Clin Neurophysiol* 2000;111:584–590.

94. Bassetti C, Bomio F, Mathis J, et al. Early prognosis in coma after cardiac arrest: a prospective clinical, electrophysiologic, and biochemical study of 60 patients. *J Neurol Neurosurg Psychiatry* 1996;61:610–615.

95. Zandbergen EG, de Haan RJ, Stoutenbeek CP, et al. Systematic review of early prediction of poor outcome in anoxic-ischaemic coma. *Lancet* 1998;352: 1808–1812.

96. Bricolo A, Turazzi S, Faccioli F. Combined clinical and EEG examinations for assessment of severity of acute head injuries. Electrophysiologic methods. *Acta Neurochir* 1979;28(suppl):35–39.

97. Valente M, Placidi F, Oliveira AJ, et al. Sleep organization pattern as a prognostic marker at the subacute stage of post-traumatic coma. *Clin Neurophysiol* 2002;113:1798–1805.

98. Hakkinen VK, Kaukinen S, Heikkila H. The correlation of EEG compressed spectral array to Glasgow Coma Scale in traumatic coma patients. *Int J Clin Monit Comput* 1988;5:97–101.

99. Steudel WI, Kruger J. Using the spectral analysis of the EEG for prognosis of severe brain injuries in the

first post-traumatic week. *Acta Neurochir* 1979;28 (suppl):40–42.

100. Theilen HJ, Ragaller M, Tscho U, et al. Electroencephalogram silence ratio for early outcome prognosis in severe head trauma. *Crit Care Med* 2000;28: 3522–3529.

101. Rae-Grant AD. Eckert N, Barbour PJ, et al. Outcome of severe brain injury: a multimodality neurophysiologic study. *J Trauma Inj Infect Crit Care* 1996;40: 40l–407.

102. Kane NM, Moss TH. Curry SH. Butler SR. Quantitative electroencephalographic evaluation of non-fatal and fatal traumatic coma. *Electroenceph Clin Neurophysiol* 1998;106:244–250.

103. Huang Z, Dong W, Yan Y, et al. Effects of intravenous mannitol on EEG recordings in *Stroke* patients. *Clin Neurophysiol* 2002;113:446–453.

104. Huang Z, Dong W, Yan Y, et al. Effects of intravenous human albumin and furosemide on EEG recordings in patients wth intracerebral hemorrhage. *Clin Neurophysiol* 2002;113:454–458.

105. Berkenbosch JW, Fichter CR, Tobias JD. The correlation of the bispectral index monitor with clinical sedation scores during mechanical ventilation in the pediatric intensive care unit. *Anesthesiol Analg* 2002;94:506–511.

106. Riess ML, Graefe C, Van Aken H, et al. Sedation assessment in critically ill patients with bispectral index. *Eur J Anesthesiol* 2002;19:18–22.

107. Frenzel D, Greim CA, Sommer C, et al. Is the bispectrral index appropriate for for monitoring the sedation level of mechanically-ventilated surgical patients? *Int Care Med* 2002;28:178–183.

108. Burrow B, McKenzie B, Case C. Do anesthetized patients recover better after Bispectral Index Monitoring? *Anesthesiol Analg* 2001;29:239–245.

109. Brocas E, Dupont H, Paugam-Burtz C, et al. Bispectral index variations during tracheal suction in mechanically-ventilated critically ill patients: effect of an alfentanil bolus. *Int Care Med* 2002;28:211–213.

110. Facco E, Munari M. The role of evoked potentials in severe head injury. *Int Care Med* 2000;26:998–1005.

111. Nuwer MR. Electroencephalograms and evoked potentials. Monitoring cerebral function in the neurosurgical intensive care unit. *Neurosurg Clin N Am* 1994;5: 647–659.

112. Chiappa KH, Ropper AIL. Long-term electrophysiologic monitoring of patients in the neurology intensive care unit. *Semin Neurol* 1984;4:469–479.

113. Guerit JM. The usefulness of EEG, exogenous evoked potentials, and cognitive evoked potentials in the acute stage of post-anoxic and post-traumatic coma. *Acta Neurol Belg* 2000;100:229–236.

114. Chiappa KH. *Evoked potentials in clinical medicine,* 3rd ed. Philadelphia: Lippincott-Raven, 1997.

115. Procaccio F, Polo A, Lanteri P, et al. Electrophysiologic monitoring in neurointensive care. *Curr Opin Crit Care* 2001;7:74–80.

116. Sacco RL, VanGool R, Mohr JP, et al. Non-traumatic coma: Glasgow coma score and coma etiology as predictors of two week outcome. *Arch Neurol* 1990;47: 1181–1184.

117. Zentner J, Rohde V. The prognostic value of somatosensory and motor evoked potentials in comatose patients. *Neurosurgery* 1992;31:429–434.

118. Goldie WD, Chiappa KH, Young RR, et al. Brainstem

auditory and short-latency somatosensory evoked responses in brain death. *Neurology* 1981;31:248–256.

119. Anderson DC, Bundlie S, Rockswold GL. Multimodality evoked potentials in closed head trauma. *Arch Neurol* 1984;41:369–374.

120. Biniek R, Ferbert A, Rimpel J, et al. The complete apallic syndrome—a case report. *Int Care Med* 1989; 15:212–215.

121. Brunko E, Zegers de Beyl D. Prognostic value of early cortical somatosensory evoked potentials after resuscitation from cardiac arrest. *Electroencephalogr Clin Neurophysiol* 1987;66:15–24.

122. Cant BR, Hume AL, Judson JA, et al. The assessment of severe head injury by short-latency somatosensory and brain-stem auditory evoked potentials. *Electroencephalogr Clin Neurophysiol* 1986;65:188–195.

123. De Meirleir LJ, Taylor MI. Prognostic utility of SEPs in comatose children. *Pediatr Neurol* 1987;3:78–82.

124. de Weerd AW, Groeneveld C. The use of evoked potentials in the management of patients with severe cerebral trauma. *Acta Neurol Scand* 1985;72:489–494.

125. Facco E, Munari M, Baratto F, et al. Somatosensory evoked potentials in severe head trauma. In: Rossini PM, Mauguiere F, eds. *New trends and advanced techniques in clinical neurophysiology.* Amsterdam: Elsevier, 1990:330–341.

126. Frank LM, Furgiuele TL, Etheridge JE Jr. Prediction of chronic vegetative state in children using evoked potentials. *Neurology* 1985;35:931–934.

127. Goodwin SR, Friedman WA, Bellefleur M. Is it time to use evoked potentials to predict outcome in comatose children and adults? *Crit Care Med* 1991;19:518–524.

128. Judson J, Cant BR, Shaw NA. Early prediction of outcome from cerebral trauma by somatosensory evoked potentials. *Crit Care Med* 1990;18:363–368.

129. Lindsay K, Pasaoglu A, Hirst D, et al. Somatosensory and auditory brainstem conduction after head in jury: a comparison with clinical features in prediction of outcome. *Neurosurgery* 1990;26:278–285.

130. Taylor MJ, Farrell EJ. Comparison of the prognostic utility of VEPs and SEPs in comatose children. *Pediatr Neurol* 1989;5:145–150.

131. Walser H, Emre M, Janzer R. Somatosensory evoked potentials in comatose patients: correlation with outcome and neuropathologic findings. *J Neurol* 1986; 233:34–40.

132. Claassen J, Hansen H-C. Early recovery after closed traumatic head injury: somatosensory evoked potentials and clinical findings. *Crit Care Med* 2001;29:494–502.

133. Facco E, Munari M, Baratto F, et al. Multimodality evoked potentials (auditory, somatosensory and motor) in coma. *Neurophysiol Clin* 1993;23:237–258.

134. Soustiel JF, Hafner H, Guilburd JN, et al. A physiologic coma scale: grading of coma by combined use of brain-stem trigeminal and auditory evoked potentials and the Glasgow Coma Scale. *Electroenceph Clin Neurophysiol* 1993;91:77–78.

135. Guerit JM, de Tourtchaninoff M, Soveges L, et al. The prognostic value of three-modality evoked potentials (TMEPs) in anoxic and traumatic comas. *Neurophysiol Clin* 1993;23:209–226.

136. Rosenberg C, Wogensen K, Starr A. Auditory brainstem and middle- and long-latency EPs in coma. *Arch Neurol* 1984;41:835–838.

137. Narayan RK, Greenberg RP, Miller JD, et al. Improved

confidence of outcome prediction in severe head injury. A comparative analysis of the clinical examination, multimodality evoked potentials, CT scanning, and intracranial pressure. *J Neurosurg* 1981;54:751–762.

138. Hume AL, Cant BR, Shaw NA. Central somatosensory conduction time in comatose patients. *Ann Neurol* 1979;5:379–384.

139. Tsubokawa T, Nishimoto H, Yamamoto T, et al. Assessment of brainstem damage by the auditory brainstem responses in acute severe head injury. *J Neurol Neurosurg Psychiatry* 1980;43:1005–1011.

140. Seales DM, Rossiter VS, Weinstein ME. Brainstem auditory evoked responses in patients comatose as a result of blunt head trauma. *J Trauma* 1979;19:347–353.

141. Ropper AH, Miller DC. Acute traumatic midbrain hemorrhage. *Ann Neurol* 1985;18:80–86.

142. Rappaport M, et al. Evoked potentials and head injury. 2. Clinical applications. *Clin Electroencephalogr* 1981;12:167–176.

143. Stern BJ, Krumholz A, Weiss H, et al. Evaluation of brainstem stroke using brainstem auditory evoked responses. *Stroke* 1982;13:705–711.

144. Symon L, Hargadine J, Zawirski M, et al. Central conduction time as an index of ischemia in subarachnoid hemorrhage. *J Neurol Sci* 1979;44:95–103.

145. Klug N. Brainstem auditory evoked potentials in syndromes of decerebration, the bulbar syndrome and in central death. *J Neurol* 1982;227:219–228.

146. Starr A. Auditory brainstem responses in brain death. *Brain* 1976;99:543-554.

147. Trojaborg W, Jorgensen EO. Evoked cortical potentials in patients with isoelectric EEGs. *Electroencephalogr Clin Neurophysiol* 1973;35:301–309.

148. Anziska B, Cracco RQ. Short latency somasensory evoked potentials in brain dead patients. *Arch Neurol* 1980;37:222–225.

149. Belsh JM, Chokroverty S. Short-latency somatosensory evoked potentials in brain-dead patients. *Electroencephalogr Clin Neurophysiol* 1987;68:75–79.

150. Miskiel E, Ozdamar O. Computer monitoring of auditory brainstem responses. *Comput Biol Med* 1987;17: 185–192.

151. Bertrand O, Garcia-Larrea L, Artru F, et al. Brain-stem monitoring. I. A system for high-rate sequential BAEP recording and feature extraction. *Electroencephalogr Clin Neurophysiol* 1987;68:433.

152. Pfurtscheller G, Schwarz G, Schroettner O, et al. Continuous and simultaneous monitoring of EEG spectra and brainstem auditory and somatosensory evoked potentials in the intensive care unit and the operating room. *J Clin Neurophysiol* 1987;4: 389–396.

153. Hilz MJ, Litscher G, Weis M, et al. Continuous multivariable monitoring in neurological intensive care patients: preliminary reports on four cases. *Int Care Med* 1991;17:87–93.

9

Persistent Vegetative State and Brain Death

The neurointensivist is called on to deal with patients in coma and varying degrees of unresponsiveness perhaps more than any other specialist. These issues arise not only in the neurological intensive care unit (neuro-ICU) but also throughout any acute care hospital and even outside the hospital in legal and societal situations where a measured and experienced opinion is requested. Although most of the information that follows in this chapter has now been well established after several decades of data collection, discussion, and colloquia, it is advisable to collect the material in one place and review current thinking as an aid to prognosis and clinical practice. Further discussion can be found in several books and monographs such as the one by Young and colleagues (1).

DEFINITIONS

Consciousness has been defined in its most simple terms as awareness of the self and the environment. Putting aside the numerous philosophical views of consciousness, for the neurologist, normal consciousness requires both *arousal* via the ascending reticular activating system of the pons, posterior hypothalamus, and thalamus, and *awareness* via the neurons of the cerebral cortex and their projections to and from the subcortical nuclei. Wakefulness is, of course, required for awareness, but wakefulness may occur without the presence of awareness. *Coma* is a condition of deep pathologic unconsciousness in which

there is no arousal and the eyes remain closed despite stimulation. (Coma is discussed throughout several chapters of this book in relation to specific disease processes.) As compared to the unconsciousness of the comatose patient who is not awake, the patient in a *vegetative state* is wakeful but lacks awareness. Of course, there is some "biologic limitation to the certainty of this definition, since we can only infer the presence or absence of conscious experience in another person" (2). A *minimally conscious state* also has been described wherein some evidence of awareness is found that precludes a diagnosis of vegetative state (3). The minimally conscious state may be considered to be part of a continuum following coma and vegetative state with perhaps a slightly higher likelihood of improvement to a fully conscious state. *Brain death* is irreversible coma and apnea with the permanent absence of all brain function, including the brainstem.

PERSISTENT VEGETATIVE STATE: DIAGNOSIS

Although well known to neurologists and neurosurgeons, several definitions bear clarification. The vegetative state is defined as a complete unawareness of self (presumed) and the environment (as observed by reactions to various stimuli) (2,4–6). Sleep–wake cycles usually are preserved, even if in rudimentary form, and there is at least partial preservation of the autonomic functions of the hypothalamus and brainstem. There should be no evidence of reproducible voluntary responses to any sensory stimuli. There is no language expression or comprehension. Sustained visual pursuit is usually absent and there is no fixation or tracking of an object, although there may be some inconsistent reflexive turning of the head or eyes toward a visual or auditory stimulus. The vegetative state almost always follows an initial period of coma lasting for days to weeks. For the vegetative state to be described as persistent, it has been suggested by several authors that it should be present for at least 1 month. If there is any evidence of voluntary responses to sensory stimuli, the diagnosis of vegetative state should not be used, and perhaps "minimally conscious state" would be a better term (3). Patients with ambiguous or inconsistent responses to sensory stimuli are not uncommon in our experience if sought by careful examination and some of them progress from an apparent vegetative state to the severe dementia of the newly defined minimally conscious state. If consciousness is fully preserved but the patient is immobile, the patient may be in a locked-in state. The locked-in syndrome generally occurs in the setting of a pontine stroke with sparing of vertical eye movements and lid elevation that are used to indicate responsiveness, but may also occur in other conditions such as severe Guillain–Barré syndrome. The clinical setting and communication through eye movement or other limited signals readily distinguishes the locked-in syndrome from the vegetative state.

Electroencephalography (EEG) of a persistently vegetative patient usually shows diffuse polymorphic delta or theta activity not affected by sensory stimulation (7). Positron emission tomography (PET) shows reduced cerebral glucose metabolism by more than 50% compared with normal and locked-in patients but comparable to normal patients dur-

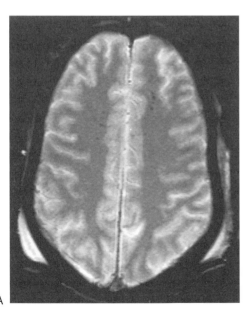
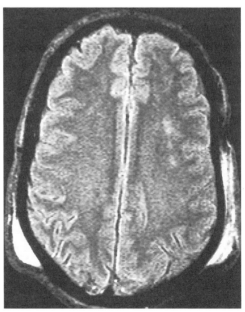

A   B

FIG. 9.1. A: A magnetic resonance imaging (MRI) gradient echo (GRE) study of the brain demonstrating bifrontal punctate hypointensities. **B:** An MRI fluid attenuation inversion recovery (FLAIR) sequence showing bifrontal hyperintensities in a 30-year-old comatose patient 1 week after an assault and prolonged hypoxic episode. The rest of the MRI showed diffuse punctate lesions throughout the white matter but predominantly in the frontal lobes. These findings are consistent with hemorrhagic diffuse axonal injury. The patient remained in persistent vegetative state 2 months after the initial injury.

ing deep general anesthesia (2,8). Whether this pattern of cerebral blood flow and metabolism can be used as a defining or diagnostic feature of the vegetative state, as indicated by several authoritative authors in the field, is not clear to us. Pathologic findings may include diffuse cortical laminar necrosis, infarcts in the hypothalamus or brainstem and, in the case of trauma, diffuse subcortical and brainstem axonal injury (2). Perhaps the most surprising aspect, concordant with our own examinations, is the high frequency of bilateral thalamic damage rather than diffuse cortical damage as the main pathologic change after both traumatic injury and ischemic–anoxic injury, as in the much-discussed case of Karen Quinlan (9). Premortem magnetic resonance imaging may or may not demonstrate some of these pathologic findings (Fig. 9.1A,B).

PERSISTENT VEGETATIVE STATE: PROGNOSIS

A number of factors in a comatose patient have been predictive of a vegetative outcome. After a traumatic brain injury, older age, ventilatory failure, and decorticate posturing have been associated with a poor outcome (10). Coma from a nontraumatic cause generally has a worse prognosis than coma from a traumatic cause. Impairment of eye opening, oculocephalic responses, and motor responses at 2 weeks after a nontraumatic brain injury is associated with a poor outcome (11). Bilateral absence of somatosensory evoked potentials 1 week after the injury is highly predictive of death or vegetative state. On the other hand, some patients with normal evoked potentials may remain in a vegetative state and some posttraumatic patients may recover slight cognitive activity despite absence of somatosensory evoked potentials (12). Prolongation of central conduction time of the somatosensory evoked response and brainstem auditory evoked potentials are not as useful predictors of poor prognosis (13). In one study of postanoxic coma, PET scanning demonstrated a 50% reduction in cerebral glucose metabolism in PVS patients compared with a

25% reduction in those who regained consciousness (14). An abnormal CT or MRI scan is more likely in PVS than in those who recover (15). There is currently not enough evidence, however, to use PET, CT, or MRI scanning for prognostication.

The prognosis for persistent vegetative state (PVS) depends in part on the etiology. The most common causes in both adults and children are head trauma and hypoxic ischemic encephalopathy (Table 9.1) (2,7). Recovery of consciousness from posttraumatic PVS is highly unlikely in an adult after 1 year. Recovery from nontraumatic PVS is unlikely after 3 months. There are, of course, exceptions but they are quite rare and the high degree of certainty of a poor prognosis should be conveyed to families of affected individuals. Young children, however, may do far better than predicted after many months of unresponsiveness. It can be said with confidence that patients that are vegetative secondary to a degenerative disease have a uniformly dismal prognosis (2). Most patients in PVS do not survive longer than 2 to 5 years. Death occurs from infection, generalized systemic failure, respiratory failure, and in some cases, sudden death of unknown etiology. It is also worth-

TABLE 9.1. *Some of the major etiologies for persistent vegetative state*

Traumatic brain injury
Nontraumatic
Hypoxic–ischemic encephalopathy
Cardiopulmonary arrest
Asphyxia
Near-drowning
Prolonged hypotension
Stroke
Meningitis
Brain abscess or tumor
Degenerative
Alzheimer disease
Parkinson disease
Creutzfeldt–Jakob disease
Developmental
Anencephaly
Hydranencephaly

From The Multi-Society Task Force on PVS. Medical aspects of the persistent vegetative state. *N Engl J Med* 1994;330:1499–1508, 1572–1579, with permission.

while noting, particularly in discussions with the family, that the Multi-Society Task Force on PVS reviewed the unusual cases of late recovery of consciousness from the literature and popular media reports and found that the total number of these patients was quite small considering the prevalence of PVS, and, perhaps more important, all were left with severe disability (2).

Management of the patient depends on accurate determination of diagnosis and prognosis. Decision-making issues regarding level of care for these patients are discussed in Chapter 23. The estimated prevalence of PVS in the United States is 10,000 to 25,000 adults and 4,000 to 10,000 children and total annual costs for the care of these patients are estimated to be between 1 and 7 billion dollars (2).

BRAIN DEATH: DIAGNOSIS

The Uniform Determination of Death Act allows that death can be diagnosed on a neurological basis, that is, brain death, in the United States (similar views are held elsewhere with minor modifications) but the United States Act does not delineate the specific criteria for the diagnosis (16). The main causes for brain death in adults are traumatic brain injury and subarachnoid hemorrhage, and in children are abuse, motor vehicle accidents, and asphyxia (17,18). Brain death generally occurs as the result of cerebral herniation with intracranial pressure simultaneously rising above mean arterial pressure and cerebral blood flow stopping.

Before performing an examination for brain death, certain confounding factors should be determined to be absent. Most important, the patient's core temperature should be at least 33°C. In actuality, the likelihood of hypothermia simulating brain death at even slightly lower levels is unlikely but some limits should be set in order to avoid a false-positive diagnosis and the difficulty that such an error produces. The patient's systolic blood pressure generally should be greater than 100 mm Hg, again, a somewhat arbitrary level but one on which there is general agreement. Certainly, entertaining the diagnosis of brain death when the blood pressure is substantially lower is tenuous. The cause and irreversibility of the coma should be known. Drug intoxication, especially with barbiturates, tricyclic antidepressants, or neuromuscular blocking agents should be ruled out by appropriate blood and urine testing, even if the source of brain injury is obvious, as in head trauma. The issue of admissible levels of therapeutic agents that may confound the neurological examination and EEG has not been satisfactorily resolved. We have taken the position that levels below those known to be soporific are acceptable but these have not been established for all barbiturate and sedative-like drugs and others have expressed the view that these drugs should be absent from the blood. There should be no significant electrolyte, acid-base, or endocrine abnormalities, but again, mild degrees of hypernatremia or hyponatremia and similar disturbances do not preclude the diagnosis. Severe metabolic abnormalities, such as hyponatremia or hypernatremia or hypophosphatemia should be corrected prior to determining brain death.

The clinical examination for brain death traditionally includes ascertainment of deep unresponsive coma, absence of brainstem reflexes, and apnea. The patient should be comatose with no responsiveness even to deep pain. Deep pain may be applied by sternal rub, supraorbital nerve compression, or nail bed pressure. There should be no eye opening or motor response present, including extensor or flexor posturing. This last item has also been a point of contention but well-formed posturing is not consistent with brain death because it most likely requires suprasegmental input from brainstem centers. Occasionally, a triple flexion response in the lower extremities or a brief flexion of the fingers may be elicited. Perhaps surprisingly, Babinski signs are uncommon in brain dead patients; instead a slow flexion and fanning of the toes is more frequent; however, there is no proscription of the diagnosis if a classic extensor toe sign is found (17,19–23).

As brain death occurs, brainstem reflexes are generally lost in a rostral to caudal direction (21). The brain death examination has been formalized to a certain degree and includes testing the reflex pathways of the midbrain, pons, and medulla. Table 9.2 outlines the examination of these brainstem reflexes.

The pupils are entirely nonreactive to a bright light. Unless there is some preexisting abnormality, they are midposition (4 to 6 mm) in size. Larger or somewhat smaller pupils (2.5 mm) may be consistent with brain death, but should prompt consideration of drug intoxication or poisoning. It is advisable to inspect the pupils with a magnifying glass, and house officers need to have emphasized that an ophthalmoscope is not an adequate light stimulus to determine loss of light reactivity. Moving the head rapidly to both sides and up and down tests oculocephalic reflexes. This test should not be performed if there is suspicion of a concomitant spinal cord injury, and oculovestibular ("caloric") reflex testing may be performed instead. Before testing the oculovestibular reflex, it has been suggested that the external auditory canal should be visualized to be certain there is no obstruction by blood or cerumen. In fact, aside from profound impaction, a cold-water stimulus still produces reflex eye movements in our experience. The head is elevated to 30 degrees to make the horizontal semicircular canal vertical. A maximal stimulus is attained with approximately 30 to 60 cc of ice water injected by syringe into each auditory canal, one at a time with an interval of a minute or more between sides. There should be no movement of the eyes with either the oculocephalic or oculovestibular maneuver. Touching a cotton swab to each cornea tests the corneal reflex and there should be no blink to the stimulus. Most neurologists include this corneal testing in the brain death examination; however, it does not appear to be necessary in that patients are not found who lose pupillary and eye movement function while preserving the corneal reflex. There should be no grimace to pain and no cough or gag both to stimulation of the back of the throat and to deep endotracheal suctioning. Other tests may be included, for example, the absence of a ciliospinal reflex, but they add little.

Apnea Testing

If these brainstem reflexes are *all* absent, then an apnea test is performed. We feel it is advisable to leave this test for last because it has little value if the other brainstem tests show preservation of function. There are several published criteria for establishing apnea. The most liberal are those of the Collabora-

TABLE 9.2. *Examination of brainstem reflexes: criteria for brain death*

Reflex	Procedure	Afferent cranial nerve	Efferent cranial nerve	Result for brain death
Pupillary	Shine bright light into each eye	Optic (I)	Oculomotor (III)	No pupillary reaction
Corneal	Touch both corneas with cotton swab	Trigeminal (V)	Facial (VII)	No eye blink
Oculocephalic	Turn head side-to-side and up and down	Vestibular (VIII)	Oculomotor (III), trochlear (IV), abducens (VI)	No eye movements
Oculovestibular	Irrigate each ear with 60 cc ice water	Vestibular (VIII)	Oculomotor (III), trochlear (IV), abducens (VI)	No eye movements
Oropharyngeal	Touch pharynx or move endotracheal tube, and deep tracheal suction	Glossopharyngeal (IX), vagus (X)	Glossopharyngeal (IX), vagus (X)	No gag or cough
Respiratory	Apneic oxygenation (see text)	Respiratory centers (medulla)	Respiratory centers (medulla)	No ventilatory effort

tive Study on brain death, which required only that the patient not show respiratory effort while being ventilated for 15 minutes (22). The guidelines of the Harvard Ad Hoc Committee require that the ventilator be disconnected for 3 minutes after the patient has been breathing room air for 10 minutes with a normal carbon dioxide tension (23). Apneic oxygenation is a more recent and reliable technique for assessing respiratory drive and is the one adopted in most neuro-ICUs with some variations. In this procedure: (a) the ventilator is first used to deliver 90% to 100% inspired oxygen for several minutes in order to replace nitrogen and provide a reservoir of oxygen and a gradient to keep the PaO_2 adequate; and (b) an endotracheal cannula is inserted to a length that ends proximal to the carina and high-flow oxygen is used to maintain the partial pressure of oxygen (apneic oxygenation). The ventilator is stopped and the $PaCO_2$ is allowed to rise to a level sufficient for inducing respiratory effort (60 mm Hg in most patients, perhaps 50 mm Hg if there is no prior lung disease). Although no large study has compared apneic oxygenation with simple disconnection, it is likely that apneic oxygenation is the safer and more reliable technique for demonstrating apnea. A "T-piece" is not appropriate as a substitute for the cannula because it does not provide oxygen replacement unless the patient is breathing and may indeed desaturate the alveoli by a Venturi effect.

Preoxygenation averts complications such as arrhythmias and hypotension during the apnea test (24). The patient is observed carefully, ideally with a hand also on the chest or abdomen, for any respiratory movements. An arterial blood gas is obtained by 8 minutes (generally no more than 6 to 8 minutes is needed) if no breathing is evident. The apnea test supports the diagnosis of brain death if there are no respirations and the arterial $PaCO_2$ has reached 60 mm Hg (or has increased by 20 mm Hg over baseline in cases of underlying pulmonary disease). The patient is placed back on the ventilator after the test is completed. Blood pressure and oxygen saturation should be monitored continuously or every minute or so during apneic oxygenation. If during testing the patient's oxygen saturation drops to less than approximately 90%, or the blood pressure drops to levels that are judged to risk cerebral ischemia, the consensus has been that the test should be aborted. The rationale for this perhaps paradoxical approach is that brain death is not documented until it has been shown that the arterial $PaCO_2$ has reached a level adequate to stimulate breathing. We find end-tidal CO_2 measurements frequently do not correlate with the arterial $PaCO_2$ and therefore do not feel they are reliable enough for use in the diagnosis of brain death.

It is advisable not to have family members present during apnea testing because occasional respiratory-like and other frightening movements occur (25). Shoulder elevation and adduction with back arching, not associated with tidal volume production, have been described and, although disconcerting to some, are spinal cord phenomena and do not preclude the diagnosis of brain death (1).

Certain conditions may cause a reversible loss of brainstem reflexes and must be excluded when declaring brain death. The pupillary reflex can be abolished with local trauma to the eye, previous eye surgery, or a prosthetic eye. Atropine, neuromuscular blocking agents, and pentobarbital can produce nonreactive pupils. Disease of the ear canals, including cerumen accumulation, can eliminate the oculovestibular reflex. Posthyperventilation apnea may abolish respiratory drive (26). Neuromuscular blockers cause paralysis and eliminate respiratory effort but a motor response elicited by the use of a train-of-four stimulator at a peripheral nerve can rule out the possibility of residual paralytic medication effect. Confirmatory tests for brain death are discussed below.

Table 9.3 summarizes the clinical criteria for brain death declaration in adults and children over the age of 5 by the President's Commission (27). In normothermic normotensive adults with a known cause of coma and no drug intoxication, an observation period of either 6 hours with or 12 hours without confir-

TABLE 9.3. *Guidelines for determining brain death: President's Commission*

An individual with irreversible cessation of all functions of the entire brain, including the brainstem, is dead.
1. *Cessation* is recognized when evaluation discloses findings of both of the following:
    a. Cerebral functions are absent.
       There must be "cortical unresponsivity and unreceptivity...."
    b. Brainstem functions are absent.
       This includes "pupillary light, corneal, oculocephalic, oculovestibular, oropharyngeal, and respiratory reflexes."
       Apnea is tested with a nasal cannula delivering oxygen and demonstrating failure of respiratory effort with $Paco_2 > 60$ mmHg
       "Spinal cord reflexes may persist after death. True decerebrate or decorticate posturing or seizures are inconsistent with the diagnosis of death."
2. *Irreversibility* is recognized when evaluation discloses all of the following:
    a. The cause of coma is established and is sufficient to account for the loss of brain functions.
    b. "The possibility of recovery of any brain function is excluded...."
    c. The cessation of all brain functions persists for an appropriate period of observation
       "confirmation of clinical findings by EEG is desirable when objective documentation is needed to substantiate the clinical findings ... complete cessation of circulation to the normothermic adult brain for more than 10 minutes is incompatible with survival of brain tissue ... absent cerebral blood flow, in conjunction with the clinical determination of cessation of all brain functions for at least 6 hours, is diagnostic of death...."
3. *Complicating conditions*
    a. Drug and metabolic intoxication
       "Drug intoxication is the most serious problem in the determination of death.... In cases where there is any likelihood of sedative presence, toxicology screening for all likely drugs is required. If exogenous intoxication is found, death may not be declared until the intoxicant is metabolized or intracranial circulation is tested and found to have ceased ... before irreversible cessation of brain functions can be determined, metabolic abnormalities should be considered and, if possible, corrected."
    b. Hypothermia
       Criteria for reliable recognition of death are not available in the presence of hypothermia (below 32.2°C core temperature).
    c. Children
       "The brains of infants and young children have increased resistance to damage and may recover substantial functions even after exhibiting unresponsiveness on neurologic examination for longer periods than do adults. Physicians should be particularly cautious in applying neurologic criteria to determine death in children younger than five years...."
    d. Shock
       "Physicians should also be particularly cautious in applying neurologic criteria to determine death in patients in shock because the reduction in cerebral circulation renders clinical examination and laboratory tests unreliable...."

From President's Commission for the Study of Ethical Problems in Medicine and Biomedical and Behavioral Research. *Defining death: medical, legal, and ethical issues in the determination of death.* Washington, DC: U.S. Government Printing Office, 1981.

matory testing is suggested (27). Some states require two physicians to declare brain death, but most states require only one. Individual hospital policies may differ from state laws, requiring more than one physician, and sometimes requiring that at least one physician is a neurologist or neurosurgeon. We recommend that, if possible, two physicians agree that brain death has been validated in a given patient, at least one of which is a neurologist or neurosurgeon. The former practice of requiring some interval between the two examinations (24 hours was used) is no longer necessary unless a question remains regarding the underlying cause of brain injury or sedative medications may play a role. Unless a patient will be an organ donor, a decision to withdraw life support without a definitive diagnosis of brain death obviates the need to fulfill all of these strict criteria.

BRAIN DEATH: CHILDREN

The history and physical examination criteria for brain death in children under the age of 5 are essentially the same as in older patients, but may include absent sucking and rooting reflexes that are not typically commented on in adults. Although, as noted, an interval between two examinations is optional in adults, there are specific recommendations regarding this in children, and they are based on age. Current recommendations are that neonates should be observed for the first 7 days of life before diagnosing brain death. Two examinations at a 48-hour interval is recommended in neonates 7 days to 2 months of age, 24 hours in those older than 2 months and younger than 1 year old, and 12 hours in children older than 1 year of age (21,28). Two sequential confirmatory tests (see the following) are recommended in neonates, one confirmatory test in those 2 months to 1 year of age, and are optional in those older than 1 year of age (28).

BRAIN DEATH: CONFIRMATORY TESTING

Supplementary tests may be helpful to confirm the diagnosis of brain death and in certain instances they are highly advisable. In cases of drug intoxication or inability to complete the apnea test owing to the occurrence of complications, a confirmatory test needs to be done. Another common scenario where a confirmatory test, such as an angiogram, may be needed is the patient who was treated with pentobarbital for raised intracranial pressure and may still have residual barbiturate effect on brainstem reflexes several days later. An EEG may need to be performed in some patients with a vertebrobasilar occlusion or massive cerebellar swelling because there may be an absence of brainstem reflexes with preserved EEG activity. Patients with severe facial trauma may be difficult to examine for absence of cranial nerve reflexes and therefore also should have a confirmatory test performed.

In the United States, the choice of confirmatory test is at the discretion of the physician but often is an EEG. Table 9.4 lists the technical recommendations for EEG diagnosis of brain death (29). Electroencephalographic monitoring for at least 30 minutes should show no electrical activity with the sensitivity set at 2 μV/mL (21). In cases of

TABLE 9.4. *Electroencephalographic diagnosis of brain death: technical recommendations*

A minimum of eight scalp electrodes with interelectrode distances at least 10 cm (may need to be proportionally smaller in small children) and ear reference electrodes.
Interelectrode resistance of 100 to 10,000 ohms.
Tested integrity of the recording system by deliberate creation of electrode artifact by manipulation.
Gains increased during most of recording to 2 μV/min.
Recording with an electrocardiogram and other monitoring devices such as a pair of electrodes on the dorsum of the hand to exclude extracerebral potentials.
Test for reactivity to pain, loud noises, or light.
Recording by a qualified technician for 30 min.

From American Electroencephalographic Society. *Guidelines in EEG.* Willoughby, OH: American Electroencephalographic Society, 1980.

suspected drug intoxication and in children, however, the EEG and clinical findings may be misleading.

Because absent blood flow to an area of the brain leads to destruction of brain tissue, an important confirmatory test in establishing brain death reliably demonstrates absent flow to the entire brain. Cerebral angiography in brain death shows a lack of filling of the intracranial arteries after injection of contrast under high pressure into each of the four neck vessels. The systolic blood pressure is not high enough to overcome the intracranial pressure, so flow stops at the foramen magnum in the posterior circulation and at the petrosal portion of the carotid artery in the anterior circulation (30). To rule out common carotid artery occlusion, the external carotid vessels should be patent (19). It should be noted that a small amount of dye often enters the very proximal vertebral arteries in the foramen magnum. Nuclear scanning with technetium should show no intracerebral uptake of the tracer on serial scanning immediately and up to 2 hours after injection (Fig. 9.2) (31). Transcranial Doppler ultrasound of the middle cerebral and vertebral arteries, another popular technique among neurointensivists, shows an absence of the diastolic or reverberating flow with only tiny systolic

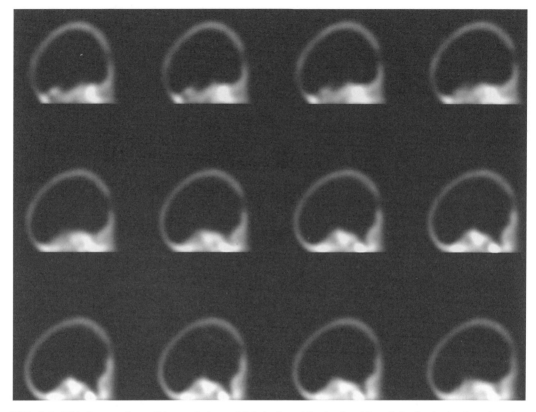

FIG. 9.2. This is a radionuclide study in a child declared brain dead by clinical criteria that demonstrates no intracerebral uptake of the tracer, confirming the diagnosis of brain death.

peaks (32). The Doppler study, however, is technologist-dependent and absence of signal owing to poor insonation must be ruled out.

Numerous other tests are of interest but infrequently used. Among these is one we have incorporated on occasion for instructive purposes; the demonstration that the pulse will not rise in response to atropine injection. This is the result of the death of vagal neurons in the medulla and the absence of vagal tone on the sinoatrial node. In essence, there is no longer acetylcholine to be blocked by atropine. It is also noteworthy that only a proportion of patients have diabetes insipidus when the criteria for brain death are demonstrated; this attests to the close approximation but not complete identity between clinical and EEG criteria and the neuropathologic state of complete brain destruction they are meant to detect.

PHYSICIAN ACTION FOLLOWING DETERMINATION OF BRAIN DEATH

Once the clinical examination and, if needed, confirmatory testing have been completed, the family is informed that diagnosis of brain death has been made. Indeed, extensive discussions should be undertaken before the testing begins so that the family is aware of the implications of the findings and the action to be taken if the criteria are met. We have found it helpful to avoid discussion of the specifics of testing but to simply indicate that a special series of highly standardized examinations will be carried out; some explanation of the apnea test may be necessary if there is likely to be a delay in obtaining the results of the final blood gas. If organ procurement is not planned, the family may want some time to see the patient prior to extubation. The issue of agonal movements and the distress they may cause the family has been mentioned and, if possible, family members should not be present when the ventilator is withdrawn.

In the troubling and not infrequent circumstance that the family refuses to allow disconnection of the ventilator, further explanation of brain death should be made. The best way to avoid this painful scene is by patient explanation beforehand as mentioned as well as by avoiding any suggestion to the family that a decision not to extubate is an option. The physician should express that medically and legally the patient is dead and that to continue would be to ventilate a dead body. Consultation by the hospital ethics committee and legal counseling may need to be obtained. In New York and New Jersey there is a religious exemption whereby physicians are required to follow the family's religious requests to continue medical care despite pronouncement of brain death. When mechanical ventilation is continued, hypotension, diffuse intravascular coagulation, pulmonary edema, and cardiac arrest usually occur within 1 to 2 weeks (33). There are, however, some notable exceptions, especially in younger patients if diabetes insipidus, hypotension, and other medical complications are aggressively treated and in cases of maternal brain death where the patient was aggressively supported for weeks to months until the fetus became viable (34,35).

BRAIN DEATH: ORGAN DONATION

With brain death, many conditions may occur that potentially might affect the viability of organs for transplantation. Hypotension, hypothermia, hypothyroidism, diabetes insipidus, and electrolyte derangements may occur. Initially there may be a brief catecholamine storm with marked hypertension followed by failure of the sympathetic nervous system with a rapid fall in blood pressure. Vasopressors and intravenous (i.v.) fluids are used to correct hypotension and hypovolemia. A systolic blood pressure of greater than 100 mm Hg and a central venous pressure (CVP) of 8 to 10 mm Hg are the goals in order to maintain organ viability. Phenylephrine (Neo-Synephrine) (starting at 50 µg/min) is preferred if there is tachycardia present and dopamine (starting at 2 to 5 µg/kg per minute) is used if there is bradycardia. Vasopressors should be titrated down as tolerated to minimize end-organ ischemia. Levophed (norepinephrine) should be avoided if possible as it can lead to vasoconstriction, thereby decreasing organ perfusion and affecting the viability of organs. Maintenance i.v. fluid of NS, D_5 NS or D_5 1/2 NS with 20 mEq/L KCl is given at rates of approximately 150 cc/h.

The hemodynamic instability may be the result of low serum levels of thyroid hormone (thyroxine). Following brain death, the hypothalamic and pituitary structures that regulate thyroid hormone production no longer function. This may manifest as metabolic acidosis and hemodynamic instability, which affect organ viability. If vasopressors and i.v. fluids have not been effective, levothyroxine sodium may be administered as a bolus of 20 µg followed by infusion at 10 µg/h (36). One ampule of 50% dextrose is given intravenously to facilitate the conversion of thyroxine (T-4) to triiodothyronine (T-3). Hormonal resuscitation also should include replacement of depleted serum levels of cortisol and insulin. Methylprednisolone (Solu-Medrol) 1g bolus and regular insulin 20 U are both given intravenously.

Diabetes insipidus begins with a marked diuresis that may result in severe hypernatremia. When urine output exceeds 300 cc/h for two consecutive hours and the urine specific gravity is less than 1.005, DDAVP should be administered as an i.v. bolus of 0.1 µg/kg. In most adults, we start with a 4 µg i.v. bolus and then repeat as needed every 6 to 8 hours to keep the urine output less than 300 cc/h. Fluids should be replaced as needed to keep the CVP 8 to 10 mm Hg.

Hypothermia may develop and should be treated with heating blankets as needed to normalize the core temperature. Arterial oxygen saturation should be maintained higher than 95% with the minimum positive end expiratory pressure (PEEP) to avoid hypotension. Common electrolyte derangements such as hypernatremia, hypokalemia, and hypophosphatemia, should be corrected.

It is federally mandated in the United States that all deaths or imminent deaths be reported to the local organ procurement organization (OPO). Their early involvement helps determine if the patient is a candidate for organ donation and therefore needs the aforementioned medical management. The OPO coordinators generally have a better rate of consent for organ donation than physicians. Therefore, it is our practice not to bring up the issue of organ donation with the family, but rather to have the OPO coordinator meet with the family separately after the physician has informed the family that the patient is brain dead. However, in the current sophisticated social environment, many families already raise the issue and it may be comforting for them to know that some great benefit may come of their tragic situation. Once the patient is pronounced brain dead and the family has consented to organ procurement, all costs are covered by the OPO.

Guidelines have been established for the diagnosis of both persistent vegetative state and brain death. Clinicians should be aware of these guidelines as well as those established at their particular institutions. Neither diagnosis should be reached quickly, but should occur after an appropriate period of observation and thorough examinations of the patient.

REFERENCES

1. Young GB, Ropper AH, Bolton CF. *Coma and impaired consciousness: a clinical perspective.* New York: McGraw-Hill, 1998.
2. The Multi-Society Task Force on PVS. Medical aspects of the persistent vegetative state. *N Engl J Med* 1994;330:1499–1508, 1572–1579.
3. American Congress of Rehabilitation Medicine. Recommendations for use of uniform nomenclature pertinent to patients with severe alterations in consciousness. *Arch Phys Med Rehab* 1995;76:205–209.
4. Jennett B, Plum F. Persistent vegetative state after brain damage: a syndrome in search of a name. *Lancet* 1972; 1:734–737.
5. President's Commission for the Study of Ethical Problems in Medicine and Biomedical and Behavioral Research. *Deciding to forego life-sustaining treatment: a report on the ethical, medical, and legal issues in treat-*
ment decisions. Washington, DC: Government Printing Office, 1983:171–192.
6. Position of the American Academy of Neurology on certain aspects of the care and management of the persistent vegetative state patient. *Neurology* 1989;39:125–126.
7. Hansotia PL. Persistent vegetative state: review and report of electrodiagnostic studies in eight cases. *Arch Neurol* 1985;42:1048–1052.
8. Levy DE, Sidtis JJ, Rottenberg DA, et al. Differences in cerebral blood flow and glucose utilization in vegetative versus locked-in patients. *Ann Neurol* 1987;22:673–682.
9. Kinney HC, Korein J, Panigrahy A, et al. Neuropathological findings in the brain of Karen Ann Quinlan. The role of the thalamus in the persistent vegetative state. *N Engl J Med* 1994;330:1469–1475.
10. Sazbon L, Fuchs C, Costeff H. Prognosis for recovery from prolonged posttraumatic unawareness: logistic analysis. *JNNP* 1991;54:149–152.
11. Levy DE, Caronna JJ, Singer BH, et al. Predicting outcome from hypoxic-ischemic coma. *JAMA* 1985;253: 1420–1426.
12. Zegers de Beyl D, Brunko E. Prediction of chronic vegetative state with somatosensory evoked potentials. *Neurology* 1986;36:134.
13. Hansotia PL. Persistent vegetative state: review and report of electrodiagnostic studies in eight cases. *Arch Neurol* 1985;42:1048–1052.
14. Devolder AG, Goffinet AM, Bol A, et al. Brain glucose metabolism in postanoxic syndrome: positron emission tomographic study. *Arch Neurol* 1990;47:197–204.
15. Levin HS, Saydjari C, Eisenberg HM, et al. Vegetative state after closed head injury: a Traumatic Coma Data Bank Report. *Arch Neurol* 1991;48:580.
16. Uniform Determination of Death Act, 12 Uniform Laws Annotated (U.L.A.) 589 (West 1993 and West Supp. 1997).
17. Wijdicks EF. Determining brain death in adults. *Neurology* 1995;45:1003–1011.
18. Ashwal S, Schneider S. Brain death in children. *Ped Neurol* 1987;3A:5–11,69–77.
19. Report of the Quality Standards Subcommittee of the American Academy of Neurology. Practice parameters for determining brain death in adults (Summary statement). *Neurology* 1995;45:1012–1014.
20. McNair NL, Meador K. The undulating toe flexion sign in brain death. *Mov Disord* 1992;7:345–347.
21. Wijdicks EFM. The diagnosis of brain death. *N Engl J Med* 2001;344:1215–1221.
22. Collaborative Study. An appraisal of the criteria of cerebral death: a summary statement. *JAMA* 1977;237: 982–986.
23. Beecher HK. A definition of irreversible coma. Report of the Ad Hoc Committee of the Harvard Medical School to Examine the Definition of Brain Death. *JAMA* 1968;205:337–340.
24. Goudreau JL, Wijdicks EF, Emery SF. Complications during apnea testing in the determination of brain death: predisposing factors. *Neurology* 2000;55:1045–1048.
25. Ropper AH. Unusual spontaneous movements in brain-dead patients. *Neurology* 1984;34:1089–1092.
26. Plum F, Posner JB. *The diagnosis of stupor and coma,* 3rd ed. Philadelphia: FA Davis, 1982.
27. President's Commission for the Study of Ethical Problems in Medicine and Biomedical and Behavioral Research. *Defining death: medical, legal, and ethical is-*

sues in the determination of death. Washington, DC: US Government Printing Office, 1981.

28. American Academy of Pediatrics Task Force on Brain Death in Children. Report of a special task force: guidelines for the determination of brain death in children. *Pediatrics* 1987;80:298–300.

29. American Electroencephalographic Society. *Guidelines in EEG.* Willoughby, OH: American Electroencephalographic Society, 1980.

30. Bradac GB, Simon RS. Angiography in brain death. *Neuroradiology* 1974;7:25–28.

31. Bonetti MG, Ciritella P, Valle G, et al. 99mTc HM-PAO brain perfusion SPECT in brain death. *Neuroradiology* 1995;37:365–369.

32. Ropper AH, Kehne SM, Wechsler L. Transcranial Doppler in brain death. *Neurology* 1987;37:1733–1735.

33. Hung TP, Chen ST. Prognosis of deeply comatose patients on ventilators. *J Neurol Neurosurg Psychol* 1995; 58:75–80.

34. Parisi JE, Kim RC, Collins GH, et al. Brain death with prolonged somatic survival. *N Engl J Med* 1982;306: 14–16.

35. Bernstein IM, Watson M, Simmons GM, et al. Maternal brain death and prolonged fetal survival. *Obstet Gynecol* 1989;74:434–437.

36. Salim A, Vassiliu P, Velmahos GC, et al. The role of thyroid hormone administration in potential organ donors. *Arch Surg* 2001;136:1377–1380.

PART II

Specific Problems in Neurological Intensive Care

=====10=====
Postoperative Neurosurgical Care

Postoperative cases account for a large number of neurological intensive care unit (neuro-ICU) admissions and in many centers there is a flexible relationship between neurosurgery recovery or postoperative wards and neuro-ICUs. Once the effects of anesthesia have receded, a neuro-ICU offers more intense surveillance for anticipated problems than is possible on the usual ward. Because few of the anticipated postoperative complications actually occur, a large number of patients produce only a few patient days. Knaus and colleagues (1) found that of all postoperative patients admitted to a neuro-ICU solely for "concentrated nursing care and intensive monitoring," only 15% actually required and received active treatment. For example, of 82 of their electively admitted neurosurgical patients, only one received specific therapy for a complication and none had abnormalities detected by physiologic monitoring. This can be only roughly translated to experience in other centers, depending on how many patients are admitted for trauma and how many early aneurysmectomies are performed. They suggested that additional staffing on general wards is a more efficient way of caring for postoperative neurosurgical patients than routinely admitting patients to a neuro-ICU. Because there will undoubtedly be increasing scrutiny of the use of neuro-ICU beds for these "anticipatory" admissions and because the disparate problems associated with each type of operation must be clearly delineated to be able to detect them, it is useful to list the main postoperative complications (Table 10.1). Knowledge of many of these is embedded in

neurosurgical operative practice because they derive from the details of the procedure; they are reviewed in neurosurgical and other textbooks (2,3), as well as in other sections of this book, particularly Chapter 16 on the neuro-ICU management of brain tumors. Some complications are generic, having to do with raised intracranial pressure (ICP), respiratory deterioration, and the general medical problems that arise during the postoperative period. Among the latter, the ones of most concern are the unpredictable difficulties that may occur after any operation, namely myocardial infarction (MI), pulmonary embolus (PE), and pneumonia. This chapter reviews the more specific postoperative neuro-ICU problems that are common to several neurosurgical operations. Less frequent ones, such as malignant hyperthermia, respiratory complications, or wound problems, are either too rare to include here, or are primarily surgical problems that are beyond the scope of the chapter but are covered well elsewhere (4).

ANESTHETIC EFFECTS IN NEUROSURGICAL PATIENTS

The main problem here is in distinguishing the residual effects of general anesthesia from the drowsiness and confusional state that are indicative of a postoperative intracranial hematoma or brain swelling. This distinction is particularly vexing because there has been a general impression in neurology that patients with cerebral diseases are excessively prone to the effects of anesthetics. However, our observation has been that there is little or

TABLE 10.1. *Neurosurgical procedures and their main postoperative complications*

	Complication		
Operation	**Immediate**	**24–48 h**	**Management**
Craniotomy/tumor (Chapter 16)	Cerebral edema Cerebral hemorrhage Subdural hemorrhage	Subgaleal cerebrospinal fluid leak Vasospasm	Avoid hypertension Slow steroid taper Fluid restriction Computed tomography and clinical follow-up Intracranial pressure monitoring when indicated
Aneurysmectomy (Chapter 15)	Stroke from vascular manipulation or clip	Vasospasm Cerebral edema	Blood pressure and aggressive fluid management (Chapter 3) Clinical monitoring
Arteriovenous malformation resection	Hemorrhage	Cerebral edema	Avoid excessive hypertension Fluid restriction if no vasospasm
Transsphenoidal hypophysectomy	Diabetes insipidus	Diabetes insipidus Nasal cerebrospinal fluid leak Visual loss	Monitoring visual acuity Preoperative endocrine evaluation and postoperative replacement (see text)
Carotid endarterectomy	Hypotension	Hypotension, myocardial infarction, neck hematoma	
Tracheotomy Gastrostomy	Hypocarbia Bleeding Airway occlusion Cuff leak	Wound drainage	Adjust ventilator Wound care
C-P angle tumor	Epidural hematoma	Hydrocephalus Apnea Aspiration	Follow-up CT Clinical monitoring

C-P, cerebellopontine; CSF, cerebrospinal fluid; CT, computed tomography.

no enhancement or prolongation of the effect of anesthesia in patients who were fully awake preoperatively. Focal neurological deficits may worsen in the first hours after anesthesia as a result of the pharmacologic agents, but it is perhaps more surprising how little anesthesia affects focal syndromes. For example, patients who have had a stroke in the past generally show little deterioration after undergoing general anesthesia. The same cannot be said for demented patients who regularly have an increase in confusion in relation to general anesthesia (5). Nonetheless, the effects of anesthesia on the nervous system are complex, often involving a combination of depressant and excitatory influences, depending on the agent used.

One of the most instructive studies on the effects of anesthesia was conducted by Rosenberg and colleagues (6). They recorded the neurological signs in patients without underlying neurological deficits who were awakening from halothane, enflurane, and nitrous oxide-narcotic ("balanced") anesthesia. Not surprisingly, the pupillary response to light and the lash reflex were eliminated under general anesthesia. Four of 27 patients had depressed pupillary responses and three had a depressed lash reflex 40 minutes after the anesthetic. Both reflexes had returned to normal by the time the patients were fully awake (able to follow verbal commands) regardless of the anesthetic. Other reflexes responded differently to various anesthetics. Unsustained clonus was seen in virtually all patients after volatile inhalation anesthesia and in about half after nitrous oxide-narcotic anesthesia, most prominently during the period of unresponsiveness immediately after anesthesia. Sustained ankle clonus was not seen after nitrous oxide-narcotic anesthesia, but occurred in half of patients after enflurane. Hyperactive quadriceps tendon reflexes occurred in 58% of patients after enflurane and in 37% after halothane but not after nitrous oxide-narcotic. Babinski signs occurred in half the patients anesthetized with Ethrane and in one fourth after halothane but not after nitrous oxide-narcotic anesthesia. The plantar response became flexor as patients awakened. Shivering, most common after enflurane anesthesia, was more frequent during periods of unresponsiveness but was not related to body temperature. A prospective study by McCulloch and Milne (7) found that transient neurological signs were more common in general surgical patients who had received enflurane–nitrous than after isoflurane–nitrous anesthesia. In their experience, quadriceps hyperreflexia and Babinski signs were most the most prevalent signs 5 to 20 minutes after anesthesia and always resolved within 1 hour in neurologically normal patients.

We have seen the following transient neurological signs in neurosurgical patients during the hours after anesthesia, all apparently related to the anesthetic rather than the procedure: Babinski signs (not previously present) up to 2 hours postoperatively; unilateral pupillary dilation in awake patients (possibly an Adie pupil phenomenon); eccentric pupil; mild worsening of previous hemiparesis for 1 to 2 hours postoperatively; worsened dysarthria; and, of course, asterixis. In contrast, rapidly increasing headache (although transient headache may occur after general anesthesia), especially with vomiting, progressive drowsiness, or evolving hemiparesis, new or worsening paresthesias, vertigo, facial paresis, or pupillary changes in a fully awake patient have almost invariably reflected neurological complications such as subdural or epidural hematoma or brain edema. It can be said in general that any progressive or fluctuating deterioration can be assumed to be from an operative complication rather than from anesthesia. Bradycardia likewise suggests a cerebral hemorrhage or brain swelling. Anticonvulsant toxicity often clouds the issue of postoperative deterioration. In our experience, the perioperative intravenous (i.v.) administration of phenytoin has caused postoperative hiccoughing and vomiting, sometimes with drowsiness or with slight agitation and mild confusion. Serum drug concentrations measured several hours later generally have been normal, but we have thought that transiently toxic levels caused the symptoms. There may be an additive effect of anticonvulsants with residual anesthetic, particularly in causing hiccoughs. Asterixis is also to be expected if anticonvulsant levels reach toxic levels and it should be kept in mind that an initial loading dose of phenytoin, even 1 g in a previously unexposed patient, may give rise to slight drowsiness and asterixis. Unilateral asterixis is indicative of a hemiparesis on the silent side or an anterior thalamic lesion on the affected side.

Another special problem arises in patients who have persistent weakness or ophthalmoplegia for hours after the administration of nondepolarizing neuromuscular blockers. Usually the remainder of the clinical state (alert, reactive pupils, flexor plantar response) make the benign nature of the weakness evident. However, ophthalmoplegia should under no circumstances be attributed to neuromuscular blocking agents or emergence from anesthesia without further consideration. We have seen four cases of basilar artery thrombosis that arose during the postoperative period, signs of which were attributed to anesthesia initially. In addition, rare cases of previously unrecognized myasthenia gravis may be uncovered by the appearance of prolonged postoperative ophthalmoplegia, weakness, or respiratory failure after the use of muscle relaxants. Problems with pseudocholinesterase deficiency are well known to practitioners and may cause similar problems after the use of succinylcholine.

In cases of prolonged unresponsiveness after anesthesia there may be concerns regarding an intraoperative ischemic or anoxic accident, or in the case of cardiac surgery, multiple cerebral emboli. Somatosensory evoked potentials can distinguish an anatomic lesion in the hemispheres or global ischemia from an anesthetic effect because these responses are relatively unaltered by anesthesia (Chapter 8). The electroencephalogram (EEG) or its several computer processed derivatives generally do not distinguish among global cerebral ischemia, anesthesia, and a metabolic encephalopathy, although subtle differences in the processed signal may be helpful. The patient who is paralyzed and has ophthalmoplegia from neuromuscular blockers will have a normal EEG, of course.

The broad issue of postoperative confusion, applicable to all surgical cases, is addressed by one of the authors in another text (5).

POSTOPERATIVE FEVER AND INFECTION

Concern regarding postoperative infection and meningitis make fever a troublesome sign during the first few postoperative days (Chapters 7 and 11). So-called central fever is extraordinarily rare in our experience and should be considered only when extremes of hyperthermia (greater than 40°C) occur in patients with lesions near the base of the brain and hypothalamus or in those with massive cerebral hemorrhage. Unsustained fever below 38.5°C is usually attributable to atelectasis, but persistence of fever beyond the first 8 hours or higher temperatures require physical examination for meningismus, chest radiograph, and sputum and urine cultures, and in appropriate circumstances (e.g., when central venous lines are present), blood cultures. Occasionally, sinusitis occurs after several days of nasal–endotracheal intubation; these sinus infections, most often ethmoidal but sometimes sphenoidal, can be appreciated on the computed tomography (CT) scan that may have been obtained for other reasons in the postoperative period.

When fever persists for 24 hours and is unexplained by overt pulmonary or urinary infection, spinal fluid examination may be advisable in cases at risk for meningitis. Several reviews have pointed out that meningismus,

headache, or drowsiness are frequently absent with infection after a neurosurgical procedure and that cerebrospinal fluid (CSF) pleocytosis is insensitive in distinguishing aseptic from bacterial meningitis (8). High fever, CSF leak, and peripheral leukocytosis generally are predictive of postoperative meningitis, in contrast to CSF glucose and the differential cell count in the spinal fluid, which have been less helpful, according to Ross and colleagues.

Drug-induced fever, most often a reaction to a newly administered antibiotic or anticonvulsant (9), or rarely, to malignant hyperthermia may also appear in the postoperative period. The diagnosis of postoperative fever in brain tumor patients is discussed in greater detail in Chapter 16. A frequent problem is the interpretation of a postoperative peripheral blood leukocytosis in the absence of a fever. Many cases can be traced to the recent institution of corticosteroids, but most remain unexplained otherwise or are found to be the harbinger of an emerging fever and pneumonia. Fever caused by multiple asymptomatic pulmonary emboli is often cited but rarely seen in neurosurgical patients.

POSTOPERATIVE BLOOD PRESSURE

Acute hypertension has been associated with increased mortality in neuro-ICU patients. Based on the same potential for damage that guides blood pressure treatment in raised ICP (Chapter 2), hypertension is usually avoided after a craniotomy. The precise levels that represent a risk for cerebral edema postoperatively are not known and depend on the size and nature of the lesion, the amount of traumatic disruption of vessels during operation, and premorbid blood pressure.

Hypertension after resection of arteriovenous malformation (AVM) or following carotid endarterectomy may pose special problems. Spetzler and colleagues (10) coined the term *normal perfusion pressure breakthrough* to describe malignant edema and hemorrhage after resection of an AVM. They postulated that the AVM created a steal phenomenon, thereby decreasing blood flow in the normal brain, and leading to reflex vasodilatation and loss of autoregulation. With the AVM resected and the steal eliminated, blood flow in surrounding brain increased far above normal. Bernstein and associates (11) and others have pointed out that the mechanism of hyperperfusion and deficient autoregulation after carotid endarterectomy is probably similar to that seen with AVM. At autopsy, changes in the hemisphere ipsilateral to an endarterectomy have resembled those seen in malignant hypertension, whereas the opposite hemisphere has been normal. This theory of dysautoregulation is supported by the observation of Sundt and coworkers (12) that hemispheric blood flow distal to the endarterectomy increases two to three times over the preoperative level after carotid artery surgery. The treatment of blood pressure problems is discussed further in Special Considerations After Carotid Endarterectomy.

Severe hypertension after tumor resection or other nonvascular lesion requires the careful administration of potent i.v. antihypertensive agents in order to prevent the exaggeration of brain edema. If abrupt in onset, the possibility of a hemorrhage at the operative site or subdural or epidural bleeding is raised. Otherwise, nitroprusside, a cerebral vasodilator (but a far better antihypertensive agent than nitroglycerin), may be a safer alternative for the treatment of severe hypertension, when mean pressure is above 110 to 120 mm Hg. The drug has the advantage of rapid titration and dependability and, in our experience, has caused minimal elevation in measured ICP. Esmolol, a rapidly acting β-blocker, can be used in a similar fashion, without the risk of raising ICP. Labetalol, a combined α- and β-antagonist, also is becoming increasingly popular when acute lowering of blood pressure is necessary in patients, particularly after craniotomy. Most calcium channel blockers cannot be currently recommended based on anecdotal reports of elevations in ICP (13), but nicardipine appears to be safe and can be used by continuous i.v. infusion (14). Angiotensin converting enzyme inhibitors are being studied for this use but most are not rapidly acting enough

to be suitable (Chapters 3 and 10 and page 96). Nitroglycerin has not been popular for this purpose because of its potential to increase ICP. Prolonged use of nitroprusside may be complicated by thiocyanate and, less commonly, by cyanide toxicity.

In patients with chronic hypertension, it seems appropriate to institute the patient's previous oral antihypertensive medications in approximately one half to two thirds of the previous dose as soon as feasible. Bedrest and sedation often reduce the antihypertensive requirements of postoperative patients but pain may increase them.

SPECIAL CONSIDERATIONS FOLLOWING CAROTID ENDARTERECTOMY

The causes of stroke that follow in the immediate postoperative period after carotid endarterectomy were well defined in the 1970s and 1980s when the procedure became routine (15–19). Most cases have been related to local thromboembolism, sometimes the result of technical inadequacy such as a residual flap of intima or a local small dissection. Some probably occur intraoperatively from the release of plaque material and only a few result from a low-flow state that occurs during clamping of the vessel. A discussion of the utility of intraoperative monitoring to prevent these complications is beyond the scope of this chapter; suffice it to say that the evidence favoring its use is scant.

More salient in the critical care unit is the problem of an abrupt change in blood pressure after endarterectomy. Postoperative hypotension, occurring in up to 40% of cases can be minimized by maintaining adequate central venous pressure preoperatively and intraoperatively, but postoperative bradycardia and hypotension requiring vasopressors still occur. Phenylephrine (Neo-Synephrine), an α-agonist vasopressor, is usually sufficient. If the pulse is below 50 beats per minute, a vasopressor can be supplemented with atropine for a brief period, or with a β-1-agonist. Bradycardia may persist for up to 36 hours postoperatively. The putative explanation for hypotension is an increased activity of the newly exposed carotid baroreceptors (20,21). These problems have been ameliorated to some degree by anesthetic blockade of the pericarotid nerves that is used prior to the procedure. Nonetheless, it seems reasonable that up to 24 hours of postoperative observation, ideally in a neuro-ICU or with frequent measurement of vital signs is justified in anticipation of hypotension.

Postoperative hypertension, occurring in 20% to 50% of various series, but far less frequently in our experience, sometimes has resulted from cerebral hemorrhage, particularly if there had been a small cerebral infarction in the weeks preceding the operation (22). The CT scan obtained postoperatively may show excessive contrast enhancement in regions that are destined to bleed postoperatively (23). Nitroprusside infusion is probably the most satisfactory treatment if the hypertension is severe, and nitroglycerin may be useful if the patient has active coronary artery disease.

Changes in the morphology of the electrocardiogram (ECG) that simulate myocardial infarction can occur after unilateral endarterectomy. (They are far more common after bilateral or rapidly sequential endarterectomy.) T-wave inversions are similar to those that occur with acute intracranial mass lesions and subarachnoid hemorrhage (Chapter 15). True myocardial ischemia probably occurs more frequently than is appreciated but most often it is minor and detectable only by a slight elevation in cardiac enzymes. However, up to 3% of routine endarterectomies reportedly have been followed by MI, with rates being highest in patients receiving vasopressors and in those with previous heart disease (24).

Also well known are infrequent cases of laryngeal paralysis from vagal nerve damage after endarterectomy, making extubation difficult, and difficulty with airway management in those few patients with neck swelling (25). Lingual palsy from injury to the hypoglossal nerve may occur concurrently or as an independent problem, but it has few implications in critical care.

CARE OF PATIENTS FOLLOWING ENDOVASCULAR PROCEDURES

The main issues that arise have to do with clinical monitoring of the neurological examination and observation of the groin puncture site and the distal vasculature of the leg. Occasional instances of brain swelling as a result of unintended cerebral infarction are evident by worsening of a preexisting focal deficit or the appearance of a new one, and by headache and unexplained systemic hypertension. Matters such as the timing of reinstitution of anticoagulation are dependent on the particular circumstances and subject to local practice.

Various methods of preventing femoral bleeding are employed, including sandbags and pressure devices (e.g., "fem-stop") but they often obscure bleeding when used after the patient has left the angiography suite. The correction of a femoral artery occlusion that causes ischemia of the distal leg and the management of retroperitoneal hematomas, most often evident by unexplained hypotension and lower abdominal pain (drop in hematocrit is a late sign), and the loss of the knee jerk, are addressed in surgical texts. Subcutaneous hematomas of the groin and upper thigh often are more unsightly than dangerous.

PROPHYLAXIS FOR VENOUS THROMBOSIS AND PULMONARY EMBOLUS

There seems to be general agreement that the use of low doses of heparin for this purpose probably represents only a slight risk for cerebral hemorrhage in patients with intracranial lesions, even postoperatively. A reduction in postoperative venous thrombosis has been shown with the use of pneumatic compression "air boots," and they are advisable in patients who are bed-bound for more than a day, especially if their mobility had been limited preoperatively. However, both heparin and pneumatic boots are documented to decrease venous thrombosis in the legs, not necessarily pulmonary embolus. Swann and colleagues found that expectant observation of known leg vein thrombosis in neurosurgical patients carries a high risk of subsequent pulmonary embolus, often fatal (26,27). They recommend interruption of the inferior vena cava as the safest course once substantial leg vein clots have been detected. However, we favor anticoagulation over a filter if the clinical circumstances permit, in part because a filter alone is prone to be associated with local thrombosis on the device and venous insufficiency in the legs. It is not known if routine surveillance for leg vein thrombosis, beyond clinical examination of the legs, is justified.

POSTOPERATIVE MONITORING OF INTRACRANIAL PRESSURE

The indications for leaving an ICP monitor in place after a craniotomy are as varied and controversial as for their initial insertion. In a retrospective study of 514 elective neurosurgeries, approximately 15% had postoperative ICP elevations greater than 20 mm Hg, particularly after glioblastoma resection or repeat tumor surgery (28). Certainly, a justification can be made for monitoring after removal of large subdural or other traumatic hematomas in which brain swelling is manifest but there is no evidence that for most types of surgery postoperative ICP monitoring improves clinical outcome or guides management in a meaningful way. Patients with severe multiple system trauma, especially if frequent fluid resuscitation or high ventilator pressures are anticipated, probably benefit most from postoperative ICP monitoring (Chapters 3 and 10). It is not even clear to the authors how randomized clinical studies resolve the issue of the appropriate use of postoperative ICP monitoring (the same can be said for the general use of monitoring) because it is difficult to establish protocols that match most clinical circumstances.

PROPHYLAXIS FOR GASTROINTESTINAL BLEEDING

The typical postoperative patient, even one receiving corticosteroids, probably does not require specific treatment to prevent gastrointestinal bleeding, but many units nonetheless use antacids, or H-2 histamine blocking drugs. In comatose patients or those who require prolonged ventilation, a reduction in gastric acidity probably is desirable; the notion being that gastric erosions are reduced and that aspiration pneumonia, should it occur, will not be complicated by acid injury. At least one study, perhaps now outdated but still worthy of attention, found that antacids were superior in this regard to cimetidine in critically ill patients (29). However, recent work suggests that the alteration in gastric acidity may remove a barrier to nosocomial infection, particularly in long-term ventilator patients, and sucralfate has been suggested as an alternative treatment (30). Increased gastric pH apparently permits bacterial growth in gastric secretions, making aspiration pneumonia more serious in long-term ventilator patients. Many debilitated patients chronically aspirate small quantities of gastric secretions despite apparently functioning endotracheal tubes. Sucralfate purportedly provides effective prophylaxis without greatly elevating gastric pH. However, the difficulty of administering sucralfate and associated reduction in absorption of anticonvulsants and other drugs administered by nasogastric tube still makes antacids or histamine blockers better alternatives for the brief postoperative period.

REFERENCES

1. Knaus WA, Draper E, Lawrence DE, et al. Neurosurgical admissions to the intensive care unit: intensive monitoring vs intensive therapy. *Neurosurgery* 1981;8: 438–442.
2. Hindman BJ, ed. *Neurological and psychological complications of surgery and anesthesia.* International Anesthesiology Clinics, vol. 24. Boston: Little, Brown, 1986.
3. Horwitz NH, Rizzoli HV. *Postoperative complications of intracranial surgery.* Baltimore: Williams & Wilkins, 1982.
4. Wirth FP, Ratcheson RA. *Neurosurgical critical care.* Baltimore: Williams & Wilkins, 1987.
5. Kaplan J, Ropper AH. Postoperative confusion. In: Grenvik A, et al., eds. *Textbook of critical care*, 4th ed. Philadelphia: WB Saunders, 2000:1825–1831.
6. Rosenberg H, Clofine R, Bialik O. Neurological changes during awakening from anesthesia. *Anesthesiology* 1981;45:125–130.

7. McCulloch PR, Milne B. Neurological phenomena during emergence from enflurane or isoflurane anesthesia. *Can J Anesthesiol* 1990;37:139–142.

8. Ross D, Rosegay H, Pons V. Differentiation of aseptic and bacterial meningitis in postoperative neurosurgical patients. *J Neurosurg* 1988;69:669–674.

9. Cunha BA, Tu RP. Fever in the neurosurgical patient. *Heart Lung* 1988;17:608–611.

10. Spetzler RF, Wilson CB, Weinstein P, et al. Normal perfusion pressure breakthrough theory. *Clin Neurosurg* 1978;25:651–672.

11. Bernstein M, Ross Fleming JF, et al. Cerebral hyperperfusion after carotid endarterectomy: a cause of cerebral hemorrhage. *Neurosurgery* 1984;15:50–56.

12. Sundt TM, Sharbrough FW, Peipgras DG, et al. Correlation of cerebral blood flow and electroencephalographic changes during carotid endarterectomy with results of surgery and hemodynamics of cerebral ischemia. *Mayo Clin Proc* 1981;56:533–543.

13. Tateishi A, Sano T, Takeshita H, et al. Effects of nifedipine on intracranial pressure in neurosurgical patients with intracranial hypertension. *J Neurosurg* 1988;69:213–215.

14. Nishiyama T, Yokoyama T, Matauyama T, et al. Continuous nicardipine infusion to control blood pressure after evacuation of acute cerebral hemorrhage. *Can J Anaesthesiol* 2000;47:1196–201.

15. Rosenthal JJ, Zeichner WD, Lamis PA, et al. Neurological deficit after carotid endarterectomy and carotid thromboendarterectomy. *Surgery* 1983;94:776–780.

16. Skillman JJ. Neurological complications of cardiovascular surgery: I. Procedures involving the carotid arteries and abdominal aorta. In: Hindman BJ, ed. *Neurological and psychological complications of surgery and anesthesia. Volume 24*. International Anesthesiology Clinics, Boston: Little, Brown, 1986:135–157.

17. Perdue GD. Management of postendarterectomy neurological deficits. *Arch Surg* 1982;117:1079–1084.

18. Steed DL, Peitzman AB, Grundy BL, et al. Causes of stroke in carotid endarterectomy. *Surgery* 1982;92:634–638.

19. Towne JB, Bernhard VM. Neurological deficit following carotid endarterectomy. *Surg Gynecol Obstet* 1982;154:849–853.

20. Bove EL, Fry WJ, Gross WS, et al. Hypotension and hypertension as consequences of baroreceptor dysfunction following carotid endarterectomy. *Surgery* 1979;85:633–637.

21. Tarlov EH, Schmidek H, Scott RM, et al. Reflex hypotension following carotid endarterectomy: mechanism and management. *J Neurosurg* 1973;39:323–327.

22. Caplan LR, Skillman R, Ojemann RG, et al. Intracerebral hemorrhage following carotid endarterectomy: a hypertensive complication? *Stroke* 1978;9:457–460.

23. Ropper AH, Kehne SM. Contrast enhancement CT scan and post-endarterectomy hemorrhage. *Stroke* 1986;17:898–899.

24. Riles TS, Kopelman I, Imparato AM. Myocardial infarction following carotid endarterectomy: a review of 683 operations. *Surgery* 1979;8:249–252.

25. O'Sullivan JC, Wells DG, Wells GR. Difficult airway management with neck swelling after carotid endarterectomy. *Anaesthesiol Int Care* 1986;14:460–464.

26. Swann KW, Black PM. Deep venous thrombosis and pulmonary embolus in neurosurgical patients: a review. *J Neurosurg* 1984;61:1055–1062.

27. Swann KW, Black PM, Baker MA. Management of symptomatic deep venous thrombosis and pulmonary emboli on a neurosurgical service. *J Neurosurg* 1986;64:563–567.

28. Constantini S, Cotov S, Rappaport ZH, et al. Intracranial pressure monitoring after elective intracranial surgery. A retrospective trial of 514 consecutive patients. *J Neurosurg* 1988;69:540–544.

29. Priebe HJ, Skillman JJ, Bushnell LS, et al. Antacid versus Cimetidine in preventing acute gastrointestinal bleeding. A randomized trial in 75 critically ill patients. *N Engl J Med* 1980;302:426–430.

30. Driks MR, Craven DE, Celli BR, et al. Rates of ventilator-associated pneumonia in patients randomized to treatment with sucralfate versus antacids or H2 blockers. *Am Rev Respir Dis* 1987;135:212.

11

Neurological Complications of Critical Medical Illnesses

There are numerous conditions encountered in intensive care that cause serious neurological dysfunction. Most are somewhat predictably associated with critical illness, or at least well defined, and several others are very infrequent and not addressed extensively in this chapter. One problem arises in that the onset of an abrupt neurological complication is frequently obscured by the effects of the primary illness (e.g., a metabolic disorder producing encephalopathy delays recognition of an intracerebral hemorrhage) or by its treatment (e.g., sedation to allow greater synchrony with a mechanical ventilator). Other neurological problems (e.g., critical illness polyneuropathy) typically develop more insidiously, and become apparent only as the patient improves. Also, the neurological problem quite often is apparent for some time, but its manifestations are inappropriately attributed to the underlying medical illness (1). To address these issues, the intensivist should be as disciplined in his interpretation of changes in level of consciousness or limb movement as he is in understanding a fall in oxygen saturation or a rising white blood cell count (2).

EPIDEMIOLOGY

The true incidence of the neurological complications of medical illness is difficult to determine but a guide sense can be obtained from the study carried out by Isensee and colleagues who evaluated 100 consecutive medical intensive care unit (MICU) patients

within 72 hours of admission to detect neurological problems (3). Their study excluded those with primarily cardiac problems. Eighteen patients were admitted for acute neurological disease and five others for encephalopathy caused by drug overdose. Of the remaining 67, fully one third had a serious neurological complication of a medical condition (11 metabolic encephalopathy, four hypoxic–ischemic encephalopathy, and seven other neurological problems). Furthermore, 59% of the patients with neurological complications died, in contrast to 20% of the nonneurological patients.

Bleck and associates have carried out a 2-year prospective study among MICU patients in order to describe the neurological complications encountered and identify their effects on mortality and length of stay (LOS) (4). As with the above-noted study, patients with a primarily neurological reason for admission to the MICU were excluded from analyses of mortality and LOS. More than half of this group had either a major ischemic stroke or intracranial hemorrhage. The others were classified as having a complication of a critical illness if they developed a neurological problem from a medical disorder or directly from its treatment. They collected the medical diagnoses into four categories for analysis: (a) sepsis, bacteremia with shock, the "sepsis syndrome," and acute respiratory distress syndrome; (b) acute coronary artery disease, including myocardial infarction (MI); (c) other cardiac problems; and (d) all others (e.g., ven-

TABLE 11.1. *Neurological complications encountered in 217 patients at risk of severe medical illnesses in the medical intensive care unit*

Complication	N (percent of patients with diagnosis)[a]
Metabolic encephalopathy	62 (28.6)
Seizures	61 (28.1)
Hypoxic–ischemic encephalopathy	51 (23.5)
Stroke	48 (22.1)
Other diagnoses	50 (23.0)

[a]A single patient could have more than one complication; therefore, the total number in this column exceeds the total number of patients.

From Bleck TP, Smith MC, Pierre-Louis SJ, et al. Neurologic complications of critical medical illnesses. *Crit Care Med* 1993;21:98–103, with permission.

tilatory failure, gastrointestinal hemorrhage, hypotension without sepsis). Patients with neurological complications were further divided into those with metabolic encephalopathies, seizures, cerebrovascular disorders, hypoxic–ischemic encephalopathy, or other global brain disorders. These neurological categories were not mutually exclusive. Patients with clinically apparent peripheral nervous system disorders were classified in the "other" group.

During the study, 1,850 patients were admitted to the MICU; of these, 92 (4.9%) were admitted for a primary neurological reason. Among the remaining 1,758 patients of prin-

cipal interest, 217 (12%) experienced neurological complications of their underlying medical disease (Table 11.1). Table 11.2 details the neurological complication rates by MICU admission category. The overall mortality rate for all MICU patients was 32%, compared to 55% for the 217 patients with neurological complications, compared to 29% for those without neurological complications. The neurological group also had significantly longer MICU and hospital stays.

Metabolic encephalopathy was the most frequent complication, occurring in 62 patients. Of these, the largest group was attributed to sepsis, without evidence for hepatic or renal dysfunction or hypoxemia. The frequencies of different metabolic encephalopathies are detailed in Table 11.3. Seizures occurred in 61 patients, most often with cerebrovascular lesions. Hypoxic–ischemic encephalopathy occurred in 51 patients, primarily because of a cardiac disorder in 27, and pulmonary disease in the remaining 24.

It is of interest (and perhaps not widely appreciated) that 48 patients had strokes while in the ICU. Thirty-two of these were infarcts, 14 were intracerebral hemorrhages, and two were subarachnoid hemorrhages. Thirteen stroke patients had an identified cause other than arteriosclerosis, including underlying connective tissue diseases and bacterial endocarditis. Stroke occurred in only 1% of patients with acute MI, a rate less than the usually cited range of 1.7% to 2.4% (5,6).

TABLE 11.2. *Neurological complication rates by primary medical intensive care unit admission category*

| Category | Percent of patients with complications | | | | |
	Seizure	Vascular	HIE	Metabolic	Other
Sepsis	11%	6%	10%	21%	11%
Other medical condition	4%	3%	4%	3%	6%
Coronary artery disease	1%	1%	1%	1%	1%
Other cardiac condition	4%	3%	3%	2%	4%

HIE, hypoxic–ischemic encephalopathy.
From Bleck TP, Smith MC, Pierre-Louis SJ, et al. Neurologic complications of critical medical illnesses. *Crit Care Med* 1993;21:98–103, with permission.

TABLE 11.3. *Etiologies of metabolic encephalopathy in a medical intensive care unit population*

Etiology	N
Sepsis	19
Hepatic	18
Renal	8
Hypertensive	7
Hyperosmolar	4
Hypoglycemic	3
Uncertain	3

From Bleck TP, Smith MC, Pierre-Louis SJ, et al. Neurologic complications of critical medical illness. *Crit Care Med* 1993;21:98–103, with permission.

SEPSIS AND SEPTIC ENCEPHALOPATHY

During the past 30 years, clinical analyses and investigations of cytokine mechanisms have contributed to our understanding of the causes and pathogenesis of sepsis (7), but the causes of the associated encephalopathy remain obscure. Although bacteremia was previously considered to be the sine qua non of systemic sepsis, occurring as a consequence of local infection, it is clear that many patients suffer the same vasomotor disturbances and organ dysfunctions without positive blood cultures. Bone has suggested that sepsis be defined as "clinical evidence of infection, tachypnea, tachycardia, and hyperthermia or hypothermia" (8). He further defined the sepsis syndrome as "sepsis with evidence of altered organ perfusion." Subsequent investigators have refined these definitions and added more quantitative factors to help guide clinical studies (9). In this current view, the crucial systemic aspects of the sepsis syndrome are altered distribution of blood flow (microcirculatory abnormalities), endothelial damage, and parenchymal injury (10). The pathogenesis of these problems is the subject of intense study, but the most convincing hypotheses regarding the systemic manifestations involve the effects of tumor necrosis factor, several interleukins, platelet activating factor, and other mediators of inflammation (11).

The epidemiologic data cited herein as well as other studies too numerous to cite, indicate that septic encephalopathy is the most frequent neurological disorder encountered in medical intensive care; it is also one of the more poorly recognized and understood. Septic encephalopathy was described in 1827 (12), but has only recently become a subject of organized neurological interest. Young and coworkers (13) should be credited with providing a thorough prospective analysis of this disorder in a large university MICU and bringing the disorder to attention in the current era. They required fever and a positive blood culture for inclusion into their study, a very restrictive definition of sepsis that nonetheless provided a homogeneous group for analysis. Patients were excluded if they had preexisting brain disease; frequent sedative or opiate administration; pulmonary, hepatic, or renal failure; endocarditis; or long bone fractures that might have produced fat embolism.

These workers identified 69 septic patients over 31 months; by clinical examination, 20 of them were not encephalopathic, 17 were mildly encephalopathic, and 32 were severely encephalopathic. The patient's age, blood pressure on entry into the study, and temperature did not vary significantly among the groups. The lowest systolic and diastolic blood pressures were statistically significantly lower (but probably not importantly so from a biological perspective) in the mildly and severely affected groups when compared with those without encephalopathy. Mortality was linked to the category of encephalopathy: None of the unaffected patients died, whereas 35% of the moderately and 53% of the severely affected patients died. It was of interest that a number of laboratory values showed a linear relationship with the severity of encephalopathy, including white blood cell count, PaO_2, blood urea nitrogen, creatinine, bilirubin, alkaline phosphatase, and potassium. The serum albumin concentration was inversely related to encephalopathy. The cerebrospinal fluid (CSF) protein content was mildly elevated (60 to 85 mg/dL).

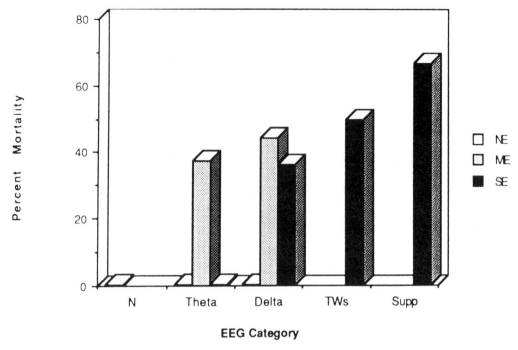

FIG. 11.1. Mortality in bacteremic patients by electroencephalography (EEG) category. The ordinate indicates the percent mortality in each category of encephalopathy as a function of the predominant EEG finding. (From Young GB, Bolton CF, Archibald YM, et al. The electroencephalogram in sepsis-associated encephalopathy. *J Clin Neurophysiol* 1992;9:145–152, with permission.)

Electroencephalography (EEG) has been found by several groups to be a more sensitive test for central nervous system (CNS) dysfunction than the clinical examination, and a correspondingly more powerful predictor of survival (Fig. 11.1) (14). Evoked potential studies in septic patients suggest that brain dysfunction is even more prevalent than detected by EEG, the evoked potentials being abnormal in 84% (15). Sprung and coworkers, reporting for the Veterans' Administration Cooperative Sepsis study, also showed that "alterations in mental status are common in septic patients, and are associated with significantly higher mortality" (16).

Eidelman and colleagues (17) studied 50 patients with severe sepsis, and showed that encephalopathy was associated with bacteremia and hepatic dysfunction. The severity of encephalopathy, measured by as simple a tool as the Glasgow Coma Scale, correlated directly with mortality. Using encephalopathy as a marker, they found that 59% of encephalopathic patients were bacteremic, whereas only 13% of patients with normal mental status were bacteremic.

Pathology and Pathophysiology

The pathologic basis of septic encephalopathy remains uncertain. Jackson and colleagues (18) reported on the autopsies of 12 patients dying after severe, prolonged sepsis. They found cerebral microabscesses in eight patients and proliferation of astrocytes and microglia in three others; these findings suggested metastatic infection. Three of these patients also had central pontine myelinolysis and three had cerebral infarcts. The remaining patient demonstrated purpuric lesions, the significance of which is uncertain. (We have experience with several patients dying with staphylococcal sepsis who had widespread brain purpura but the clinical correlation was not certain because all were comatose prior to death.) Eight of the patients had EEGs, three of which showed multifocal epileptiform activity.

Pendlebury and associates (19) identified 35 patients with multiple CNS microabscesses among 2,107 consecutive autopsies. All these patients had chronic, usually immunocompromising, diseases, and were frequently septic before death. The most common organisms implicated were *Staphylococcus aureus* and *Candida albicans.* In contrast, the study by Bleck and colleagues did not find microabscesses in the four patients autopsied of 14 fatal cases with septic encephalopathy; therefore, the importance and frequency of this finding cannot be stated with confidence (4).

Regarding the pathophysiology of septic encephalopathy, a number of the systemic mediators of inflammation alluded to earlier have been implicated, most of which are capable of damaging the blood–brain barrier (BBB) (20). Such disruption has been documented in an animal model early in sepsis (21). The behavioral effects of cytokines vary with the neuroanatomic structures affected but include thermogenic behaviors (e.g., shivering) in the hypothalamus (22) and somnolence in relation to the locus ceruleus (23). Interferons also alter individual cortical and hippocampal neuronal functions, suggesting potential effects on memory and emotion (24). Brain catecholamine concentrations are decreased in experimental sepsis, but this is not easily interpreted (25).

Cerebral blood flow (CBF) and cerebral oxygen extraction decrease in septic encephalopathy (26), and parallel to some extent the development of cerebral edema and a disruption of the BBB (27). Failure of cerebrovascular autoregulation is likely to compound these disorders (28), potentially producing cerebral ischemia. Both cerebral edema and BBB disruption appear to correlate with damage to astrocyte foot-processes (29). The cause of the changes in CBF and oxygen extraction are less well understood, and the clinical meaning of many of these physiologic changes, although provocative, cannot be interpreted. Focal elevations in intracellular free calcium may cause neuronal dysfunction and also contribute to apoptotic or necrotic cell loss (30). Activation of adenosine A_1 receptors may be important in the development of a local CNS inflammatory response (31). Although cytokines have been suggested as mediators, a study of the effects of tumor necrosis factor was unable to confirm its role in this regard (32). A decline in CSF ascorbic acid concentration found in one study (33) may reflect difficulty in safely handling the oxygen-derived free radicals potentially resulting from both cytokine and nitric oxide excess.

It has been proposed that abnormal systemic metabolism in sepsis may contribute to CNS dysfunction. For example, Mizock and associates (34) (as have others) demonstrated altered phenylalanine metabolism (elevated blood and CSF levels, and elevated phenylalanine metabolites) in 11 patients with septic encephalopathy; in contrast, patients with hepatic encephalopathy had elevated CSF concentrations of many other aromatic amino acids. Sprung and coworkers found elevated serum levels of phenylalanine, ammonia, and tryptophan in encephalopathic patients compared with infected patients with a normal sensorium, along with lower concentrations of isoleucine (35). Other studies have confirmed this, and find that these changes are linked also to concentrations of calcitonin precursors and interleukin-6 (36). As with most of the other biochemical and immune findings, the significance of these correlative studies for the pathogenesis of encephalopathy is uncertain but they provide a basis for study of the condition. Several authors have tried to implicate abnormal hepatic and muscular metabolism of aromatic amino acids in both hepatic and septic encephalopathies, but this hypothesis has been challenged as commented on in the following section.

Septic patients are prey to a wide variety of other metabolic disorders and intoxications that cause encephalopathy apart from the direct effects of sepsis on the brain and on cerebral blood flow (37). Nonconvulsive status epilepticus is an under-recognized problem in the population at risk (38). There is neither a diagnostic test to discriminate it from other causes of encephalopathy, nor a specific treatment for the CNS disturbance. In summary, from a clinical standpoint, the diagnosis of septic encephalopathy remains one of exclusion (39).

HEPATIC FAILURE AND THE CENTRAL NERVOUS SYSTEM

The current debate over the pathogenesis of hepatic encephalopathy is of great importance to clinical neuroscientists. In fulminant hepatic failure, increased intracranial pressure (ICP) has become a major cause of death in patients awaiting transplantation (40). Patients whose ICP has been elevated may survive a transplant but be left with CNS deficits (41).

The mechanism of the cerebral edema that develops in fulminant hepatic failure is unknown (42), but it requires aggressive treatment (43). Steroids are not effective, but mannitol has been useful in some series, along the lines discussed in Chapter 3 (44). Hyperventilation had previously been thought to increase mortality in this condition, but a controlled trial has demonstrated its benefit, albeit slight (45). Based on clinical experience, high-dose barbiturates may be used if mannitol and hyperventilation fail to control ICP (46). Interestingly, as mentioned in Chapter 3, the effect of posture on ICP is unpredictable (47). Computed tomographic (CT) scanning has turned out to be an uncertain indicator of the severity of intracranial hypertension (48,49). Attempts to lower ICP by reducing extracellular volume through hemofiltration have not been effective (50). There is no current substitute for invasive ICP monitoring in patients with fulminant hepatic failure who are in grade 3 (stuporous) or grade 4 (comatose). The need for monitoring extends through the period of the transplant operation into at least the first postoperative day (51).

Patients with acute liver failure have elevated levels of so-called endogenous 1,4-benzodiazepines (52), which some authorities offer as an explanation for stupor or coma in patients who do not have ICP elevations. An interaction between γ-aminobutyric acid (GABA) and elevated concentrations of ammonia may be important in both the acute condition and in more chronic forms of hepatic encephalopathy (53).

Chronic hepatic encephalopathy does not appear to cause ICP elevation unless intracranial bleeding supervenes. As in acute hepatic disease, endogenous benzodiazepine-like compounds ($GABA_A$ agonists) likely play a role (54), and the use of GABA antagonists is being actively investigated but has not yet become standard practice to reverse stupor and coma. About 70% of chronic hepatic encephalopathy patients awaken rapidly when given flumazenil (but transiently, for the duration of the drug's effect) (55,56). These patients have numerous other metabolic abnormalities that may contribute to their encephalopathy, including abnormalities in the Krebs cycle (57) and of methionine metabolism (58).

OTHER CAUSES OF ENCEPHALOPATHY IN THE INTENSIVE CARE UNIT SETTING

Renal and hypoxic encephalopathies, of course, are quite common in the ICU environment. Details of their diagnosis and management are beyond the scope of this chapter, but have been reviewed (59).

Iatrogenic causes of encephalopathy are particularly common in MICU settings and should be excluded before attributing reduced alertness to more ambiguous causes, such as septic encephalopathy. Hypnosedative drugs and narcotic analgesics are the most common agents in this category. Flumazenil and naloxone reverse these drug-induced encephalopathies, and can be used as diagnostic tests, but the degree of dependability of the former as an indicator of excessive benzodiazepine dose is not known. The need to reverse the effects of these drugs in an individual ICU patient should be carefully assessed, because the emergence of agitation or severe pain may be detrimental. If these drugs are used to determine whether encephalopathy is owing to medications, doses much smaller than those to reverse respiratory depression should be used initially. Flumazenil, 0.1 to 0.2 mg intravenously (i.v.) over 15 seconds, may be given every 60 seconds to a maximum of 1.0 mg. Naloxone, 0.04 to 0.08 mg i.v., may be given every 60 seconds to a total dose of 0.8 mg. Barbiturates are not antagonized by available agents. It should also be apparent from the preceding section on hepatic encephalopathy that a response to flumazenil is not specific for a benzodiazepine overdose.

With increasing numbers of patients with cancer benefiting from critical care, a study of the causes and outcome of altered mental status in these patients provides a useful guide to their evaluation and management. In an analysis of 140 patients, two of three had more than one cause contributing to their alteration in mentation (60). Drugs, metabolic abnormalities, infection, and recent surgery were the most commonly detected antecedents. One fourth of these patients died within 30 days.

Other encephalopathic conditions may arise during the course of ICU treatment. One that bears emphasis because it is regularly missed is that of Wernicke's encephalopathy that may be precipitated by seemingly innocuous treatments such as the dextrose administered as the vehicle for a lidocaine infusion to treat ventricular arrhythmias after an acute MI.

SEIZURES IN THE INTENSIVE CARE UNIT

In the epidemiologic study referred to earlier, 34 patients had simple partial seizures (with or without secondary generalization), and six had complex partial seizures (with or without secondary generalization) (4). Twenty patients had seizures that appeared to be generalized at onset, and six patients developed status epilepticus in the MICU; all required at least two agents to terminate their status (usu-

ally a benzodiazepine and phenytoin). Two of these patients developed refractory status epilepticus and were treated with pentobarbital coma. As often happens, three patients required admission to the MICU for refractory hypotension after receiving phenytoin infusions at rates between 25 and 50 mg/minute. The blood pressures of these patients did not improve with fluid resuscitation alone; all required dopamine infusions for several hours to maintain blood pressure and systemic perfusion.

In contrast to our experience in other hospitalized patients, the focal onset of partial seizures with secondary generalization was usually noted and adequately described. This was a useful guide to management, because patients with partial seizures generally experienced seizure recurrence and thus probably benefited from anticonvulsant treatment (61).

The diagnosis and management of seizures should be pursued differently in ICU patients than in other patients (Chapter 20). We had hoped to develop rules to predict which patients having seizures in the ICU might be evaluated without imaging procedures, but were unable to do so because most patients had vascular or infectious causes for their seizures. All patients experiencing a single seizure in the ICU were treated with some form of anticonvulsant therapy; this was often justified by the argument that their underlying medical condition might be adversely affected by subsequent seizures. We believe that this constitutes excessively aggressive management and that it postpones an appropriate search for etiology. For example, all three patients with recurrent seizures caused by nonketotic hyperglycemia were treated with at least two anticonvulsants; these drugs are known to be ineffective in this condition (62).

Phenytoin remains a reasonable first choice when ICU patients do require treatment. However, a second agent, usually phenobarbital, was required in most patients. Lorazepam was useful for the suppression of breakthrough seizures, but the use of this drug was often continued without adequate attention to optimal use of phenytoin or phenobarbital.

Pentobarbital coma had been considered the treatment of choice for refractory status epilepticus in ICU patients, as discussed in Chapter 20. We have adopted instead the use of high-dose midazolam in this circumstance (63). This method appears to be more rapidly effective and to have substantially fewer and less severe adverse effects than pentobarbital, thiopental, or propofol (64).

NEUROMUSCULAR COMPLICATIONS OF SEPSIS

Although recognized by earlier authors such as Osler, the modern era of interest in this problem began with the independent reports of three groups reported by Rivner (four patients) (65), Bolton (17 patients) (16,66), and others. Bolton's group followed their initial description with a series of papers that characterized the clinical (67), electrophysiologic (68), and pathologic (69) aspects of critical illness polyneuropathy. Although many other groups have made significant contributions to this area (e.g., Op de Coul and coworkers), the work of Bolton, Young, and colleagues is in great measure responsible for the recognition of this problem among intensivists.

These neuromuscular complications can be categorized anatomically. *Critical illness polyneuropathy* is an axonal disorder affecting both sensory and motor nerves (69). Electrophysiologic evidence of this condition, as noted earlier, is present in about 70% of septic patients, but the percentage with weakness sufficient to impede ventilator weaning or ambulation is less. The phrenic nerves are typically the most severely involved. *Neuromuscular junction dysfunction* in the setting of critical illness is typically a consequence of a prolonged effect of neuromuscular junction (NMJ) blocking agents, usually because of impaired clearance (70). Myopathy in critically ill patients is most commonly seen in those who have received NMJ blocking agents and corticosteroids in the treatment of severe asthma (71). Although this disorder has been reported most commonly after ve-

curonium use, it also occurs after NMJ blocking agents that do not depend on renal or hepatic excretion (e.g., atracurium) (72). Myopathy also may occur in the setting of some viral infections (e.g., influenza) and there is no doubt that underlying neuromuscular illnesses such as myasthenia gravis may become apparent during the course of another illness or treatment in the ICU with precipitating drugs such as neuromuscular blocking agents. A syndrome of disseminated pyogenic myopathy has also been described (73), presumably as a consequence of bacteremic seeding of muscles.

Critical illness polyneuropathy has also been noted after organ transplantation without sepsis (74).

Although most of the patients reported to have critical illness polyneuropathy have been adults, this condition has been recognized with increasing frequency in children as well (75).

In contrast to the body of experimental work on septic encephalopathy, very little is understood about the pathogenesis of the neuromuscular complications of sepsis (76). Hyperglycemia correlates with the development of critical illness polyneuropathy, but these may be independent markers of the severity of the underlying illness. The neuronal microenvironment of peripheral nerves is similar to that of the extracellular space of the brain; therefore, it is possible that the same alterations that produce septic encephalopathy may be responsible for critical illness polyneuropathy. Critical illness myopathy may result from the functional denervation induced by NMJ blockade; it does not appear to be simply a severe form of steroid myopathy.

Diagnosis, Differential Diagnosis, and Prognosis

Recognition of a neuromuscular complication of sepsis generally occurs as the patient begins to recover from the critical illness that first required ventilatory support. Critical illness polyneuropathy is usually first suspected when the patient's pulmonary mechanics, clinical state, and gas exchange suggest that weaning should be possible, but the patient is unable to tolerate removal of the ventilator (77). There is commonly some evidence of both proximal and distal weakness on examination but the degree varies and our experience is that there are numerous instances that do not come to attention because they cause only mild weakness. Tendon reflexes are often absent or diminished, but critical illness polyneuropathy may be present without alteration in reflexes (78). The degree of sensory loss tends to be slight and the facial and ocular muscles are not affected to any great degree. These rules become difficult to apply when the patient has an underlying diabetic or other chronic neuropathy.

The diagnosis depends in part on electrophysiologic studies, which demonstrate an axonal disorder. Electromyographic studies of the diaphragm confirm the presence of denervation (79). The differential diagnosis is usually limited to consideration of the axonal form of the Guillain–Barré syndrome (80); this latter condition usually causes much more severe generalized weakness than critical illness polyneuropathy, and typically displays an elevated CSF protein concentration, whereas the protein concentration in critical illness neuropathy is normal or only slightly elevated. Antecedent infection with *Campylobacter jejuni* is frequently noted in patients with the axonal form of Guillain–Barré (81). Other differential diagnostic concerns are botulism, which impairs presynaptic acetylcholine release, and myasthenia gravis, in which the motor end plate is damaged. These conditions also have characteristic nerve conduction and electromyographic characteristics that serve to distinguish them from critical illness neuropathy.

No specific treatment for critical illness polyneuropathy is available. Anecdotal evidence does not favor the use of plasma exchange or i.v. immunoglobulin, but there have been no definitive trials. Almost all patients recover eventually, but this may require 6 months or more of ventilatory support in the worst cases. A recent patient of ours was ventilator-dependent for over 10 months but recovered to walk with a walker; the precipitating illness was a sternal wound infection after coronary bypass.

The prolonged effect of NMJ blocking agents is suspected on the basis of suppressed or absent tendon reflexes and an inability to produce muscle contraction with a bedside neuromuscular stimulator or electromyogram machine. If the diagnosis is in question, it can be confirmed by nerve conduction studies that show either complete block to stimulation or a decremental response as in myasthenia. There is no specific treatment, but the condition will resolve when the agent in question has cleared.

Critical illness myopathy is often accompanied by substantial elevation of the serum creatine kinase (CK) concentration, which serves to distinguish this condition from steroid myopathy in which the CK is usually normal. Electromyography is usually an adequate diagnostic study, and muscle biopsy is only rarely required (82). Again, no specific treatment is available, but the condition will resolve; whether it will resolve faster if systemic steroids are reduced or discontinued is uncertain. Definitive diagnosis can be obtained by a muscle biopsy and this can be performed at the bedside with a needle technique unless the history suggests a more chronic myopathic disorder preceding the acute illness. We recently saw a 45-year-old patient for postoperative difficulty in weaning from mechanical ventilation, who then gave a history of progressive proximal muscle weakness, in whom a muscle biopsy confirmed the diagnosis of acid maltase deficiency. Biopsies in such patients require the more exotic studies performed on open biopsy material. We resort to biopsy only in that modest proportion of cases that have equivocal CK tests and in which the context (use of NMJ blocking agents and/or steroids) is unclear.

There are many other neurological problems that arise during the course of an intensive care unit stay that may impede weaning from mechanical ventilation. Kelly and Matthay (82) prospectively studied 66 consecutive adult patients requiring mechanical ventilation for more than 48 hours to determine the reasons for their ventilatory problems. Neurological problems, primarily encephalopathies, were held responsible for the continuing need for ventilatory support in 32% of the patients, and contributed to this problem in another 41%. Although this study was not directed at patients who failed to wean after resolution of their presenting disease, it does highlight the role of neurological problems early in critical illness. Spitzer and colleagues (83) studied 21 patients who failed to wean after their presenting disease had improved to the point that their intensivists believed that mechanical ventilation should no longer have been necessary. Thirteen (62%) of these patients had a neuromuscular disorder that was either the major cause of or contributed substantially to their ventilatory problems. Only seven of these 13 patients had critical illness polyneuropathy; other neuropathic conditions and unsuspected motor neuron disease were also uncovered. Most intensivists are also familiar with the less common acute myopathies that may complicate critical illnesses, especially in patients who have received neuromuscular junction blockade (71).

Traditionally, nutritional factors and hypokalemia were said to be the main cause of failure to wean, and they should not be neglected when this problem or generalized weakness arises.

A more recently described syndrome of so-called acute quadriplegic myopathy is also probably associated with steroids; in this condition, muscle is electrically inexcitable even with direct stimulation (84). Nerves are histologically normal, but muscles show thick filament loss (85). Although no treatment is known, the prognosis for this condition is for more rapid recovery than is typical for that for critical illness polyneuropathy or myopathy.

REFERENCES

1. Bleck TP. Why isn't this patient awake? *J Int Care Med* 1993;8:155–156.
2. Wijdicks EF. Neurological complications in critically ill patients. *Anesthesiol Analg* 1996;83:411–419.
3. Isensee LM, Weiner LJ, Hart RG. Neurological disorders in a medical intensive care unit: a prospective survey. *J Crit Care* 1989;4:208–210.
4. Bleck TP, Smith MC, Pierre-Louis SJ, et al. Neurological complications of critical medical illnesses. *Crit Care Med* 1993;21:98–103.
5. Komrad MS, Coffey CE, Coffey KS, et al. Myocardial infarction and stroke. *Neurology* 1984;34:1403–1409.
6. Thompson PL, Robinson JS. Stroke after acute myocardial infarction: relation to infarct size. *Br Med J* 1978;2:457–459.
7. Nathan BR, Bleck TP. Central nervous system complications of critical medical illness. In: Miller DH, Raps EC, eds. *Critical care neurology.* Boston: Butterworth-Heinemann, 1999:331–340.
8. Bone RC. Systemic inflammatory response syndrome: a unifying concept of systemic inflammation. In: Fein AM, Abraham EM, Balk RA, et al, eds. *Sepsis and multiorgan failure.* Baltimore: Williams & Wilkins, 1997:3–10.
9. Abraham E, Matthay MA, Dinarello CA, et al. Consensus conference definitions for sepsis, septic shock, acute lung injury, and acute respiratory distress syndrome: time for a reevaluation. *Crit Care Med* 2000;28:232–235.
10. Bone RC. The pathogenesis of sepsis. *Ann Intern Med* 1991;115:457–469.
11. Strassheim D, Park JS, Abraham E. Sepsis: current concepts in intracellular signaling. *Int J Biochem Cell Biol* 2002;34:1527–1533.
12. Bright R. *Reports of medical cases selected with a view of illustrating the symptoms and cure of diseases, with a reference to morbid anatomy.* London: Longman, Rees, Orme, Brown and Green, 1827.
13. Young GB, Bolton CF, Austin TW, et al. The encephalopathy associated with septic illness. *Clin Invest Med* 1990;13:297–304.
14. Young GB, Bolton CF, Archibald YM, et al. The electroencephalogram in sepsis-associated encephalopathy. *J Clin Neurophysiol* 1992;9:145–152.
15. Zauner C, Gendo A, Kramer L, et al. Impaired subcortical and cortical sensory evoked potential pathways in septic patients. *Crit Care Med* 2002;30:1136–1139.
16. Sprung CL, Peduzzi PN, Shatney CH, et al. Impact of encephalopathy on mortality in the sepsis syndrome. The Veterans Administration Systemic Sepsis Cooperative Study Group. *Crit Care Med* 1990;18:801–806.
17. Eidelman LA, Putterman D, Putterman C, et al. The spectrum of septic encephalopathy. Definitions, etiologies, and mortalities. *JAMA* 1996;275:470–473.
18. Jackson AC, Gilbert JJ, Young GB, et al. The encephalopathy of sepsis. *Can J Neurol Sci* 1985;12:303–307.
19. Pendlebury WW, Perl DP, Munoz DG. Multiple microabscesses in the central nervous system: a clinicopathologic study. *J Neuropathol Exp Neurol* 1989;48:290–300.
20. Quagliarello VJ, Wispelwey B, Long WJ Jr, et al. Recombinant human interleukin-1 induces meningitis and blood–brain barrier injury in the rat. Characterization and comparison with tumor necrosis factor. *J Clin Invest* 1991;87:1360–1366.
21. du Moulin GC, Paterson D, Hedley-Whyte J, et al. *E. coli* peritonitis and bacteremia cause increased blood–brain barrier permeability. *Brain Res* 1985;340:261–268.
22. Dinarello CA, Cannon JG, Wolff SM. New concepts on

the pathogenesis of fever. *Rev Infect Dis* 1988;10: 168–189.

23. De Sarro GB, Masuda Y, Ascioti C, et al. Behavioural and ECoG spectrum changes induced by intracerebral infusion of interferons and interleukin 2 in rats are antagonized by naloxone. *Neuropharmacology* 1990;29: 167–179.

24. Reyes-Vazquez C, Prieto-Gomez B, Georgiades JA, et al. Alpha and gamma interferons' effects on cortical and hippocampal neurons: microiontophoretic application and single cell recording. *Int J Neurosci* 1984;25:113–121.

25. Kadoi Y, Saito S, Kunimoto F, et al. Impairment of the brain beta-adrenergic system during experimental endotoxemia. *J Surg Res* 1996;61:496–502.

26. Maekawa T, Fujii Y, Sadamitsu D, et al. Cerebral circulation and metabolism in patients with septic encephalopathy. *Am J Emerg Med* 1991;9:139–143.

27. Papadopoulos MC, Davies DC, Moss RF, et al. Pathophysiology of septic encephalopathy: a review. *Crit Care Med* 2000;28:3019–3024.

28. Terborg C, Schummer W, Albrecht M, et al. Dysfunction of vasomotor reactivity in severe sepsis and septic shock. *Int Care Med* 2001;27:1231–1234.

29. Papadopoulos MC, Lamb FJ, Moss RF, et al. Faecal peritonitis causes oedema and neuronal injury in pig cerebral cortex. *Clin Sci (Lond)* 1999;96:461–466.

30. Zhan RZ, Fujiwara N, Shimoji K. Regionally different elevation of intracellular free calcium in hippocampus of septic rat brain. *Shock* 1996;6:293–297.

31. Weeks SG, Silva C, Auer RN, et al. Encephalopathy with staphylococcal endocarditis: multiple neuropathological findings. *Can J Neurol Sci* 2001;28:260–264.

32. Moller K, Strauss GI, Qvist J, et al. Cerebral blood flow and oxidative metabolism during human endotoxemia. *J Cereb Blood Flow Metab* 2002;22:1262–1270.

33. Voigt K, Kontush A, Stuerenburg HJ, et al. Decreased plasma and cerebrospinal fluid ascorbate levels in patients with septic encephalopathy. *Free Radic Res* 2002; 36:735–739.

34. Mizock BA, Sabelli HC, Dubin A, et al. Septic encephalopathy. Evidence for altered phenylalanine metabolism and comparison with hepatic encephalopathy. *Arch Intern Med* 1990;150:443–449.

35. Sprung CL, Cerra FB, Freund HR, et al. Amino acid alterations and encephalopathy in the sepsis syndrome. *Crit Care Med* 1991;19:753–757.

36. Basler T, Meier-Hellmann A, Bredle D, et al. Amino acid imbalance early in septic encephalopathy. *Int Care Med* 2002;28:293–298.

37. Kunze K. Metabolic encephalopathies. *J Neurol* 2002; 249:1150–1159.

38. Towne AR, Waterhouse EJ, Boggs JG, et al. Prevalence of nonconvulsive status epilepticus in comatose patients. *Neurology* 2000;54:340–345.

39. Bleck TP. Sepsis on the brain. *Crit Care Med* 2002;30: 1176–1177.

40. Nora PM, Bleck TP. Increased intracranial pressure complicating acute hepatic failure. *J Crit Illness* 1989; 4:87–96.

41. O'Brien CJ, Wise RJ, O'Grady JG, et al. Neurological sequelae in patients recovered from fulminant hepatic failure. *Gut* 1987;28:93–95.

42. Zaki AE, Ede RJ, Davis M, et al. Experimental studies of blood brain barrier permeability in acute hepatic failure. *Hepatology* 1984;4:359–363.

43. Bleck TP. Neurological consequences of fulminant hepatic failure. *Mayo Clin Proc* 1995;70:195–196.

44. Canalese J, Gimson AE, Davis C, et al. Controlled trial of dexamethasone and mannitol for the cerebral oedema of fulminant hepatic failure. *Gut* 1982;23:625–629.

45. Ede RJ, Gimson AE, Bihari D, et al. Controlled hyperventilation in the prevention of cerebral oedema in fulminant hepatic failure. *J Hepatol* 1986;2:43–51.

46. Forbes A, Alexander GJ, O'Grady JG, et al. Thiopental infusion in the treatment of intracranial hypertension complicating fulminant hepatic failure. *Hepatology* 1989;10:306–310.

47. Davenport A, Will EJ, Davison AM. Effect of posture on intracranial pressure and cerebral perfusion pressure in patients with fulminant hepatic and renal failure after acetaminophen self-poisoning. *Crit Care Med* 1990;18: 286–289.

48. Munoz SJ, Robinson M, Northrup B, et al. Elevated intracranial pressure and computed tomography of the brain in fulminant hepatocellular failure. *Hepatology* 1991;13:209–212.

49. Wijdicks EF, Plevak DJ, Rakela J, et al. Clinical and radiologic features of cerebral edema in fulminant hepatic failure. *Mayo Clin Proc* 1995;70:119–124.

50. Davenport A, Will EJ, Losowsky MS. Rebound surges of intracranial pressure as a consequence of forced ultrafiltration used to control intracranial pressure in patients with severe hepatorenal failure. *Am J Kidney Dis* 1989;14:516–519.

51. Keays R, Potter D, O'Grady J, et al. Intracranial and cerebral perfusion pressure changes before, during and immediately after orthotopic liver transplantation for fulminant hepatic failure. *Q J Med* 1991;79:425–433.

52. Basile AS, Hughes RD, Harrison PM, et al. Elevated brain concentrations of 1,4-benzodiazepines in fulminant hepatic failure. *N Engl J Med* 1991;325:473–478.

53. Jones EA, Basile AS. Does ammonia contribute to increased GABA-ergic neurotransmission in liver failure? *Metab Brain Dis* 1998;13:351–360.

54. Basile AS, Jones EA. The involvement of benzodiazepine receptor ligands in hepatic encephalopathy. *Hepatology* 1994;20:541–543.

55. Bansky G, Meier PJ, Rieder E, et al. Effects of the benzodiazepine receptor antagonist flumazenil in hepatic encephalopathy in humans. *Gastroenterology* 1989;97: 744–750.

56. Grimm G, Ferenci P, Katzenschlager R, et al. Improvement of hepatic encephalopathy treated with flumazenil. *Lancet* 1988;2:1392–1394.

57. Bessman SP, Wang W, Mohan C. Ammonia inhibits insulin stimulation of the Krebs cycle: further insights into the mechanism of hepatic coma. *Neurochem Res* 1991;16:805–811.

58. Blom JH, Ferenci P, Grimm G, et al. The role of methanethiol in the pathogenesis of hepatic coma. *Hepatology* 1991;13:445–454.

59. Bleck TP. Metabolic encephalopathy. In: Weiner WJ, Shulman LM, eds. *Emergent and urgent neurology,* 2nd ed. Philadelphia: Lippincott, 1999:223–253.

60. Tuma R, DeAngelis LM. Altered mental status in patients with cancer. *Arch Neurol* 2000;57:1727–1731.

61. Frucht MM, Bleck TP. Seizures in the intensive care unit patient. In: Delanty M, ed. *Seizures: medical causes and management.* Totowa, NJ: Humana Press, 2002:309–318.

62. Singh BM, Strobos RJ. Epilepsia partialis continua associated with nonketotic hyperglycemia: clinical and biochemical profile of 21 patients. *Ann Neurol* 1980;8: 155–160.

63. Kumar A, Bleck TP. Intravenous midazolam for the treatment of refractory status epilepticus. *Crit Care Med* 1992;20:483–488.

64. Prasad A, Worrall BB, Bertram EH, et al. Propofol and midazolam in the treatment of refractory status epilepticus. *Epilepsia* 2001;42:380–386.

65. Rivner MH, Kim S, Greenberg M, et al. Reversible generalized paresis following hypotension: a new neurological entity. *Neurology* 1983;33(Suppl 2):164.

66. Bolton CF, Brown JD, Sibbald WJ. The electrophysiologic investigation of respiratory paralysis in critically ill patients. *Neurology* 1983;33(Suppl 2):186.

67. Bolton CF, Gilbert JJ, Hahn AF, et al. Polyneuropathy in critically ill patients. *J Neurol Neurosurg Psychiatry* 1984;47:1223–1231.

68. Bolton CF, Laverty DA, Brown JD, et al. Critically ill polyneuropathy: electrophysiologic studies and differentiation from the Guillain-Barre syndrome. *J Neurol Neurosurg Psychiatry* 1986;49:563–573.

69. Zochodne DW, Bolton CF, Wells GA, et al. Critical illness polyneuropathy: a complication of sepsis and multiple organ failure. *Brain* 1987;110:819–842.

70. Segredo V, Caldwell JE, Matthay MA, et al. Persistent paralysis in critically ill patients after long-term administration of vecuronium. *N Engl J Med* 1992;327:524–528.

71. Zochodne DW, Ramsay DA, Saly V, et al. Acute necrotizing myopathy of intensive care: electrophysiological studies. *Muscle Nerve* 1994;17:285–292.

72. Hoffman TA, Ruiz CJ, Counts GW, et al. Waterborne typhoid fever in Dade County, Florida. Clinical and therapeutic evaluation of 105 bacteremic patients. *Am J Med* 1975;59:481–487.

73. Young GB. Neurological complications of systemic critical illness. *Neurol Clin* 1995;13:645–658.

74. Rezaiguia-Delclaux S, Lefaucheur JP, Zakkouri M, et al. Severe acute polyneuropathy complicating orthotopic liver allograft failure. *Transplantation* 2002;74: 880–882.

75. Sheth RD, Bolton CF. Neuromuscular complications of sepsis in children. *J Child Neurol* 1995;10:346–352.

76. Bolton CF. Sepsis and the systemic inflammatory response syndrome: neuromuscular manifestations. *Crit Care Med* 1996;24:1408–1416.

77. Bleck TP. The expanding spectrum of critical illness polyneuropathy. *Crit Care Med* 1996;24:1282–1283.

78. Hund EF, Fogel W, Krieger D, et al. Critical illness polyneuropathy: clinical findings and outcomes of a frequent cause of neuromuscular weaning failure. *Crit Care Med* 1996;24:1328–1333.

79. Bolton CF. AAEM minimonograph 340: clinicl neurophysiology of the respiratory system. *Muscle Nerve* 1993;16:809–818.

80. Feigin RD, Dodge PR. Bacterial meningitis: newer concepts of pathophysiology and neurological sequelae. *Pediatr Clin North Am* 1976;23:541–556.

81. Griffin JW, Li CY, Ho TW, et al. Pathology of the motor-sensory axonal Guillain-Barre syndrome. *Ann Neurol* 1996;39:17–28.

82. Kelly BJ, Matthay MA. Prevalence and severity of neurological dysfunction in critically ill patients. Influence on need for continued mechanical ventilation. *Chest* 1993;104:1818–1824.

83. Spitzer AR, Giancarlo T, Maher L, et al. Neuromuscular causes of prolonged ventilator dependency. *Muscle Nerve* 1992;15:682–686.

84. Rich MM, Teener JW, Raps EC, et al. Muscle is electrically inexcitable in acute quadriplegic myopathy. *Neurology* 1996;46:731–736.

85. Sander HW, Golden M, Danon MJ. Quadriplegic areflexic ICU illness: selective thick filament loss and normal nerve histology. *Muscle Nerve* 2002;26:499–505.

12

Head Injury

Head trauma remains a major health predicament despite extensive preventive efforts. The magnitude of the problem can be appreciated by pointing out that approximately 2 million people suffer head injuries in the United States each year. Of these, approximately 100,000 die and almost as many are left with long-term disabilities. The cost of caring for these patients in the United States approaches $25 billion each year.

Over the past three decades general developments in the field of critical care have helped reduce mortality in patients with severe traumatic brain injury (TBI) (1). More recently, a number of developments that have focused specifically on the treatment of intracranial injuries have paralleled the growth of the field of neurological critical care. Evidence-based guidelines were developed in an effort to define and standardize the treatment of patients with severe TBI (2). Also, new devices have become available to monitor head-injured patients. Currently, our understanding of the pathophysiology of head injury is evolving. For example, the concept that ischemia is a major cause of ongoing injury in severe TBI is being questioned and mitochondrial dysfunction has been proposed as the cause of metabolic suppression of neuronal function after injury (3,4).

This chapter focuses on the intensive care unit (ICU) treatment of patients with severe head injury, defined generally as comprising those patients with a Glasgow Coma Scale (GCS) score less than 9 after initial resuscitation (the well-known GCS is shown in Table 12.1). Throughout the chapter reference is made to the TBI guidelines, which were developed jointly by the Brain Trauma Foundation, American Association of Neurological Surgeons, Congress of Neurological Surgeons, and Joint Section on Neurotrauma and Critical Care (2) and updated in 2000 (5–10). This effort was undertaken to establish an evidence-based approach to guidelines for the treatment of patients with severe head injury. The literature was reviewed and the recommendations of these groups were classified as a:

> 1) Standard of care: high degree of clinical certainty, usually class I (prospective randomized controlled trial) evidence; 2) Guideline: moderate degree of clinical certainty, class II (observational, cohort, prevalence, and case-control studies) evidence; and 3) Options: unclear clinical certainty, class III (retrospective case series, registries, case reports, and expert opinion) evidence.

This approach, although perhaps omitting some nuances that should be known to neurointensivists and others interested in head trauma, is nonetheless the most comprehensive and well-considered summary of current thinking on the subject. Use is also made of the traumatic Coma Data Bank [a National Institutes of Health (NIH)–funded multicenter project to study patients with severe TBI] that should be familiar to all intensivists (11–15).

PRIMARY AND SECONDARY CEREBRAL INJURY

Primary injuries, those that occur at the time of the trauma, can only be ameliorated

TABLE 12.1. *Glasgow coma scale*

Eye opening	
Spontaneous	4
To voice	3
To pain	2
None	1
Verbal response	
Oriented	5
Confused	4
Inappropriate	3
Incomprehensible sounds	2
None	1
Motor response	
Obeys commands	6
Localizes pain	5
Withdraws to pain	4
Flexion response to pain	3
Extension response to pain	2
None	1

by prevention. These include crushing or laceration of the brain and large hematomas. Secondary injury refers to the intracranial and systemic factors that cause ongoing and potentially reversible injury. In some instances the delineation is not quite so clear; for example, brain contusion and vascular injury have irreversible mechanical or necrotic, and partly reversible subcellular components, the latter being subsumed by the currently fashionable term "apoptosis" (16–18). In order to provide rational and effective care, it is essential to understand the mechanisms responsible for secondary injury. To date, most ICU treatment has focused on the control of elevated intracranial pressure (ICP) and on maintaining adequate cerebral perfusion pressure (CPP) and there have been several unsuccessful trials of neuroprotective agents (19,20). The latter address the somewhat controversial concept that ischemia is an important cause of secondary damage after head injury. From these approaches we have learned that extremes of high ICP and low CPP are clearly harmful, but the importance of other factors within those other pressure limits remains uncertain. As we gain an understanding of the cause of metabolic depression in the pathophysiology of head injury, we may advance our ability to treat severe cases.

Intracranial Pressure and Cerebral Perfusion Pressure

Intracranial hypertension occurs in approximately 40% of patients suffering persistent traumatic loss of consciousness (21), and mortality rises with increased ICP (22) (Chapters 2 and 3). These observations have led to the logical (but not necessarily valid) assumption that lowering ICP leads to improved outcome.

The manner in which elevated ICP causes neurological injury is incompletely understood. As discussed in Chapter 2, elevated ICP in the setting of low or normal blood pressure can result in a critical reduction in CPP and inadequate delivery of oxygen and glucose to maintain neuronal viability. The definition of this CPP threshold is discussed in the following. If this were the only manner by which elevated ICP caused injury, however, the problem could be overcome by simply raising blood pressure to sufficient levels. Analysis of the Traumatic Coma Databank supports the concept that intracranial hypertension is harmful even in the setting of adequate CCP. In a multiple regression analysis, elevated ICP remained an independent predictor of poor outcome after controlling for CPP, age, GCS motor score, and other factors (23,24).

One mechanism, albeit indirect, through which elevated ICP may cause damage is by the creation of pressure gradients. When bilateral ICP monitors were placed in patients with unilateral mass lesions the difference in ICP between hemispheres was as high as 15 mm Hg (25,26). These gradients develop as a result of the dural reflections that divide the intracranial space into a number of compartments, and occasionally by asymmetric ventricular enlargement. These pressure gradients can produce tissue shifts and eventually herniation and coma.

Cerebral Blood Flow and Metabolism

Ischemia

Disturbances of cerebral blood flow (CBF) following severe TBI has been the focus of considerable attention and has led to the assumption that ischemia was a major cause of secondary brain injury. This concept should be viewed in the context of pathologic studies performed in the 1970s; ischemic neuronal damage was a common finding in the brains of patients who died following TBI (27,28). However, the population studied was skewed because only patients whose initial injury was severe enough to be fatal were included. In addition, the pathologic findings could have resulted from systemic hypotension, hypoxia, or aggressive hyperventilation. Some regions of ischemia were attributed to vasospasm, a phenomenon that has been difficult to corroborate and is not reflected in the more global reduction in flow summarized below. Thus, the frequency of ischemia in patients who survive with present-day treatment, the time period during which it occurs, its contribution to secondary injury, and its impact on outcome are not known.

Physiologic studies performed 20 or more years ago found hemispheric CBF to be moderately reduced in most patients 1 to 2 days after TBI (29,30), whereas others reported hyperemic hemispheric flow (normal or elevated CBF in comatose patients) in over 50% of patients studied within 96 hours of trauma. More recent studies performed during the first few hours after injury found hemispheric CBF to be low in most cases (24,31). In studies performed very early after injury (average of 3.1 hours), Bouma and coworkers (32) reported global or regional CBF of <18 mL/100 g per minute (considered to be a critical level for ischemic damage) in one third of patients. Subsequent studies that included patients with mass lesions (33) also found regional CBF below this threshold in almost 30% of patients studied within 4 hours, and in 20% of patients studied 4 to 8 hours after injury. Furthermore, low blood flow was associated with poor outcome (34).

Several studies of global cerebral metabolic rate for oxygen ($CMRO_2$) using simultaneous sampling of arterial and jugular venous blood have reported low global $CMRO_2$ (29,34–36). $CMRO_2$ also was found to corre-

late with the level of consciousness (35,36) and outcome (23).

The oxygen/lactic acid index, derived from arterial and jugular venous blood, also has been used to define cerebral ischemia (37,38). Some caution needs to be exercised in the interpretation of lactate levels because increased brain lactate production can occur in the presence of adequate CBF and oxygen delivery (39,40). In addition, increased levels of lactate also may result from the accumulation of white blood cells following TBI (41–43), or reduced clearance of lactate caused by low CBF.

The arteriovenous difference in oxygen content ($a\text{-}vDO_2$) has been used to assess for global ischemia following TBI. Normal values for $a\text{-}vDO_2$ range from approximately 4.5 vol% to 9 vol% (44–47). When ischemia was defined as $a\text{-}vDO_2$ <10 vol% Obrist found evidence of ischemia in only one of 75 TBI patients (35).

Recently, a number of studies have suggested an alternative explanation for reduced CBF following TBI. There is a growing body of evidence that following TBI, subarachnoid hemorrhage (48), and intracerebral hemorrhage (49), metabolic suppression may be the primary event and this is followed by a passive fall in CBF. Using a number of experimental models of TBI, investigators have found impaired mitochondrial function (4,50), which results in diminished ATP production. Preliminary positron emission tomography (PET) studies in TBI patients have suggested that there may be a compensatory rise in glucose use (51). Recently, biopsies from a small series of patients with severe TBI also demonstrated impaired mitochondrial function, and some have proposed that mitochondrial function may be used as a surrogate efficacy measure for preclinical studies of head injury (50).

If it is confirmed that mitochondrial function is impaired following TBI, it will fundamentally affect how TBI patients are treated. Current approaches to treatment focus on improving CBF and delivery of energy substrates (oxygen and glucose). If the limiting factor in ATP synthesis is the inability of the

TABLE 12.2. *Computed tomography classification system of head injury*

Diffuse injury I	No visible pathology seen on computed tomography
Diffuse injury II	Cisterns are present with shift 0–5 mm. No high- or mixed-density lesion >25 cc. May include bone fragments and foreign bodies
Diffuse injury III (swelling)	Cisterns compressed or absent. Shift 0–5 mm. No high- or mixed-density lesion >25 cc
Diffuse injury IV (shift)	Shift >5 mm. No high- or mixed-density lesion >25 cc
Evacuated mass lesion	Any lesion surgically evacuated
Nonevacuated mass lesion	High- or mixed-density lesion >25 cc not surgically evacuated

From Marshall SB, Klauber MR, Van Berkum C, et al. The diagnosis of head injury requires a classification based on computed axial tomography. *J Neurotrauma* 1992;9:S287–S292, with permission.

mitochondria to use oxygen, then improving delivery may not have much impact. Instead treatment strategies should be directed toward improving mitochondrial function.

The question of ischemia remains unresolved at present. If present it is most likely limited to the first few hours following injury. During that period maintaining adequate blood pressure is essential (see the following) and management of elevated ICP is appropriate. Whether continuing to aggressively treat ICP and CPP in the subsequent days is useful is uncertain; such efforts should be integrated with the patient's overall clinical status.

PROGNOSTICATING AND CLASSIFYING HEAD TRAUMA

Computed Tomography Classification

Early classifications of computed tomography (CT) findings in TBI separated patients with intracerebral clots or large contusions

from those with little or no obvious intracranial pathology. The hematomas were further classified as epidural, subdural, or intracerebral. It appears, however, that patients without intracerebral mass lesions are a not homogeneous group and that examination of the cisterns and the position of normally midline structures yields additional prognostic information. A new scheme (52), which has become widely adopted, categorizes CT finding by the six categories listed in Table 12.2.

When applied to the Traumatic Coma Databank population this classification provides prognostic information as summarized in Table 12.3.

Early Prognostic Factors

Systemic insults that occur prior to the patient's arrival in the Emergency Department have a profound influence on outcome. A prospective multicenter study (53) of 717 TBI

TABLE 12.3. *Outcome based on computed tomography (CT) classification of head injury*

Intracranial diagnosis	Percent of category	Discharge Glasgow outcome score		
		Good/moderate	Vegetative	Dead
Diffuse injury I	7.0	62	29	10
Diffuse injury II	24	35	52	14
Diffuse injury III	21	16	50	34
Diffuse injury IV	4	6	38	56
Evacuated mass	37	23	38	39
Nonevacuated mass	5	11	36	53
Brainstem injury	1	0	33	67
TOTAL	100	26	42	33

From Marshall SB, Klauber MR, Van Berkum C, et al. The diagnosis of head injury requires a classification based on computed axial tomography. *J Neurotrauma* 1992;9:S287–S292, with permission.

patients identified the impact of prehospital hypoxia or hypotension on outcome. The major findings are summarized in Table 12.4. The special attention that should be afforded to early hypotension and hypoxia have been corroborated by other studies. To a large extent these problems occur prior to hospitalization and it has never been clarified if they are avoidable or simply reflect the degree of injury and parallel systemic injuries. Nonetheless, these systemic alterations should be attended to as quickly as possible.

A number of clinical and x-ray features that can be assessed shortly after arrival in the Emergency Department also provide important prognostic information. Three clinical variables have been consistently identified (not surprisingly) as independent predictors of outcome in severe TBI: age, postresuscitation GCS motor score, and pupillary reactivity (54,55). Analyses using a prediction tree (56) and neural network (57) have produced similar results. Radiologic factors that provide prognostic information include the condition of the basal cisterns (normal, partial, or complete obliteration) and the presence of mass lesions and midline shift (58,59). In patients with civilian gunshot wounds, additional poor prognostic factors include presence of subarachnoid or intraventricular blood (12).

SPECIFIC CRANIAL INJURIES

Skull Fracture

Skull fractures are classified as simple (linear), comminuted, depressed, or basilar. They are considered either closed or open, depending on whether there is an overlying scalp laceration. Skull fractures seen on plain radiographs suggest significant underlying pathology and should be followed up with a CT scan. Most skull fractures are linear and usually are located in the temporoparietal region, overlying the middle meningeal artery. Open depressed skull fractures usually are surgically debrided. When appropriate, this is accompanied by elevation of the depressed skull fragments, repair of any underlying dural laceration, and evacuation of any accompanying hematoma.

Hemotympanum, raccoon eyes (bilateral periorbital ecchymosis), Battle's sign (superficial ecchymosis over the mastoid process), otorrhea, or rhinorrhea usually indicate a basilar skull fracture. It is important to note that Battle's sign generally takes more than 12 hours to appear. Rhinorrhea is seen with fractures of the frontal bone and otorrhea with fractures of the middle fossa that extend into the middle ear. It is important not to plug the external ear but rather to allow free egress of CSF to reduce the risk of infection. Prophylactic antibiotics are not generally recommended because they can select for more aggressive organisms (60,61). Most CSF leaks resolve spontaneously in 7 to 10 days; otorrhea resolves spontaneously in a higher percentage of cases than rhinorrhea. Basilar skull fractures may be confirmed on the routine CT cuts traversing the base of the skull, but definitive diagnosis often requires thin cuts through that region.

TABLE 12.4. *Impact of prehospital hypotension and hypoxia on outcome*

Secondary insult	n	Good or moderate disability (%)	Severe disability or vegetative (%)	Dead (%)
None	456	11	22	27
Hypoxia (PaO$_2$ <60)	78	45	22	33
Hypotension (SBP <90)	113	26	14	60
Both	52	6	19	75
TOTAL CASES	699	43	20	37

SBP, systolic blood pressure.
From Chesnut RM, Marshall LF, Klauber MR, et al. The role of secondary brain injury in determining outcome from severe head injury. *J Trauma* 1993;34:216–222, with permission.

The petrous bone may be involved in fractures of the skull base. Longitudinal fractures are more common and account for approximately 50% of facial palsies seen in basilar skull fracture. They can cause delayed facial paresis 5 to 7 days after the injury, perhaps caused by swelling of the perineural tissues. This pattern of nerve injury has an excellent prognosis for full recovery. Longitudinal fractures also are more often associated with disruption of the dura and subsequent leak of CSF into the middle ear. Otorrhea may result if the tympanic membrane is also torn.

Cerebral Contusion

Hemorrhagic cerebral contusions are very common in severely head-injured patients. Contusions may result from direct external forces (e.g., those underlying depressed skull fractures), the brain's contact with rough intracranial surfaces (often occurring in the deep frontal and anterior temporal regions), or pure acceleration/deceleration injuries (e.g., the contrecoup injury seen opposite from the site of direct impact). Contusions generally are evident on CT scans and may be a source of significant mass effect. They may occur initially or appear over the ensuing 24 to 72 hours as the small hemorrhages coalesce and edema forms. Contusions in the temporal poles pose a significant threat of sudden deterioration because of their direct proximity to the upper brainstem. These patients may show signs of herniation at ICP levels that are considered normal otherwise.

Intracranial Hematomas

Early CT scanning of patients with abnormal neurological examinations, fractures on skull films, or injury with substantial force is now routine. The management of subdural and intracerebral hematomas depends on their mass effect. Such lesions often are removed or drained if they cause a shift in the midline of greater than 5 mm or are associated with intracranial hypertension. A more complete accounting of this subject can be found in standard neurosurgical textbooks.

Delayed Traumatic Intracerebral Hematoma

Delayed traumatic intracerebral hemorrhage is defined as a hemorrhage that develops in brain regions that appeared normal or nearly so on the initial CT scan. They are reported to occur in 1% to 8% of patients with severe head injury (62,63) and usually develop within 48 hours of trauma but can occur rarely as late as 2 weeks (64). Neurological deterioration is common at the time of these hemorrhages; thus any neurological worsening not clearly referable to other factors should be investigated with a CT scan. The pathogenesis of these hematomas may include coagulation abnormalities, necrosis of blood vessels, impaired autoregulation, and release of the tamponade effect with evacuation of extraaxial hematomas but most are unexplained.

Diffuse Axonal Injury

There are a number of patients with clinically severe head injury but a relatively unremarkable CT scan. Although the "classic" image of diffuse axonal injury (DAI) shows multiple petechial white matter hemorrhages, particularly in the corpus callosum and brainstem, CT scans may be normal. One explanation for the condition is shearing of nerve fibers at the time of head injury (65,66). Pathologic findings consist of focal hemorrhages or lacerations in the corpus callosum, deep white matter, and brainstem. It may well be that CT scanning is not sensitive to the changes in these patients. Magnetic resonance imaging shows many more scattered small regions of white matter damage than CT (see Fig. 9.1, page 155). Patients with DAI characteristically present with coma. About half develop intracranial hypertension with CT evidence of diffuse edema and compressed cisterns and have a poor prognosis (67).

PREHOSPITAL MANAGEMENT AND INITIAL STABILIZATION

Initial stabilization of trauma patients always should begin with the ABCs. Because of the deleterious effects of hypoxia on head injuries particular attention must be paid to the airway. Premedication should be provided for intubation. Etomidate (Chapter 3) is especially useful because it is short-acting, may be neuroprotective (by suppressing metabolism), and has less tendency than other agents to produce hypotension. Often it is possible to achieve adequate visualization of the airway using sedatives alone, in which case paralytic agents should be avoided so as not to make assessment of neurological function impossible. If necessary, short-acting agents should be used.

At the same time, any existing hypotension should be aggressively corrected. To achieve a rapid correction of blood pressure, vasopressors should be administered while giving intravenous (i.v.) fluids and blood products as needed. The TBI guidelines (2,5,9,22) recommend maintaining mean arterial blood pressure above 90 mm Hg.

No data exist regarding the empiric treatment of raised ICP immediately following severe TBI. Intracranial pressure is usually not elevated initially, except when there is diffuse edema or a mass lesion. The TBI guidelines recommend that no specific treatment should be directed at intracranial hypertension unless there are signs of transtentorial herniation or progressive neurological deterioration not attributable to extracranial causes. Patients who show a dilated pupil and asymmetric posturing on presentation, or have neurological deterioration not owing to extracranial causes, should be empirically treated for presumed intracranial hypertension. The usual measures (discussed in greater detail in Chapter 3) include hyper-

ventilation to a P_{CO_2} of approximately 25 mm Hg and mannitol (1 to 1.5 g/kg) rapidly administered with special attention to providing adequate volume replacement in order to avoid hypotension. A CT scan must be obtained urgently to identify any mass lesion amenable to surgical resection.

Sedation may be essential in the early evaluation and management of agitated or combative patients. Again, the ideal agents should be short-acting and easily controlled and have no risk of hypotension. Several agents are available with varying degrees of these characteristics, including morphine, fentanyl, lorazepam, midazolam, etomidate, and propofol. On the other hand, the prolonged routine use of neuromuscular blocking agents should be avoided. Use of paralytic agents has been shown to increase ICU length of stay and result in a higher incidence of pneumonia with no change in neurological outcome (68).

Once the patient has been stabilized, a CT scan should be obtained as soon as possible. The patient is taken directly to the operating room if the CT scan demonstrates a surgical intracranial lesion; otherwise, the patient is transported to the ICU. The indications for surgery are beyond the scope of this book. The reader is referred to standard neurosurgical texts.

INTENSIVE CARE UNIT MANAGEMENT

The ICU is central to the treatment of patients with severe TBI. Although the primary focus is on detecting and treating worsening neurological function, a number of systemic factors must be addressed in order to optimize outcome. Cardiopulmonary function may be disturbed because of trauma or preexisting medical conditions. Extracranial injuries can be multiple and serious and require close management in conjunction with trauma surgeons. Traumatic brain-injured patients enter a catabolic state requiring supplemental calories and protein. They are prone to a number of complications, including coagulopathy, gastrointestinal bleeding, deep venous thromboses, pulmonary emboli, and frequent pulmonary and urinary tract infections.

Monitoring of Neurological Status

The mainstay of neurological monitoring is serial assessment of neurological function. For patients with severe TBI, this typically includes hourly, or every other-hourly assessment of the ability to follow commands, orientation, pupillary reactivity, corneal reflexes, motor strength, and the GCS.

Often the ability to detect clinical deterioration is limited in these patients by their depressed level of neurological function and the use of sedative medications. Therefore, the neurological examination is supplemented with monitoring of cerebral physiology.

Intracranial Pressure Monitoring

Intracranial pressure monitoring can be useful for a number of purposes, but controversies regarding its use abound and differing opinions can be found even within major institutions, as noted in Chapters 2 and 3 and further commented on in the following. A steadily rising ICP should generally prompt a CT scan in order to detect delayed hematomas or expanding edema surrounding a contusion. This is especially important in patients who are difficult to examine because of sedation. In addition, monitoring ICP helps avoid the indiscriminate use of measures to reduce ICP, all of which have deleterious side effects. If a ventriculostomy is being used, drainage of CSF also can be used to help control elevated pressure. Finally, ICP monitoring provides prognostic information.

A prospective randomized controlled study of the impact of ICP monitoring has not been performed. Uncontrolled data collected shortly after the introduction of ICP monitoring indicated that mortality was lower following the institution of routine ICP monitoring when compared to historical controls (22,69). However, use of historical controls does not take into account the possibility that other changes in management occurred at the time the institution introduced routine ICP monitoring. In addition, it is argued that treatment of ICP improves outcome because patients who respond to treatment of elevated ICP have lesser degrees of injury than patients in whom ICP could not be controlled (70). Comparing responders to nonresponders does not take into account the possibility that patients with less severe injury (and a better prognosis) are more likely to respond to treatment. Despite a paucity of data, ICP monitoring is considered the standard of care in selected patients with severe TBI and is used in most patients who are unresponsive or stuporous after injury if for no other reason than to avoid iatrogenic causes of raised ICP.

In general, the decision to place an ICP monitor is based on the patient's risk for intracranial hypertension. The TBI guidelines recommend that ICP monitoring is appropriate in severe head injury patients with: (a) an abnormal admission CT scan (presence of hematoma, contusions, edema, or compressed basal cisterns); and (b) a normal CT scan if they have at least two of the following: age greater than 40, unilateral or bilateral motor posturing, systolic blood pressure (BP) less than 90.

Jugular Bulb Catheters

Some trauma centers routinely place a fiberoptic catheter in the jugular bulb to allow for continuous monitoring of jugular venous saturation ($SjvO_2$) as well as collection of blood samples for direct measurement of jugular venous oxygen content. These values can be used to monitor how closely CBF and oxygen metabolism are matched. The relationship between arterial and cerebral-venous blood is expressed as the absolute difference in oxygen content ($a\text{-}vDO_2$). A widened $a\text{-}vDO_2$ (less than 10 vol%) indicates a relative deficiency in CBF in relation to metabolic needs.

When $CMRO_2$ is stable, any fall in cerebral oxygen delivery (reduced CBF or oxygen content) results in a fall in $SjvO_2$. Thus, a fall in SjvO$_2$ (or widening of a-vDO$_2$) indicates CBF/CMRO$_2$ mismatch but does not identify its cause. One study found that falls in SjvO$_2$ were almost always owing to reduced CPP (intracranial hypertension or systemic hypotension), arterial hypoxia, or hypocarbia (71).

Several issues can complicate the interpretation of SjvO$_2$ values. In one study, almost two thirds of the falls in SjvO$_2$ identified by a fiberoptic catheter were not confirmed when blood samples were measured with a cooximeter (71). Contamination with extracerebral blood also can lead to erroneous information (72). In addition, when bilateral jugular bulb catheters were placed in TBI patients the differences in saturation were as high as 15% in almost half the patients studied (73). Finally, TBI often results in focal cerebral injury and SjvO$_2$ measurements give no information about regional changes such as might occur in contused brain or surrounding hematomas.

Jugular venous desaturations to less than 50% for greater than 10 minutes are more common in patients with low CBF and are associated with poor neurological outcome (74). Frequent causes of desaturations in that study were intracranial hypertension, systemic hypotension, hypocarbia, and arterial hypoxia. It is not known if these desaturations indicate ongoing damage or are a manifestation of an already damaged brain.

Computed Tomography Scanning

The possibility of a surgically accessible intracranial lesion should be constantly kept in mind. Hydrocephalus, infarction, coalescence of an area of contusion, or delayed intraaxial or extraaxial hematomas can exacerbate intracranial hypertension (75,76). Patients with difficult-to-control intracranial hypertension or unexpected elevations in ICP should be considered for repeat CT scanning.

Brain Tissue Oxygen Tension

Recently, an oxygen electrode has become available that measures oxygen tension within the brain substance. The probe is placed either alone or in conjunction with an ICP monitor. Several studies in TBI patients have attempted to determine the relationship between "brain tissue" oxygen tension (PbtO$_2$) and outcome. In 101 patients with severe TBI, the depth and duration of low PbtO$_2$ was an independent predictor of poor outcome (77). The threshold for mortality was identified by the duration of a PbtO$_2$ of less than 15 mm Hg or any PbtO$_2$ less than 7 mm Hg (78). More recent studies have suggested that the value of PbtO$_2$ best correlates with CBF (79,80).

It is important to recognize that the probe only gives information about a small focal region of brain. Thus, unlike jugular bulb catheters they give regional not global information (78). Oxygen electrodes have become a very useful research tool; however, their role, if any, in the routine treatment of TBI patients has yet to be defined.

Brain Specific Treatments

The relative role of intracranial hypertension and reduced CPP in causing secondary brain injury are incompletely understood. Even assuming that CPP can be accurately measured, what remains unclear are the ICP and CPP thresholds for global hypoperfusion, and the likelihood that elevated ICP causes injury if CPP remains adequate. Without definitive answers to these questions, competing management strategies have evolved; namely, "ICP" and "CPP" management. In the former, aggressive treatment of ICP is given paramount importance and elevated BP may be lowered to prevent cerebral edema associated with hyperperfusion (81,82). In the latter approach, BP is raised using vasopressors to maintain CPP greater than 70 mm Hg (2,83) and measures to reduce ICP are instituted if ICP exceeds 25 mm Hg.

There is no clear answer as to which of these approaches is more appropriate, but two recent studies have addressed this issue. One study randomized over 300 patients to "ICP" versus "CBF" management. In the ICP management group, measures (sedation, osmotic agents, hyperventilation) were used to treat elevated ICP and blood pressure was only raised if CPP fell below 50 mm Hg. In the CBF management group, CPP was maintained over 70 mm Hg at all times and ICP was treated if it exceeded 20 mm Hg. The primary end point of the study was the number of jugular venous desaturations (less than 50%). The investigators found that although the frequency of jugular bulb catheter desaturations was lower in the CPP-managed group, clinical outcome was no different. Those authors suggest that this result arose because measures were taken to correct jugular bulb catheter desaturation, thus preventing any negative impact on outcome (84).

A second study had opposite results. In a retrospective analysis of the placebo arm of a trial (85) in severe head injury, the relative contributions of ICP and CPP to outcome were assessed. The analysis indicated that the most powerful predictor of neurological deterioration was an ICP greater than 20 mm Hg and that there was no relationship between CPP and outcome when CPP was greater than 60 mm Hg.

Until these issues are resolved, it seems appropriate to treat ICP and CPP simultaneously. Cerebral perfusion pressure should be maintained above a minimal value, independent of ICP. Taken together, recent studies suggest that this threshold is about 50 to 60 mm Hg. It also seems prudent to avoid excessively high CPP that can exacerbate edema and hemorrhage. This upper limit is harder to define based on our current state of knowledge, but 90 to 100 mm Hg seems reasonable. At the same time, ICP should be treated if it exceeds 20 to 25 mm Hg (see the following).

Management of Elevated Intracranial Pressure

A threshold for initiating treatment must be established in order to make sensible use of ICP monitoring (Chapter 3). To determine this level, the impact of raised ICP on outcome was examined in 5-mm Hg increments (0 to 80 mm Hg) while controlling for multiple potential confounding factors. An analysis of prospectively collected data on 426 patients found that the proportion of hourly ICP values greater than 20 was a strong predictor of poor outcome (86). This, of course, does not address the impact of treatment. In fact, different centers in this study used different thresholds for treatment, confounding the interpretation. Another study found that mortality was reduced following a change in the threshold for treatment from 20 to 25 mm Hg to 15 mm Hg (87). However, there were other protocol changes that confound the data. The current TBI guidelines suggest that: (a) ICP treatment should be initiated at an upper threshold of 20 to 25 mm Hg (Guideline) and (b) interpretation and treatment of ICP based on any particular threshold should be corroborated by frequent clinical examination and CPP data (Option).

The rationale for and principles of treatment of intracranial hypertension are discussed extensively in Chapter 3. This discussion reviews the application of those principles to the treatment of patients with severe TBI.

Cerebrospinal Fluid Drainage

Drainage of cerebrospinal fluid (CSF) through a ventricular catheter, even in the presence of normal- or small-sized ventricles, can rapidly reduce ICP. Many centers routinely use CSF drainage as the first intervention in treating intracranial hypertension in TBI patients (8). Even in patients who are monitored by means other than ventricular access, the placement of a ventricular drain should be considered when other modalities cease to provide adequate control of ICP. One difficulty with drainage of CSF in the presence of small ventricles, however, is ventricular collapse around the catheter, which halts the flow of CSF and temporarily or permanently occludes the catheter. The risks of ventricular drainage, particularly infection, are discussed in Chapter 3.

Sedation

The obvious drawback of sedatives is their effect on clinical neurological assessment. In some situations short-acting agents may reasonably be used in order to allow periodic cessation of sedation to facilitate neurological assessment. In others, it may be more prudent to continue sedation and rely on an examination limited to cranial nerve and motor function in conjunction with ICP monitoring, serial imaging studies, and possibly other monitoring tools.

The utility and wisdom of periodically "awakening" TBI patients for neurological assessment are debated. On "awakening" some patients may become wildly agitated and have marked rises in ICP that become difficult to control. On the other hand, such an approach has been reported to reduce the duration of mechanical ventilation and ICU length of stay and to reduce the number of other tests required to assess neurological function (88). The choice of approach should be standardized in a given ICU and should take into account the patient's response to a trial of discontinued medication, the intracranial compliance, and the nature of the underlying traumatic injuries. Thus, in patients who become agitated, difficult to manage and have a significant rise in ICP when sedation is reduced should remain sedated and not undergo periodic "awakening."

Pharmacologic Neuromuscular Paralysis

In the absence of severely compromised pulmonary function, there is little need for paralytic agents in the management of elevated ICP or brain tissue shifts. Although they are effective in controlling agitation and "bucking" the ventilator, these benefits can be achieved with appropriate doses of sedatives and use of alternate modes of ventilation (pressure support) without complicating the situation by complete loss of the motor and cranial nerve examinations. These agents also eliminate coughing, can accumulate in the presence of liver or renal disease, and have

been linked to critical illness polyneuropathy (89,90) as discussed in Chapter 11. The routine use of paralytic drugs in head injury patients has been associated with longer length of stay and a higher incidence of pneumonia (91). However, their intermittent use may serve a purpose when a patient must remain absolutely motionless during radiologic or other procedures or to absolutely eliminate muscle artifact from an EEG study that is difficult to interpret. Paralytic agents should not be administered without sedatives unless there is a high certainty that there is a deep coma from the injury.

Hyperventilation

Hyperventilation has long been a mainstay for ICP reduction (Chapter 3). It is clear that in many situations acute hyperventilation can lower ICP and briefly reverse the signs of herniation. What is not clear is whether there is an impact on outcome. Hyperventilation improves CPP by lowering ICP and thus is presumed to raise CBF. On the other hand, hyperventilation reduces ICP through cerebral vasoconstriction, which reduces CBF. Monitoring of jugular bulb saturation has been proposed as a means to monitor whether hyperventilation is potentially causing injury from hypoperfusion because repeated desaturations below 50% have been associated with poor outcome in TBI patients (74).

Hyperventilation also may act in another way to ameliorate injury. When initiated solely in response to clinical indications of "herniation" (coma, dilated pupil, motor posturing), hyperventilation can reverse these signs. The mechanisms responsible for this response are not clear but might include local improvement of CBF in compressed tissues or regional reduction in the volume of the herniating brain with reversal of tissue shifts.

Despite a considerable number of studies of hyperventilation in head injury, there is only one prospective controlled outcome study (92). That study compared chronic prophylactic hyperventilation to a $PaCO_2$ of 25 mm Hg for 5 days after severe head injury to normocapnia. At 6 months it was found that the subgroup with GCS motor scores of 4 to 5 had a worse outcome; however, the difference did not persist at 1 year. Overall, the conclusion was that prophylactic hyperventilation was of little benefit if used for a prolonged period and is potentially harmful.

The TBI guidelines recommend that:

> 1) In the absence of increased ICP, chronic prolonged hyperventilation ($PaCO_2$ less than 35 mm Hg) should be avoided after severe head injury (Standard); 2) the use of prophylactic hyperventilation ($PaCO_2$ less than 35 mm Hg) during the first 24 hours after severe head injury should be avoided because it can compromise cerebral perfusion when CBF is reduced (Guideline); 3) hyperventilation may be necessary for brief periods when there is acute neurological deterioration, or for longer periods if there is intracranial hypertension refractory to sedation, paralysis, CSF drainage, and osmotic diuretics (Option); (see p. 189) 4) jugular venous saturation, arterial–jugular oxygen content differences, and CBF monitoring may help to identify cerebral ischemia if hyperventilation, resulting in $PaCO_2$ values less than 30 mm Hg, is necessary (Option).

A more recent prospective PET study found that acute hyperventilation to a $PaCO_2$ of 30 within 24 hours of head injury lowered CBF without changing cerebral metabolism (93). This indicates that oxygen delivery was adequately maintained with this degree of hyperventilation. In a subsequent study of patients with severe TBI, the regional change in metabolism was determined before and after hyperventilation to $PaCO_2$ of 25 mm Hg (94). $CMRO_2$ did not fall even in regions where CBF fell below 10 mL/100 g per minute (well below the threshold for injury in ischemic stroke). Thus, acute hyperventilation appears safe from the perspective of causing ischemia. However, this study did not address overall outcome.

In our view, in patients who demonstrate signs of herniation or sudden neurological deterioration, hyperventilation appears to be a safe means of temporarily lowering ICP while further evaluation takes place and other measures are instituted to control ICP. In addition, transient hyperventilation can be used during plateau waves to help reduce ICP.

Osmotic Agents

It is widely accepted that mannitol can reduce ICP, improve CPP, and reverse neurological deterioration. It also appears to reduce blood viscosity and raise CBF (95). As discussed in Chapter 3, mannitol establishes an osmotic gradient between the intracellular and extracellular compartments of the brain that results in movement of water from the former to the latter and improves brain compliance. Mannitol acts as an osmotic diuretic when excreted in the urine, reducing body water and increasing serum osmolality.

There are no studies that prove that the use of mannitol improves outcome in TBI patients. One prospective randomized study comparing mannitol to barbiturates as the initial intervention for ICP control and found no difference in overall mortality (96). However, mortality was higher in those receiving barbiturates in the subgroup with diffuse injury on CT scan. The use of pentobarbital was associated with significant hypotension, which could have increased mortality in that group.

The TBI guidelines recommend that:

> 1) Mannitol is effective for control of raised ICP. Limited data suggest that intermittent boluses may be more effective than continuous infusion. Effective doses range from 0.25 to 1 g/kg (Guideline), 2) The indication for the use of mannitol prior to the institution of ICP monitoring include signs of transtentorial herniation or progressive neurological deterioration not attributable to systemic pathology (Option), 3) Serum osmolality should be kept below 320 mOsm because of concern for renal failure (Option), 4) Euvolemia should be maintained by adequate fluid replacement (Option).

Barbiturate Therapy

Approximately 10% to 15% of patients with severe head injury demonstrate sustained intracranial hypertension despite aggressive conventional medical and surgical therapy (2). In these situations, controversial therapies such as induced barbiturate coma sometimes are used. There is evidence that barbiturates can lower ICP (97), yet they have not been shown to improve overall outcome in head injury (98).

Barbiturates have been used in two ways: as an early intervention to control elevated ICP or, in patients who are refractory, on an ongoing basis as conventional management of intracranial hypertension. Two studies have addressed the early use of barbiturates. The first (mentioned in the preceding) found increased mortality with barbiturate therapy, possibly because of its hypotensive effects. The second was a randomized trial of pentobarbital versus standard treatment that found no difference in 1-year outcome but noted a much higher rate (54% versus 7%) of hypotension in the group given pentobarbital (99).

A randomized trial of pentobarbital for ongoing refractory ICP in patients with GCS 4 to 8 found that survival was higher in responders than in nonresponders but not in the overall intention-to-treat analysis (97). This study was confounded in that it allowed crossovers between groups; therefore, 32 of 36 controls eventually received pentobarbital.

It is important to keep in mind that barbiturates have significant and potentially profound side effects, the most detrimental being hypotension. This results from systemic vasodilation and myocardial depression. There is an increased incidence of infection that appears to result from suppression of the immune response in patients undergoing prolonged high-dose barbiturate therapy. Patients are also at increased risk of the complications associated with prolonged immobilization such as gastrointestinal (GI) bleeding, deep venous thrombosis, pulmonary emboli, and skin breakdown.

The TBI guidelines recommend:

High-dose barbiturate therapy may be considered in hemodynamically stable salvageable severe head injury patients with intracranial hypertension refractory to maximal medical and surgical ICP lowering therapy (Guideline).

Despite this recommendation, many centers have abandoned the use of barbiturates in the treatment of intracranial hypertension. Others continue their use based on a local perception of efficacy. Pentobarbital is no longer easily available. Alternative agents (e.g., propofol, midazolam, and lorazepam) have never been studied in TBI but are presumed to work through the same mechanism. When used for this purpose, these drugs are administered in much higher doses than typically used for sedation and have significant potential side effects, including respiratory depression, hypotension, and prolonged sedation. Other side effects of the prolonged use of propofol have led many to avoid this agent except for brief periods.

Corticosteroids

There is substantial evidence that steroids are ineffective in controlling intracranial hypertension or improving outcome in severe head injury. Several prospective randomized controlled trials failed to demonstrate any benefit of high-dose dexamethasone (100–105). Despite preliminary evidence that high-dose administration of a 21-amino steroid (tirilazad) was useful, it was not effective in a large randomized controlled trial. The TBI guidelines state: "The use of glucocorticoids is not recommended for improving outcome or reducing ICP in patients with severe head injury" (Standard).

Hypothermia

The use of hypothermia has been studied extensively in head injury. Case series were reported as early as 1943, and small controlled trials appeared more recently. The study by Marion and coworkers (106) was the first to report a significant improvement in outcome. The benefit, however, was limited to patients with a GCS of 5 to 7 on presentation and did not persist at 12 months. The lack of demonstrated efficacy was thought to result from insufficient power. However, a recently completed larger NIH–sponsored multicenter trial of early therapeutic hypothermia in severe TBI did not even show a trend toward efficacy (107).

New techniques for inducing hypothermia are being introduced. The use of cooling blankets and gastric lavage are cumbersome and ineffective at rapid cooling. A cooling vest that increases contact with skin has been introduced, and intravascular devices that cool the body by circulating cold saline around a central venous catheter are under development. Whether or not these new methods are applied to head injury in an effort to provide more rapid cooling remains uncertain at this time; it cannot be routinely recommended.

Decompressive Craniectomy

The traditional goal of surgery for TBI patients is decompression of the intracranial vault by removal of hematomas and sometimes the adjacent necrotic brain. This allows the cranium to better accommodate swelling with less of a rise in ICP. Craniectomy and duraplasty, on the other hand, are performed in order to increase the size of the intracranial vault, provide space for expansion of edematous brain tissue, and reduce shift of brain tissue. A number of small case series address its use as a last ditch effort to control refractory intracranial hypertension.

More recently, it has been suggested that early craniectomy and duraplasty in conjunction with the initial decompressive surgery would improve outcome and shorten length of stay (108). Currently, a prospective randomized trial of early craniectomy in TBI patients with CT signs of early edema is underway. The circumstances may (or may not) be comparable to the adoption of decompressive craniectomy for large cerebral infarctions with brain edema, as detailed in Chapter 13.

Other Measures and Complications in Severely Injured Patients

Anticonvulsants

Anticonvulsants are typically administered to patients with TBI to prevent early and late seizures. The rationale for and data to support their use differs for these two indications. Early seizure activity can exacerbate intracranial hypertension. Additionally, seizure activity may go unrecognized in patients who are pharmacologically sedated or paralyzed and intracranial surgery is associated with an increased risk of seizures. For delayed seizures the putative rationale is to prevent the development of chronic epileptic foci.

Three prospective randomized study have indicated that both phenytoin and carbamazepine are effective in preventing early seizures, and a number of prospective randomized trials of anticonvulsants to prevent delayed seizures have been performed (109). Phenytoin, phenobarbital, and carbamazepine were all ineffective in preventing late seizures. The TBI guidelines recommend:

1) prophylactic use of phenytoin, carbamazepine, or phenobarbital is not recommended for preventing late posttraumatic seizures (Standard), 2) Anticonvulsants may be used to prevent early posttraumatic seizures in patients at high risk for seizure following head injury (Option). In most centers, patients with severe TBI are loaded with phenytoin (15 to 18 mg/kg) intravenously and the drug is continued for 1 week.

Nutrition

The nutritional and metabolic impacts of serve TBI are substantial and include negative nitrogen balance, loss of lean body mass, compromised vital organ function, and diminished immunity. The serum concentrations of certain catabolic hormones (epinephrine, norepinephrine, cortisol, glucagon) rise after head injury and result in the mobilization of amino acids from skeletal muscle for increased gluconeogenesis. This leads to wasting of muscle and negative nitrogen balance. In addition, a hyperdynamic cardiac state exists after head injury with tachycardia, increased cardiac output, and increased calorie consumption.

When these metabolic perturbations were appreciated 20 years ago, focused efforts at nutritional support began to be accepted for TBI patients. In early trials of the effects of enteral nutrition, high-protein feedings reduced negative nitrogen balance. The importance of early adequate feeding was demonstrated in a randomized trial of parenteral nutrition versus standard tube feedings. Those receiving parenteral nutrition had much higher protein and calorie intake and a significantly lower mortality, emphasizing the importance of aggressive nutritional support. Later, roughly equivalent enteral and parenteral feeding were compared and enteral feeding were found to be superior in terms of preservation of gut integrity, incidence of sepsis, and use of nutrients (110–114).

Recommendations for severe TBI patients include early enteral feedings that provide 40% to 70% above basal caloric needs and approximately 2 g/kg per day of protein. Most patients can be fed via a nasogastric or orogastric tube into the stomach. Elevating the head of the bed and the administration of GI motility agents (metoclopramide) usually are effective in emptying the stomach. Patients who have persistent residual gastric feedings should have a feeding tube passed into the small bowel. Parenteral nutrition is necessary if that is not possible or fails to meet metabolic needs.

Coagulopathy and Disseminated Intravascular Coagulation

Disorders of coagulation occur frequently in patients with severe TBI and increase the risk of delayed hematomas (76). Disseminated intravascular coagulation (DIC), the consequence of widespread intravascular activation of the coagulation and fibrinolytic systems, is not common but may be seen in patients with overwhelming systemic or cranial injury and greatly increase complications. In patients with systemic injuries, coagulation

disorders lead to uncontrolled hemorrhage. Another important risk of coagulopathy in patients with severe TBI is the increased incidence of bleeding with the placement of a ventricular catheter (115).

The underlying mechanism of the coagulation disorders appears to be a massive release of tissue thromboplastin into the circulation from the brain. Concentration of circulating fibrinogen degradation products roughly correlates with magnitude of brain parenchymal injury (116).

Disseminated intravascular coagulation normally is treated by correcting the underlying pathologic process if possible. Because this is generally not possible in the setting of brain injury, supportive therapy is the mainstay of treatment. Disseminated intravascular coagulation associated with head injury appears to be self-limited, correcting in hours if the patient survives. Replacement of clotting factors and maintenance of adequate blood volume are important in the few protracted cases. Fresh-frozen plasma (FFP) or cryoprecipitate should be given to replenish circulating coagulation factors if there is persistent coagulopathy. Thrombocytopenia should be corrected with the administration of platelets. The administration of heparin for the treatment of DIC is not supported in head injury.

REFERENCES

1. Jennett B, Teasdale G, Galbraith S, et al. Severe head injuries in three countries. *J Neurol Neurosurg Psychiatry* 1977;40:291–298.
2. Bullock R, Chesnut RM, Clifton G, et al. *Guidelines for the management of severe head injury.* New York: Brain Trauma Foundation, 1995.
3. Clausen T, Zauner A, Levasseur JE, et al. Induced mitochondrial failure in the feline brain: implications for understanding acute posttraumatic metabolic events. *Brain Res* 2001;908:35–48.
4. Verweij BH, Muizelaar JP, Vinas FC, et al. Impaired cerebral mitochondrial function after traumatic brain injury in humans. *J Neurosurg* 2000;93:815–820.
5. The Brain Trauma Foundation. The American Association of Neurological Surgeons. The Joint Section on Neurotrauma and Critical Care. Critical pathway for the treatment of established intracranial hypertension. *J Neurotrauma* 2000;17:537–538.
6. The Brain Trauma Foundation. The American Association of Neurological Surgeons. The Joint Section on

Neurotrauma and Critical Care. Guidelines for cerebral perfusion pressure. *J Neurotrauma* 2000;17:507–511.

7. The Brain Trauma Foundation. The American Association of Neurological Surgeons. The Joint Section on Neurotrauma and Critical Care. Intracranial pressure treatment threshold. *J Neurotrauma* 2000;17:493–495.

8. The Brain Trauma Foundation. The American Association of Neurological Surgeons. The Joint Section on Neurotrauma and Critical Care. Recommendations for intracranial pressure monitoring technology. *J Neurotrauma* 2000;17:497–506.

9. The Brain Trauma Foundation. The American Association of Neurological Surgeons. The Joint Section on Neurotrauma and Critical Care. Resuscitation of blood pressure and oxygenation. *J Neurotrauma* 2000;17:471–478.

10. The Brain Trauma Foundation. The American Association of Neurological Surgeons. The Joint Section on Neurotrauma and Critical Care. Use of mannitol. *J Neurotrauma* 2000;17:521–525.

11. Aldrich EF, Eisenberg HM, Saydjari C, et al. Predictors of mortality in severely head-injured patients with civilian gunshot wounds: a report from the NIH Traumatic Coma Data Bank. *Surg Neurol* 1992;38:418–423.

12. Aldrich EF, Eisenberg HM, Saydjari C, et al. Diffuse brain swelling in severely head-injured children. A report from the NIH Traumatic Coma Data Bank. *J Neurosurg* 1992;76:450–454.

13. Eisenberg HM, Gary HE Jr, Aldrich EF, et al. Initial CT findings in 753 patients with severe head injury. A report from the NIH Traumatic Coma Data Bank. *J Neurosurg* 1990;73:688–698.

14. Levin HS, Gary HE Jr, Eisenberg HM. Duration of impaired consciousness in relation to side of lesion after severe head injury. NIH Traumatic Coma Data Bank Research Group. *Lancet* 1989;1:1001–1003.

15. Poca MA, Sahuquillo J, Baguena M, et al. Incidence of intracranial hypertension after severe head injury: a prospective study using the Traumatic Coma Data Bank classification. *Acta Neurochir Suppl (Wien)* 1998;71:27–30.

16. Hutchison JS, Derrane RE, Johnston DL, et al. Neuronal apoptosis inhibitory protein expression after traumatic brain injury in the mouse. *J Neurotrauma* 2001;18:1333–1347.

17. Lin X, Zhi D, Zhang S. Inhibiting effect of moderate hypothermia on cell apoptosis after diffuse brain injury in rats. *Chin J Traumatol* 2001;4:14–19.

18. Vink R, Nimmo AJ, Cernak I. An overview of new and novel pharmacotherapies for use in traumatic brain injury. *Clin Exp Pharmacol Physiol* 2001;28:919–921.

19. Bullock R. Strategies for neuroprotection with glutamate antagonists. Extrapolating from evidence taken from the first stroke and head injury studies. *Ann NY Acad Sci* 1995;765:272–278.

20. Morris GF, Bullock R, Marshall SB, et al. Failure of the competitive N-methyl-D-aspartate antagonist Selfotel (CGS 19755) in the treatment of severe head injury: results of two phase III clinical trials. The Selfotel Investigators. *J Neurosurg* 1999;91:737–743.

21. Miller JD, Becker DP, Ward JD, et al. Significance of intracranial hypertension in severe head injury. *J Neurosurg* 1977;47:503–516.

22. Marshall LF. The outcome with aggressive treatment in severe head injuries. *J Neurosurg* 1979;50:20–25.

23. Jaggi JL, Obrist WD, Gennarelli TA, et al. Relationship of early cerebral blood flow and metabolism to outcome in acute head injury. *J Neurosurg* 1990;72:176–182.

24. Marion DW, Bouma GJ. The use of stable xenon-enhanced computed tomographic studies of cerebral blood flow to define changes in cerebral carbon dioxide vasoresponsivity caused by a severe head injury. *Neurosurgery* 1991;29:869–873.

25. Mindermann T, Gratzl O. Interhemispheric pressure gradients in severe head trauma in humans. *Acta Neurochir Suppl (Wien)* 1998;71:56–58.

26. Sahuquillo J, Poca MA, Arribas M, et al. Interhemispheric supratentorial intracranial pressure gradients in head-injured patients: are they clinically important? *J Neurosurg* 1999;90:16–26.

27. Adams JH, Graham DI. The pathology of blunt head injury. In: Critchley M, O'Leary JL, Jennett B, eds. *Scientific foundations of neurology.* London: Heinemann, 1972:488–491.

28. Graham DI, Adams JH, Doyle D. Ischaemic brain damage in fatal non-missile head injuries. *J Neurol Sci* 1978;39:213–234.

29. Bruce DA, Langfitt TW, Miller JD. Regional cerebral blood flow, intracranial pressure and brain metabolism in comatose patients. *J Neurosurg* 1973;38:131–144.

30. Enevoldsen E, Jensen F. Compartmental analysis of regional cerebral blood flow in patients with acute severe head injuries. *J Neurosurg* 1977;47:699–712.

31. Bouma GJ, Muizelaar JP. Cerebral blood flow, cerebral blood volume, and cerebrovascular reactivity after severe head injury. *J Neurotrauma* 1992;9:S333–348.

32. Bouma GJ, Muizelaar JP. Evaluation of regional cerebral blood flow in acute head injury by stable xenon-enhanced computerized tomography. *Acta Neurochirurg Suppl* 1993;59:34–40.

33. Bouma GJ, Muizelaar JP, Stringer WA, et al. Ultra-early evaluation of regional cerebral blood flow in severely head-injured patients using xenon-enhanced computerized tomography. *J Neurosurg* 1992;77:360–368.

34. Bouma GJ, Muizelaar JP, Choi SC, et al. Cerebral circulation and metabolism after severe traumatic brain injury: the elusive role of ischemia. *J Neurosurg* 1991;75:685–693.

35. Obrist WD, Langfitt TW, Jaggi JL, et al. Cerebral blood flow and metabolism in comatose patients with acute head injury. Relationship to intracranial hypertension. *J Neurosurg* 1984;61:241–253.

36. Muizelaar JP, Marmarou A, DeSalles AA, et al. Cerebral blood flow and metabolism in severely head-injured children. Part 1: Relationship with GCS score, outcome, ICP, and PVI. *J Neurosurg* 1989;71:63–71.

37. Cruz J, Hoffstad OJ, Jaggi JL. Cerebral lactate-oxygen index in acute brain injury with acute anemia: assessment of false versus true ischemia. *Crit Care Med* 1994;22:1465–1470.

38. Holzschuh M, Metz C, Woertgen C, et al. Brain ischemia detected by tissue-PO_2 measurement and the lactate-oxygen index in head injury. *Acta Neurochir Suppl (Wien)* 1998;71:170–171.

39. Prichard J, Rothman D, Novotny E, et al. Lactate rise detected by 1H NMR in human visual cortex during

physiologic stimulation. *Proc Natl Acad Sci USA* 1991;88:5829–5831.

40. Sappey-Marinei D, Calabrese G, Fein G, et al. Effect of photic stimulation on human visual cortex lactate and phosphates using 1H and 31P magnetic resonance spectroscopy. *J Cereb Blood Flow Metab* 1992;12: 584–592.

41. McIntosh TK. Neurochemical sequelae of traumatic brain injury: therapeutic implications. *Cerebrovasc Brain Metab Rev* 1994;6:109–162.

42. Kaczorowski SL, Schiding JK, Toth CA, et al. Effect of soluble complement receptor-1 on neutrophil accumulation after traumatic brain injury in rats. *J Cereb Blood Flow Metab* 1995;15:864.

43. Clark RSB, Schiding JK, Kaczorowski SL, et al. Neutrophil accumulation after traumatic brain injury in rats: comparison of weight drop and controlled cortical impact models. *J Neurotrauma* 1994;11:499–506.

44. Finnerty F, Witkin L, Fazekas J. Cerebral hemodynamics during cerebral ischemia induced by acute hypotension. *J Clin Invest* 1954;33:1227–1232.

45. Gibbs E, Lennox W, Nims L, et al. Arterial and cerebral venous blood. *J Biol Chem* 1942;144:325–332.

46. Kety S, Schmidt C. The effects of active and passive hyperventilation on cerebral blood flow, cerebral oxygen consumption, cardiac output, and blood pressure of normal young men. *J Clin Invest* 1946;25:107–119.

47. Scheinberg P, Stead E. The cerebral blood flow in male subjects as measured by the nirous oxide technique. Normal values for blood flow, oxygen utilization, glucose utilization, and peripheral resistance, with observations on the effect of tilting and anxiety. *J Clin Invest* 1949;28:1163–1171.

48. Carpenter DA, Grubb RL Jr, Tempel LW, et al. Cerebral oxygen metabolism after aneurysmal subarachnoid hemorrhage. *J Cereb Blood Flow Metab* 1991; 11:837–844.

49. Zazulia AR, Diringer MN, Videen TO, et al. Hypoperfusion without ischemia surrounding acute intracerebral hemorrhage. *J Cereb Blood Flow Metab* 2001;21: 804–810.

50. Verweij BH, Muizelaar JP, Vinas FC, et al. Improvement in mitochondrial dysfunction as a new surrogate efficiency measure for preclinical trials: dose-response and time-window profiles for administration of the calcium channel blocker Ziconotide in experimental brain injury. *J Neurosurg* 2000;93:829–834.

51. Bergsneider M, Hovda DA, Shalmon E, et al. Cerebral hyperglycolysis following severe traumatic brain injury in humans: a positron emission tomography study. *J Neurosurg* 1997;86:241–251.

52. Marshall LF, Marshall SB, Klauber MR, et al. The diagnosis of head injury requires a classification based on computed axial tomography. *J Neurotrauma* 1992;9:S287–S292.

53. Chesnut RM, Marshall LF, Klauber MR, et al. The role of secondary brain injury in determining outcome from severe head injury. *J Trauma* 1993;34:216–222.

54. Fearnside MR, Cook RJ, McDougall P, et al. The Westmead Head Injury Project outcome in severe head injury. A comparative analysis of pre-hospital, clinical and CT variables. *Br J Neurosurg* 1993;7:267–279.

55. Quigley MR, Vidovich D, Cantella D, et al. Defining the limits of survivorship after very severe head injury. *J Trauma* 1997;42:7–10.

56. Choi SC, Muizelaar JP, Barnes TY, et al. Prediction tree for severely head-injured patients. *J Neurosurg* 1991;75:251–255.

57. Lang EW, Pitts LH, Damron SL, et al. Outcome after severe head injury: an analysis of prediction based upon comparison of neural network versus logistic regression analysis. *Neurol Res* 1997;19:274–280.

58. Alberico AM, Ward JD, Choi SC, et al. Outcome after severe head injury. Relationship to mass lesions, diffuse injury, and ICP course in pediatric and adult patients. *J Neurosurg* 1987;67:648–656.

59. Toutant SM, Klauber MR, Marshall LF, et al. Absent or compressed basal cisterns on first CT scan: ominous predictors of outcome in severe head injury. *J Neurosurg* 1984;61:691–694.

60. Einhorn A, Mizrahi EM. Basilar skull fractures in children. The incidence of CNS infection and the use of antibiotics. *Am J Dis Child* 1978;132:1121–1124.

61. Ignelzi RJ, VanderArk GD. Analysis of the treatment of basilar skull fractures with and without antibiotics. *J Neurosurg* 1975;43:721–726.

62. Cooper PR. Delayed traumatic intracerebral hemorrhage. *Neurosurg Clin N Am* 1992;3:659–665.

63. Oertel M, Kelly DF, McArthur D, et al. Progressive hemorrhage after head trauma: predictors and consequences of the evolving injury. *J Neurosurg* 2002;96: 109–116.

64. Alvarez-Sabin J, Turon A, Lozano-Sanchez M, et al. Delayed posttraumatic hemorrhage. "Spat-apoplexia." *Stroke* 1995;26:1531–1535.

65. Bigler ED. Quantitative magnetic resonance imaging in traumatic brain injury. *J Head Trauma Rehabil* 2001;16:117–134.

66. Wallesch CW, Curio N, Galazky I, et al. The neuropsychology of blunt head injury in the early postacute stage: effects of focal lesions and diffuse axonal injury. *J Neurotrauma* 2001;18:11–20.

67. Kampfl A, Franz G, Aichner F, et al. The persistent vegetative state after closed head injury: clinical and magnetic resonance imaging findings in 42 patients. *J Neurosurg* 1998;88:809–816.

68. Hsiang JK, Chesnut RM, Crisp CB, et al. Early, routine paralysis for intracranial pressure control in severe head injury: is it necessary? *Crit Care Med* 1994;22: 1471–1476.

69. Saul TGDTB. Effect of intracranial pressure monitoring and aggresive treatment on mortality in severe head injury. *J Neurosurg* 1982;56:498–503.

70. Eisenberg HM, Frankowski RF, Contant CF, et al. High-dose barbiturate control of elevated intracranial pressure in patients with severe head injury. *J Neurosurg* 1988;69:15–23.

71. Sheinberg M, Kanter MJ, Robertson CS, et al. Continuous monitoring of jugular venous oxygen saturation in head-injured patients [see comments]. *J Neurosurg* 1992;76:212–217.

72. Cruz J. Jugular venous oxygen saturation monitoring. *J Neurosurg* 1992;77:162–163.

73. Stocchetti N, Paparella A, Bridelli F, et al. Cerebral venous oxygen saturation studied with bilateral samples in the internal jugular veins. *Neurosurgery* 1994;34: 38–43.

74. Gopinath SP, Robertson CS, Contant CF, et al. Jugular venous desaturation and outcome after head injury. *J Neurol Neurosurg Psychiatry* 1994;57:717–723.

75. Bullock R, Hanemann CO, Murray L, et al. Recurrent hematomas following craniotomy for traumatic intracranial mass. *J Neurosurg* 1990;72:9–14.

76. Kaufman HH, Moake JL, Olson JD, et al. Delayed and recurrent intracranial hematomas related to disseminated intravascular clotting and fibrinolysis in head injury. *Neurosurgery* 1980;7:445–449.

77. van den Brink WA, van Santbrink H, Steyerberg EW, et al. Brain oxygen tension in severe head injury. *Neurosurgery* 2000;46:868–876.

78. Gopinath SP, Valadka AB, Uzura M, et al. Comparison of jugular venous oxygen saturation and brain tissue Po_2 as monitors of cerebral ischemia after head injury [see comments]. *Crit Care Med* 1999;27:2337–2345.

79. Doppenberg EM, Watson JC, Bullock R, et al. The rationale for, and effects of oxygen delivery enhancement to ischemic brain in a feline model of human stroke. *Ann NY Acad Sci* 1997;825:241–257.

80. Hemphill JC III, Knudson MM, Derugin N, et al. Carbon dioxide reactivity and pressure autoregulation of brain tissue oxygen. *Neurosurgery* 2001;48:377–383.

81. Asgeirsson B, Grande PO, Nordstrom CH. A new therapy of post-traumatic brain oedema based on haemodynamic principles for brain volume regulation. *Intern Care Med* 1994;20:260–267.

82. Grande PO, Asgeirsson B, Nordstrom CH. Physiologic principles for volume regulation of a tissue enclosed in a rigid shell with application to the injured brain. *J Trauma* 1997;42(5 Suppl):S23–S31.

83. Rosner MJ, Daughton S. Cerebral perfusion pressure management in head injury. *J Trauma* 1993;30:933–940.

84. Robertson CS, Valadka AB, Hannay HJ, et al. Prevention of secondary ischemic insults after severe head injury. *Crit Care Med* 1999;27:2086–2095.

85. Juul N, Morris GF, Marshall SB, et al. Intracranial hypertension and cerebral perfusion pressure: influence on neurological deterioration and outcome in severe head injury. The Executive Committee of the International Selfotel Trial. *J Neurosurg* 2000;92:1–6.

86. Marmarou A, Anderson R, Ward J. Impact of ICP instability and hypotension on outcome in patients with severe head injury. *J Neurosurg* 1991;75:S59–S66.

87. Saul TG, Ducker TB. Effect of intracranial pressure monitoring and aggressive treatment on mortality in severe head injury. *J Neurosurg* 1982;56:498–503.

88. Mayer SA, Copeland D, Bernardini GL, et al. Cost and outcome of mechanical ventilation for life-threatening stroke. *Stroke* 2000;31:2346–2353.

89. Bolton CF, Young GB, Zochodne DW. The neurological complications of sepsis. *Ann Neurol* 1993;33:94–100.

90. Garnacho-Montero J, Madrazo-Osuna J, Garcia-Garmendia JL, et al. Critical illness polyneuropathy: risk factors and clinical consequences. A cohort study in septic patients. *Int Care Med* 2001;27:1288–1296.

91. Hsiang JK, Chesnut RM, Crisp CB, et al. Early, routine paralysis for intracranial pressure control in severe head injury: is it necessary? *Crit Care Med* 1994;22:1471–1476.

92. Muizelaar JP, Marmarou A, Ward JD, et al. Adverse effects of prolonged hyperventilation in patients with severe head injury: a randomized clinical trial. *J Neurosurg* 1991;75:731–739.

93. Diringer MN, Yundt K, Videen TO, et al. No reduction in cerebral metabolism as a result of early moderate hyperventilation following severe traumatic brain injury. *J Neurosurg* 2000;92:7–13.

94. Diringer MN, Videen TO, Yundt K, et al. Regional cerebrovascular and metabolic effects of hyperventilation following severe traumatic brain injury. *J Neurosurg* 2001;96:103–108.

95. Muizelaar JP, Lutz HA, III, Becker DP. Effect of mannitol on ICP and CBF and correlation with pressure autoregulation in severely head-injured patients. *J Neurosurg* 1984;61:700–706.

96. Schwartz ML, Tator CH, Rowed DW, et al. The University of Toronto head injury treatment study: a prospective, randomized comparison of pentobarbital and mannitol. *Can J Neurol Sci* 1984;11:434–440.

97. Eisenberg HM, Frankowski RF, Contant CF, et al. High-dose barbiturate control of elevated intracranial pressure in patients with severe head injury. *J Neurosurg* 1988;69:15–23.

98. Roberts I. Barbiturates for acute traumatic brain injury. *Cochrane Database Syst Rev* 2000;CD000033.

99. Ward JD, Becker DP, Miller JD, et al. Failure of prophylactic barbiturate coma in the treatment of severe head injury. *J Neurosurg* 1985;62:383–388.

100. Cooper PR, Moody S, Clark WK, et al. Dexamethasone and severe head injury. A prospective double-blind study. *J Neurosurg* 1979;51:307–316.

101. Dearden NM, Gibson JS, McDowall DG, et al. Effect of high-dose dexamethasone on outcome from severe head injury. *J Neurosurg* 1986;64:81–88.

102. Gudeman SK, Miller JD, Becker DP. Failure of high-dose steroid therapy to influence intracranial pressure in patients with severe head injury. *J Neurosurg* 1979;51:301–306.

103. Bruno A, Biller J, Adams HP Jr, et al. Acute blood glucose level and outcome from ischemic stroke. Trial of ORG 10172 in Acute Stroke Treatment (TOAST) Investigators. *Neurology* 1999;52:280–284.

104. Donnan GA, Davis SM, Chambers BR, et al. Streptokinase for acute ischemic stroke with relationship to time of administration: Australian Streptokinase (ASK) Trial Study Group. *JAMA* 1996;276:961–966.

105. Pantano P, Caramia F, Bozzao L, et al. Delayed increase in infarct volume after cerebral ischemia: correlations with thrombolytic treatment and clinical outcome. *Stroke* 1999;30:502–507.

106. Marion DW, Penrod LE, Kelsey SF, et al. Treatment of traumatic brain injury with moderate hypothermia. *N Engl J Med* 1997;336:540–546.

107. Clifton GL, Miller ER, Choi SC, et al. Lack of effect of induction of hypothermia after acute brain injury. *N Engl J Med* 2001;344:556–563.

108. Coplin WM, Cullen NK, Policherla PN, et al. Safety and feasibility of craniectomy with duraplasty as the initial surgical intervention for severe traumatic brain injury. *J Trauma* 2001;50:1050–1059.

109. Schierhout G, Roberts I. Anti-epileptic drugs for preventing seizures following acute traumatic brain injury. *Cochrane Database Syst Rev* 2001;CD000173.

110. Haider W, Benzer H, Krystof G, et al. Urinary catecholamine excretion and thyroid hormone blood level in the course of severe acute brain damage. *Eur J Int Care Med* 1975;1:115–123.

111. Rapp RP, Young B, Twyman D, et al. The favorable ef-

fect of early parenteral feeding on survival in head-injured patients. *J Neurosurg* 1983;58:906–912.

112. Twyman D, Young AB, Ott L, et al. High protein enteral feedings: a means of achieving positive nitrogen balance in head-injured patients. *J Parenter Enteral Nutr* 1985;9:679–684.

113. Young B, Ott L, Haack D, et al. Effect of total parenteral nutrition upon intracranial pressure in severe head injury. *J Neurosurg* 1987;67:76–80.

114. Young B, Ott L, Phillips R, et al. Metabolic management of the patient with head injury. *Neurosurg Clin N Am* 1991;2:301–320.

115. Narayan R, Kishore K, Pulla RS, et al. Intracranial pressure: to monitor or not to monitor? *J Neurosurg* 1982;56:650–659.

116. Miner ME, Kaufman HH, Graham SH, et al. Disseminated intravascular coagulation fibrinolytic syndrome following head injury in children: frequency and prognostic implications. *J Pediatr* 1982;100 687–691.

13

Critical Care of Acute Stroke

The intensivist is in a position to make substantial contributions to the care of stroke patients. The problem of clinically serious and anatomically large stroke has several aspects that must be considered simultaneously; the most pressing are restoration of blood flow and the emergence of a particularly aggressive form of brain edema and swelling that often has a fatal outcome. Also addressed in the intensive care unit (ICU) are treatments that potentially spare neurons from irreversible death, and a number of more mundane medical issues such as the prevention of aspiration.

GENERAL PRINCIPLES IN STROKE

Treatment of stroke traditionally has focused on anatomic localization, modification of risk factors, and secondary prevention after a transient ischemic attack (TIA) or minor stroke (1). Efforts to limit infarct size after an acute ischemic event have been hampered by the short interval between cessation of blood flow and the cascade of irreversible changes that lead to cell death. With complete global ischemia, this interval may be as short as 4 minutes, essentially precluding any possibility of clinical intervention (2), but the human cerebral circulation provides collateral pathways that allow residual perfusion in portions of the territory of an occluded vessel. Therefore, partial ischemia is probably common in typical stroke that arises from occlusion of large arteries. Experimental models of acute ischemic stroke suggest that partial ischemia affords a longer interval before irreversible ischemic changes occur.

Reduction in cerebral blood flow from normal levels of 50 to 100 mL/100 g per minute to less than 18 mL/100 g per minute results in cessation of brain electric activity, but important cellular functions that maintain neuronal viability may continue (3). When blood flow falls below 10 mL/100 g per minute, basic cellular functions can no longer be maintained, leading to a series of events that result in cell death (4,5). Clinical deficits appear at an early stage, but because irreversible changes may not yet have occurred, the ischemic process should be reversible by raising blood flow above the critical threshold. Both the absolute level of cerebral blood flow and the duration of ischemia determine the development of cerebral infarction (6). Restoration of blood flow within 1 to 3 hours reverses ischemia and reduces infarction in some animal models. In human strokes, the length of time reduced levels of blood flow can be tolerated is unknown and almost certainly varies from case to case as well as between focal and global ischemia. The clinical and biologic features of global ischemia are reviewed in Chapter 17.

Clinical experience shows that ischemic deficits occasionally improve rapidly, within minutes to hours after onset. Experimental and some clinical studies indicate that cellular functions may return toward normal levels after transient brain ischemia and that neuronal death is not determined for up to 24 to 48 hours. The thrust of modern stroke intervention is predicated on this potential reversibility (7,8). In addition to enhancing standard medical care, two innovative strategies have been pursued in this regard; decreasing neuronal vulnerability to ischemia and improving blood flow.

Maximizing Standard Medical Management

Maintenance of adequate blood pressure is a tenet of acute stroke care. In patients with fluctuating basilar or carotid artery syndromes, most neurologists have had the experience that rapid lowering of blood pressure leads to clinical deterioration in some patients. The problem of how to approach the larger group of patients with fixed stroke deficits and hypertension has been addressed by several studies. Wallace and Levy (9) found that 84% of 334 consecutive stroke patients had elevated pressure, only half with a hypertensive history, which declined an average of 20 mm Hg systolic and 10 mm Hg diastolic in the 10 days after stroke. Patients with cerebral hemorrhage had a more variable blood pressure course, as expected. A subsequent case-controlled study by Britton and colleagues (10) found that 69% of stroke patients and 36% of controls had acute hypertension after admission and that a spontaneous decline occurred over the first few days of hospitalization, similar to the Wallace and Levy study. Other studies (11–13) have given similar results and have led to the admonition that all but the most extreme hypertension after acute stroke should be left untreated unless there is acute angina, hypertensive encephalopathy, or progressive renal failure (10). Rapid reductions in cerebral perfusion pressure in the setting of ischemia can markedly decrease blood flow and enlarge the ischemic area. We have generally used a threshold of systolic pressures above 200 mm Hg or diastolic pressures over 110 mm Hg before beginning treatment. Rapidly acting agents such as intravenous labetalol are useful, with angiotensin converting enzyme inhibitors favored for more long-acting therapy.

Present knowledge about the pathophysiology of infarction suggests that fever, seizure activity, and hyperglycemia are detrimental to stroke outcome. Human and animal data indicate that neuronal susceptibility to ischemic death is very temperature-dependent. Metabolic energy requirements and many of the enzyme systems that participate in cell dissolution are strictly temperature dependent. This is typified by patients suffering cold water drowning who sustain prolonged anoxia and arrest yet have good recovery of neurological function. Improved outcome in several animal studies has resulted from lowering brain temperature 4°C to 5°C, and profound hypothermia is used successfully in vascular neurosurgery to allow almost complete diversion of blood from the brain. Conversely, seizure activity increases the requirements for metabolic energy and, if sustained, promotes neuronal death even under normal metabolic circumstances. Studies in animals and clinical work also suggest that hyperglycemia may adversely affect infarct size; therefore, maintenance of blood glucose in the normal range has been suggested as an ancillary therapy for acute stroke.

Decreasing Neuronal Vulnerability

Ischemia initiates a series of biochemical and cellular events resulting in irreversible changes in essential cell functions and eventually cell death. Three particular biochemical events have been identified as potentially important in leading to ischemic death: (a) elevated intracellular calcium; (b) production of free radical compounds; and (c) lactic acidosis. During ischemia, diminishing energy supplies compromise the function of the Na^+/K^+ pump, leading to neuronal depolarization and indiscriminate release of all neurotransmitters. Depolarization and transmitter actions cause massive flux of ions and water; cells swell, extracellular K^+ and intracellular Ca^{2+} rise, and pH falls.

Intracellular free calcium concentration is normally kept almost 10,000 times lower inside than outside neurons. The precipitous rise in intracellular calcium during ischemia may be an important factor in the cascade of metabolic derangements that eventuate in neuronal death. The endoplasmic reticulum and mitochondria release calcium, causing an increase in intracellular Ca^{2+}, in turn exacerbating calcium influx caused by membrane depolarization (14). High intracellular calcium further depletes energy stores by activation of energy-dependent ion exchanges that attempt to move calcium into mitochondria.

Strategies designed to limit free radical concentrations may also prove to be of benefit in patients with brain injury and cerebral edema. Increasing the levels of superoxide dismutase, a free radical scavenger, has been shown to limit infarction in animal stroke models (15). Newly developed modified steroid compounds, termed *lazaroids*, inactivate iron-related free radicals and have some protective effect in animal stroke models.

The interest in neuroprotection has led to dozens of clinical trials over the last decade, although no agent has yet been clearly demonstrated to improve neurological outcome following ischemic stroke. Various calcium antagonists, free radical scavengers and other novel agents have appeared much less effective in clinical trial than early work in animal models of stroke. There are many possible reasons to explain the early disappointing trial results, and also many reasons to be optimistic that the strategy will eventually prove beneficial (16).

Improving Cerebral Blood Flow

Induced Hypertension

Induced hypertension has been proposed as one strategy to increase cerebral blood flow in acute ischemic stroke. Although many patients have elevated blood pressures at presentation, others may benefit from pharmacologic elevation of pressure. The concept is similar to induced hypertension for ischemia related to vasospasm following subarachnoid hemorrhage. Induced hypertension in an animal model appeared to decrease lactate accumulation following middle cerebral artery occlusion, although edema formation may have been enhanced (17). Rordorf and coworkers (18) reported on a group of patients with

acute stroke treated with induced hypertension and indicated that 10 of 30 patients had rapid and clinically apparent improvement in neurological deficits when the pressure was increased. The systolic pressure threshold for improvement ranged from 120 to 190 mm Hg, with a mean of 156 mm Hg. The treatment may be reasonable for those patients with relatively low pressures at presentation.

Thrombolysis

Acute revascularization with thrombolytic therapies has been demonstrated to improve outcome in stroke (19). The most commonly used strategy is intravenous systemic t-PA used within the first 3 hours after stroke symptom onset. Drug infusion frequently begins in the emergency department, but most patients are monitored and cared for in an ICU setting. An intraarterial strategy also has been pursued, and a recent randomized trial demonstrated improved outcome with a 6-hour treatment window (20). The intraarterial approach may be most useful with more proximal large vessel occlusions. A combination strategy is also under study, using an initial intravenous dose followed by angiography and intraarterial therapy as needed. Further clinical study will be needed to establish the optimal timing and route of administration of lytic therapy.

Stroke patients treated with thrombolytic therapy should remain in a monitored setting for at least 24 hours. Blood pressure should be carefully monitored and controlled as needed to maintain systolic pressures less than 185 mm Hg and diastolic pressures less than 110 mm Hg. Although one would not usually intervene at this pressure level, the risks of excessive hemorrhage lead to a more aggressive approach to blood pressure control in this group of patients. Serious systemic hemorrhages are uncommon, although they can be life threatening if not rapidly detected. Retroperitoneal hemorrhage often presents with lower abdominal pain, and must be treated with volume replacement. There is not a rapidly effective reversal of the coagulopathy associated with thrombolytic agents, although some degree of hemostasis may be restored with the administration of cryoprecipitated clotting factors.

BRAIN EDEMA FOLLOWING LARGE HEMISPHERIC STROKE

Patients with large hemispheric stroke are at high risk for neurological deterioration and thus are frequently seen in the neurological intensive care unit (neuro-ICU). When the condition of a patient with a large hemispheric stroke worsens the initial evaluation should address both neurological and systemic factors that could cause such deterioration. The primary neurological causes of deterioration are cerebral edema, hemorrhage into the infarct and, rarely, recurrent stroke. Systemic causes include fever, infection, hypotension, hypoxia, and hypercarbia. Brain edema in patients with small strokes often has no or minimal impact on clinical status. On the other hand, edema following large hemispheric strokes can have devastating consequences. Considerable effort recently has been directed toward determining the best management of massive hemispheric swelling following ischemic stroke.

Infarction of the entire middle cerebral artery (MCA) territory is almost always caused by occlusion of the distal internal carotid artery or the proximal middle cerebral artery trunk. The presence of well-developed leptomeningeal collateral vessels may help limit infarct size. These strokes usually are caused by emboli from cardiac or arterial sources. About 10% to 20% of ischemic stroke patients suffer infarction of the complete MCA territory. Midline shift following MCA stroke begins during the first 3 days, peaks at 3 to 5 days, and subsides by 2 weeks.

Some patients with complete MCA territory stroke deteriorate dramatically over the next 24 to 72 hours and on repeat CT scanning demonstrate massive edema with severe midline shift and compression of the basal cisterns. This has been described as the "malignant MCA syndrome" with a reported historical mortality rate as high as 80% (21). More recent series suggest the mortality rate is closer to 50% (22).

There appears to be a subset of patients who develop very rapid and massive edema over the first day following stroke. This occurs frequently in patients who receive thrombolytics (23,24) and may be the result of reperfusion of a large area of already infarcted brain.

Early Identification of Patients Likely to Develop Massive Cerebral Edema

It is important to identify as early as possible patients who are likely to develop massive edema because of their high risk for deterioration and poor outcome. Early identification will facilitate timely discussions of whether the patient has executed an advanced directive or expressed their wishes regarding health care. The early identification of patients likely to develop massive cerebral edema also helps define what level of monitoring is necessary, when aggressive measures should be instituted, and what the outcome is likely to be. Although better methods are needed to identify this population a number of clinical and radiographic signs have been found to provide some guidance.

Clinical signs typically include a hemispheric syndrome with hemiparesis, hemianesthesia, and eye deviation. Early respiratory disturbances occur and some patients require intubation for airway protection. Global aphasia is almost always present if the dominant hemisphere is involved. Some patients are somnolent. Although these signs are almost always present in patients who develop massive hemispheric edema, not all patients with these signs go on to develop massive hemispheric edema.

Early radiographic signs occur more frequently in patients who develop massive hemispheric swelling. Computed tomography (CT) findings within the first 6 hours after stroke include large early hypodensity of the affected territory, loss of gray/white matter distinction, the "hyperdense MCA sign," and early loss of definition of cortical sulci. Computed tomography scan 24 hours after onset almost always shows mass effect with compression of the lateral ventricle. A study of computed tomography scan within the first 6 hours after onset of symptoms in patients with MCA occlusion indicated that hypodensity involving greater than 50% of the MCA territory and local brain swelling (effacement of sulci, compression of the lateral ventricle) were strong predictors of mortality with a high specificity (94%) but only moderate sensitivity (61%) (25). Similarly, in the ECASS (European Cooperative Acute Stroke Study) trial, these signs were associated with mass effect and death caused by herniation (26).

Management of "Malignant" Ischemic Brain Edema

When considering intervention, it is important to reassess the patient's and family's wishes regarding the degree of medical intervention because treatment involves a number of invasive and as-of-yet not established, interventions.

Airway

Deterioration in patients with massive MCA infarction is always associated with a decline in level of consciousness, which should prompt reassessment of the patient's airway. Reduced tone in the pharyngeal musculature and tongue, as well as impaired gag and cough reflexes, contribute to upper airway obstruction and inability to manage oral secretions. It is important to recognize, however, that the use of mechanical ventilation following a large ischemic stroke is controversial. Case series of stroke patients undergoing mechanical ventilation report mortality rates of 50% to 90% (27–30). Factors associated with higher mortality include Glasgow Coma Scale (GCS) score less than 10, absent brainstem reflexes, male gender, age greater than 65, and intubation owing to coma. Unfortunately, statistical models developed to date lack sufficient power to reliably predict

mortality with a high degree of certainty early in the hospitalization. Therefore, in some patients who exhibit many of the above risk factors, intubation may be withheld based on the patient's and family's preferences. In others owing to the uncertainly involved, mechanical ventilation may be provided initially until the neurological course is more clearly established.

If intubation is necessary, it is important to administer medication to provide adequate relaxation of the jaw while avoiding hemodynamic instability, preventing a rise in intracranial pressure (ICP), and minimizing the duration of the period of sedation. Etomidate is an ideal agent because it is short-acting and has minimal cardiovascular effects (31). Thiopental also is effective but is more likely to cause hypotension. Lidocaine helps minimize coughing and the rise in ICP. Benzodiazepines should be avoided because they frequently do not provide adequate sedation unless larger doses are used that can frequently cause hypotension. Use of neuromuscular blocking agents is usually unnecessary and should be avoided because it limits the ability to perform serial neurological examinations. Short-acting agents are preferred if needed.

Monitoring

In patients showing signs of deterioration owing to cerebral edema from a large hemispheric stroke it is important to monitor progression in order to determine if and when more aggressive interventions should be considered. The use of serial clinical assessments is fairly insensitive because deterioration is difficult to detect in a patient who is already poorly responsive until frank uncal herniation occurs. Serial CT scans are helpful in following the course of mass effect and the anatomic response to interventions; however, the use of frequent CT scans is logistically difficult and repeatedly exposes the patient to potential complications of transport to and from the CT scanner.

In the past ICP monitoring has been proposed as a useful adjunct to monitoring these patients. However, several studies have suggested that ICP monitoring is not particularly helpful in the setting of large hemispheric stroke. In a group of patients admitted to a neuro-ICU because of deterioration after a large hemispheric stroke, the majority of patients who suffered clinical herniation did so with a normal ICP (32). Another study found that ICP greater than 30 mm Hg was a poor prognostic factor but that routine ICP monitoring was not helpful in patient management (33). By the time the ICP has risen to critical values, both clinical and radiographic signs of herniation already are present.

Threshold for Initiation of Treatment

The decision about if and when to proceed with intervention requires careful consideration of the potential risks and benefits of the treatment and how those risks and benefits change over time. This analysis is particularly complicated in these patients. Interventions such as hemicraniectomy and induced hypothermia are very invasive and carry significant risk. The benefit of performing any aggressive intervention is debated, especially in patients who have multiple comorbid conditions or have dominant hemisphere infarction. Additionally, delaying treatment with aggressive measures until the clinical signs of herniation occur limits their effectiveness. In order to use invasive therapies early after stroke onset more specific predictive criteria of clinical deterioration are needed. Currently no standard criteria exist for identifying patients at risk for deterioration. Many centers have established local protocols based on the criteria discussed.

Treatment of Mass Effect Caused by Edema

The management of mass effect is discussed in detail in Chapter 3. This discussion focuses on the application of those techniques to the management of patients with large hemispheric infarct and cerebral edema.

Hyperventilation

There are very little data that address the use of hyperventilation in this clinical setting. That hyperventilation, at least transiently, can reverse clinical signs of herniation is not debated. Whether hyperventilation causes additional injury by reducing cerebral blood flow in ischemic brain regions is not known (see also Chapters 3 and 12). Lacking clinical outcome data, it is reasonable to base treatment on what is known about the physiologic response to the intervention. Thus, it is important to recognize that the effect of hyperventilation on blood flow and ICP is transient, lasting only a matter of hours (34–36). This is in contradistinction to the duration of ischemic cerebral edema, which lasts several days. Additionally, the rapid weaning of sustained hyperventilation can cause a rebound increase in ICP. Based on these observations, it appears appropriate that the use of hyperventilation should be limited to a temporizing measure in acute deteriorations while other measures are being instituted. A $PaCO_2$ of 25 to 30 mm Hg probably is a reasonable target.

Osmotic Agents

The administration of osmotic agents is also well known to reverse the clinical signs of herniation (37). Their use in the treatment of ischemic edema is based on what is known about their use in head injury. Classic teaching has long been that mannitol acts by extracting water only from brain regions where the blood–brain barrier is intact. Additionally, the potential for mannitol accumulation in injured brain and increase in edema has long been a concern (although without any sound basis). Based on these factors it has been hypothesized that administration of mannitol in the setting of ischemic edema could result in an increase in midline shift (32). This concern was not supported by two carefully performed magnetic resonance imaging (MRI) studies of the effect of a single very large dose (1.5 g/kg) of mannitol administered to patients with hemispheric stroke, edema, and midline shift. There was a small reduction in the volume of the normal but not the infarcted hemisphere (38), which could only be detected using complex postimaging analysis. Despite this, there was no measurable effect on midline shift on standard MRI (39).

Even less is known about appropriate timing, dosage, monitoring, and duration of therapy. Typically, 1.0 to 1.5 g/kg i.v. of mannitol are given for a sudden neurological deterioration. Such a dose can easily produce sufficient diuresis to result in volume depletion and hypotension; this can be avoided by administering sufficient intravenous normal saline. The timing and magnitude of subsequent doses must be based on the clinical and radiographic response. Typical doses range from 0.25 to 1.0 g/kg every 4 to 6 hours. Excessive diuresis and urinary loss of potassium, magnesium, and phosphate should be anticipated and corrected.

Hypertonic saline is another osmotic agent that is being used more frequently. The results of treatment of raised intracranial pressure in head injury using hypertonic saline have been encouraging. In one study reporting its use in ischemic stroke a 3% hypertonic saline/acetate solution was administered to six patients with cerebral infarction. The mean GCS worsened in this group after treatment and there was no improvement in midline shift or intracranial pressure (40).

Decompressive Craniectomy

There has been renewed interest over the past 10 to 15 years in the use of decompressive craniectomy in patients with large hemispheric stroke. Hemicraniectomy and dural augmentation allows expansion of the edematous tissue outside the cranial vault, reversing tissue shifts and reducing intracranial pressure.

In a case series from Heidelberg of decompressive craniectomy in patients with space-occupying hemispheric stroke, outcome among surgically treated patients was compared to that of medically treated historical controls. Medically treated patients had 76% mortality, and all survivors were moderately disabled. Surgically treated patients had only 32% mortality with two out of three of the survivors independent or mildly to moderately disabled (41).

In a subsequent series from the same center, craniectomy was performed earlier, less than 24 hours after stroke onset (42). Mortality was 16% in this cohort, and functional outcome was better than in the previous series. The lack of randomized controls makes this difficult to interpret. The improved outcome may result from inclusion of patients who may have done well without surgical intervention and younger patients. More recent multicenter data comparing medically and surgically treated patients reported mortality rates of approximately 50% and 40%, respectively, which were not statistically different. The issue remains controversial (43–45). Numerous questions remain regarding patient selection, the appropriate timing for craniectomy, patients with dominant hemisphere stroke, and whether it improves outcome but we endorse it in younger otherwise healthy patients (see page 45).

Hypothermia

There are considerable data that indicate that mild hypothermia (32°C to 33°C) reduces experimental infarct volume (46), even when instituted 90 minutes after a focal ischemic insult (47,48). Possible mechanisms responsible for this protective effect include reduction of metabolism and levels of excitatory amino acids, and stabilization of the blood–brain barrier and cell membranes (49,50).

Fever is associated with a poor outcome following stroke. In a prospective study of 183 patients a temperature of greater than 37.9°C in the first 7 days after an acute stroke was an independent predictor of poor outcome (51). Another study found that hyperthermia is independently related to larger infarct volume and a worse outcome, but only if hyperthermia occurs within 24 hours of the stroke onset (52). On the other hand patients with mild hypothermia on admission had a lower mortality and better outcome (53). Although it has not been definitively established that reducing fever in patients improves outcome, treating elevated temperature and avoiding hyperthermia seems warranted.

Body and/or brain temperature can be lowered to subnormal levels to induce therapeutic hypothermia. A feasibility and safety study of modest hypothermia (35.5°C to 36.5°C) in acute stroke found that hypothermia could be achieved without significant complications using external or internal cooling devices (54). In another study moderate hypothermia (body core temperature 33°C to 34°C) was induced in 25 stroke patients using a cooling blanket. Hypothermia was maintained for 48 to 72 hours followed by gradual rewarming. Intracranial pressure fell in all patients with initiation of hypothermia and increased with rewarming. Mortality was 44% in this group of patients (55).

The use of hypothermia is potentially very invasive, requiring mechanical ventilation, sedation, neuromuscular paralysis, and frequent use of vasopressors. These measures make it impossible to clinically examine patients on a regular basis. Side effects include pneumonia and coagulopathy, electrocardiographic abnormalities, and elevation of serum amylase and lipase. Fortunately, most of these abnormalities have not been clinically significant (56). There was a rebound increase in ICP during rewarming; a slow rewarming rate may minimize this rebound.

In the end, a coordinated approach that takes each of these elements and potential therapies into account is required. Certainly, the state of current knowledge will be expanded by further clinical inquiry and laboratory studies. Past experience has shown that adoption of novel ideas into clinical practice for stroke should occur only after careful scrutiny and testing in the ICU.

REFERENCES

1. Kistler JP. Therapy of ischemic cerebral vascular disease due to atherothrombosis. *N Engl J Med* 1984;311: 100–105.
2. Plum F, Posner JB. The diagnosis of stupor and coma. *Contemp Neurol Ser* 1972;10:1– 286.
3. Astrup J. Energy-requiring cell functions in the ischemic brain. Their critical supply and possible inhibition in protective therapy. *J Neurosurg* 1982;56:482–497.
4. Siesjo BK. Cell damage in the brain: a speculative synthesis. *J Cereb Blood Flow Metab* 1981;1:155–185.
5. Choi DW. Excitotoxic cell death. *J Neurobiol* 1992;23:1261–1276.
6. Jones TH. Thresholds of focal cerebral ischemia in awake monkeys. *J Neurosurg* 1981;54:773–782.
7. Petito CK. Delayed hippocampal damage in humans following cardiorespiratory arrest. *Neurology* 1987;37: 1281–1286.
8. Pulsinelli WA. Temporal profile of neuronal damage in a model of transient forebrain ischemia. *Ann Neurol* 1982;11:491–498.
9. Wallace JD, Levy LL. Blood pressure after stroke. *JAMA* 1981;246:2177–2180.
10. Britton M, deFaire U, Helmers C. Hazards of therapy for excessive hypertension in acute stroke. *Acta Med Scand* 1980;207:253–257.
11. Carlberg B, Asplund K, Hagg E. Factors influencing admission blood pressure levels in patients with acute stroke. *Stroke* 1991;22:527–530.
12. Jansen PA. Course of blood pressure after cerebral infarction and transient ischemic attack. *Clin Neurol Neurosurg* 1987;89:243–246.
13. Loyke HF. Lowering of blood pressure after stroke. *Am J Med Sci* 1983;286:2–11.
14. Raichle ME. The pathophysiology of brain ischemia. *Ann Neurol* 1983;13:2–10.
15. Liu TH. Polyethylene glycol-conjugated superoxide dismutase and catalase reduce ischemic brain injury. *Am J Physiol* 1989;256:H589–H593.
16. Martinez-Vila E, Sieria PI. Current status and perspectives of neuroprotection in ischemic stroke treatment. *Cerebrovasc Dis* 2001;11:60–70.
17. Aspey BS, Ehteshami S, Hurst CM, et al. The effect of increased blood pressure on hemispheric lactate and water content during acute cerebral ischaemia in the rat and gerbil. *J Neurol Neurosurg Psychiatry* 1987;50: 1493–1498.
18. Rordorf G, Cramer SC, Efird JT, et al. Pharmacological elevation of blood pressure in acute stroke. Clinical effects and safety. *Stroke* 1997;28:2133–2138.
19. Tissue plasminogen activator for acute ischemic stroke. The National Institute of Neurological Disorders and Stroke rt-PA Stroke Study Group. *N Engl J Med* 995; 333:1581–1587.
20. Furlan A, Higashida R, Wechsler L, et al. Intraarterial prourokinase for acute ischemic stroke. The PROACT II study: a randomized controlled trial. Prolyse in Acute Cerebral Thromboembolism. *JAMA* 1999;282: 2003–2011.
21. Hacke W, Schwab S, Horn M, et al. 'Malignant' middle cerebral artery territory infarction: clinical course and prognostic signs. *Arch Neurol* 1996;53:309–315.
22. Wijdicks EF, Diringer MN. Middle cerebral artery territory infarction and early brain swelling: progression and effect of age on outcome. *Mayo Clin Proc* 1998;73: 829–836.
23. Cruz-Flores S, Thompson DW, Boiser JR. Massive cerebral edema after recanalization post-thrombolysis. *J Neuroimaging* 2001;11:447–451.
24. Koudstaal PJ, Stibbe J, Vermeulen M. Fatal ischaemic brain oedema after early thrombolysis with tissue plasminogen activator in acute stroke. *BMJ* 1988;297: 1571–1574.
25. von Kummer R, Meyding-Lamade U, Forsting M, et al.

Sensitivity and prognostic value of early CT in occlusion of the middle cerebral artery trunk. *AJNR Am J Neuroradiol* 1994;15:9–15.

26. Davalos A, Toni D, Iweins F, et al. Neurological deterioration in acute ischemic stroke: potential predictors and associated factors in the European cooperative acute stroke study (ECASS) I. *Stroke* 1999;30: 2631–2636.

27. Gujjar AR, Deibert E, Duff S, et al. Mechanical ventilation for ischemic stroke and intracerebral hemorrhage: indications, timing, and outcome. *Neurology* 1998;51: 447–451.

28. Berrouschot J, Rossler A, Koster J, et al. Mechanical ventilation in patients with hemispheric ischemic stroke. *Crit Care Med* 2000;28:2956–2961.

29. el-Ad B, Bornstein NM, Fuchs P, et al. Mechanical ventilation in stroke patients–is it worthwhile? *Neurology* 1996;47:657–659.

30. Mayer SA, Copeland D, Bernardini GL, et al. Cost and outcome of mechanical ventilation for life-threatening stroke. *Stroke* 2000;31:2346–2353.

31. Deibert E, Diringer MN. Intensive care management of acute ischemic stroke. *Neurologist* 2001;5:313–325.

32. Frank JI. Large hemispheric infarction, deterioration, and intracranial pressure. *Neurology* 1995;45: 1286–1290.

33. Steiner T, Weber R, Krieger D. Increased intracerebral pressure following stroke. *Curr Treat Options Neurol* 2001;3:441–450.

34. Albrecht RF, Miletich DJ, Ruttle M. Cerebral effects of extended hyperventilation in unanesthetized goats. *Stroke* 1987;18:649–655.

35. Cain SM. An attempt to demonstrate cerebral anoxia during hyperventilation of anesthetized dogs. *Am J Physiol* 2001;204:323–326.

36. Christensen MS. Acid-base changes in cerebrospinal fluid and blood and blood volume changes following prolonged hyperventilation in man. *Br J Anaesthesiol* 1974;46:348–357.

37. Qureshi AI, Geocadin RG, Suarez JI, et al. Long-term outcome after medical reversal of transtentorial herniation in patients with supratentorial mass lesions. *Crit Care Med* 2000;28:1556–1564.

38. Manno EM, Adams RE, Derdeyn CP, et al. The effects of mannitol on cerebral edema after large hemispheric cerebral infarct. *Neurology* 1999;52:583–587.

39. Videen TO, Zazulia AR, Manno EM, et al. Mannitol bolus preferentially shrinks non-infarcted brain in patients with ischemic stroke. *Neurology* 2001;57:2120–2122.

40. Qureshi AI, Suarez JI, Bhardwaj A, et al. Use of hypertonic (3%) saline/acetate infusion in the treatment of cerebral edema: effect on intracranial pressure and lateral displacement of the brain. *Crit Care Med* 1998;26: 440–446.

41. Rieke K, Schwab S, Krieger D, et al. Decompressive surgery in space-occupying hemispheric infarction: results of an open, prospective trial. *Crit Care Med* 1995; 23:1576–1587.

42. Schwab S, Steiner T, Aschoff A, et al. Early hemicraniectomy in patients with complete middle cerebral artery infarction. *Stroke* 1998;29:1888–1893.

43. Auer RN. Hemicraniectomy for ischemic stroke: temerity or death cure? *Can J Neurol Sci* 2000;27:269.

44. Demchuk AM. Hemicraniectomy is a promising treatment in ischemic stroke. *Can J Neurol Sci* 2000;27: 274–277.

45. Wijdicks EF. Management of massive hemispheric cerebral infarct: is there a ray of hope? *Mayo Clin Proc* 2000;75:945–952.

46. Busto R, Globus MYT, Dietrich WD, et al. Effect of mild hypothermia on ischemia-induced release of neurotransmitters and free fatty acids in rat brain. *Stroke* 1989;20:904–910.

47. Colbourne F, Corbett D, Zhao Z, et al. Prolonged but delayed postischemic hypothermia: a long-term outcome study in the rat middle cerebral artery occlusion model. *J Cereb Blood Flow Metab* 2000;20:1702–1708.

48. Maier CM, Sun GH, Kunis D, et al. Delayed induction and long–term effects of mild hypothermia in a focal model of transient cerebral ischemia: neurological outcome and infarct size. *J Neurosurg* 2001;94:90–96.

49. Ginsberg MD, Busto R. Combating hyperthermia in acute stroke: a significant clinical concern. *Stroke* 1998; 29:529–534.

50. Zhao W, Alonso OF, Loor JY, et al. Influence of early posttraumatic hypothermia therapy on local cerebral blood flow and glucose metabolism after fluid-percussion brain injury. *J Neurosurg* 1999;90:510–519.

51. Azzimondi G, Bassein L, Nonino F, et al. Fever in acute stroke worsens prognosis. A prospective study. *Stroke* 1995;26:2040–2043.

52. Castillo J, Davalos A, Marrugat J, et al. Timing for fever-related brain damage in acute ischemic stroke [see comments]. *Stroke* 1998;29:2455–2460.

53. Reith J, Jorgensen HS, Pedersen PM, et al. Body temperature in acute stroke: relation to stroke severity, infarct size, mortality, and outcome [see comments]. *Lancet* 1996;347:422–425.

54. Schwab S, Georgiadis D, Berrouschot J, et al. Feasibility and safety of moderate hypothermia after massive hemispheric infarction. *Stroke* 2001;32:2033–2035.

55. Schwab S, Spranger M, Aschoff A, et al. Brain temperature monitoring and modulation in patients with severe MCA infarction. *Neurology* 1997;48:762–767.

56. Steiner T, Friede T, Aschoff A, et al. Effect and feasibility of controlled rewarming after moderate hypothermia in stroke patients with malignant infarction of the middle cerebral artery. *Stroke* 2001;32:2833–2835.

14

Management of Nontraumatic Brain Hemorrhage

The third most common cause of death in the United States is cerebrovascular disease, and 10% to 15% of strokes are intracerebral hemorrhages (ICH). There are approximately 65,000 cases of ICH each year in the United States, occurring more commonly in men, Asians, African Americans, and older individuals (1). Intracerebral hemorrhage is even more common in Japan and Southeast Asia, constituting 30% of all strokes annually. However, there may be a lower incidence of ICH in Japanese men who have emigrated to the United States (2). African Americans have a higher risk of ICH than Whites in the United States, but this difference may be accounted for by a higher incidence of hypertension in that group (3). Hispanics in the United States also may have a higher risk of stroke compared with Whites, but it has been suggested (on limited data) that this results from the higher prevalence of cavernous angiomas in the Hispanic population (4).

Most relevant to intensive care unit (ICU) practice, mortality for ICH is much higher than for ischemic stroke or even for subarachnoid hemorrhage, with up to 50% of patients dying within 1 month of the bleeding; furthermore, up to 80% of survivors have severe neurological deficits (5,6). Consequently, a large number of patients with ICH require intensive care services. The main issues that arise are the control of intracranial hypertension (Chapters 2 and 3) and decisions regarding surgical treatment. Despite the critical nature of ICH, only a few small randomized trials of medical and surgical treatments have been performed, none of which has demonstrated significantly improved outcome.

ETIOLOGY

Intracranial hemorrhage can be classified by etiology and location. One case control study found that a history of hypertension increased the risk of ICH by 3.9-fold (7). Hypertension, the presumed cause of hemorrhage in 70% to 90% of patients, causes bleeding that arises from penetrating vessels of 80- to 300-μm diameter that are derived from the main vessels of the circle of Willis or the basilar artery (8). This pathoanatomic factor accounts for the characteristic locations of hypertensive hemorrhages: basal ganglia (35 to 45%), subcortical white matter (25%), thalamus (20%), cerebellum (15%), and pons (5%). Chronic hypertension leads to fibrinoid necrosis, which reduces the tensile strength of the vessel wall (9,10). Classic neuropathologic studies suggest that most hemorrhages arise from small "Charcot–Bouchard" aneurysms. Although the precise factor that finally precipitates the hemorrhage is unknown, it has been speculated that transient increases in blood pressure are the proximate cause of the hemorrhage in many patients (11).

In the 10% to 30% of patients with ICH in whom there is no evidence of hypertension, the bleeding is often centered in the subcortical white matter of one of the lobes, termed lobar, subcortical, white matter, or slit hemorrhage, the latter describing the pathologic appearance of the hemosiderin-stained cavity years after the stroke (12,13). In patients older than 65 years, amyloid angiopathy may exceed hypertension as a cause for hemorrhages, particularly multiple and recurrent lobar or cortical–subcortical brain hemorrhages (14). Amyloid deposition is usually related to aging in the brain, because 60% of individuals older than 90 years have pathologic evidence of amyloid deposition (15). Amyloid angiopathy results from the deposition of amyloid in the media and adventitia of small- and medium-sized arteries located near the surface of the cerebral cortex and in the leptomeninges; among the several theories of causation it has been suggested that there is abnormal catabolism of γ-trace protein in the cerebrospinal fluid (16). The epsilon 2 and 4 alleles of apolipoprotein E are associated with increased β-amyloid protein deposition, fibrinoid necrosis, and increased risk of recurrent bleeding among patients with ICH secondary to amyloid angiopathy (17).

More bloody, nontraumatic brain hemorrhages are associated with the etiologic factors listed in Table 14.1. Of course, a thorough history excludes a traumatic etiology. Besides chronic hypertension, inquiry should be made about alcoholism, use of illicit drugs, and use of anticoagulants. Heavy alcohol use can impair coagulation and affect the integrity of the intracerebral vessels,

thereby increasing the risk of hemorrhage (18). Intracerebral hemorrhage in patients taking sympathomimetic drugs may be related to acute hypertension, arteriovenous malformations, aneurysms, or drug-induced vasculitis. An increasingly common type arises as a result of anticoagulant drugs or an endogenous coagulopathy. Coagulopathy owing to hepatic failure, thrombocytopenia, and leukemia can all lead to brain hemorrhage. Aspirin and dipyridamole use also have been associated with ICH. Although low serum cholesterol has been reported to be a risk factor for ICH, the data need to be confirmed with a larger prospective study (19–21). Clinical trials of lipid-lowering statin medications more recently have shown a reduction in risk of stroke without an increase in rate of ICH (22,23).

CLINICAL FEATURES

The clinical syndrome of brain hemorrhage is one of abrupt onset and rapid evolution of symptoms and signs over minutes or hours. Generally, no prodromal symptoms occur to herald the stroke. Headache, nausea, and vomiting are often the initial symptoms and are attributed to increased intracranial pressure (ICP). A few patients have a seizure at the onset of bleeding, but this is rarely a persistent management issue. Meningismus may result from intraventricular blood that travels to the subarachnoid space but it is surprising how often this sign is absent. Acute hypertension and a diminished level of consciousness are frequent. It has become apparent that expansion of the hematoma may occur, particularly in the first few hours after onset, and the progression of neurological signs during this period is often caused by this ongoing bleeding and enlargement of the hematoma (24). Surrounding edema begins to develop immediately, possibly from the release of osmotically active proteins from the hematoma. This brain swelling worsens over the next several days and can persist for 2 or more weeks (25). This is followed by secondary distortion of the dien-

TABLE 14.1. *Etiologies of nontraumatic intracerebral hemorrhage*

Hypertension
Aneurysm
Vascular malformation
Amyloid angiopathy
Abnormal coagulation
Use of anticoagulants or thrombolytics
Heavy alcohol use
Sympathomimetic drugs (cocaine, amphetamines, pseudoephedrine, phenylpropanolamine)
Tumor
Arteritis
Hemorrhagic infarction, especially from venous occlusion
Reperfusion (after recanalization of occluded vessel or after carotid endarterectomy)
Central nervous system infection (fungal, herpes simplex virus)
Others

cephalon and upper-midbrain, resulting in progressive loss of consciousness and pupillary enlargement. Nearly two thirds of patients with ICH have a smooth progression of neurological symptoms, unlike ischemic stroke and subarachnoid hemorrhage where over 80% of patients present with symptoms maximal at onset (26). A low Glasgow Coma Scale (GCS) score (less than 9), a large hematoma, and intraventricular blood each increase the risk of neurological deterioration and poor outcome (27,28).

Despite the ease with which hemorrhages are demonstrated on computed tomography (CT) scanning, it is necessary to identify the clinical syndrome in order to suspect the diagnosis and distinguish it from an ischemic stroke. Although headache (and vomiting) is a frequent but nonspecific accompaniment of ICH, it may help delineate the site of a *lobar hemorrhage* (13). Frontal lobe hemorrhage is associated with frontal headache and contralateral weakness. Temporal lobe hemorrhage causes pain anterior to the ipsilateral ear and, when in the dominant hemisphere, a fluent aphasia with poor auditory comprehension. Hemorrhage in the parietal lobe is also associated with ipsilateral anterior temporal headache but causes signs of a hemisensory deficit. Occipital lobe hemorrhage causes severe ipsilateral eye pain and dense hemianopia. The clinical syndromes of lobar hemorrhage sometimes are difficult to distinguish from emboli to the same regions. Computed tomography scanning allows rapid distinction between the two.

During the evolution of a *putaminal hemorrhage,* the signs of raised intracranial pressure rapidly blend with progressive contralateral hemiparesis and hemisensory loss. The eyes deviate away from the side of the paretic limbs. Visual field defects are common if the level of consciousness allows accurate testing. Hemorrhages in the dominant hemisphere may result in significant nonfluent aphasia (or fluent, if located more posteriorly), and those in the nondominant hemisphere may cause dysprosody of speech and anosognosia. Large hemorrhages produce al-most immediate coma, and smaller hemorrhages can lead to more gradual impairment of consciousness and signs of upper brainstem compression.

Thalamic hemorrhage also produces a contralateral hemiplegia and hemisensory deficit. However, the hemisensory deficit is often more pronounced than with a putaminal hemorrhage. Visual field deficits, aphasia, and contralateral neglect also may be seen as with putaminal hemorrhages. Because of the near midline location of thalamic hemorrhages, they are more likely to lead to pupil abnormalities, ocular palsies, and alteration of consciousness than are putaminal hemorrhages of similar size. The classical presentation of obtundation associated with downward and inward deviation of the eyes is well known to clinicians.

Cerebellar hemorrhage is often associated with repeated vomiting, vertigo, and the inability to walk, but without limb ataxia in many patients. It is most often mistaken for "labyrinthitis" or confused with basilar artery occlusion. Therefore, it is imperative to test gait in patients with vomiting and dizziness. As the hemorrhage enlarges, conjugate gaze palsy develops such that the patient cannot look toward the side of the hemorrhage. Sometimes a sixth cranial nerve palsy precedes the conjugate gaze palsy. Dysarthria and a mild ipsilateral facial weakness may be present. As these signs of brainstem dysfunction occur, mentation is altered. Although this alteration may be subtle initially, it can progress rapidly to frank coma, pinpoint pupils, and decerebration.

Pontine hemorrhage is the most likely to lead to rapid onset of deep coma and bilateral signs of brainstem dysfunction (Fig. 14.1). The pupils are pinpoint, but light reaction is often preserved if the pupils are observed with a magnifying glass. Bilateral horizontal conjugate gaze paresis is usually present and a skew deviation also may be present. Ocular bobbing frequently is observed. Quadriplegia and bifacial weakness are the most common motor findings. Progression of the hemorrhage may lead to cessation of respiration.

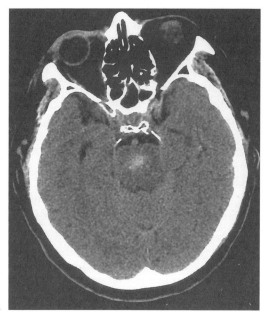
A

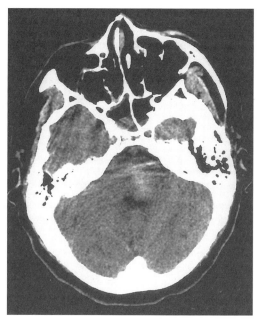
B

FIG. 14.1. This 45-year-old man with hypertension and heavy alcohol use developed sudden headache and dizziness followed by unresponsiveness. He was intubated and transferred to our medical center comatose with small but reactive pupils, an absent corneal reflex on the right, ocular bobbing, skew deviation, and bilateral extensor posturing. **A,B:** The head computed tomography demonstrated a 2- by 2.5-cm pontine intracranial hemorrhage. An angiogram showed no arteriovenous malformation or aneurysm. Over the next month he became fully alert, had a tracheostomy for secretion management but no longer required mechanical ventilation, was able to swallow, had ophthalmoparesis in all directions of gaze, and had bifacial weakness and right hemiparesis.

RADIOLOGIC EVALUATION

After an initial clinical assessment, the patient is taken to the radiology suite for a plain CT scan to confirm the diagnosis of brain hemorrhage and to assess the size of the clot. The characteristic CT picture of ICH is an area of increased density in the parenchyma measuring 40 to 90 Hounsfield units, which is related to the hemoglobin content of the extravasated blood (29). Therefore, it must be remembered that blood may appear virtually isodense to brain on the CT scan if the patient has a significant anemia (30). The scan allows the clinician to assess the topography of the hemorrhage and the extent of concomitant ventricular, subarachnoid, or subdural blood. The pattern of these features may suggest an etiology for the hemorrhage. Additionally, the CT scan

demonstrates secondary complications such as hydrocephalus and herniation. In the authors' experience, the level of consciousness in ICH is closely associated with the degree of horizontal displacement of midline structures: a 4- to 6-mm shift of the pineal calcification corresponds to drowsiness, 6- to 8-mm with stupor, and greater than 8- to 9-mm with coma (31). Compression of the basal cisterns is also a dependable sign of serious mass effect and is likely to be associated with moderately or greatly raised ICP.

If the hemorrhage is in an unusual location or has unusual features, a contrast-enhanced CT scan can be performed to assess for an underlying aneurysm, vascular malformation, or tumor. Initially, however, the hemorrhage itself may obscure the recognition of these pathologic entities. Often, a contrast-enhanced CT scan yields more information if performed at least 1 week after the hemorrhage. An arteriovenous malformation or aneurysm should be suspected if subarachnoid blood is present.

Although angiography is not currently part of the routine evaluation of ICH, it continues to be the mainstay for identifying an underlying vascular abnormality. Of paramount importance initially is identifying hemorrhages that have occurred secondary to aneurysmal rupture. These clots usually appear on CT scan as lobar hemorrhages in the frontal or temporal lobes, or largely within the sylvian fissure. In most cases the parenchymal hemorrhage is accompanied by subdural or subarachnoid hemorrhage. Parenchymal hemorrhage secondary to aneurysmal rupture is associated with a high rate of rehemorrhage and mortality. Therefore, early identification of these patients with angiography allows the clinician to plan timely surgical intervention. Angiography is useful in delineating vascular malformations as well. However, an angiogram performed within several days of the hemorrhage may fail to identify the lesion because of compression by the hemorrhage and surrounding edema. In this situation, a repeat angiogram is indicated 2 to 3 weeks after the hemorrhage. Vascular malformations may not be visualized even by an angiogram performed after the hemorrhage has resolved and the edema has subsided (32). These angiographically occult lesions may be the sites of recurrent hemorrhage. A prospective study of cerebral angiography in ICH indicated that it had a low yield in identifying an underlying vascular abnormality in patients older than 45 years with a history of hypertension and a putaminal, thalamic, pontine, or cerebellar ICH (33). Patients with lobar ICH, isolated intraventricular hemorrhage, normotensive, or who are younger than 45, were more likely to have diagnostic angiographic abnormalities.

Although magnetic resonance imaging (MRI) is not routinely obtained during the initial evaluation, it may be particularly helpful in identifying small brainstem hemorrhages and revealing vascular malformations that cannot be seen with angiography. Acute blood on MRI generally appears isointense to hypointense on T1-weighted imaging and hypointense on T2-weighted imaging. Although it may miss small aneurysms and vascular malformations, MRI is superior to CT and angiography in detecting cavernous malformations and can give information regarding the time course of the hemorrhage (34).

INITIAL MANAGEMENT

The initial goals for management are to prevent subsequent neural damage from rebleeding, edema, or hypoxia; localize the location and extent of the hemorrhage; and determine its etiology. The initial assessment includes evaluation of airway, breathing, and circulation, neurological examination, and searching for signs of trauma or rhabdomyolysis if the patient is found some time after the ICH occurred.

Correct identification of the location and etiology of the hemorrhage begins by obtaining as many details as possible about the prior medical history and about the initial onset of neurological symptoms. Frequently, a characteristic pattern and progression of symptoms and signs identify the location of the hemorrhage. These patients then receive a thorough neurological examination. Although brief, requiring 5 to 10 minutes, the initial evaluation must be comprehensive because it is the basis for judging subsequent improvement or deterioration in neurological function. The most important aspect of the initial examination is an assessment of the level of consciousness. The level of consciousness at the onset and the rate of progression of obtundation are important for assessing prognosis as well as guiding subsequent management decisions. Patients presenting to the hospital in coma or becoming comatose before definitive intervention have a mortality rate exceeding 50% (35,36).

While the patient is assessed clinically, simultaneous management must be oriented toward preventing neurological deterioration. Abnormalities in electrolytes and coagulation parameters are identified and corrected. Elevated serum glucose should be treated aggressively. If a coagulopathy is present and hepatic disease is suspected, liver function studies should be performed. Fresh-frozen plasma and vitamin K may need to be administered if the prothrombin time is elevated. If the patient had received heparin recently, protamine 1 mg per 100 units of heparin may be administered, watching for anaphylaxis and hypotension. Following the use of thrombolytic agents, treatment with platelets, fresh-frozen plasma, and cryoprecipitate should be initiated. Laboratory testing might include a toxicology screen in younger patients, or if there is any suspicion of illicit drug use. Phenytoin may be administered to prevent seizures, particularly for lobar hemorrhages, although there are little data to support doing this. The authors do not routinely start anticonvulsant medications unless the patient has had a seizure. Mannitol is generally given if the patient is stuporous or comatose (see the following and Chapter 3).

Patients with poor airway control, imminent ventilatory insufficiency, or a GCS score less than 9 are intubated and ventilated to maintain an arterial PCO_2 between 30 and 35 mm Hg. Endotracheal intubation should be performed with preoxygenation and administration of drugs such as a combination of either thiopental [up to 2.5 to 4.5 mg/kg intravenously (i.v.)], etomidate (0.3 mg/kg i.v.), succinylcholine (1 mg/kg i.v.), lidocaine (1 to 2 mg/kg i.v.), midazolam, propofol, or atropine, to avoid reflex arrhythmia or hypertension that might result in recurrent hemorrhage (34,37). Short-acting anesthetic agents are preferred before intubation to prevent rises in ICP. Patients requiring intubation are also managed with a nasogastric tube to prevent gastric distention and aspiration of gastric contents.

Blood Pressure Management

Most patients are hypertensive immediately after a hemorrhage. An important goal of initial management is to reduce the blood pressure below a level that is likely to precipitate another hemorrhage or exaggerate edema. Because the precise value for this level of blood pressure is uncertain, the authors arbitrarily attempt to maintain the systolic blood pressure below 160 mm Hg or the mean arterial blood pressure

(MAP) below 110 mm Hg in the conscious patient. One of the authors, with the AHA Stroke Council, has recommended treating only for a MAP greater than 130 mm Hg in patients with a history of hypertension (34,37). We have found this to be most easily accomplished initially using labetalol, a competitive α-1, β-1, and β-2 antagonist, administered intravenously by repeated boluses of 10 to 40 mg per hour or, less commonly, by continuous infusion at 2 to 8 mg/minute (34). It appears safer than hydralazine in the older patient with ischemic coronary artery disease because there is no reflex tachycardia. If there is bradycardia, however, hydralazine 10 to 20 mg every 4 hours as needed may be preferable. Enalaprilat (i.v. enalapril) 0.625 to 1.2 mg boluses every 6 hours as needed is another option (34). Continuous nitroprusside is reserved for uncontrollable blood pressure and should be used cautiously because of the vasodilatory effects and the theoretical risk of increased cerebral blood volume and thereby increased ICP. Some studies have suggested that lowering blood pressure may lead to worsening ischemia around the ICH. However, one study with positron emission tomography scanning demonstrated no increase in cerebral ischemia in hypertensive ICH patients with a MAP lowered by 15% (38).

Intracranial Pressure

Based in our current conceptualization of cerebral hemodynamics, patients with large hemorrhages or those whose brainstem function is compromised by the mass of the hemorrhage require higher blood pressure to maintain a cerebral perfusion pressure. The selection of appropriate antihypertensive therapy in these patients requires concomitant measurement and control of ICP. Patients with a GCS score of less than 9 or a rapid decline in level of consciousness are assumed to have elevated ICP. In this situation, monitoring with either an intraparenchymal fiberoptic or intraventricular ICP device is often used in the authors' neurological intensive care units (neuro-ICUs) to guide subsequent therapy, as described in Chapter 3 (39). A ventricular catheter may be used in patients with evidence of blood within the ventricular system because intermittent drainage of CSF may be more helpful in lowering ICP in these patients. We and a number of other neurointensivists have found ICP monitoring helpful in guiding medical therapy and deciding when to implement surgical therapy (13,40,41), although we recognize that only anecdotal experience supports the notion that monitoring improves outcome (Chapter 2). Intracranial pressure should ideally be maintained at less than 20 mm Hg and cerebral perfusion pressure maintained above 70 mm Hg.

Osmotic therapy and hyperventilation are recommended in those with clinical signs of impending brain herniation. Mannitol is usually the first-line treatment for raised ICP and is given every 4 hours as needed for an ICP greater than 20 mm Hg in boluses of 0.25 to 0.5 g/kg (Chapter 3). A furosemide bolus is used sometimes as an adjunctive treatment. Electrolytes and serum osmolarity should be monitored periodically and the mannitol should be discontinued if the serum osmolarity approaches 320 mOsm/L. The authors have also used hypertonic saline boluses in an attempt to reduce cerebral edema; however, there is concern that edema may be exacerbated by the potential sequestration of sodium in the injured brain tissue, although the same theoretical concern may be raised regarding sequestered mannitol.

Hyperventilation to establish a $PaCO_2$ of 30 to 35 mm Hg should be maintained as necessary until ICP is normalized. If ICP is controlled, hyperventilation can be reduced slowly avoiding rebound intracranial hypertension by normalizing $PaCO_2$ over the course of at least 48 hours. Pentobarbital is an optional treatment for refractory elevated ICP but should be used cautiously with i.v. fluids and vasopressor medication readily available for the induced hypotension.

Other Medical Management

This should include prophylaxis for deep venous thrombosis with pneumatic compression devices. Euvolemia is the goal in fluid management, and maintenance of normothermia is preferred. Agitated patients may require short-acting benzodiazepines or propofol for sedation to avoid rebleeding. Additionally, consideration should be given to the possibility of drug or alcohol withdrawal as a cause for otherwise unexplained agitation. Older patients with ICH often have coexisting coronary artery disease with increased risk for myocardial infarction and should be monitored for chest pain or cardiovascular insufficiency. In some patients with ICH, as with subarachnoid hemorrhage, there may be electrocardiographic changes without myocardial ischemia, such as prolongation of the QT interval, ST segment changes, and U waves (42,43).

SPECIFIC TREATMENT AND SURGICAL EVACUATION

Corticosteroids are currently not recommended in the management of brain hemorrhage on the basis of one prospective, double-blind, randomized study of 93 patients that studied the efficacy of dexamethasone in primary supratentorial ICH (44). The death rate was identical in patients receiving dexamethasone and in those receiving placebo. However, the study was terminated early when it became apparent that the rate of infectious complications was higher in the dexamethasone-treated group. Similarly, glycerol has not been shown to improve outcome in a randomized trial (45). Intravenous infusion of activated recombinant coagulation factor VIIa, used in the treatment of hemophilia, is now being studied in noncoagulopathic patients with ICH in an effort to prevent hematoma expansion.

It has been estimated that 7,000 surgeries are performed each year in the United States for ICH even though there has been no proven benefit to evacuation of the hematoma (46). Only a few small randomized studies of surgical evacuation of ICH have been published in the post-CT era and none has shown benefit as discussed in the following (47–49). There is general agreement that surgery is not recommended for a small ICH (less than 10 cm^3) or if the neurological deficit is mild. However, cerebellar hemorrhages that are causing brainstem compression or hydrocephalus or neurological deterioration generally are evacuated surgically as soon as possible, as discussed further on. Also in young patients who are worsening neurologically with a lobar hemorrhage, surgery often is performed, based on anecdotal experience. The optimal treatment for the rest of ICH cases is not clear (34). Alternatives to conventional craniotomy such as CT-guided stereotactic or ultrasound-guided aspiration, and instillation of thrombolytics into the hematoma combined with aspiration have not been investigated in a large randomized study. Thrombolytic instillation via an external ventricular drainage device has been used in ICH and is currently being studied in a multicenter randomized trial that includes some of the authors' neuro-ICUs.

Definitive management of a brain hemorrhage varies with the location, size, and etiology of the hemorrhage. Small hemorrhages with mild to moderate focal deficit require only careful observation and intermittent therapy to reduce cerebral edema. Conversely, large hemorrhages, particularly the large putaminal hemorrhages, are unlikely to benefit from any therapy. Hemorrhages within the brain parenchyma that are secondary to aneurysmal rupture are managed with early surgical intervention at the time of clipping of the aneurysm, whereas hemorrhages that are secondary to bleeding from an arteriovenous malformation are managed initially with aggressive medical therapy to prevent increased ICP. We prefer to delay surgery on operable arteriovenous malformations until 2 to 3 weeks after the hemorrhage. At that time the clot has liquefied, and a definitive operation to remove the arteriovenous malformation may be planned. If increasing ICP or worsening neurological deficit necessitates earlier surgical intervention, this is limited to drainage of the clot itself with the provisions noted in the following section. A definitive operation to remove the arteriovenous malformation is performed after the cerebral edema has subsided. Traditional teaching has been to avoid surgery in patients with known or suspected amyloid angiopathy because of the high rate of postoperative hemorrhage. However, two studies suggest that this risk may not be as high as once thought (50,51).

Therapy for supratentorial ICH has been evaluated by three prospective randomized studies (47–49). One of these trials was conducted in Helsinki and prospectively randomized 52 patients who were mostly stuporous or comatose to receive either emergency surgery or conservative treatment (47). All patients were randomized within 48 hours of the ictus. The median time from bleeding to operation was 14.5 hours in the surgical group. At 6 months after the ICH there was no statistically significant difference in the numbers of patients able to conduct independent activities of daily living between the two groups. The mortality rates among the semicomatose or stuporous patients were lower in the surgical group. However, all of these patients remained severely disabled. Therefore, this study concluded that surgical intervention does not offer any advantage over conservative medical care.

Auer and coworkers (48) conducted a randomized prospective trial in Austria comparing the effectiveness of surgical endoscopic evacuation of supratentorial brain hemorrhages with medical therapy in 100 patients. Surgical patients with subcortical hematomas showed a significantly lower mortality rate compared with medical treatment (30% versus 70%). In addition, more of the surgically treated patients in this group had a good outcome (40%) than did those treated with medical therapy (25%; $P < 0.01$). The outcome of surgical patients with putaminal or thalamic hemorrhage was no better than for those patients who received medical therapy; however, there was a trend toward a better chance and quality of survival in the surgically treated patients.

Batjer and associates (49), in a smaller randomized trial of putaminal ICH in the United States, attempted to compare best medical therapy, best medical therapy with ICP monitoring, and surgical evacuation of the hematoma without ICP monitoring. This 6-year study only included patients with severe deficits and hematoma diameter greater than 3 cm; the trial was stopped after 21 patients were enrolled. Seven of nine patients in the medical group died or were severely disabled compared with six of eight patients who received craniotomy and hematoma evacuation. Although this study has been interpreted as a negative surgical trial, the study design (i.e., including only severely impaired patients with a large putaminal ICH) and the small number of patients included, make any conclusions difficult to apply to the wide range of patients that present with ICH.

In a metaanalysis of the three randomized studies (47–49), craniotomy for ICH was associated with a nonsignificant trend toward increased death and disability compared to medical treatment (6). Stereotactic endoscopic evacuation has been associated with a reduced risk of death and a nonsignificant trend toward reduced disability, but more randomized controlled trials are needed. A more recent nonrandomized small study found that rebleeding complicated ultra-early (within 4 hours of symptom onset) craniotomy and evacuation of hematoma, but that maximum removal of blood was a predictor of good outcome (52). They suggest that either more aggressive lowering of blood pressure or less invasive surgical techniques might improve outcome. Several small series have reported favorable results with aspiration combined with thrombolytic infusion into the clot (53,54). There are several ongoing trials of craniotomy, stereotactic endoscopic evacuation, and thrombolysis combined with stereotactic evacuation. Techniques that maximize the amount of hematoma removed, minimize invasiveness and damage to normal brain tissue, and minimize postoperative rebleeding are needed.

Many patients with brain hemorrhage do not fit into the aforementioned discrete categories. Thus, it may be more valuable to consider the definitive management of hemorrhages by their location.

Putamen

The putamen is the most common site for hypertensive ICH. It is of some interest that recommendations for management of hemorrhage in this location have undergone considerable evolution. Small- to moderate-sized hemorrhages up to 2 to 3 cm in diameter produce mild to moderate focal deficits. A good recovery is expected with medical therapy alone. However, hemorrhages larger than 3 cm are often associated with stupor or coma. One small randomized study of these larger putaminal hemorrhages found no difference in outcome between medical and surgical treatment (49). However, Kaneko and colleagues (55,56), in a nonrandomized trial, concluded that stuporous or "semicomatose" patients without evidence of brainstem herniation had a better overall outcome if subjected to aggressive microsurgical removal of the hemorrhage within 7 hours of the ictus. Patients presenting with evidence of coma and brainstem herniation are not often helped by acute surgery. We generally have avoided urging our surgeons to evacuate putaminal hemorrhages, but there have been notable exceptions in young patients who are deteriorating with teardrop-shaped clots that cannot be easily distinguished from frontal or parietal lobar hematomas. An angiogram usually is undertaken first. Intracranial pressure monitoring may play a role in identifying surgical candidates after the first day because patients with an ICP who cannot be contained by medical therapy do very poorly (39).

Cerebellum

Hemorrhage within the cerebellum produces life-threatening neurological dysfunction, primarily by compressing the brainstem and secondarily by inducing obstructive hydrocephalus. The outcome in these patients is related in most studies directly to the level of consciousness. Comatose patients are more likely to die or be left impaired neurologically than are patients who are alert or only drowsy. Because hematomas of increasing size produce more brainstem compression and thus more impairment in consciousness, the size of the hematoma on CT scan is important in planning management. The literature supports the notion that hematomas less than 2 cm in diameter usually can be managed medically in an ICU in the alert patient (57–60). Conversely, the consensus has evolved that hematomas larger than 3 cm in diameter should be evacuated emergently, even in patients who are alert or minimally drowsy. Hematomas between 2 and 3 cm can be managed medically if the patient is awake and does not demonstrate any evidence of brainstem compression (58). However, if evidence of brainstem dysfunction is present or appears, these hematomas should be evacuated surgi-

cally. Ventricular drainage alone has a limited role in the nonsurgical management of these patients because it treats only the secondary hydrocephalus without addressing the primary brainstem compression. However, we place a ventricular catheter at the time of surgical intervention in these patients to allow for monitoring of ICP and drainage of CSF postoperatively.

Patients presenting in deep coma with minimal evidence of remaining neurological function usually are not considered to be surgical candidates. However, we have seen patients who recover from this state after evacuation of a cerebellar hemorrhage (Fig. 14.2).

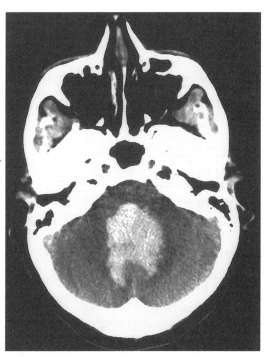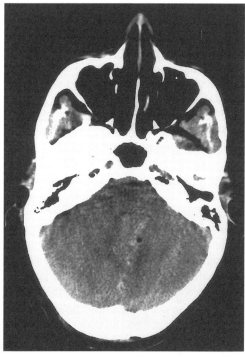

A   B

FIG. 14.2. This 41-year-old woman was transferred to our medical center after developing sudden left hemisensory loss, occipital headache, and difficulty ambulating. She arrived comatose, pupils were small and nonreactive, corneal reflexes were absent, all extremities were flaccid, but a cough was still present. **A:** The head computed tomography (CT) demonstrated a large fourth ventricular and cerebellar vermian intracranial hemorrhage with blood extending into the third and lateral ventricles with moderate hydrocephalus. She was taken immediately to the operating room for a suboccipital craniotomy, clot evacuation, and ventriculostomy. An arteriovenous malformation was found and resected. **B:** The postoperative CT scan showed successful evacuation of the hematoma. She regained consciousness during the first postoperative week and the intraventricular catheter was removed. She was extubated and transferred to a rehabilitation hospital with dysarthria, dysphagia, horizontal gaze paresis, bifacial weakness, and mild quadriparesis. She continues to recover well.

Therefore, recent coma and poor neurological function do not disqualify an appropriate patient with a cerebellar hemorrhage from aggressive surgical intervention. The patient's age, general medical condition, and the length of time since the ictus must be considered before making a decision to operate.

Pons

Most brainstem hemorrhages occur within the pons and are related to chronic hypertension. Because of the compact anatomic arrangement of the brainstem, small hemorrhages can produce devastating neurological impairment. Hematomas larger than 1 cm are almost always associated with a poor outcome (61). However, the excellent neurological outcome seen in the patient described in Figure 14.1 despite the initial presence of poor prognostic signs underscores that dramatic recovery is possible in some patients with pontine hemorrhage. Medical management for these lesions includes support of blood pressure and respiration. Increased ICP usually is not a problem, although hydrocephalus requires ventricular drainage in some patients (62). Brainstem hemorrhages have been evacuated surgically, although the precise indications for surgery remain entirely unclear (63,64). Some argue against surgical evacuation of these lesions (62). Our practices do not include the routine surgical evacuation of brainstem hemorrhages caused by hypertension. However, surgical evacuation of brainstem hemorrhages caused by vascular anomalies, particularly cavernous angiomas, is becoming more common. We have been favorably impressed that such surgery can improve long-term outcome in these patients. Surgery for these brainstem hemorrhages can be performed using microsurgical or stereotactic techniques and can be used in almost all areas of the brainstem.

Thalamus

The thalamus is another area where the compact anatomic organization allows small hemorrhages to cause substantial neurologi-

cal dysfunction. Small hemorrhages without alterations in consciousness or ventricular hemorrhage are managed medically to reduce cerebral edema. Moderate hemorrhages (1 to 3 cm) usually are associated with third ventricular hemorrhage. In addition to medical management, these patients receive a ventriculostomy to allow drainage of CSF and monitor ICP. Large hemorrhages (larger than 3 cm in diameter) usually are associated with a fatal outcome despite therapy (65,66). The role of surgical therapy remains controversial. One review suggests that surgical evacuation is indicated for thalamic hemorrhage with extension into the internal capsule or subthalamus if the patient is drowsy or has increased ICP (67).

Lobar

Management of lobar hemorrhages depends on size, location, and etiology and few good studies are available to guide treatment. More of these hemorrhages are from a nonhypertensive cause than are hemorrhages in other areas. The management of some of these specific underlying causes, such as coagulopathy, has been outlined already. As in other areas of the brain, the size of the hemorrhage determines if medical therapy alone will be successful, or if surgical evacuation is reasonable. However, the subcortical white matter is able to accommodate larger hemorrhages without secondary brainstem compression than clots in the previously discussed deeper regions. Furthermore, the precise region of the cerebrum that is involved is important in this regard. For instance, a large hemorrhage may be accommodated by the occipital lobes, whereas the same size hemorrhage in the temporal lobe produces brainstem compression (Chapter 2). Therefore, it is difficult to provide management guidelines on the basis of size alone. Intracranial hemorrhage volume is estimated on the CT scan by the formula ABC/2, where A is the largest ICH diameter, B is the diameter 90 degrees to A, and C is the number of CT slices with hemorrhage multiplied by the thickness of each slice (68). It has been suggested that hemorrhages larger than 30 mL in volume are likely to produce brainstem compression and should be subjected to surgical intervention (69). In patients presenting with focal deficits but who are awake or drowsy, we prefer to initiate intensive medical management, usually with ICP monitoring. If the clinical deficits worsen or consciousness becomes depressed, the patient is rescanned with CT (usually showing an appropriate increase in horizontal displacement of the midline structures) and if there has been enlargement or the appearance of marked surrounding edema, we have generally favored surgical evacuation. Patients presenting with stupor, severe drowsiness, or pupillary enlargement are candidates for immediate surgical intervention. We do not delay surgery in these patients to obtain an angiogram. An aneurysm or arteriovenous malformation may be suspected from the preoperative CT scan. The surgical procedure is planned to deal with these entities, if they are encountered. If an aneurysm is suspected, the anterior circulation vessels are explored after removal of the hematoma.

Hemorrhages in the deep white matter lead to neurological dysfunction by destroying some fiber pathways and compressing adjacent pathways. An important, but unresolved issue in the management of these hemorrhages is whether removal of the offending mass allows for more complete neurological recovery than occurs spontaneously as the hemorrhage is reabsorbed. Our general experience has been that the rationale for removal of the clot is to prevent further upper brainstem compression and contain ICP but that the focal deficit is not greatly improved. An answer to this question, through large randomized trials, will continue to shape our ideas on the management of intracerebral hemorrhage.

In summary, nontraumatic ICH is most commonly caused by hypertension; however, other potential etiologies exist and may be distinguished by history, localization on clinical examination, and radiologic evaluation. Hematoma expansion and surrounding edema result in raised intracranial pressure; and intubation, mechanical ventilation, and placement of an ICP monitor should be considered. Although as many as 10% to 15% of strokes are ICHs, up until now only small studies have investigated treatment efficacy. More randomized trials are needed to definitively determine the optimal management of the patient with ICH. Several trials are in progress to determine efficacy of both medical and surgical interventions, including craniotomy, stereotactic endoscopic evacuation, and stereotactic evacuation combined with thrombolysis.

ACKNOWLEDGMENT

The authors thank Dr. Lawrence Borges for the use of material from his chapter in the third edition of the book.

REFERENCES

1. Sacco RL, Mayer SA. Epidemiology of intracerebral hemorrhage. In: Felmann E, ed. *Intracerebral hemorrhage.* Armonk, NY: Futura, 1994:3–23.
2. Takeya Y, Popper JS, Shimizu Y, et al. Epidemiologic studies of coronary heart disease and stroke in Japanese men living in Japan, Hawaii, and California: incidence of stroke in Japan and Hawaii. *Stroke* 1984;15:15–23.
3. Quereshi AI, Giles WH, Croft JB. Racial differences in the incidence of intracerebral hemorrhage: effects of blood pressure and education. *Neurology* 1999;52: 1617–1621.
4. Bruno A, Carter S. Possible reason for the higher incidence of spontaneous intracerebral hemorrhage among Hispanics than non-Hispanic whites in New Mexico. *Neuroepidemiology* 2000;19:51–52.
5. Broderick J, Brott T, Tomsick T, et al. Intracerebral hemorrhage is more than twice as common as subarachnoid hemorrhage. *J Neurosurg* 1993;78:188–191.
6. Hankey GJ, Hon C. Surgery for primary intracerebral hemorrhage: is it safe and effective? A systematic review of case series and randomized trials. *Stroke* 1997; 28:2126–2132.
7. Brott T, Thalinger K, Hertzberg V. Hypertension as a risk factor for spontaneous intracerebral hemorrhage. *Stroke* 1986;17:1078–1083.
8. Mohr JP, Caplan LR, Melski JW, et al. The Harvard Cooperative Stroke Registry: a prospective registry. *Neurology* 1978;28:754–762.
9. Feigin I, Prose P. Hypertension fibrinoid arteritis of the brain and gross cerebral hemorrhage. *Arch Neurol* 1959;1:98–110.
10. Fisher CM. Pathological observations in hypertensive cerebral hemorrhage. *J Neuropathol Exp Neurol* 1971; 24:536–550.
11. Zulch KJ. Pathological aspects of cerebral accidents in arterial hypertension. *Acta Neurol Belg* 1974;71: 196–221.
12. Kase CS, Williams JP, Wyatt DA, et al. Lobar intracerebral hematomas: clinical and CT analysis of 22 cases. *Neurology* 1982;32:1146–1150.

13. Ropper AH, Davis KR. Lobar cerebral hemorrhages: Acute clinical syndrome in 26 cases. *Ann Neurol* 1980; 8:141–147.

14. Okazaki H, Whisnant JP. Clinical pathology of hypertensive intracerebral hemorrhage. In: Mizukami M, Kogine K, Kanaya H, et al., eds. *Hypertensive intracerebral hemorrhage.* New York: Raven, 1983:177–180.

15. Vinters HV, Gilbert JJ. Cerebral amyloid angiopathy: Incidence and complications in the aging brain II. Distribution of amyloid vascular changes. *Stroke* 1983;14: 924–928.

16. Grugg A, Jensson O, Gudmundsson G, et al. Abnormal metabolism of γ-trace alkaline microprotein: the basic defect in hereditary cerebral hemorrhage with amyloidosis. *N Engl J Med* 1984;34:1547–1549.

17. O'Donnell HC, Rosand J, Knudsen KA, et al. Apolipoprotein E genotype and the risk of recurrent lobar intracerebral hemorrhage. *N Engl J Med* 2000;342: 240–245.

18. Gorelick PB. Alcohol and stroke. *Stroke* 1987;18: 268–271.

19. Yano K, Reed DM, MacLean CJ. Serum cholesterol and hemorrhagic stroke in the Honolulu Heart Program. *Stroke* 1989;20:1460–1465.

20. Iribarren C, Jacobs DR, Sadler M, et al. Low total serum cholesterol and intracerebral hemorrhagic stroke: is the association confined to elderly men? The Kaiser Permanente Medical Care Program. *Stroke* 1996;27: 1993–1998.

21. Segal AZ, Chiu RI, Eggleston-Sexton PM, et al. Low cholesterol as a risk factor for primary intracerebral hemorrhage: a case control study. *Neuroepidemiology* 1999;18:185–193.

22. Plehn JF, Davis BR, Sacks FM, et al. Reduction of stroke incidence after myocardial infarction with pravastatin: the Cholesterol and Recurrent Events (CARE) study. *Circulation* 1999;99:216–223.

23. White HD, Simes RJ, Anderson NE, et al. Pravastatin therapy and risk of stroke. *N Engl J Med* 2000;343: 317–326.

24. Brott T, Broderick J, Kothari R, et al. Early hemorrhage growth in patients with intracerebral hemorrhage. *Stroke* 1997;28:1–5.

25. Zazulia AR, Diringer MN, Derdeyn CP, et al. Progression of mass effect after intracerebral hemorrhage. *Stroke* 1999;30:1167–1173.

26. Caplan LR. General symptoms and signs. In: Kase CS, Caplan LR, eds. *Intracerebral hemorrhage.* Boston: Butterworth-Heinemann, 1994:31–43.

27. Mayer SA, Sacco RL, Shi T, et al. Neurological deterioration in noncomatose patients with supratentorial intracerebral hemorrhage. *Neurology* 1994;44:1379–1384.

28. Broderick JP, Brott TG, Duldner JE, et al. Volume of intracerebral hemorrhage: a powerful and easy-to-use predictor of 30-day mortality. *Stroke* 1993;24:987–993.

29. Scott WR, New PFH, Davis KR, et al. Computerized axial tomography of intracerebral and intraventricular hemorrhage. *Radiology* 1974;112:73–79.

30. Kasdon DL, Scott RM, Adelman LS, et al. Cerebellar hemorrhage with decreased absorption values on computed tomography. A case report. *Neuroradiology* 1977;131:265–267.

31. Ropper AH. Lateral displacement of the brain and level of consciousness in patients with acute hemispheral masses. *N Engl J Med* 1986;314:953–958.

32. Becker DH, Townsend JJ, Kramer RA, et al. Occult cerebrovascular malformations. A series of 18 histologically verified cases with negative angiography. *Brain* 1979;102:249–287.

33. Zhu XL, Chan MS, Poon WS. Spontaneous intracranial hemorrhage: which patients need diagnostic cerebral angiography? A prospective study of 2206 cases and review of the literature. *Stroke* 1997;28:1406–1409.

34. Broderick JP, Adams HP, Barsan W, et al. Guidelines for the management of spontaneous intracerebral hemorrhage: a statement for health care professionals from a special writing group of the Stroke Council, American Heart Association. *Stroke* 1999;30:905–915.

35. Hier DB, Davis KR, Richardson EPJ, et al. Hypertensive putaminal hemorrhage. *Ann Neurol* 1977;1:152–159.

36. Paillas JE, Alliez B. Surgical treatment of spontaneous hemorrhage: Immediate and long-term results in 250 cases. *J Neurosurg* 1973;39:145–151.

37. Diringer MN. Intracerebral hemorrhage: pathophysiology and management. *Crit Care Med* 1993;21:1591–1603.

38. Powers WJ, Zazulia AR, Videen TO, et al. Autoregulation of cerebral blood flow surrounding acute (6 to 22 hours) intracerebral hemorrhage. *Neurology* 2001;57:18–24.

39. Ropper AH, King RB. Intracranial pressure monitoring in comatose patients with cerebral hemorrhage. *Arch Neurol* 1984;41:725–728.

40. Marshall LF, El-Hefnami M. Spontaneous intracranial hemorrhage. *Semin Neurol* 1984;4:422–429.

41. Janny P, Colnet G, Georget AM, et al. Intracranial pressure with intracranial hemorrhages. *Surg Neurol* 1978; 10:371–375.

42. Golbasi Z, Selcoki Y, Eraslan T, et al. QT dispersion. Is it an independent risk factor for in-hospital mortality in patients with intracerebral hemorrhage? *Jpn Heart J* 1999;40:405–411.

43. Oppenheimer SM, Cechetto DF, Hachinski VC. Cerebrogenic cardiac arrhythmias. Cerebral electrocardiographic influences and their role in sudden death. *Arch Neurol* 1990;47:513–519.

44. Poungvarin N, Bhoopat W, Viriyavejakul A, et al. Effects of dexamethasone in primary supratentorial intracerebral hemorrhage. *N Engl J Med* 1987;316: 1229–1233.

45. Yu YL, Kumana CR, Lauder IJ, et al. Treatment of acute cerebral hemorrhage with intravenous glycerol: a double-blind, placebo-controlled, randomized trial. *Stroke* 1992;23:967–971.

46. Broderick J. Intracerebral hemorrhage. In: Gorelick PB, Alter M, eds. *Handbook of neuroepidemiology.* New York: Marcel Dekker, 1994:141–167.

47. Juvela S, Heiskanen O, Poranen A, et al. The treatment of spontaneous intracerebral hemorrhage: a prospective randomized trial of surgical and conservative treatment. *J Neurosurg* 1989;70:755–758.

48. Auer L, Deinsberger W, Niederkorn K, et al. Endoscopic surgery versus medical treatment for spontaneous intracerebral hematoma: a randomized study. *J Neurosurg* 1989;70:530–535.

49. Batjer HH, Reisch JS, Allen BC, et al. Failure of surgery to improve outcome in hypertensive putaminal hemorrhage: a prospective randomized trial. *Arch Neurol* 1990;47:1103–1106.

50. Greene GM, Godersky JC, Biller J, et al. Surgical experience with cerebral amyloid angiopathy. *Stroke* 1990; 21:1545–1549.

51. Leblanc R, Preul M, Robitaille Y, et al. Surgical considerations in cerebral amyloid angiopathy. *Neurosurgery* 1991;29:712–718.

52. Morganstern LB, Demchuck AM, Kim DH, et al. Rebleeding leads to poor outcome in ultra-early craniotomy for intracerebral hemorrhage. *Neurology* 2001; 56:1294–1299.

53. Mohadjer M, Braus DF, Myers A, et al. CT-stereotactic fibrinolysis of spontaneous intracerebral hematomas. *Neurosurg Rev* 1992;15:105–110.

54. Montes JM, Wong JH, Fayad PB, Awad IA. Stereotactic computed tomographic-guided aspiration and thrombolysis of intracerebral hematoma. Protocol and preliminary experience. *Stroke* 2000;31:834–840.

55. Kaneko M. Timing of surgery for hypertensive intracerebral hemorrhage. In: Mizukami M, ed. *Hypertensive intracerebral hemorrhage*. New York: Raven, 1983: 249–253.

56. Kaneko M, Tanaka M, Shimada T, et al. Long term evaluation of ultra-early operation for hypertensive intracerebral hemorrhage in 100 cases. *J Neurosurg* 1983; 58:838–842.

57. Heimann TD, Satya-Murti S. Benign cerebellar hemorrhages. *Ann Neurol* 1978;3:366–368.

58. Ito Z, Nakajima K. Surgical treatment of acute cerebellar hemorrhage. In: Mizukami M, ed. *Hypertensive intracerebral hemorrhage*. New York: Raven, 1983:215–223.

59. Little JR, Tubman DE, Ethier R. Cerebellar hemorrhage in adults. Diagnosis by computerized tomography. *J Neurosurg* 1978;48:575–579.

60. Oh KH, Kase CS, Ojemann RG, et al. Cerebellar hemorrhage: diagnosis and treatment. A review of 56 cases. *Arch Neurol* 1974;31:160–167.

61. Sano K, Ochiai C. Brainstem hematomas: clinical aspects with reference to indications for treatment. In: Pia HW, Lanjmaid C, Zierski J, eds. *Spontaneous intracerebral hematomas*. New York: Springer-Verlag, 1980:366–371.

62. Tanaka Y, Nishiya M, Svematsu K, et al. Pontine hemorrhage. In: Mizukami M, ed. *Hypertensive intracerebral hemorrhage*. New York: Raven, 1983:205–214.

63. O'Laoire SA, Crockard HA, Thomas DGT, et al. Brainstem hematoma: a report of six surgically treated cases. *J Neurosurg* 1982;56:222–227.

64. Durward QJ, Barnett HIM, Barr HWK. Presentation and management of mesencephalic hematoma. *J Neurosurg* 1982;56:123–127.

65. Walshe TM, Davis KD, Fisher CM. Thalamic hemorrhage: a computed tomographic-clinical correlation. *Neurology* 1977;27:217–222.

66. Barraguer-Bordas L, Illa A, Escartin J, et al. Thalamic hemorrhage. A study of 23 patients with diagnosis by computed tomography. *Stroke* 1981;12:524–527.

67. Kagawa M. Thalamic hemorrhage. In: Mizukami M, ed. *Hypertensive intracerebral hemorrhage*. New York: Raven, 1983:225–231.

68. Kothari RU, Brott T, Broderick JP, et al. The ABCs of measuring intracerebral hemorrhage volumes. *Stroke* 1996;27:1304–1305.

69. Marshall LF, El-Hefnami M. Spontaneous intracranial hemorrhage. *Semin Neurol* 1984;4:422–429.

15

Subarachnoid Hemorrhage

Subarachnoid hemorrhage (SAH) represents a small portion of cerebrovascular disease, but accounts for a significant amount of stroke morbidity and mortality. The annual incidence of nontraumatic SAH is estimated at 10 to 15 per 100,000, with over 30,000 cases per year in the United States. Acute mortality of SAH has been estimated at 25% to 50%, depending on allowances for the likelihood of underdiagnosis in cases of sudden death. Additionally, SAH represents about 4.5% of stroke mortality, but because it occurs at younger ages than ischemic stroke, it accounts for over 25% of all stroke-related years of potential life lost before age 65 (1). For the most part, the management of ruptured intracranial aneurysm is shared between neurosurgeons and neurointensivists and offers one of the most fruitful areas for clinical investigation in neurocritical care.

Traumatic head injury is the most common cause of SAH, with bleeding related to cortical contusions, hematomas, and vessel injury. Vascular malformations are responsible for a small number of SAH cases, with arteriovenous malformation (AVM) responsible for 5% to 10%. Studies have inconsistently associated hypertension with SAH (2), and 10% to 20% have no vascular lesion identified on angiography. A small number of these patients have SAH related to bleeding dyscrasias and malignancy.

Rarely, intracranial vertebral dissections can lead to dissecting aneurysms with subsequent rupture and SAH (3). The subject of this chapter, spontaneous SAH, is for all intents and purposes caused by rupture of an in-

tracerebral aneurysm. Although developmental abnormalities of the vessel wall may be the fundamental cause of berry aneurysms, they are only rarely present at birth, but rather develop over time, increasing in prevalence with increasing age. It is estimated that the population prevalence among adults approaches 3% to 5% (4,5). Most saccular aneurysms occur at the bifurcations of the large arteries at the base of the brain and rupture into the subarachnoid space of the basal cisterns (Fig. 15.1). Less commonly, they rupture into the

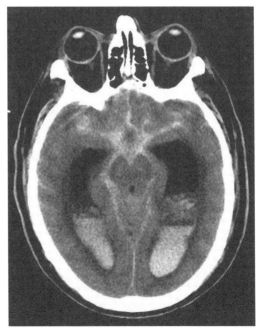

FIG. 15.1. Computed tomography without contrast demonstrates blood in the basal cisterns.

brain or ventricular system or both, resulting in intracerebral hemorrhage or acute hydrocephalus. In contrast, mycotic aneurysms occur at distal branch points of the middle, anterior, posterior cerebral, vertebral, or basilar arteries and rupture into the subarachnoid space over the cortical surface rather than into the basal cisterns.

The sites of the aneurysm and subsequent subarachnoid, intraventricular, or intracerebral clot determine the clinical features of the rupture and to some degree, the risks of subsequent development of vasospasm and hydrocephalus. As is well known, the most common sites of saccular aneurysms are the junction of the anterior communicating artery and the anterior cerebral artery, the junction of the posterior communicating artery and the internal carotid artery, the bifurcation of the middle cerebral artery, and the top of the basilar artery. Approximately 85% of cases occur in the anterior circulation. Furthermore, 12% to 31% of patients have multiple aneurysms, and in some 10% to 20% the aneurysms have bilateral identical locations (6). Aneurysms are slightly more common in women, and smoking has been identified as a risk factor.

Current data suggest that many aneurysms remain asymptomatic throughout life. The natural history risk of these so-called "incidental aneurysms" has long been a topic of debate. A recent retrospective review of a large cohort of patients with unruptured aneurysms suggested that small, incidental aneurysms have a bleeding risk less than 0.1% per year (7). This study and a related prospective study demonstrated that larger aneurysms (over 7 to 8 mm in diameter), have higher risks of hemorrhage. In addition, patients with residual aneurysms following rupture of the first aneurysm have the highest risks of rupture of the second incidental one. These and other studies also have demonstrated that the complication rate for surgical treatment of unruptured aneurysm is higher than previously thought, ranging from 5% to 30% for combined morbidity and mortality depending on the age of the patient and aneurysm size and location (7,8). The recent

development of aneurysm treatment with endovascular techniques may well be safer but the long-term prevention of rupture remains to be demonstrated.

Management of subarachnoid hemorrhage has become a complex issue, with numerous treatment options and putative benefits of various aspects of neurocritical care. It is apparent that centers that have more experience with the care of this group of patients appear to have significantly better outcomes as judged by in-hospital death and disability (9).

CLINICAL PRESENTATION, EVALUATION, AND MANAGEMENT

Prodromal Symptoms

Prodromal symptoms may betray the location of an unruptured aneurysm and, at times, suggest progressive enlargement. The onset of a third cranial nerve palsy—particularly when associated with pupillary dilation, loss of light reflex, and focal pain above and behind the eye—points to an expanding aneurysm at the junction of the posterior communicating artery and internal carotid artery (10). Involvement of the third cranial nerve usually signifies acute aneurysmal enlargement or a small focal hemorrhage. Sixth cranial nerve palsy suggests a cavernous sinus aneurysm and visual field defects can result from an expanding supraclinoid carotid aneurysm. Occipital and posterior cervical pain suggest a posterior inferior cerebellar artery or anterior inferior cerebellar artery aneurysm; pain in or behind the eye and in the low temple suggests an expanding middle cerebral aneurysm. Sudden severe headache may result from a small leakage of blood from an aneurysm, and has been termed a sentinel headache. Indeed, a sudden unexplained headache in any location should arouse suspicion of subarachnoid hemorrhage, although the majority of sudden headaches turn out to be benign. Many patients presenting with subarachnoid hemorrhage have sought medical attention for headache in the preceding days. Although this likely reflects "sentinel hemorrhage" pain related to expansion of an aneurysm has been postulated. Whatever the mechanism, the importance of rapid recognition and intervention is clear. A review of referrals to tertiary centers that see large numbers of patients with aneurysms revealed that 25% of patients had been seen earlier and not diagnosed with subarachnoid hemorrhage (11). Not surprisingly, the risk of misdiagnosis was greatest (38%) in those with no or minimal neurological deficit at the time of evaluation.

Initial Clinical Presentation

Acute Major Subarachnoid Hemorrhage

For the brief moment of aneurysmal rupture, when acute major subarachnoid hemorrhage occurs, intracranial pressure (ICP) approaches the mean arterial pressure and cerebral perfusion pressure falls (12). These changes may account for the sudden but transient decrease in consciousness that occurs in most cases. Although the change in level of consciousness may be preceded by a brief moment of excruciating headache, most patients first complain of headache on regaining consciousness. In about 45% of patients, severe headache, usually associated with exertion, but without loss of consciousness, is the presenting complaint (13). The headache is often described by the patient as "the worst headache of my life." Words such as *explode* or *burst* may be used. Often it is described as all over or in the back of the head and neck. Whatever the nature of the onset, vomiting is a prominent symptom, and vomiting with sudden headache, of course, should raise the question of acute subarachnoid hemorrhage.

Although sudden severe headache in the absence of focal neurological symptoms is the hallmark of aneurysmal rupture, not infrequently neurological deficits emerge. Unilateral third cranial nerve palsy strongly suggests a posterior communicating artery aneurysm. Sixth nerve palsy is common and does not have great significance as a localizing sign, although it often corresponds to an infratentorial aneurysmal rupture. A middle cerebral artery bifurcation aneurysm may rupture into the subdural space and present as a subdural hematoma. Anterior communicating artery aneurysms sometimes rupture into the basal cisterns of the subarachnoid space and form a clot that is large enough to produce localized mass effect. Any aneurysm can rupture into the brain parenchyma and result in intracerebral hemorrhage (14). The common resulting deficits include hemiparesis, aphasia, anosognosia, memory loss, and abulia. Cerebral edema often follows, resulting in progressive mass effect and deterioration, sometimes requiring surgical evacuation.

Occasionally, acute unilateral hemispheric swelling and associated focal neurological signs occur immediately after aneurysmal rupture. The reasons for such swelling are uncertain. Acute vasospasm has been proposed as an explanation for transient interruption of the cerebral circulation in an arterial territory. Unwitnessed hypotension or hypoxia may have accompanied the initial bleeding with secondary global brain injury. Acute hydrocephalus also may occur independently of acute cerebral edema and account for the persistence of a stuporous or comatose state. Often there is no adequate explanation for the initial neurological deficits, and in many cases they gradually improve over a matter of days.

Careful documentation of the initial neurological deficit, attempting to establish its cause, and closely following its course is of utmost importance for further decisions in the management of such patients. A clinical grading system devised by Hunt and Hess is widely used to categorize the clinical status of patients with acute subarachnoid hemorrhage (15). Although the scale (Table 15.1) is useful and used routinely in patient management, it does not adequately quantitate the clinical deficit, nor account for the pathophysiologic nature of the deficit. Restated, diagnostic and therapeutic decisions regarding these patients are best made with an accurate, serial, quantitative documentation of the neurological deficit and its pathophysiologic nature.

TABLE 15.1. *Hunt and Hess Scale for clinical grading in subarachnoid hemorrhage*

I   Asymptomatic, mild headache
II Cranial nerve palsy, severe headache
III Drowsy, confused, mild deficit
IV Stupor, moderate to severe hemiparesis, early posturing
V   Coma, decerebrate posturing

Initial Evaluation

Computed Tomography Scan

Noncontrast computed tomography (CT) of the head has become the initial diagnostic study of choice for suspected subarachnoid hemorrhage. Approximately 95% of patients have evidence of subarachnoid blood on a plain CT scan obtained within the first 48 hours after aneurysmal rupture (16). Inexperienced radiologists frequently miss small amounts of subarachnoid blood and a "negative" scan in a suggestive case is worth reviewing. A plain CT scan should be performed first because contrast may show enhancement in the basal cisterns that may be mistaken for clotted blood. A later contrast CT scan including CT angiography, may demonstrate an aneurysm or an unsuspected arterial venous malformation (17). If the CT scan neither establishes the diagnosis of subarachnoid hemorrhage nor demonstrates a mass lesion or obstructive hydrocephalus, a lumbar puncture should be performed to establish the diagnosis of subarachnoid hemorrhage. Lumbar puncture may be indicated before CT scanning if the imaging study is not available at the time of the suspected subarachnoid hemorrhage and the patient has no lateralizing neurological deficits or evidence of papilledema. The extent and location of subarachnoid blood generally points to the location of the aneurysm and identifies the cause of an initial neurological deficit. The CT scan also has found great use in predicting which patients are destined to develop delayed ischemic neurological deficits caused by cerebral vasospasm (4,18,19).

Laboratory Evaluation

Routine laboratory studies should include electrolytes, blood urea nitrogen, and creatinine, as well as white blood count, hematocrit, and platelet count. Clotting studies of prothrombin time (INR) and partial thromboplastin time also should be checked. Toxicology screens may be helpful if cocaine and amphetamine use is suspected. Baseline electrolytes are of value because hyponatremia may develop, most commonly probably related to a salt wasting syndrome, which causes loss of salt and water in the urine with subsequent volume depletion and dilutional hyponatremia (Chapter 6) (20,21). Platelet count, bleeding time, and other clotting parameters should be documented again before invasive procedures. Serum viscosity increases significantly when the hematocrit is greater than 40% or when the serum fibrinogen levels are greater than 250 mg%. Adjustment of the serum viscosity becomes important in patients at risk for symptomatic cerebral vasospasm but its significance has not been studied systematically and it is not often attended to in most units.

A baseline electrocardiogram (ECG) is important and often shows ST changes similar or identical to ischemic abnormalities or a prolonged QRS complex or Q-T interval, and perhaps most characteristically, tall T waves (22). These changes have been linked to elevated blood catecholamine levels as a result of hypothalamic dysfunction that in turn stimulates the α-adrenergic receptors in the myocardium. Catecholamine excess, either via stimulation by norepinephrine-containing nerve terminals or circulating epinephrine, results in prolonged muscle fiber contraction, and leads to myofibrillar necrosis. This topic is reviewed extensively in Chapter 5. Serum markers of myocardial ischemia, creatine kinase, and troponin, are frequently elevated and found more frequently in larger hemorrhages. The distinction from an associated myocardial infarction is then difficult. Echocardiography is indicated in those patients presenting with hypotension and signs of left ventricular failure. Hypokinesis in a diffuse global pattern or predominantly affecting the cardiac base is consistent with an initial catecholamine stress injury and suggests that recovery of cardiac function will occur over several days. Focal wall motion abnormalities or apical hypokinesis is more suggestive of coronary ischemia. Cardiac catheterization may be useful in the setting of continued and/or recurrent ischemic injury as indicated by ECG changes or serum markers.

Angiography

Cerebral angiography is usually planned as part of the acute evaluation to identify the source of the hemorrhage and localize and characterize the anatomy of any aneurysm. Angiography should also be performed without delay if an arteriovenous malformation or mycotic aneurysm is suspected because of the presence of intraparenchymal blood or subarachnoid blood located over the hemisphere rather than in the basal cisterns. Another possible indication for acute angiography is an intracerebral hematoma secondary to aneurysmal rupture presenting with mass effect, a combination that may make emergency surgical evacuation necessary. This most frequently occurs when a middle cerebral bifurcation aneurysm ruptures and produces a large intratemporal or sylvian fissure hematoma. Documenting the location and anatomy of the aneurysm before such surgery is imperative because it is almost always preferable to clip the aneurysm at the time of clot evacuation. Some centers now use CT and CT angiography in this scenario to shorten the evaluation time so that emergency surgical intervention can be more quickly carried out.

If no aneurysm is found on the initial selective cerebral angiogram, the likelihood of rebleeding from subarachnoid hemorrhage is low (1% to 2%) (23). However, even selective cerebral angiography can miss a small or partially thrombosed aneurysm, particularly of the anterior communicating artery or in the posterior circulation. Therefore, we repeat four-vessel angiography several days or up to several weeks after the hemorrhage. Possible explanations for the absence of an aneurysm include a ruptured small superficial cortical artery (24), a spinal cord intramedullary or extramedullary AVM, or the obliteration of the aneurysm during the acute hemorrhage and a fortuitous smooth healing vascular wall at the site.

Occasionally, a spinal cord AVM and an aneurysm of a cervical artery appear together. In most of these rare cases, back pain or paraparesis with minimal headache and subarachnoid blood suggests the diagnosis. A syndrome of perimesencephalic subarachnoid hemorrhage has been defined, almost always without vasospasm or rebleeding, and with a good prognosis. In this group of patients the subarachnoid blood is confined to the peripontine or midbrain cisterns, and aneurysms are rarely found (25). The bleeding mechanism is not clear, but the low risk of recurrent hemorrhage argues against undiscovered aneurysm, and venous bleeding has been postulated (26). Angiogram negative subarachnoid hemorrhage with more extensive cisternal blood not conforming to the definition of benign perimesencephalic hemorrhage may not share the favorable low risk of recurrent hemorrhage (27).

Initial Management

Seizure related to subarachnoid hemorrhage is reported frequently in the prehospital setting, but a seizure witnessed in the hospital is uncommon (28). There are no clear data to guide decisions about the need for acute anticonvulsant therapy. It may be reasonable to treat with an anticonvulsant acutely until any aneurysm has been identified and obliterated, although there is little consensus on this issue. We do not institute anticonvulsants unless a seizure is observed during the few days after hemorrhage. The brief tonic seizure that accompanies the cessation of cerebral blood flow with aneurysm rupture is certainly not a justification for the use of anticonvulsants. The choice of anticonvulsant, if one is required, is somewhat arbitrary, despite theoretical considerations that favor one or another.

Corticosteroids have been used commonly in acute subarachnoid hemorrhage, and it has been hypothesized that the meningeal irritation and scarring may be reduced and therefore therapy may reduce hydrocephalus. High-dose steroids in this group of patients complicate infectious risks, and we cannot support its routine use without data demonstrating benefit.

The initial neurological condition significantly affects prognosis. The most commonly used aforementioned clinical grading scale is that of Hunt and Hess, and although originally devised as a predictor of surgical risk, it has gained wide use because of the correlation with overall outcome (Table 15.1) (15). Not surprisingly, patients in grades I through III have significantly better chances for survival than grade IV and V patients. Although some have advocated delay of aggressive treatment of higher-grade patients because of poor prognosis, any delay increases the risks of rebleeding and other complications. The acute evaluation should attempt to define the mechanism responsible for the neurological dysfunction, and include the potential reversibility of that injury in the overall decision. For example, hydrocephalus can be present at initial evaluation accounting for obtundation, and ventricular drainage can lead to marked clinical improvement. A patient with massive midbrain destruction from rupture of a basilar tip aneurysm, however, may have no reasonable chance for recovery of function. Initial decision making should include more than simple clinical grade, because some poor-grade patients can have excellent outcomes (29,30). Our approach with these patients is to rapidly evaluate patients with grade IV and V SAH and most receive ventriculostomy drainage acutely. We offer no treatment to those with massive tissue injury or sustained ICP greater than 25 mm Hg. Those judged to have potential for recovery are treated aggressively with early angiography and aneurysm treatment. This is a group well suited to endovascular treatment, because surgery may be more difficult in grade IV and V patients. We try to avoid the "wait and see" strategy, because the risk of rerupture and vasospasm is high in this group.

In addition to facilitating an expeditious evaluation, early management must begin to focus on the major sources of morbidity and mortality in patients with subarachnoid hemorrhage: rebleeding, hydrocephalus, and vasospasm.

Rerupture

The incidence of aneurysmal rerupture may be as high as 30% (for some reason it has been lower in our experience in the last few years, even discounting for early surgery) and it carries a significant initial morbidity and mortality (31,32). Sixty-two percent of patients in one series who were drowsy or had headache but no other neurological deficit sustained a major neurological deficit as a result of rerupture, and 31% of these patients died (32). Although the incidence of rerupture is high during the first 4 weeks, evidence clearly shows that the highest incidence of rebleeding is within the first 24 hours, over which period 4% or more of patients deteriorate as a result of recurrent hemorrhage (33).

It has been argued, but not proved, that controlling blood pressure may reduce early rebleeding. Our clinical impression accords with this view. Blood pressure control can be initiated in the emergency room, and a β-blocker such as labetalol is an ideal intravenous agent. In patients who are awake, ICP is unlikely to exceed 25 to 30 mg/Hg; therefore, the mean arterial pressure can be lowered below 100 mm Hg without compromising cerebral perfusion. Patients with impaired consciousness may have markedly elevated ICP and aggressive lowering of blood pressure could compromise cerebral perfusion. Such patients likely need emergent ventriculostomy, which allows measurement of ICP, and blood pressure can then be lowered as much as tolerated by ICP. It is reasonable to maintain cerebral perfusion pressures of 50 to 70 mm Hg because vasospasm should not be an issue for several days. The initial hypertension can be difficult to control, and additional medications are needed in many instances. Enalaprilat 0.625 to 1.25 mg given intravenously or captopril 6.25 to 12.5 mg sublingually can be useful. Although nitroprusside may not be ideal on theoretic grounds, it is often the most convenient effective agent, and has not been frequently associated with ICP complications in our experience.

Early aneurysm treatment, whether by surgical clipping or endovascular coiling, is the most powerful tool in reducing the rebleeding risk. Although data from clinical trials have been inconclusive in supporting early treatment (34), most centers now proceed with definitive treatment within the first 24 to 48 hours in an effort to decrease the morbidity related to rerupture. Decisions about the treatment choice (surgical or endovascular) should be based largely on the skills of available operators and on the patient's condition and aneurysm configuration, but always with the goal of aneurysm treatment relatively early. A recent clinical trial compared outcomes of death or severe disability in patients with acutely ruptured aneurysms felt to be amenable to treatment by either surgical or endovascular technique. This randomized study demonstrated improved outcomes in acutely ruptured aneurysms treated by endovascular technique compared to surgical clipping with a relative risk reduction of death or disability at 1 year exceeding 20%. Despite this, significant controversy persists regarding the relative merits of surgical clipping and endovascular coiling of aneurysms. The procedural morbidity associated with treatment of acutely ruptured aneurysm is likely less with an endovascular technique than surgical treatment, but the long-term efficacy of coil treatment remains to be demonstrated.

Hydrocephalus

Hydrocephalus after subarachnoid hemorrhage is most appropriately divided into three categories: acute, subacute, and delayed. Each has its own characteristic mechanism of production, timing of onset, symptomatology, and management. Acute hydrocephalus usually develops after intraventricular hemorrhage or from the disposition of an excessive amount of blood in the basal cisterns of the posterior fossa. It is most commonly seen with ruptured anterior communicating artery aneurysms or top of the basilar aneurysms. It is most commonly noted in the first 24 hours, but can be seen immediately after aneurysmal rupture. Acute hydrocephalus is seen in 10% to 20% of patients at initial presentation, and contributes to the clinical state in many of these (35). The abrupt onset of stupor or the persistence of coma after the initial rupture suggests hydrocephalus, and urgent intervention with ventriculostomy and external drainage is indicated. The ventricular drainage system initially can be left open to drain at 10 cm above the external auditory meatus, preventing excessive CSF drainage. Bilateral ventriculostomy may be required in cases with extensive intraventricular blood or thick clot in the third ventricle. In some patients, ventricular drainage results in dramatic improvement, whereas in other cases improvement may be gradual.

A subacute form of communicating hydrocephalus may develop in the first few days to a week after subarachnoid hemorrhage. Although it too may present with the precipitous onset of coma, most often its onset is gradual. Progressive drowsiness accompanied by inability to look up is a suggestive finding. The quiet abulic state that is associated with the onset of symptomatic cerebral vasospasm in the anterior communicating artery complex is often difficult to distinguish from this subacute form of hydrocephalus. The CT with comparison by measurement (in mm) of the ventricular span at the level of the frontal horns may help make the diagnosis. However, a change as small as 1 mm in ventricular span may be all that is required to produce a stuporous state.

Significant ventricular dilation can occur in hydrocephalus related to subarachnoid hemorrhage despite relatively low or normal intraventricular pressures. This increase in brain compliance may relate to the effects of the hemorrhage and is most often noted in older patients. Symptomatic hydrocephalus relates to ventricular dilation, not necessarily to raised ICP. Effective treatment of hydrocephalus in this setting may require lowering the ventricular drainage system to 5 cm or less above the external auditory meatus to achieve CSF drainage and reduction in ventricular size.

Last, delayed hydrocephalus may appear 10 or more days after the hemorrhage while a patient seemingly is recovering well from surgery. Gait difficulty and difficulty getting out of bed then appear, sometimes with a quiet behavior. The lumbar pressure often is normal but nonetheless a spinal tap may result in clinical improvement during the following day. Permanent ventriculoperitoneal drainage is almost always needed in this setting and is associated with a high rate of improvement.

Cerebral Vasospasm

Vasospasm represents the next major threat and the management of vasospasm begins with the initial evaluation of the patient. Vasospasm is a transient pathology of the basal segments of intracerebral arteries leading to narrowing of the vessel lumen (36). This process is triggered by blood pooling around the basal segments of vessels, and the severity of the spasm is related closely to the amount of blood and the duration of exposure of the outer vessel wall to the blood. Hemoglobin and its breakdown products, particularly oxyhemoglobin, are the most likely spasmogens in this setting (37). The precise nature of the vascular lesion is not well understood, and probably consists of prolonged and intense smooth muscle contraction. There are associated changes in the vessel wall that include smooth muscle cell proliferation, fibrosis, and inflammatory changes (38). Localized inflammatory responses, including the release of cytokines, may lead to hemodynamic changes (39). There is thickening of the vessel wall, although the contribution of this effect to luminal narrowing probably is modest.

Symptomatic cerebral vasospasm is the major cause of delayed morbidity or death, occurring in approximately 30% of patients (40). The clinical course is quite predictable. The first signs of regional ischemia rarely appear before day 4, and the process increases in severity through days 10 to 14, with rapid spontaneous resolution thereafter. Early studies by Fisher (18) were able to correlate site and severity of vasospasm with CT localization of persistent clot in the subarachnoid space adjacent to a basal vessel. This is most reliable when using a CT from 24 to 48 hours following hemorrhage (19). Patients at high risk for severe vasospasm based on the CT scan appearance (Table 15.2) should probably be treated more aggressively from the outset with the approaches detailed in the following, but particularly with fluid administration to support blood pressure and intravascular volume. The presence of a basal clot does not preclude early surgery, but established symptomatic vasospasm increases the likelihood of a focal deficit after surgery.

Nimodipine has been a standard treatment for the prevention of ischemia from vasospasm for nearly a decade, and is used at 60 mg every 4 hours. Numerous studies have demonstrated a modest effect in improved neurological outcome, although no clear angiographic demonstration of reduced spasm has been found (41,42). It is speculated that the effect is at the cellular level, acting perhaps as a neuronal protectant. This is consistent with the modest evidence that nimodipine has a beneficial effect in acute ischemic stroke when used in the first hours. The clinical trials of nimodipine were carried out before aggressive neurocritical care management with induced hypertension had been introduced, and it is unclear if the benefits

TABLE 15.2. *Fisher Scale for grading computed tomography predictors of vasospasm*

I No subarachnoid blood
II Diffuse or thin sheet
III Clot or thick layer
IV Diffuse or no subarachnoid blood, with intraventricular clot

of nimodipine and fluid administration or vasopressors are additive. Given all this, the use of nimodipine seems reasonable as long as the ability to treat with induced hypertension is not compromised. Should nimodipine lead to unmanageable drops in blood pressure the dose can be split or reduced, or the drug eliminated.

Transcranial Doppler (TCD) insonation has been, in many units, an effective tool for the monitoring of vasospasm (43). The ultrasound study is noninvasive, rapidly interpretable, and can be done daily to guide therapy. Like all ancillary studies, one must understand the limitations of the technology in order to gain the most reliable benefits. High flow velocities by TCD are highly predictive for severe vasospasm in the affected vessel (44). Transcranial Doppler gives flow velocities in the basal segments of the cerebral vessels, and elevations in velocities may be seen in states of increased perfusion or with narrowing of the basal segments. For example, generalized increased flow velocities can be seen with fever and sepsis and need to be differentiated from focal narrowing. Coincident flow velocities can be measured in the extracranial ICA, and the ratio of velocities in the middle cerebral artery (MCA) to extracranial artery (Lindegaard ratio) helps distinguish vasospasm from hyperperfusion. It is difficult to precisely correlate ischemic symptoms with absolute TCD velocities, in part because of the variability of collateral supply. Table 15.3 provides guidelines for the interpretation of vasospasm severity with TCD. Vasospasm affecting the anterior cerebral artery and MCA are in our experience symptomatic at lower velocities than isolated MCA vasospasm. As TCD velocities increase, the intensity of medical management can be correspondingly increased.

Standard medical management for vasospasm is traditionally referred to as "triple H" (hemodilution, hypervolemia, and hypertension), and this approach has been shown consistently to increase cerebral perfusion and reduce ischemia (45). Hemodilution is considered to be effective because of the rheologic improvement it causes in blood flow in small channels as a result of reduced viscosity. The balance of oxygen carrying capacity and viscosity is optimized at hematocrit in the range of 30% to 35%. It is rare for a patient who is days into the ICU course to have a hematocrit high enough to require therapeutic phlebotomy, because diagnostic phlebotomy and intravenous fluids usually have accomplished this goal.

Hypervolemia is useful in so far as increased volume facilitates efforts to increase blood pressure. However, hypervolemia per se likely does not increase cerebral perfusion. Perfusion is largely determined by the pressure gradient across the segment of vessel that is in severe vasospasm. The goal then is adequate volume to facilitate mild hypertension, and driving volume to a specific wedge pressure is usually not helpful. Our practice has been to use crystalloid solutions such as normal saline at 100 to 200 mL/hour, without a central venous pressure or wedge pressure goal. Several recent studies have suggested that increasing cardiac output without increasing blood pressure can benefit cerebral perfusion in vasospasm. Perhaps the agent used for this purpose (e.g., dobutamine) leads to arterial dilation in the cerebral circulation and favorably alters cerebral vascular resistance. Pressure management is probably simpler and associated with fewer risks than attempting to raise cardiac output. Much of the morbidity associated with "triple H" therapy comes from volume overload and may be avoidable without sacrifice of efficacy. Volume support usually can be provided with isotonic crystalloid, 0.9% NaCl, or blood when appropriate. Colloid such as albumin generally is not necessary and adds significantly to cost.

TABLE 15.3. *Interpretation of transcranial Doppler velocities in the anterior circulation in subarachnoid hemorrhage*

Mean velocity	Spasm	IC/EC ICA ratio
120–139 cm/sec	Mild	3.0–3.99
140–179 cm/sec	Moderate	4.0–5.99
>180 cm/sec	Severe	>6.0

As vasospasm progresses, proximal vessels narrow and the normal autoregulatory mechanisms lead to distal vasodilatation. As focal ischemia develops, autoregulation and dilatation is at maximum and cerebral blood flow then becomes proportional to the pressure gradient across the cerebral capillary bed. Induced hypertension increases flow across the narrowed segments by increasing mean arterial blood pressure. Hypertension is the major tool in increasing brain perfusion in the setting of vasospasm. We have found the most useful pressor to be phenylephrine, because it is well tolerated without tachycardia or ectopy. Occasionally, inotropic agents such as dopamine are also required, but are most useful in the setting of significant left ventricular failure.

Many patients have significant acute hydrocephalus and require external ventriculostomy drainage; this has occurred in about 25% of SAH patients in our unit. Given that cerebral perfusion pressure is defined as MAP–ICP, it is clear that one can gain some small advantage by lowering ICP. In severe vasospasm it can be easier to lower ICP by 5 to 10 mm Hg than to raise MAP an additional 10 mm Hg; therefore, draining the ventriculostomy to a lower pressure can be a helpful maneuver in difficult cases. This can be a temporizing measure while moving to a more definitive treatment, such as angioplasty.

In our view, the optimal management depends on a careful "spasm watch" relying on serial TCD and clinical signs to monitor the severity of spasm, and then responding with an intensity of medical therapy (mainly fluid administration and pressors to raise blood pressure) gauged to avoid the onset of ischemic symptoms. In the ideal setting, quantitative blood flow measurements guide appropriate therapy. Technology such as near infrared spectroscopy, bedside Xenon CT, or CT and magnetic resonance perfusion studies have not yet replaced clinical judgment.

Angiography with the intention of angioplasty and/or the infusion of intraarterial vasodilators such as papaverine can be an extremely useful adjunct to hypertension in precluding an ischemic deficit from vasospasm (46). Microcatheters and high-compliance balloons can access the vertebral, basilar, internal carotid and proximal middle cerebral arteries. Gentle angioplasty restores a normal vessel caliber with a durable effect that persists without recurrence through the course of vasospasm. As experience is gained with this technique, it is being applied earlier in the course of vasospasm. Many centers now perform angioplasty when severe spasm is predicted by TCD, even before clinical signs of ischemia appear. The goal is to undertake invasive therapy prior to prolonged clinical deficits in order to maximize neurological function. We have moved to earlier intervention with angioplasty, and now treat many patients before the onset of any ischemic symptoms. This is especially useful in those patients with cardiac injury or preexisting disease where the risks of profound induced hypertension may be significant.

Medical Complications of Subarachnoid Hemorrhage

These patients benefit greatly from vigilant intensive care and are vulnerable to all the complications associated with a prolonged intensive care unit (ICU) stay. Several specific issues arise commonly in this group and merit special discussion.

Subarachnoid hemorrhage is commonly associated with cardiac effects. The acute hemorrhage causes a profound catecholamine release, leading in susceptible patients to cardiac dysrhythmias and subendocardial ischemia as well as transiently diminished cardiac contractility. These effects are reviewed in Chapter 5. Although evidence of ischemic myocardial injury is common, both by electrocardiogram and serum markers, the cardiac injury usually recovers over days. Even those patients who present with marked hypotension and require inotropic agents and pressors usually recover ventricular contractility and function rapidly. Although low-dose β-blocker therapy seems reasonable given the likely mechanism of injury, no data yet exist to guide treatment.

Hyponatremia also is a characteristic feature of patients in the ICU with subarachnoid hemorrhage. Details of the phenomenon are reviewed in Chapter 6. It seems likely that in some cases this represents true salt wasting, and fluid restriction is associated with worsened outcomes (47). The controversy regarding the relative roles of atrial natriuretic factor, other undiscovered causes of salt wasting and inappropriate secretion of antidiuretic hormone are discussed in that chapter. It is only reemphasized here that the reduction in intravascular volume associated with natriuresis increases the risk of cerebral infarction from vasospasm (47).

Enteral sodium and intravenous hypertonic saline are very effective at replacing lost sodium and stabilizing serum sodium levels. It has been been demonstrated also that treatment with fludrocortisone can decrease the natriuresis and facilitate efforts to achieve hypervolemia (48,49).

Fever is commonplace in the subarachnoid hemorrhage patient, and is often (sometimes incorrectly) attributed to a central fever related to blood in the cerebrospinal fluid. No specific infectious agent is identified in many of these patients (50). Elevated peripheral white blood counts are suggestive of infection, but can be the result of steroid therapy. Hyperthermia is almost certainly harmful to injured brain tissue, and efforts at temperature control are important. Acetaminophen is modestly effective at best. Cooling blankets are helpful, although the associated shivering can be a problem. Intravascular cooling devices may soon be available and may be very useful in this patient group.

REFERENCES

1. Johnston SC, Selvin S, Gress DR. The burden, trends, and demographics of mortality from subarachnoid hemorrhage. *Neurology* 1998;50:1413–1418.
2. Mayberg MR, et al. Guidelines for the management of aneurysmal subarachnoid hemorrhage. A statement for healthcare professionals from a special writing group of the Stroke Council, American Heart Association. *Circulation* 1994;90:2592–2605.
3. Provenzale JM, Morgenlander JC, Gress D. Spontaneous vertebral dissection: clinical, conventional angio-graphic, CT, and MR findings. *J Comput Assist Tomogr* 1996;20:185–193.
4. Chason JM, Hindman WM. Berry aneurysms of the circle of Willis. *Neurology* 1958;8:41–44.
5. Housepian EM, Poll JL. A systematic analysis of intracranial aneurysms from the autopsy files of the Presbyterian Hospital, 1914 to 1956. *J Neuropathol Exp Neurol* 1958;17:409–423.
6. Wilkins RH. Update-subarachnoid hemorrhage and saccular intracranial aneurysms. *Surg Neurol* 1981;15:92–101.
7. Unruptured intracranial aneurysms—risk of rupture and risks of surgical intervention. International Study of Unruptured Intracranial Aneurysms Investigators. *N Engl J Med* 1998;339:1725–1733.
8. Johnston SC, et al., Endovascular and surgical treatment of unruptured cerebral aneurysms: comparison of risks. *Ann Neurol* 2000;48:11–19.
9. Bardach NS, et al. Association between subarachnoid hemorrhage outcomes and number of cases treated at California hospitals. *Stroke* 2002;33:1851–1856.
10. Soni SR. Aneurysms of the posterior communicating artery and oculomotor paresis. *J Neurol Neurosurg Psychiatry* 1974;37:475–484.
11. Mayer PL, et al. Misdiagnosis of symptomatic cerebral aneurysm. Prevalence and correlation with outcome at four institutions. *Stroke* 1996;27:1558–1563.
12. Nornes H, Magnaes B. Intracranial pressure in patients with ruptured saccular aneurysm. *J Neurosurg* 1972;36:537–547.
13. Fisher CM. Clinical syndromes in cerebral thrombosis, hypertensive hemorrhage, and ruptured saccular aneurysm. *Clin Neurosurg* 1975;22:117–147.
14. Crompton MR. Intracerebral hematoma complicating ruptured cerebral aneurysm. *J Neurol Neurosurg Psychiatry* 1962;25:378–386.
15. Hunt WE, Hess RM. Surgical risk as related to time of intervention in the repair of intracranial aneurysms. *J Neurosurg* 1968;28:14–20.
16. Fontanarosa PB. Recognition of subarachnoid hemorrhage. *Ann Emerg Med* 1989;18:1199–1205.
17. White PM, et al. Intracranial aneurysms: CT angiography and MR angiography for detection. Prospective blinded comparison in a large patient cohort. *Radiology* 2001;219:739–749.
18. Fisher CM, Kistler JP, Davis JM. Relation of cerebral vasospasm to subarachnoid hemorrhage visualized by computerized tomographic scanning. *Neurosurgery* 1980;6:1–9.
19. Kistler JP, et al. The relation of cerebral vasospasm to the extent and location of subarachnoid blood visualized by CT scan: a prospective study. *Neurology* 1983;33:424–436.
20. Nelson PB, et al. Hyponatremia and natriuresis following subarachnoid hemorrhage in a monkey model. *J Neurosurg* 1984;60:233–237.
21. Wijdicks EF, et al. Atrial natriuretic factor and salt wasting after aneurysmal subarachnoid hemorrhage. *Stroke* 1991;22:1519–1524.
22. Goldman MR, Rogers EL, Rogers MC. Subarachnoid hemorrhage. Association with unusual electrocardiographic changes. *JAMA* 1975;234:957–958.
23. Beguelin C, Seiler R. Subarachnoid hemorrhage with normal cerebral panangiography. *Neurosurgery* 1983;13:409–411.

24. Hochberg FH, Fisher CM, Roberson GH. Subarachnoid hemorrhage caused by rupture of a small superficial artery. *Neurology* 1974;24:319–321.

25. van Gijn J, et al. Perimesencephalic hemorrhage: a nonaneurysmal and benign form of subarachnoid hemorrhage. *Neurology* 1985;35:493–497.

26. Watanabe A, et al. Perimesencephalic nonaneurysmal subarachnoid haemorrhage and variations in the veins. *Neuroradiology* 2002;44:319–325.

27. Canhao P, et al. Perimesencephalic and nonperimesencephalic subarachnoid haemorrhages with negative angiograms. *Acta Neurochir* 1995;132:14–19.

28. Rhoney DH, et al. Anticonvulsant prophylaxis and timing of seizures after aneurysmal subarachnoid hemorrhage. *Neurology* 2000;55:258–265.

29. Rordorf G, et al. Patients in poor neurological condition after subarachnoid hemorrhage: early management and long-term outcome. *Acta Neurochir* 1997;139: 1143–1151.

30. Le Roux PD, et al. Predicting outcome in poor-grade patients with subarachnoid hemorrhage: a retrospective review of 159 aggressively managed cases. *J Neurosurg* 1996;85:39–49.

31. Winn HR, Richardson AE, Jane JA. The long-term prognosis in untreated cerebral aneurysms: I. The incidence of late hemorrhage in cerebral aneurysm: a 10-year evaluation of 364 patients. *Ann Neurol* 1977;1: 358–370.

32. Sundt TM Jr, Whisnant JP. Subarachnoid hemorrhage from intracranial aneurysms. Surgical management and natural history of disease. *N Engl J Med* 1978;299: 116–122.

33. Kassell NF, Torner JC. Aneurysmal rebleeding: a preliminary report from the Cooperative Aneurysm Study. *Neurosurgery* 1983;13:479–481.

34. Kassell NF, et al. The International Cooperative Study on the Timing of Aneurysm Surgery. Part 2: Surgical results. *J Neurosurg* 1990;73:37–47.

35. Graff-Radford NR, et al. Factors associated with hydrocephalus after subarachnoid hemorrhage. A report of the Cooperative Aneurysm Study. *Arch Neurol* 1989;46: 744–752.

36. Findlay JM, Macdonald RL, Weir BK. Current concepts of pathophysiology and management of cerebral vasospasm following aneurysmal subarachnoid hemorrhage. *Cerebrovasc Brain Metab Rev* 1991;3: 336–361.

37. Mayberg MR, Okada T, Bark DH. The role of hemoglobin in arterial narrowing after subarachnoid hemorrhage. *J Neurosurg* 1990;72:634–640.

38. Findlay JM, et al. Arterial wall changes in cerebral vasospasm. *Neurosurgery* 1989;25:736–745; 745–746.

39. Fassbender K, et al. Inflammatory cytokines in subarachnoid haemorrhage: association with abnormal blood flow velocities in basal cerebral arteries. *J Neurol Neurosurg Psychiatry* 2001;70:534–537.

40. Biller J, Godersky JC, Adams HP Jr. Management of aneurysmal subarachnoid hemorrhage. *Stroke* 1988;19: 1300–1305.

41. Pickard JD, et al. Effect of oral nimodipine on cerebral infarction and outcome after subarachnoid haemorrhage: British aneurysm nimodipine trial. *BMJ* 1989; 298:636–642.

42. Allen GS, et al. Cerebral arterial spasm—a controlled trial of nimodipine in patients with subarachnoid hemorrhage. *N Engl J Med* 1983;308:619–624.

43. Sloan MA, et al. Sensitivity and specificity of transcranial Doppler ultrasonography in the diagnosis of vasospasm following subarachnoid hemorrhage. *Neurology* 1989;39:1514–1518.

44. Vora YY, et al. Role of transcranial Doppler monitoring in the diagnosis of cerebral vasospasm after subarachnoid hemorrhage. *Neurosurgery* 1999;44:1237–1247; 1247–1248.

45. Origitano TC, et al. Sustained increased cerebral blood flow with prophylactic hypertensive hypervolemic hemodilution ("triple-H" therapy) after subarachnoid hemorrhage. *Neurosurgery* 1990;27:729–739; 739–740.

46. Mechanical and pharmacologic treatment of vasospasm. *AJNR Am J Neuroradiol* 2001;22:S26–27.

47. Wijdicks EF, et al. Hyponatremia and cerebral infarction in patients with ruptured intracranial aneurysms: is fluid restriction harmful? *Ann Neurol* 1985;17: 137–140.

48. Hasan D, et al. Effect of fludrocortisone acetate in patients with subarachnoid hemorrhage. *Stroke* 1989;20: 1156–1161.

49. Mori T, et al. Improved efficiency of hypervolemic therapy with inhibition of natriuresis by fludrocortisone in patients with aneurysmal subarachnoid hemorrhage. *J Neurosurg* 1999;91:947–952.

50. Oliveira-Filho J, et al. Fever in subarachnoid hemorrhage: relationship to vasospasm and outcome. *Neurology* 2001;56:1299–1304.

16

Intensive and Postoperative Care of Intracranial Tumors

Although patients who have just been operated on for tumor occupy a large proportion of beds in many neurological intensive care units (neuro-ICUs), little attention has been given to the subject. The main critical care problems that are associated with cerebral tumors relate to the postoperative state and clinical signs of mass effect and raised intracranial pressure (ICP). Some of these issues are addressed in general terms in Chapter 3. Here, it must be acknowledged that the intensivist largely acts as an agent for the neurosurgeon and to some extent, for the neuroanesthesiologist. In a few instances, complications of a large tumor may justify critical care attention on their own, particularly when manifestations of increased intracranial pressure, hydrocephalus, or status epilepticus bring the brain tumor to attention. Numerous medical complications of neurological disease, such as a pulmonary embolus and gastric hemorrhage, also require critical care at different stages of the disease. Certain cerebral neoplasms call for special attention as well; for example, pituitary apoplexy or tumors in the posterior fossa involve structures that affect breathing and swallowing. Tumor recurrence after treatment by surgery, radiation therapy, and chemotherapy, in most cases, is viewed as a less critical circumstance and is usually addressed on the ward, but the intensivist can provide valuable aid in the way of advice on the management of raised intracranial pressure in these cases.

Intracranial tumors can arise from any structure within the intracranial cavity (Tables 16.1 and 16.2). Most begin in the brain, but the pituitary, pineal, cranial nerves, and leptomeninges are additional sites of origin. Furthermore, any intracranial structure may be the site of metastatic spread from tumors that begin outside the nervous system. Patients with parenchymal brain tumors (i.e., gliomas, lymphomas, brain metastases) are the most likely candidates for intensive care management; these tumors are considered in this chapter. The concepts of critical care management presented also apply to patients with other intracranial tumors who develop serious complications.

In adults, most primary brain tumors arise in the cerebrum; the commonest of these are gliomas: astrocytomas (25%); high-grade gliomas (including glioblastoma) (20%); meningiomas (25%; more common in women than men); and a number of miscellaneous tumors, including primary central nervous system (CNS) lymphomas, which follow in frequency (1,2). The incidence of virtually all adult tumors increases with age, gliomas being more likely to be of higher grade with increasing age.

It has been recognized in recent years that the incidence of primary lymphomas of the CNS has increased markedly (3). Part of the increase is the result of the acquired immunodeficiency syndrome (AIDS) epidemic, but independent of this, there has been at least a threefold increase in primary CNS lymphomas in immunocompetent patients over the past decade. At the Sloan-Kettering Hospital the frequency of primary CNS lym-

TABLE 16.1. *Major intracranial tumors in adults by percent*

Metastatic	%	Primary brain tumor	%	Other intracranial tumors	%
Lung	40	Glioblastoma	40	Meningioma	80
Breast	20	Anaplastic astrocytoma	20	Acoustic neuroma	10
Melanoma	20	Astrocytoma	15	Pituitary adenoma	5
Miscellaneous	20	Lymphoma	10	Miscellaneous	5
		Oligodendroglioma	5		
		Miscellaneous	10		

phomas in immunocompetent patients has gone from less than 1% of primary brain tumors to 15% (4).

According to some authorities, there is also evidence that other primary brain tumors may be increasing in incidence, at least in the elderly. There has been an apparent twofold increase in "brain cancer" (primarily high-grade gliomas) in patients 75 to 79 years old, fourfold in patients 80 to 84 years old, and fivefold in patients 85 years old and upward between 1973 and the current era (5). It is unclear whether this represents a real increase, better ascertainment because of better diagnostic techniques, or both.

In children, brain tumors arise largely in the posterior fossa and include cerebellar astrocytomas (20%), medulloblastomas (20%), brainstem gliomas (15%), and ependymomas (10%). Their peak age incidence is 5 to 10 years (6,7).

As mentioned, metastatic intracranial tumors are more common than primary ones, occurring in about 25% of cancer patients who come to autopsy (8,9). Of these, more than half are symptomatic making patients with them likely to appear regularly in any large general intensive care unit (8,10,11). All primary cancers can metastasize to the nervous system, but the common ones, well known to clinicians, are lung, breast, and malignant melanoma. In approximately 50% of patients, the brain metastasis is single; in another 20% there are two brain metastases. Approximately 10% of patients with lung cancer present with a brain metastasis before the lung cancer is diagnosed.

CLINICAL FINDINGS

Pathophysiology of Peritumoral Brain Edema

Intracranial tumors tend to cause signs and symptoms while still relatively small when compared with tumors in other organs. The tumor itself may invade, replace, or compress cranial tissues, leading either to failure of function or to seizures. The tumor usually causes an opening of the blood–brain barrier (BBB), with resulting brain edema. The combination of the tumor mass and the surrounding edema produces mass effect that shifts normal structures from their usual position and may interfere with cerebrospinal fluid (CSF) flow, leading to increased intracranial pressure (ICP)

TABLE 16.2. *Major intracranial tumors in children by percent*

	Primary (% of total brain tumors)	Supratentorial (% by compartment)	Infratentorial (% by compartment)
Pilocytic astrocytoma	19	23	29
Medulloblastoma	17	2	32
Ependymoma	8	5	12
Craniopharyngioma	7	15	2
Anaplastic astrocytoma	6	13	2
Others	45	52	23

with or without hydrocephalus (Chapter 2). The result may be symptoms that are only indirectly related to the presence of the tumor itself, so-called false localizing signs.

The edema associated with brain tumors is considered to be largely of the "vasogenic" type, meaning a leakage of water and plasma ultrafiltrate through the vascular BBB (12). In part, it results also from neovascularization engendered by the tumor. Some edema fluid also may arise from breakdown of the BBB in the edematous area immediately surrounding the brain tumor. The edema is distributed more readily through the white matter extracellular space in comparison to the gray matter, possibly because of a lower mechanical resistance. This pattern of distribution is apparent on scans and in autopsy specimens in which the fluid follows white matter tracts more or less radially outward from the site of the tumor. The edema often creates more mass effect than the tumor itself and may be correspondingly responsible for more symptoms than is the mass of the tumor. Whether focal neurological symptoms are attributable to edema *per se* has not been satisfactorily resolved, but the clinical improvement that usually accompanies a reduction in edema in response to corticosteroids suggests that there is a relationship.

The breakdown of the BBB within the tumor probably results from a number of factors, including the aforementioned angiogenesis, particularly because these new vessels do not possess tight junctions that are usually found at sites of the BBB in normal cerebral vasculature. Factors such as vascular endothelial growth factor that are elaborated by cerebral tumors are currently proposed to be the cause of angiogenesis. Furthermore, metastatic tumors appear to contain fenestrated endothelium, as in vessels elsewhere in the body. Both lead to the passage of large molecules (e.g., albumin) into the tumor interstitial space, resulting in a loss of intravascular oncotic pressure. Primary brain tumors also secrete permeability factors that promote vasogenic edema. The exact nature of these factors is not known, but a variety of substances such as metabolites of arachidonic acid, especially

the leukotrienes (13–15), glutamate (16), and so-called vascular permeability factor (17) have been implicated. Some investigators have found a correlation between the degree of macrophage infiltration and peritumoral edema. Macrophages secrete enzymes, platelet-activating factors, and free radicals that may contribute to the development of edema (18). Finally, and perhaps most salient for the ICU, pressure on the cortex from intraoperative brain retraction and brain manipulation, as well as reperfusion at the end of surgery, may exacerbate cerebral edema (19–23).

Symptoms and Signs of Brain Tumor

As a general rule, low-grade cerebral tumors are more likely to present with seizures, whereas higher-grade and more rapidly growing gliomas typically cause early focal signs (e.g., hemiparesis) or signs of generalized dysfunction (e.g., headache and diminished consciousness). Lymphomas rarely produce seizures but may produce behavioral changes. Slowly growing tumors such as meningiomas, particularly those that arise in relatively silent areas of the brain (e.g., frontal pole), are more likely to cause false localizing signs than are rapidly growing ones (24).

The site of the lesion, of course, also plays an important role. Frontal tumors cause behavioral changes, whereas tumors closer to the motor strip and in the parietal lobe are more likely to cause seizures, focal weakness, or sensory change. Posterior fossa tumors often cause cranial nerve or cerebellar signs, but because they also obstruct the ventricular system, generalized symptoms and signs include headache, nausea, vomiting, and papilledema, often occurring early in the course of the disease.

Focal or generalized seizures occur in 20% to 50% of patients with tumors and are the usual presenting complaint in patients with low-grade gliomas. When focal, the seizure localizes the site of the tumor. Seizures represent a threat in patients with brain tumors beyond the usual risks of aspiration, respiratory arrest, and physical injury from convulsion, because the increased blood flow caused by either a focal or generalized seizure further increases ICP and may lead to exaggeration of brain edema.

Seizures appear to be more common in patients with metastatic melanoma than other brain metastases, probably because the gray matter is more frequently involved in this tumor than in other types. Seizures are a common presenting problem in meningiomas as well and may be more common in the postoperative period than after removal of other tumors (25,26).

Focal seizures may be difficult to diagnose in patients with brain tumors. They frequently last longer and are more complex than in patients with other intracranial lesions. They are also more likely to be associated with headache and to produce "negative" than "positive" symptoms. As a result, they may be mistaken either for transient ischemic attacks or late-life migraine and not recognized as focal seizures.

TREATMENT

Patients with brain tumors may require intensive care treatment in the preoperative period, usually to treat seizures or increased ICP with herniation and in the immediate postoperative period to treat the complications of surgery. Many of the critical care problems associated with brain tumors are similar to those associated with other CNS disorders and are discussed in detail in Chapters 3 and 10.

Preoperative and Perioperative Period

Seizures

Seizures, either focal or generalized, can occur at any time during the course of a brain tumor but are most frequent as the presenting complaint before the diagnosis is established. Most are individual focal or generalized seizures, but in occasional patients, repetitive focal seizures and status epilepticus may be the central problem (Chapter 20). If seizures

raise intracranial pressure, as mentioned, they may in turn lead to herniation or permanent brain damage.

The choice of anticonvulsants for brain tumor patients is not straightforward. Phenytoin, the one most commonly used, increases the metabolism of dexamethasone and some chemotherapeutic agents, often rendering them less effective (27). Furthermore, patients on phenytoin whose steroids are to be tapered and who are being treated with radiation therapy within a month after beginning the drug may have a slightly increased risk of Stevens–Johnson syndrome (27). Carbamazepine also induces microsomal enzymes in the liver, leading to increased metabolism of other drugs, and also may lead to Stevens–Johnson syndrome when combined with brain radiation therapy. Furthermore, carbamazepine suppresses the white count, a potentially undesirable effect in patients who receive myelosuppressive chemotherapy (27). Phenobarbital causes excessive sedation in patients already lethargic from their brain tumors and, in up to 20% of patients with brain tumors, leads to a rheumatic disorder with pain and often limited mobility in the shoulder contralateral to the brain tumor (27). Valproate is a generally effective drug, but its effect on the liver is problematic when used in conjunction with multiple chemotherapeutic agents.

Nonetheless, most intensivists begin the treatment of seizures with phenytoin. If the patient is having frequent seizures, 1.0 to 1.25 g intravenously (i.v.) is administered at a rate not exceeding 50 mg/minute with cardiac monitoring during the loading dose. A maintenance dose of approximately 5 mg/kg maintains serum levels at 10 to 20 mg/L in most patients. Stable blood levels are often difficult to maintain because of interactions with other medications. Oral loading, 1 g over 24 hours followed by 300 to 400 mg daily, is safer than i.v. loading and indicated for most patients not having repetitive seizures.

Treatment of generalized repetitive seizures or status epilepticus follows the lines given in Chapter 20. The initial situation should be controlled with i.v. midazolam, diazepam (5 to 10 mg over 1 to 2 minutes) or lorazepam (1 to 3 mg over 1 to 2 minutes). If the patient was not previously treated with a conventional anticonvulsant, 15 to 18 mg/kg phenytoin is begun and then the patient is placed on a maintenance dose. If these measures fail to abort repetitive seizures, the further measures used in an intensive care unit setting are discussed in Chapter 20.

The patient with a brain tumor who is having seizures, of course, should be evaluated for metabolic derangements that lower the seizure threshold, particularly hypocalcemia, hyponatremia, hypoglycemia, and renal or hepatic failure (which may be manifestations of metastatic disease) or alcohol withdrawal.

Preoperative *prophylactic anticonvulsants* may be considered in patients with *primary brain tumors* who have not had previous seizures but several recent trials have failed to show a clear benefit. One prospective controlled study of supratentorial operations in 281 patients showed a reduction in seizure incidence in patients given prophylactic phenytoin (25,26). The protective effect was most dramatic in the first month, but 75% of seizures in both groups occurred within the first 3 months. These authors recommended phenytoin prophylaxis for 3 months in most cases. Meningiomas have a higher postoperative seizure rate than other tumors and it has been suggested that they should be prophylactically treated for 12 months. Therapeutic anticonvulsant levels must be attained for the drug to be effective after surgery.

The use of *prophylactic anticonvulsants for metastatic tumors* is more complicated. There are several prospective studies that have been summarized by Glantz and colleagues (28). The summary of their analysis is that there is no advantage to prophylactic anticonvulsants in patients with metastatic tumors for which reason our approach has generally been not to use these drugs except with malignant melanoma, which has a higher overall seizure rate than other metastatic tumors.

Patients with primary or metastatic tumors who receive iodinated contrast materials for CT scanning are at slightly increased risk for seizures, and a prophylactic dose of diazepam 5 to 10 mg orally 30 to 60 minutes before the injection of contrast reduces the incidence of seizures; however, we often do not use this approach (29).

Increased Intracranial Pressure

The treatment of intracranial hypertension is discussed in detail in Chapter 3 and only a few aspects specifically related to brain tumors are discussed here. Glucocorticoids are particularly effective in the management of patients with brain tumors and peritumoral edema. With one exception (see the following), once a diagnosis of intraparenchymal brain tumor with cerebral edema or shift is made, we start most patients on dexamethasone (or an equivalent steroid) in a dose of approximately 8 to 16 mg/day. In many patients, the symptoms caused by the tumor resolve within 48 hours. Generalized symptoms such as headache respond better than focal symptoms. If symptoms persist, the dose of steroids can be doubled every 48 hours until a clinical response has been achieved or until no response occurs at a dose of 100 mg/day.

For acutely decompensating patients, dexamethasone may be given as a 100-mg bolus followed by 100 mg/day in divided doses. When combined with i.v. hyperosmolar agents (mannitol) and, if necessary, hyperventilation, most patients herniating from the effects of brain tumor stabilize and improve.

The exception to the early use of steroids referred to above is in patients suspected of harboring brain lymphoma (4) because the oncolytic and antiedema effects of corticosteroids cause the tumor to become temporarily inapparent on scans in as many as 40% of patients. This may prevent definitive diagnosis by needle biopsy.

Corticosteroids are continued in the postoperative period (see the following) and during the course of radiation therapy if that modality is indicated. They can be tapered gradually during radiation therapy but should not be discontinued until the radiation has been completed. We usually begin radiation therapy while the patient is on a dose of 12 to 16 mg dexamethasone per day and taper by approximately 2 mg a week such that the patient ends the steroid course soon after the radiation is completed. If the symptoms of the tumor are exacerbated during the course of the taper, the dose is raised temporarily and the taper begun again. Others have reported a more rapid taper to be equally effective and safe (30).

Steroids may induce hyperglycemia or exacerbate diabetes. Management of diabetes in the perioperative period is important, and we typically check blood glucose levels every 4 hours when the patient is not eating in preparation for surgery. The evening before surgery, patients receiving intermediate-acting insulin (NPH, Lente, Monotaid) should have this dose decreased to one third with short-acting insulin kept at the same preoperative dose. After an i.v. line has been started with a dextrose infusion just before surgery, the intermediate-acting insulin should be administered at one half the normal dose, with the regular insulin given at one third the normal dose. Glucose determinations should be taken hourly during surgery. Postoperatively, the patient may be managed on sliding scale regular insulin every 6 hours, until able to take a regular diet. During a steroid taper, adjustments in insulin dosage are also required.

Patients on oral hypoglycemics should usually be maintained on an appropriate diet until surgery. Oral hypoglycemics should be withheld the day of surgery and until the patient is taking the normal preoperative diet.

Patients on steroids are at risk for developing gastrointestinal perforation. The problem is particularly common in patients who are severely constipated. The classical peritoneal signs caused by the inflammation may be masked by the steroids, but the diagnosis generally can be made by detection of free air under the diaphragm on upright films of the abdomen. Prevention of constipation, which includes laxatives, enemas, and manual disimpaction, often prevents this serious side effect (31).

Gastritis, peptic ulceration, and gastrointestinal bleeding are serious consequences of steroid administration but are much less common than generally believed. There is little evidence to support the widespread use of gastric acid prophylaxis in patients on corticosteroids. There is evidence suggesting that patients on respirators in ICUs may have a decreased incidence of gastrointestinal bleeding if treated prophylactically (32). Histamine H_2 receptor blockers have been used routinely, but their occasional side effects of psychosis and thrombocytopenia may limit their usefulness in patients with brain tumors. Their tendency to raise gastric pH may lead to an increased incidence of pneumonia because of colonization of the stomach by bacteria that are then aspirated into the lungs. Antacids and sucralfate are good alternatives, but these drugs must be given orally or by nasogastric tube.

Corticosteroids increase the susceptibility of a patient with brain tumor to infection. A particular problem has occurred with Pneumocystis carinii (Pneumocystis jiroveci) infection occurring during the tapering of steroids in patients with brain tumors (33). Some investigators have recommended prophylaxis with trimethoprim/sulfamethoxazole using one double-strength tablet twice a day for 3 days per week. No controlled trials have demonstrated the effectiveness of this method in patients with brain tumors, although it appears to be useful in preventing Pneumocystis carinii infection in patients with leukemia.

Other side effects of steroids, many associated with prolonged use, are detailed in Table 16.3.

Steps taken in the perioperative period can decrease or eliminate many complications that otherwise occur during surgery or the immediate postoperative period. Dexamethasone 4 mg q6h should be administered in most patients starting 48 hours before surgery. If the patient has not received dexamethasone within 24 hours of surgery, a

TABLE 16.3. *Potential side effects of corticosteroids in brain tumor patients in the intensive care unit*

Gastrointestinal bleeding
Gastrointestinal perforation
Diabetes-hyperosmolar state
Adrenocortical insufficiency
Myopathy
Insomnia
Hallucinations
Psychosis
Seizures
Avascular necrosis of the hip
Cataracts
Opportunistic infections

TABLE 16.4. *Treatment of air embolism*

Surgeon
  Flood surgical field with saline
  Coagulate all bleeding points
  Wax bone
Anesthesia
  Change nitrous oxide to 100% O_2
  Aspirate air from Swan–Ganz
  Vasopressors for blood pressure
  Place patient in left lateral recumbent position

loading dose of 10 mg may be given on admission to the hospital, followed by 6 mg every 6 hours. (These doses are arbitrary and pharmacokinetic data are lacking, but our impression is that they work clinically.) To reduce the effects of brain retraction in edematous regions before the dural incision, mannitol is given in a dose of 0.5 to 1.0 g/kg. After intubation, patients are hyperventilated to a $Paco_2$ of 30 mm Hg or an end-tidal CO_2 of approximately 25 mm Hg. Cerebrospinal fluid drainage by lumbar puncture, indwelling subarachnoid catheter, or ventriculostomy is used just before the dural incision in selected patients. (If spinal drainage is used, postoperative headache may be from that procedure and not a direct result of the surgery.)

Air Embolism

The incidence of air embolism may be as high as 25% in patients operated on in the sitting position, the result of entry of air through tears in the cortical veins, dural sinuses, or diploic veins. A major embolus causes right heart failure with hypotension and tachycardia. Precordial (or transcranial) Doppler detects air embolism, as does the measurement of end-tidal Pco_2, which decreases when air embolism occurs.

To treat embolism, the surgeon floods the field with saline, coagulates all bleeding points, and occludes the exposed bone with wax. Aspiration of air from a Swan–Ganz catheter or right atrial line is both diagnostic and therapeutic (34,35). The breathing gas is switched to 100% O_2 to decrease the effect of nitrogen (and nitrous oxide if it was used) in expanding the volume of the embolism (36). Vasopressors are given to maintain the blood pressure. The patient may also be turned in the left lateral recumbent position. Most patients survive air embolism, but it can have important sequelae including ischemic stroke if a patent foramen ovale is present (37,38) (Table 16.4).

Coagulopathy

Some patients with recurrent primary brain tumors or brain metastasis are thrombocytopenic from the myelosuppressive effects of chemotherapy, which causes the greatest degree of platelet reduction approximately 3 weeks after administration of the last dose. Ranitidine and heparin may also induce thrombocytopenia. For major craniotomies, the platelet count should preferably be greater than 100,000 and the prothrombin time or international normalized ration (INR) and partial thromboplastin time (PTT) should be in the normal range. There is little evidence that the bleeding time is a useful marker of adequate hemostasis. Coumadin should, of course, be stopped several days before craniotomy to ensure that the INR normalizes. An elevated INR, whether from coumadin, liver disease, or nutritional deficiency, is corrected acutely with vitamin K and fresh-frozen plasma (FFP). Vitamin K can be given intravenously, a total dose of 2.5 to 25 mg, at a rate of 1 mg/minute. Repeat INR testing can be performed every 4 to 6 hours to ensure normalization. If a patient requires anticoagulation, such as for a prosthetic heart valve, heparin can be started after the coumadin has been discontinued. The PTT should normalize 6 hours after the heparin has been turned off. Protamine sulfate can be given for urgent reversal of heparin-induced anticoagulation. Protamine should be given at a dose of no greater than 50 mg over a 10-minute period. The usual dose is 1.0 to 1.5 mg for each 100 units of heparin. One half hour after injection of the heparin bolus, the protamine reversal dose is reduced to 0.5 mg per 100 units. If any abnormality in coagulation is documented, a full coagulation study is obtained to determine the presence of factor deficiencies or DIC.

One of the indications that a total resection of brain tumor has not been achieved is the inability to maintain hemostasis. Oxidized cellulose (Surgicel) is the most effective hemostatic agent used intraoperatively, although thrombin-soaked Gelfoam and microfibrillary collagen (Avitene) also can be used (39). These pledgets normally become saturated with blood and may be confused with an intraparenchymal hematoma on postoperative computed tomography (CT) scan; however, the saturated hemostatic agents generally produce no mass effect, as opposed to a hematoma. Loose dural closure with a closed drainage system in either the subgaleal or epidural space may prevent accumulation of a clot or assist in early detection.

Postoperative Period (See also Chapter 10)

Once the patient arrives in the ICU, several postoperative complications may be anticipated. *Deterioration of consciousness in the postoperative period is usually related to: (a) mass effect and elevated intracranial pressure; (b) various drugs used in the intraoperative period; (c) subclinical seizures; or (d) electrolyte imbalance, specifically hyponatremia from water overload.* The CT scan usually differentiates the first of these. If there is a large amount of edema, general measures to reduce the ICP (e.g., mannitol, hyperventilation) should be started and a CT scan obtained. An MRI is preferable if the operation was in the posterior fossa.

Additional problems relate to *abnormalities of blood gases, deep venous thromboses, electrolyte changes and fever* (with or without infection). Careful monitoring and postoperative care avoid many of these complications.

Head Elevation

The appropriate head position for patients in the postoperative period is as controversial for other patients with raised ICP (Chapter 2). An elevated head position lowers ICP and may help avoid some of the potential consequences of the inevitable brain edema in the postoperative period. However, elevation of the head potentially decreases arterial pressure in the brain, lowering the cerebral perfusion pressure. Studies from head-injured patients have suggested that the supine position (zero degrees) is optimal, although others have recommended head elevations of 15 to 30 degrees (40,41). Whether these studies are applicable to patients with brain tumors is uncertain and the controversy suggests that there is not a great deal of difference among these head positions, or that the ideal position must be determined by ICP measurement in an individual patient. It is our practice to keep the head elevated in the immediate postoperative period about 15 degrees unless there is a risk for tension pneumocephalus.

Intracranial Hypertension

The most important sources of postoperative intracranial hypertension include bleeding, edema, hydrocephalus, tension pneumocephalus, and cerebral infarction (Table 16.5). Intracranial hypertension may be heralded by failure to recover consciousness in the immediate postsurgical period, a subsequent change in the level of consciousness after initial recovery, or the development of an unexpected change or loss of neurological function (Chapter 10).

TABLE 16.5. *Risk factors, prevention, and treatment of postoperative neurological complications*

Complications	Hematoma	Edema	Hydrocephalus	Tension pneumocephalus	Infarction
Time	Immediate	36–72 H	Variable	2–4 D	Immediate to 5 D
Risk factors Intraparenchymal	Subtotal resection Tumor type (melanoma, chorio) Hypertension	Excessive brain retraction Tumor type (e.g., meningioma)	Posterior fossa lesions Intraventricular hemorrhage	Base of skull surgery Excessive cerebrospinal fluid drainage	Arterial ligation Excessive brain retraction Ligation of posterior 2/3 of sagittal sinus Ligation of major draining veins
Subdural	Acute brain decompression Sitting position		Intraventricular tumor (e.g., colloid cyst)		
Epidural	Dura stripped from skull Middle meningeal artery				
Prevention	Intraoperative cauterization of bleeding points Use of hemostatic agents (surgical) Epidural drains Epidural tenting sutures Blood pressure <160	Preoperative steroids Minimal brain retraction	Venticulostomy Ventriculoperitoneal shunts Ommaya reservoir	Dural closure Reconstruction of skull base Reexpansion of intracranial contents Epidural drains Head of bed flat 48–72 h	Preoperative imaging to determine relationship of tumor to major vessels and to determine the patency of the sinuses
Treatment	General Evacuation of hematoma	General Increased steroid dosage	Same as prevention	70–100% O_2 administration Needle or catheter aspiration Water-seal drainage	General, as in Chapter 13

Hematomas

Postoperative hematomas are usually intra-parenchymal, occurring at the site of the tumor resection, but they can occur epidurally, subdurally, or rarely distant from the operative site. In a large series from the Cleveland Clinic, the postoperative hemorrhage rate was 0.8% with meningioma, the most commonly implicated tumor (42). Aside from tumor type, the extent of resection also affects the rate of postoperative hematoma formation. From a study at Sloan-Kettering, gross total resection of malignant gliomas did not result in postoperative hematomas, but subtotal resection resulted in 5.5% incidence of clinically significant clots (43).

Hypertension also places the patient at risk for developing an intraparenchymal hematoma (42). Surgeons prefer to maintain postoperative systolic blood pressure less than 160 mm Hg; however, patients who were previously hypertensive may require postoperative blood pressures in their usual range for adequate cerebral perfusion pressure. Antihypertensive agents should be given judiciously to avoid an acute decrease in the blood pressure and a concomitant fall in the cerebral perfusion pressure (Chapter 3). The antihypertensive agents most frequently used are labetalol and nitroprusside, although there are theoretic reasons to avoid the latter. Parenteral administration of labetalol is given in 10- to 20-mg boluses every 5 to 10 minutes until the blood pressure is brought to the desired level.

Epidural hematomas result from inadequately cauterized middle meningeal vessels or the stripping of the dura from the inner table of the skull. Epidural tenting sutures can be used, particularly where the dura is pulled away from the inner table of the skull, to decrease this potential risk. Subdural hematomas may result from acute brain decompression by mannitol or spinal or ventricular drainage. Surgery performed in the sitting position also places the patients at increased risk for subdural hematomas because of traction on bridging veins, particularly after posterior fossa surgery (44). Brain edema generally peaks postoperatively at 36 to 72 hours; however, clinical signs of edema may be encountered in the first 6 to 12 hours after surgery. Intracranial pressure monitoring has revealed that in a small group of patients with an uneventful postoperative course and small amount of edema, the mean ICP at 1 to 2 hours was 7 mm Hg; plateau waves as high as 10 to 30 mm Hg occurred at 12 hours and again at 24 to 48 hours. Patients with clinically significant edema in the postoperative period experienced plateau waves between 30 to 50 mm Hg at 12 hours, with a second rise to 50 mm Hg at 24 to 48 hours. Postoperative hematomas caused a more acute rise than did edema in ICP during the early hours after surgery (45).

Patients who develop significant postoperative brain tumor edema usually appear normal when they awaken from anesthesia, but between 6 and 36 hours they gradually become more lethargic or develop new neurological deficits. If the CT scan excludes a clinically significant hematoma, the recommended treatment is to increase the steroid dose and reduce any free water administration.

Acute Hydrocephalus

Posterior fossa and intraventricular surgery, the most likely procedures to introduce blood into the subarachnoid space and interfere with CSF absorption, are occasionally associated with postoperative hydrocephalus. Patients with symptomatic third ventricular tumors also may acutely decompensate and require ICU attention.

Ventriculostomy is effective in treating hydrocephalus caused by posterior fossa tumors and may be better than permanent preoperative shunting for two reasons. First, in most patients the hydrocephalus resolves with steroids and surgical excision of the posterior fossa mass. In a series of 62 children and adolescents, 41 had total removal of posterior fossa lesions with only 25% requiring permanent shunts (46). Second, upward herniation has been documented in 3% to 10% of patients (46,47) after external drainage. The drainage pressure should be kept at 140 to 165 mm H_2O to avoid this. If permanent shunting is felt to be necessary preoperatively, an on–off valve may help control the pressure in an acceptable range to prevent upward herniation.

Routine ventriculostomy is performed frequently after excision of an intraventricular tumor such as craniopharyngiomas or giant pituitary tumors that invade the third ventricle. Bleeding from the tumor resection site into the ventricle can cause hydrocephalus and an acute rise in intracranial pressure. The ventricular catheter serves both diagnostic and therapeutic purposes.

Patients with third ventricular tumors (e.g., colloid cysts, astrocytomas, papillary ependymomas, and subependymomas) may rarely suffer coma or sudden death (48). The phenomenon probably results from plateau waves. A patient with a third ventricular tumor and signs of increased ICP should be closely monitored with early placement of a ventriculostomy or a biventricular shunt. Lumbar puncture is contraindicated in these patients.

Cerebral Infarction

Postoperative cerebral infarction can occur as a result of ligation of a vessel during tumor excision or from excessive retraction on cortical vessels, probably through the mechanism of vasospasm. Venous infarctions occur by acute occlusion of the superior sagittal sinus in the posterior two thirds or by sacrifice of a major draining vein. Acute occlusion of a major venous sinus can result in catastrophic hemispheric swelling and death. If there is tumor compression of the sinus in the anterior two thirds, the sinus usually can be safely ligated and removed at that site because collateral venous circulation develops. Preoperative magnetic resonance imaging or angiogram delineates the patency of the sinus and may help determine the safety of sacrificing the sinus.

In the postoperative period, blood volume should be sufficient to keep arterial pressure and central venous pressures at normal levels. Hypovolemia from diuresis and severe fluid restriction may lead to development of cerebral infarction in patients with vasospasm.

Tension Pneumocephalus

The incidence of tension pneumocephalus has increased with the increase in skull base surgery. Efflux of CSF from the intracranial space during surgery creates a negative pressure that is filled by the entry of air, the "inverted pop bottle" phenomenon (49,50). Intraoperative measures to prevent the development of tension pneumocephalus include closure of the dura, reconstruction of the skull base, reexpansion of the intracranial contents, and epidural drain placement.

Patients at risk should be positioned postoperatively with the head of bed flat for 48 to 72 hours. Clinical signs of tension pneumocephalus usually occur 2 to 4 days postoperatively when the intracranial air causes mass effect, which can clinically mimic a space-occupying lesion. However, the air may appear months to years after the procedure. The CT scan differentiates tension pneumocephalus from hematoma or edema. Patients should breathe 100% oxygen, which may stabilize them for up to 48 hours by replacing the nitrogen component of the intracranial air with oxygen, which is more readily absorbed into the bloodstream. This treatment is less effective after 48 hours. If the patient is rapidly decompensating, needle aspiration or placement of a catheter into the pocket may be required. To prevent reaccumulation, a water-seal drainage system can be used similar to the system used in pneumothorax. This system has been used successfully in persistent cases of tension pneumocephalus (51). Finally, surgery may be required to repair a skull base fracture or CSF leak.

Fluid and Electrolyte Abnormalities (See also Chapter 6)

Careful attention is required to prevent fluid and electrolyte abnormalities in the postoperative and ICU period. It is important to recognize that hyponatremia in the postoperative period is not always a manifestation of inappropriate secretion of antidiuretic hormone and water retention. Failure to recognize hypovolemic hyponatremia in postoperative patients with tumor, similar to subarachnoid hemorrhage, may lead to cerebral infarction from vasospasm, as discussed in Chapter 15 (44).

A compromise is required between hypoosmolality, which may lead to brain edema, and dehydration, which can decrease blood volume and blood flow and increase blood viscosity. Unfortunately, simple measurement of the serum sodium, which is often used as a benchmark in the postoperative period to determine administration of fluids, does not adequately distinguish hyponatremia with an increased blood volume requiring fluid restriction from a hyperosmolar state with decreased blood volume that requires fluid and electrolyte replacement. Nor does simple "1-to-1" fluid replacement of output suffice if the patient is dehydrated by the time he reaches the ICU. The goal in the immediate postoperative period should be to keep the patient normovolemic and normoosmolar or slightly hyperosmolar.

Mannitol and furosemide are often administered during surgery to induce brain relaxation and reduce intracranial pressure. Both alter the electrolyte balance in the postoperative period, particularly causing hypokalemia. Furthermore, patients may already be mildly dehydrated from being without liquids before surgery and from glucose-induced diuresis as a result of steroid therapy. These issues are discussed in detail in Chapter 6. The syndrome of inappropriate antidiuretic hormone (SIADH) is characterized as a euvolemic hyponatremia state with a low plasma osmolality and a high urine osmolality. Retention of water results in increases of blood and tissue volume (and probably brain edema) and in decreased serum sodium. Treatment of SIADH consists of water restriction to 500 cc/day if the sodium is less than 120 mEq/L and to 1 L/day if the sodium is between 120 and 130

mEq/L. If the sodium is less than 115 mEq/ L or the patient is seizing or comatose as a result of hyponatremia, 3% NaCl solution may be used to raise the serum sodium. Demeclocycline (600 to 1,200 mg/day) or oral furosemide with salt replacement (3 g/day) also may be used.

Hyponatremia characterized by hypovolemic hyponatremia results from diuretics, mineralocorticoid deficiency, vomiting, or diarrhea or any disorder in which both fluid and sodium are lost but only replaced by hypoosmolar solution (48). Arterial blood pressure, urine output, and urine osmolality may all be low, but blood urea nitrogen and creatinine are elevated (52).

Neurogenic diabetes insipidus (DI) is a state of in hypernatremia and hyperosmolarity with decreased extracellular fluid volume, resulting from a decreased secretion of antidiuretic hormone and a concomitant increase in urinary output. Patients are placed at risk for DI with surgery of the hypothalamic–pituitary axis, direct injury to the hypothalamus, or diffuse injury to the brain. Fifteen percent to 20% of patients undergoing transsphenoidal resection of pituitary adenomas experience DI in the immediate postoperative period, usually resolving within 2 to 4 days (53). Diagnosis is made by a urine specific gravity of less than 1.005 for 2 hours with urine output 250 cc greater than fluid intake for any 1-hour period or greater than 1 L for any 4-hour period. The serum osmolarity may be greater than 300 mOsm/kg, and the urine osmolarity may be less than 200 mOsm/kg. Serum sodium is generally greater than 150 mg/L (Chapter 6).

The hypernatremia resulting from fluid loss is often well tolerated, but altered levels of consciousness may be seen at serum osmolarities greater than 340 mOsm/L. Decreased blood volume may lead to dehydration and hypotension. As long as the thirst mechanism is intact, patients with mild DI remain euvolemic by drinking augmented by the administration of i.v. fluids. If the DI is severe, aqueous pitressin (5 to 10 units subcutaneously) or pitressin tannate in oil (5 units i.m.) can be used to decrease the fluid loss. For prolonged DI, patients may be given DDAVP (10 to 20 µg intranasally), which may be started on the third postoperative day after transphenoidal surgery. Other causes of hypernatremia and hyperosmolarity in the brain tumor patient include failure to replace insensible fluid losses from fever or oxygen delivery through tracheostomy without humidification over a number of days. Also, excessive solute loading in tube feeds and high-output renal failure from acute tubular necrosis may result in hypernatremia (54).

Peripheral Venous Occlusions

Deep venous thrombosis (DVT) and pulmonary embolism (PE) are major sources of morbidity and mortality in patients with brain tumors. The common risk factors include preoperative or postoperative leg weakness with inability to ambulate, extracranial malignancy, obesity, length of surgery greater than 4 hours, and varicose veins (55–58). Brain tumors may release thrombogenic factors such as plasmin inhibitors (42) or thromboplastin-like substances (59,60). There is a slight association between suprasellar tumors and the later occurrence of DVT (61,62). In a study from Sloan-Kettering, malignant glioma patients had a 37% risk of developing DVT, with 60% showing signs within the first 6 weeks after surgery (63). Low-dose heparin prophylaxis and pneumatic compression boots have both been shown to decrease the incidence of DVT in neurosurgical patients, without unduly raising the rate of intracranial bleeding (55,57,64–67). When DVT is suspected, venous Doppler studies and venogram establish the diagnosis. In another large series, the risk of pulmonary embolism was as high as 75% in patients with symptomatic DVT above the knee (57).

The safety of anticoagulation with full-dose heparin in patients harboring intracranial tumors or use in the perioperative period is controversial. The recommendations regarding institution of anticoagulation vary from 5 days to 3 weeks after craniotomy (20,68). Five days to a week is probably a safe interval if anticoagulation is necessary.

Inferior vena cava filters are as effective as anticoagulation in the prevention of PE. Percutaneous placement of filters can be performed at the time of diagnostic venogram in patients confirmed to have DVT or in PE in patients who cannot be anticoagulated. The placement of percutaneous inferior vena cava filters has been shown to be more accurate in placement and as effective as those placed through the internal jugular vein at surgery (69). There is a high patency rate with these devices and less than a 1% risk of subsequent PE. (See Chapters 10 and 12 for a discussion of these problems in the head-injured patient.)

Fever

Fever in the postoperative period is common from atelectasis, pneumonia, craniotomy infection, or aseptic meningitis. Other minor factors include anemia, subgaleal fluid or hematoma collections, acute adrenal insufficiency, inflammation of the salivary glands, DVT, fecal impaction, and medication allergy (e.g., penicillin or vancomycin reaction are the most common) (Table 16.6). Nadir sepsis from chemotherapy may complicate the postoperative care of treated brain tumor patients. Manipulation of the CNS or removal of large blocks of brain may rarely result in fevers as high as 41°C. Another rare cause of unregulated hyperther-

TABLE 16.6. *Causes of fever in the postcraniotomy patient*

Atelectasis
Pneumonia
Urinary tract infection
Aseptic meningitis
Bacterial meningitis
Medication reaction
Craniotomy infection
Anemia
Subgaleal fluid or hematoma
Inflammation of the salivary gland
Deep vein thrombosis
Fecal impaction
Surgery of the anterior hypothalamus

mia is surgical injury to the anterior hypo-thalamus (70). Measures in addition to treating the inciting cause of the fever, should be used to reduce very high fevers. These steps include acetaminophen, alcohol rubs, and a cooling blanket.

Atelectasis is responsible for up to 90% of postoperative pulmonary complications and is probably the most frequent cause of mild early postoperative fever, within 24 to 48 hours after surgery. It is the result of inspiratory insufficiency and may be treated by incentive spirometry, deep suctioning, and bronchodilators. Humidified oxygen may be important for function of the respiratory cilia. Patients should be instructed to stop smoking at least 2 weeks before surgery and to practice abdominal deep breathing.

Pneumonia may result from obstruction caused by persistent atelectasis or aspiration. Airway protection should be a priority to prevent this complication. Extubation is delayed until patients are fully awake and able to protect their airways. Cranial neuropathies from surgery or tumor invasion of the brainstem may result in loss of a gag reflex, which may lead to aspiration. A swallowing evaluation is essential in these patients before starting feeding.

Postoperative craniotomy infections are uncommon. Risk factors for infection include diabetes mellitus, hematologic disorders, myelosuppressive or immunosuppressive medications, multiple craniotomies, scalp dermatologic disorders, and long-term phenytoin therapy (71). Drains, long operative time, and hemostatic clips that are too tight may also increase the risk of infections. Surgical infections may be superficial, such as stitch abscess, or deep bone flap infections, meningitis, or ventriculitis. The most common organisms are *Staphylococcus aureus* and *Staphylococcus epidermidis,* but in one series 80% of postoperative meningitis were the result of Gram-negative bacilli (72). (See Chapter 7 for a complete discussion of postsurgical nosocomial infections.)

Prophylactic antibiotics have been effective in reducing the number of postoperative infections in several series of clean craniotomies (73–76). Effective regimens have included i.m. tobramycin or gentamicin, i.v. vancomycin and streptomycin irrigating solution, and cefazolin and gentamicin. Submerging the bone plate in bacitracin during the operative period may additionally reduce the infection rate. However, there is still some controversy in this field, as noted in Chapter 7.

Aseptic meningitis presents a special problem but can be anticipated with certain tumors. It usually presents with moderate temperature elevation, but fever may be as high as 39.5°C. The process has been attributed to blood or necrotic tumor in the subarachnoid space and is most common with posterior fossa surgery in children where it occurs in up to 70% of cases (77). Epidermoid tumors may cause chemical aseptic meningitis by leakage of the tumor contents into the subarachnoid space (78). This disorder may begin postoperatively or be delayed until steroids are tapered, allowing inflammation to develop. Patients are febrile with headache but appear less ill than those with bacterial meningitis. A CT scan should be performed to determine if mass effect is present, and if not, a lumbar puncture should be performed. The CSF pressure is usually high, the cell count varies from a few hundred white blood cells to thousands of white blood cells, initially dominated by neutrophils, which are then replaced by lymphocytes; the protein concentration is raised and the glucose concentration remains in the normal range, although hypoglycorrhachia sometimes occurs. The CSF cultures are negative but we institute antibiotics for 2 or 3 days until this is clarified. The lumbar puncture may be therapeutic in relation to headache, and sometimes to fever, but aseptic meningitis is treated specifically by increasing the steroid dose followed by a slow steroid taper.

The major risk factor for bacterial meningitis after craniotomy is a persistent CSF leak. Patients usually have fever, stiff neck, and photophobia and appear more ill systemically than those with aseptic meningitis. The CSF shows an elevated white blood cell count with predominant neutrophils. An elevated protein concentration and hypoglycorrhachia are the rule. CSF Gram stain and cultures should reveal the offending organism. The leading causes of postoperative meningitis are *S. aureus* and Gram-negative bacilli. Nafcillin or vancomycin and a third-generation cephalosporin is started and then tailored once the organism has been identified. Cultures for Gram-negative bacilli in the CSF may remain positive for 1 to 2 weeks even with satisfactory treatment (79).

Cerebrospinal fluid fistulae result from either nontraumatic erosion of the meninges by the tumor through bone and meninges, or surgical damage after base of skull surgery, such as suboccipital craniectomy for acoustic neuromas or transphenoidal surgery for pituitary adenomas. Fluid draining from the nose or ears should be tested for glucose; CSF contains glucose, but mucus does not. However, the glucose oxidase test is only 45% to 75% specific (80). A laboratory glucose value of greater than 30 mg/mL identifies CSF. The prevention of CSF fistula begins with good dural closure and sealing off of the sinuses or mastoid air cells with wax, pericranial graft, or adipose tissue. If a leak subsequently develops, the wound should be reinforced by oversewing or by the application of collodion and cotton, which can sometimes temporize the leak. This tactic occasionally leads to an acute rise in intracranial pressure. Ventricular or lumbar drainage may be necessary to divert CSF away from the fistula, giving it time to gradually heal. Overdrainage may lead to pneumocephalus. The head is elevated 0 to 30 degrees to reduce the CSF pressure on the leak. Prophylactic antibiotics probably are not indicated.

In summary, several problems in the ICU relate more or less specifically to the care of patients with cerebral tumors, for which reason the anticipation and identification of these complications is an important part of neuro-ICU practice.

ACKNOWLEDGMENT

The authors thank Drs. Mark Bilsky and Jerome Posner for use of large portions of their chapter in the third edition of the book.

REFERENCES

1. Levi AD, Wallace MC, Bernstein M, et al. Venous thromboembolism after brain tumor surgery: a retrospective review. *Neurosurgery* 1980;6:859–863.
2. Posner JB. Neurological complications of systemic cancer. *Med Clin North Am* 1979;63:783–800.
3. Eby NL, Grufferman S, Flannelly DM, et al. Increasing incidence of primary brain lymphoma in the US. *Cancer* 1988;62:2461–2465.
4. DeAngelis L, Yahalom J, Heinemann MH. Primary CNS lymphoma: combined treatment with chemotherapy and radiotherapy. *Neurology* 1990;40:80–86.
5. Boyle P, Maisonneuve P, Saracci R, et al. Is the increased incidence of primary malignant brain tumors in the elderly real? *J Natl Cancer Inst* 1990;82:1594–1596.
6. Childhood Brain Tumor Consortium. A study of childhood brian tumors based on surgical biopsies from the North American institutions: sample description. *J Neurol Oncol* 1988;6:9–23.
7. Walker RW, Allen JC. Pediatric brain tumors. *Pediatr Ann* 1983;12:383–394.
8. Papo I, Caruselli G, Luongo A. External ventricular drainage in the management of posterior fossa tumors in children and adolescents. *Neurosurgery* 1982;10:13–15.
9. Silverberg E, Lubera JA. Cancer statistics, 1988. *CA Cancer J Clin* 1988;38:5–22.
10. Byrne TN, Cascino TL, Posner JB. Brain metastasis from melanoma. *J Neurooncol* 1983;1:313–317.
11. Smith HP, Challa VR, Moody DM, et al. Biological features of meningiomas that determine the production of cerebral edema. *Neurosurgery* 1981;8:428–433.
12. Kalfas IH, Little JR. Postoperative hemorrhage: a survey of 4992 intracranial procedures. *Neurosurgery* 1988;23:343–347.
13. Black KL, Hoff JT, McGillicuddy JE, et al. Increased leukotriene C6 and vasogenic edema surrounding brain tumors. *Ann Neurol* 1985;19:592–595.
14. Gaetani P, Baena RR, Marzatic F, et al. *"Ex vivo"* release of eicosanoid from human brain tissue: its relevance in the development of brain edema. *Neurosurgery* 1991;28:853–858.
15. Unterberg A, Schmidt W, Wahl M, et al. Evidence against leukotrienes as mediators of brain edema. *J Neurosurg* 1991;74:773–780.
16. Baethamnn A, Maier-Hauff K, Schurer L, et al. Release of glutamate and of free fatty acids in vasogenic brain edema. *J Neurosurg* 1989;70:578–591.
17. Criscuolo GR, Merill MJ, Oldfield EH. Further characterization of malignant glioma-derived vascular permeability factor. *J Neurosurg* 1988;69:254–262.
18. Sawaya R, Decourteen-Meyers G, Copeland B. Massive preoperative pulmonary embolism and suprasellar brain tumor: report and review of the literature. *Neurosurgery* 1984;15:566–571.
19. Albin MS, Bunegin L, Bennett MH, et al. Clinical and experimental brain retraction pressure monitoring. *Acta Neurol Scand* 1977;56:522–523.
20. Albin MS, Bunegin L, Dujovny M, et al. Brain retraction pressure during intracranial procedures. *Surg Forum* 1975;26:499–500.
21. Albin MS, Carroll RG, Maroon JC. Clinical considerations concerning detection of venous air embolism. *Neurosurgery* 1963;3:810–811.

22. Allen MB, Johnston KW. Preoperative evaluation: complications, their prevention and treatment. In: Youmans JR, ed. *Neurological surgery,* 3rd ed. Philadelphia: WB Saunders, 1990:833–900.

23. North JB, Penhall RK, Hanieh A, et al. Phenytoin and postoperative epilepsy. A double-blind study. *J Neurosurg* 1983;58:672–677.

24. Gassel MM. False localizing signs. A review of the concept and analysis of the occurrence in 250 cases of intracranial meningioma. *Arch Neurol* 1960;122:70–98.

25. Narins RG, Jones ER, Stom MC, et al. Diagnostic strategies in disorders of fluid, electrolyte, and acid-base homeostasis. *Am J Med* 1982;72:496–521.

26. North X, et al. The prevention of postoperative epilepsy. *Lancet* 1980;1:384–386.

27. Weissman DE. Glucocorticoid treatment for brain metastases and epidural spinal cord compression: a review. *J Clin Oncol* 1988;6:543–551.

28. Glantz MJ, Cole BF, Forsyth PA, et al. Anticonvulsant prophylaxis in patients with newly diagnosed brain tumors. *Neurology* 2000;54:1886–1893.

29. Ommaya AK. Spinal fluid fistulae. *Clin Neurosurg* 1976;23:363–392.

30. Weissman DE, Janjan NA, Erikson B. Twice daily tapering dexamethasone treatment during cranial radiation for newly diagnosed brain metastases. *J Neurol Oncol* 1991;11:235–239.

31. Fadul CE, Lemann W, Thaler HT, et al. Perforation of the gastrointestinal tract in patients receiving steroids for neurological disease. *Neurology* 1988;38: 348–362.

32. Cook DJ, Witt LG, Cook RJ. Stress ulcer prophylaxis in the critically ill: a meta-analysis. *Am J Med* 1991;91: 519–528.

33. Haft H, Liss H, Mount LA. Massive epidural hemorrhage as a complication of ventricular drainage. *J Neurosurg* 1960;17:49–54.

34. Maroon JC, Edmonds-Seal J, Campbell RL. An ultrasonic method for detecting air embolism. *J Neurosurg* 1969;31:196–201.

35. Michenfelder JD, Martin IT, Altenburg BM, et al. Air embolism during neurosurgery: an evaluation of right-atrial catheters for diagnosis and treatment. *JAMA* 1969; 208:1353–1358.

36. Higashi H. Tissue coagulation system and fibrinolytic activity of brain tumors. *Neurol Med Chir* 1979;19: 509–516.

37. Durant TM, Long J, Oppenheimer MJ. Pulmonary (venous) air embolism. *Am Heart J* 1947;33:269–281.

38. Malis Li. Prevention of neurosurgical infection by intraoperative antibiotics. *Neurosurgery* 1979;5:339–343.

39. Higazi I. Epidural hematoma as complication of ventricular drainage: report of a case and review of literature. *J Neurosurg* 1963;20:527–528.

40. Feldman Z, Kanter MJ, Robertson CS, et al. Effect of head elevation on intracranial pressure, cerebral perfusion pressure, and cerebral blood flow in head-injured patients. *J Neurosurg* 1992;76:207–211.

41. Rosner MJ, Becker DP. Origin and evolution of plateau waves. Experimental observation and a theoretical model. *J Neurosurg* 1984;50:312–324.

42. Joffe SN. Incidence of postoperative deep vein thrombosis in neurosurgical patients. *J Neurosurg* 1975;42: 201–203.

43. Fadul CE, Wood J, Thaler H, et al. Morbidity and mortality of craniotomy for excision of supratentorial gliomas. *Neurology* 1988;38:1374–1379.

44. Gurtner P, Ramina R, Stoppe G, et al. Postoperative observation at the neurosurgical intensive care unit after surgery the posterior fossa. In: Wenker H, Klinger M, Brock M, et al., eds. *Advances in neurosurgery I.* Berlin: Springer-Verlag, 1986:352–358.

45. Munson ES, Paul WL, Perry JC, et al. Early detection of venous air embolism using a Swan-Ganz catheter. *Anesthesiology* 1975;42:223–226.

46. Pagani JJ, Hayman LA, Bigelow RH, et al. Diazepam prophylaxis of contrast media-induced seizures during computed tomography of patients with brain metastases. *AJR Am J Roentgenol* 1983;140:787–792.

47. Epstein F, Murali R. Pediatric posterior fossa tumors: hazards of the preoperative shunt. *Neurosurgery* 1978; 3:348–350.

48. Ruff R, Posner J. Incidence and treatment of peripheral venous thrombosis in patients with glioma. *Ann Neurol* 1983;13:334–336.

49. Klatzo I. Pathophysiologic aspects of brain edema. In: Reuben HJ, Schurmann K, eds. *Steroid and brain edema.* New York: Springer-Verlag, 1972:1–8.

50. Lownie S, Wu X, Karlik S, et al. Brain retractor edema during induce hypotension: the effect of the rate of return of blood pressure. *Neurosurgery* 1990;27:901–906.

51. Arbit Ehud, Shah J, Bedford R, et al. Tension pneumocephalus: treatment with controlled decompression via a closed water-seal drainage system. Case report. *J Neurosurg* 1991;74:139–142.

52. Nakagawa Y, Yada K, Mitsuo T. Clinical significance of ICP measurements following intracranial surgery. In: Lundberg N, Ponten U, Brock M, eds. *Intracranial pressure II.* Berlin: Springer-Verlag, 1975:350–354.

53. Tindall GT, McLanahan CS. Hyperfunctional pituitary tumors: pre- and postoperative management considerations. *Clin Neurosurg* 1980;27:48–82.

54. Chou SN, Erickson DL. Craniotomy infections. *Clin Neurosurg* 1976;23:357–362.

55. Cerrato D, Ariano C, Fiacchino F. Deep vein thrombosis and low-dose heparin prophylaxis in neurosurgical patients. *J Neurosurg* 1987;49:378–381.

56. Kofman S, et al. Treatment of cerebral metastases from breast carcinoma with prednisone. *JAMA* 1957;163: 1473–1476.

57. Swann KW, Black McLP. Deep vein thrombosis and pulmonary emboli in neurosurgical patients: a review. J *Neurosurg* 1984;61:1055–1062.

58. Valledares JB, Hankinson J. Incidence of lower extremity deep vein thrombosis in neurosurgical patients. *Neurosurgery* 1980;6:138–141.

59. Henson JW, Jalaj KJ, Walker RW, et al. *Pneumocystis carinii* pneumonia in patients with primary brain tumors. *Arch Neurol* 1991;48:406–409.

60. Tovi D, Pandolfi M, Astedt B. Local haemostasis in brain tumours. *Experientia* 1975;31:977–978.

61. Brisman R, Mandell J. Thromboembolism and brain tumors. *J Neurosurg* 1973;38:337–388.

62. Ryder JW, Kleinschmidt-Demasters BK, Keller TS. Sudden deterioration and death in patients with benign tumors of the third ventricle area. *J Neurosurg* 1986; 64:216–223.

63. Rosner MJ, Coley IB. Cerebral perfusion pressure, intracranial pressure and head elevation. *J Neurosurg* 1986;65:636–641.

64. Barnett HG, Clifford J, Llewellyn RC. Safety of mini-dose heparin administration for neurosurgical patients. *J Neurosurg* 1977;47:27–30.

65. Black PM, Baker MF, Snook CP. Experience with external pneumatic calf compression in neurology and neurosurgery. *Neurosurgery* 1986;18:440–444.

66. Posner JB. Brain metastases: a clinician's view. In: Weiss L, Gilbert HA, Posner JB, eds. *Brain metastases.* Boston: GK Hall, 1980;22–29.

67. Skillman JJ, Collins REC, Coe NP, et al. Prevention of deep vein thrombosis in neurosurgical patients: a controlled randomized trial of external pneumatic compression boots. *Surgery* 1978;83:354–358.

68. Swann KW, Black McLP, Baker MF. Management of symptomatic deep venous thrombosis and pulmonary embolism on a neurosurgical service. *J Neurosurg* 1986;64:563–567.

69. Horwitz NH, Rizzoli HV. Introduction. In: Horwitz NH, Rizzoli HV, eds. *Postoperative complications of intracranial neurological surgery.* Baltimore: Williams & Wilkins, 1982:1–30.

70. Carmel PW. Surgical syndromes of the hypothalamus. *Clin Neurosurg* 1980;27:133–159.

71. Wright RL. A survey of possible etiologic agents in postoperative craniotomy infections. *J Neurosurg* 1966; 25:125–132.

72. Bridges SL, Ebersole JS. Incidence of seizures with phenytoin toxicity. *Neurology* 1985;35:1767–1768.

73. Geraghty J, Feely M. Antibiotic prophylaxis in neurosurgery. *J Neurosurg* 1984;60:724–726.

74. Mahaley SM, Metlin C, Natarjan N, et al. National survey of patterns of care for brain tumor patients. *J Neurosurg* 1989;71:826–836.

75. Powers SK, Edwards MSB. Prophylaxis of thromboembolism in neurosurgical patient: a review. *Neurosurgery* 1982;10:509–513.

76. Salcman M. *Neoplastic emergencies from neurological emergencies.* New York: Raven, 1990:117–134.

77. Carmel PW, Fraser RA, Stein BM. Aseptic meningitis following posterior fossa surgery in children. *J Neurosurg* 1974;41:44–48.

78. Berger MS, Wilson CB. Epidermoid cysts of the posterior fossa. *J Neurosurg* 1989;21:1051–1058.

79. Durack DT, Perfect JR. Bacterial infections. *Neurosurgery* 1985;3:1921–1927.

80. Numoto M, Donaghy RMP. Effects of local pressure on cortical electrical activity and cortical vessels in the dog. *J Neurosurg* 1970;33:381–387.

17

Hypoxic–Ischemic Cerebral Injury

The cerebral effects of cardiac arrest are not strictly a neurological intensive care unit (neuro-ICU) problem; neurologists and intensivists are called on to give authoritative opinions regarding the treatment and outcome in these cases. In many ways, the clinical and scientific problems presented by this condition reflect the central challenge to neurointensivists, namely, the sparing and salvaging of damaged neurons. Coma, brain death, and the vegetative state are often derivatives of cardiac arrest. Furthermore, in comparison to the classic problems of critical care neurology such as raised intracranial pressure (ICP) and neuromuscular respiratory failure (which occupy much of the rest of this book), the frequency of cardiac arrest is considerably higher. The dimensions of the problem can be appreciated in that according to recent Centers for Disease Control data: Over 700,000 cardiac deaths occur in the United States every year, with half estimated to be related to cardiac sudden death.

RESUSCITATION

Some of the factors that adversely influence survival and recovery have been identified: advanced age, history of myocardial infarction, and the presence of congestive heart failure (1,2). The prognosis of the cardiac arrest victim depends mostly on how quickly appropriate resuscitation is initiated. Several studies indicate that mortality increases approximately 3% during each minute before cardiopulmonary resuscitation is initiated and continues to increase 4% during each additional minute until the first defibrillatory

shock is administered (3). Therefore, increased survival rates after out-of-hospital cardiac arrest should be attainable by reducing the time to cardiopulmonary resuscitation (CPR) and defibrillation (4). The goal of neurologists, nonetheless, has been to attempt to reduce secondary cerebral damage. This is driven by experimental evidence that neurons may not be irrevocably damaged for minutes or hours after exposure to hypoxia–ischemia.

In a patient with cardiac arrest caused by ventricular fibrillation, closed chest massage is at best only a "holding" procedure until defibrillation can be administered. When patients who develop cardiac arrest are defibrillated immediately, as in a supervised cardiac rehabilitation program, 100% survival has been reported. In the future, widespread use of automatic defibrillators in heart attack victims may eliminate delays in defibrillation (5–7). This device does not require that the user be skilled in the recognition of dysrhythmias and, therefore, permits an individual trained only in basic first aid to deliver the initial countershocks almost immediately after cardiac arrest. These devices are becoming more widely available, and are now commonly found in large workplaces and public areas such as airports and office buildings.

In addition to rapid defibrillation, effective perfusion of vital organs during CPR is critical for recovery (8). Conventional CPR provides only marginal cerebral perfusion, and cerebral blood flow (CBF) during resuscitation attains only a fraction (2% to 11%) of prearrest values. Both pharmacologic and mechanical attempts have been made to increase cerebral perfusion. Epinephrine in doses greater than 0.2 mg/kg has increased CBF in animal models of cardiac arrest (9), and therefore has been emphasized in guidelines in patient resuscitation. "New" CPR (now over a decade old), which uses simultaneous chest and abdominal compression and negative intrathoracic pressure, provides greater CBF than present methods of manual CPR, but requires mechanical devices.

Once spontaneous effective cardiac function has been restored, attention must be directed toward assessing the ischemic damage to other organs of the body, which vary in their tolerance to ischemia. Renal tubular cells and myocardial cells can survive periods of circulatory arrest of up to 30 minutes; liver cells can survive up to 1 or 2 hours; and lung tissue can survive more than 2 hours. However, the brain's ability to tolerate no more than a few minutes of circulatory arrest is the major factor limiting the success of CPR (10,11).

PHYSIOLOGIC ASPECTS OF HYPOXIC–ISCHEMIC BRAIN INJURY

It should be pointed out that ischemia, although difficult to separate from hypoxia in many circumstances, is probably the primary cause of neuronal damage after cardiac arrest. Hypoxia alone arises as a result of strangulation, suffocation, or anesthesia accident and gives rise to somewhat different patterns of neuropathologic damage. In both instances, the rapidity of decline in blood flow or blood oxygen content is a major factor in the degree of damage; this is perhaps truer for hypoxia insofar as we have observed patients to be awake and with minimal cognitive disruption with PaO_2 of 35 mm Hg. In the case of hypotension, however, certain approximate limits seem to be common to all individuals and below which consciousness is lost.

The brain does not store oxygen; therefore, it functions only for seconds and survives only for minutes after its oxygen supply is reduced below critical levels. The extent of tissue injury is a product of both the degree of hypoxia and hypoperfusion, and the duration of exposure to inadequate oxygen delivery. The term "hypoxia" is necessarily ambiguous, because untreated anoxia is a complex state of decreased oxygen availability, systemic acidosis, hypercapnia, and eventual circulatory collapse.

As discussed later, it should be emphasized that the neuropathologic pattern of low blood flow is either heterogeneous infarction in the border zones between major cerebral vessels ("watershed infarction") or global damage throughout the cerebrum, mainly in layers 3 and 6 of the cortex but also in the lenticular nuclei; by contrast, severe hypoxia causes preferential damage in special vulnerable areas, mainly the medial temporal lobes. To the extent that widespread cortical infarction typical of reduced blood flow also occurs at times from hypoxia, and the extraordinary medial temporal lobe Korsakoff syndrome that is typical of hypoxia can also result from cardiac arrest, the distinctions are not pure, but a differentiation between the various pathologic patterns serves a useful purpose. For brevity, "anoxia" is sometimes used in the following discussion as shorthand for the combined ischemia–hypoxia that is necessarily part of a cardiac arrest. Some of these issues are detailed in the following.

NEUROLOGICAL SYNDROMES AFTER CARDIAC ARREST

A spectrum of clinical disorders can result, depending on the severity of cerebral ischemia or anoxia (12,13) (Table 17.1).

Transient or Mild Neurological Deficits

Global ischemia can result in both metabolic dysfunction and structural injury to the central nervous system (CNS). Brief episodes of cerebral anoxia generally are well tolerated, and patients usually awaken promptly. Patients with slightly longer episodes of systemic circulatory arrest suffer mild degrees of cerebral anoxia and have a reversible metabolic encephalopathy. Drowsiness in these patients, if present, lasts only a few hours, usually less than 12.

TABLE 17.1. *Neurological syndromes after cardiac arrest*

Transient central nervous system (CNS) deficits after brief coma (<12 h)
Pathology	No damage or scattered ischemic neurons
Clinical	Transient confusion often followed by antegrade amnesia
Outcome	Rapid, complete recovery; delayed deterioration (rare)

Persistent focal CNS deficits after coma (>12 h)
  Cerebral syndrome
Pathology	Focal or multifocal infarcts of cortex, especially in boundary zones
Clinical	Amnesia
	Dementia
	Bibrachial or quadriparesis
	Cortical blindness, visual agnosia
	Also may occur: seizures, myoclonus (acute state); ataxia, intention myoclonus, parkinsonism (chronic stage)
Outcome	Slow, often incomplete, recovery

  Spinal cord syndrome (may occur in isolation or accompany cerebral syndrome)
Pathology	Focal or multifocal infarcts of spinal cord, especially in the lower thoracic boundary zone
Clinical	Flaccid paralysis of lower limbs
	Urinary retention
	Loss of pain and temperature sense
	Preserved touch and position sense
Outcome	No or incomplete recovery

Global CNS damage (no recovery of consciousness)
  Destruction of hemispheres alone
Pathology	Laminar necrosis of cortex
Clinical	Vegetative state (awake but unaware)
Outcome	Prolonged survival in vegetative state

  Brain death
Pathology	Necrosis of cortex + brainstem ± spinal cord
Clinical	No evidence of cortical activity, no brainstem reflexes, reflexes of purely spinal origin may persist
Outcome	Systemic death within days

Residual signs of confusion or amnesia may persist for hours to days. In general, recovery is rapid and complete, and these patients are able to resume their previous occupations.

Amnestic Syndrome

An amnestic syndrome may follow a brief period of postanoxic confusion or may occur as an isolated phenomenon. Finklestein and Caronna (14) followed 16 patients after cardiac arrest, none of whom remained in coma after resuscitation, but developed an amnestic syndrome as their only neurological sequel. All had severe antegrade amnesia and variable retrograde memory loss with preservation of immediate and remote memory, resembling Korsakoff psychosis, and a bland, unconcerned affect, with confabulation. Recovery was complete within 7 to 10 days in 12 of the 16 patients; amnesia persisted for a month or longer in the other four; all later recovered. The time required for recovery and the occasional instances of incomplete recovery distinguished this syndrome from transient global amnesia and the postictal state, from which recovery is rapid and complete. Electroencephalograms (EEGs) and computed tomography (CT) scans failed to identify a cerebral lesion, although changes in the hippocampal region are almost always appreciated nowadays with magnetic resonance imaging (MRI). In view of the vulnerability of the hippocampal regions to anoxia, transient post–cardiac arrest amnesia is thought to represent partially reversible bilateral damage to the hippocampi. Subtle but more permanent cognitive impairment may also follow cardiac arrest. Individuals with anoxic–ischemic coma of more than 6 hours' duration but with unremarkable cranial MRI and CT have demonstrated persistent poor learning and recall of paired associations when compared with controls matched for age and intelligence quotient (IQ). Impaired neurotransmitter synthesis may be responsible for these mild amnestic syndromes of anoxic amnesia, possibly through impairment of cholinergic memory circuits (15).

After apparently recovering from the immediate effects of an anoxic insult to the brain, rare patients develop a progressive cerebral disorder and relapse into unconsciousness (16). In fatal cases, pathologic lesions have been primarily restricted to the deep white matter of the parietal and occipital lobes. The clinical syndrome of this delayed anoxic leukoencephalopathy is distinctive: Days to weeks after a period of improvement or recovery from global anoxia, patients suffer progressive neurological deterioration and often die or remain comatose. Occasional cases are encountered that have a slow recovery (17). Delayed neurological deterioration has been reported after all types of anoxic insults but follows no more than one or two of each thousand arrests and is not predictable by the type of insult, duration of anoxia, period of coma, or any identifiable clinical feature (18).

Syndromes of Persistent Central Nervous System Damage

Focal Cerebral Syndromes

Several types of strokelike focal structural brain lesions occur after severe or prolonged hypotension (19). Patients in this group usually remain in coma for 12 hours or more and on awakening have lasting focal or multifocal motor, sensory, and intellectual deficits. Among the focal signs clinically manifest in this group of patients are three main syndromes: partial or complete *cortical blindness, bibrachial paresis, and quadriparesis.*

Cortical blindness, often transient (20) but occasionally permanent, probably results from disproportionate ischemia of both occipital poles as a result of their location in an arterial border zone, as alluded to in the preceding (21). The visual syndromes are commonly seen in children following hypoxic events. Magnetic resonance imaging has demonstrated injury in the striate and parastriate cortices and the regions of the optic radiations (22). The extent of visual recovery is most related to the age at insult and extent of injury demonstrated in the optic radiations.

Bilateral infarction of the cerebral motor cortex in the region that innervates the shoulder in the border zone between the anterior and middle cerebral arteries appears to be responsible for the syndrome of bibrachial paresis sparing the face and legs. The deficit of more proximal than distal pyramidal weakness has been described as "man in a barrel," and in one report was seen in 11 of 34 comatose patients following hypoxic injury (23). Many of those patients were severely affected and did not survive. The "man in a barrel" syndrome can be seen with less severe injury, and has been reported in a hypoperfused cardiac patient who never lost consciousness (24). Recovery often is incomplete and delayed over a period of weeks to months. Some of these patients eventually are able to lead a relatively independent existence at home (25), whereas others remain in nursing homes, severely disabled and dependent.

Spinal Cord Syndromes

The spinal cord generally is more resistant to transient ischemia than more rostral parts of the CNS. Nevertheless, rare cases of isolated spinal cord infarction after cardiac arrest occur without evidence of cerebral injury. Necrosis of central structures of the spinal cord can occur in the periphery of the territory supplied by a main contributory artery. These border zones or "watersheds" in the upper thoracic and lumbar regions of the spinal cord are at risk from any profound drop in perfusion pressure. The syndrome of spinal stroke from hypotension is characterized by flaccid paralysis of the lower limbs, urinary retention, and a sensory level in the thoracic region, with pain and temperature more affected than light touch or position sense.

Syndromes of Global Cerebral Damage

A third group of resuscitated patients has more widespread destruction of the brain, progressing to either a vegetative state or brain death. Some patients with severe irreversible brain damage who survive for more than 1 week regain eye opening, sleep–wake cycles, spontaneous roving eye movements, and other reflex activities at brainstem and spinal cord levels but remain in a functionally decorticate state of wakefulness without awareness. This state, distinct from the sleeplike condition of coma, is referred to as (perhaps unfortunately) the "vegetative state" (26). In rare instances, recovery of cognition has occurred after prolonged unconsciousness (see later).

Extrapyramidal tract dysfunction after anoxia can produce a clinical syndrome with elements of parkinsonism. It has been reported particularly after carbon monoxide poisoning but may follow an episode of anoxia or ischemia. In some cases, parkinsonian features are only a small part of widespread cerebral injury, whereas in others, the signs of parkinsonism (i.e., rigidity, akinesia, and tremor) are the only neurological disability. Some patients have responded to treatment with L-dopa, but this is exceptional in our experience (27).

Myoclonus

Myoclonic jerks and convulsions may acutely follow episodes of acute cerebral ischemia, especially when they are severe enough to cause coma. Myoclonus refers to irregular, asynchronous shocklike jerks of one or more limbs, and it is a relatively common manifestation of disturbance in function of diverse regions of the CNS. The acute myoclonus has not been well understood, although the brainstem is likely involved in the origin of the movement disorder (28). The myoclonic activity may resolve rapidly over the first 24 to 48 hours, and specific treatment is difficult. There is only an inconsistent relationship to paroxysmal EEG activity, and traditional anticonvulsants have little effect. Nonetheless, if the movements are upsetting to the family or interfere with ventilation they can sometimes be suppressed by large doses of a benzodiazepine or by morphine. When severe and protracted, the myoclonic movements are associated with a dis-

mal prognosis. In a report of 107 consecutive patients comatose after cardiac arrest, myoclonic status was seen in over one third, and associated with burst suppression on EEG, cerebral edema, and infarctions on CT imaging (29). Mortality was 100% in that series.

An entirely different "action myoclonus" syndrome described by Lance and Adams has been recognized after recovery from coma secondary to cerebral ischemia (30). Here, the awake patient is incapacitated by jerking during attempted use of the limbs. Jerks in this condition may also be stimulus-activated and brought on by light, sound, or touch. Thus, these involuntary jerks can incapacitate the patient in walking, eating, and using the upper limbs for carrying out other activities of daily living. Some control of this intention myoclonus has been reported with a combination of 5-hydroxytryptophan (31), clonazepam (32), and valproic acid (33). We have found benefit from piracetam and more recently with levetiracetam. The anatomic origin of this syndrome is a matter of debate. Chronic posthypoxic myoclonus is most commonly considered a type of cortical reflex myoclonus, but reticular reflex myoclonus and an exaggerated startle response also may occur (28). In at least some cases the evidence favors a diffuse cerebellar cortical lesion, rather than or in addition to the more commonly proposed cerebral cortical lesion (34).

Cerebellar ataxia is another, albeit infrequent postanoxic syndrome that appears to be related to the selective vulnerability of Purkinje cells to ischemia. These patients are ataxic in all movements and gait but tend not to have nystagmus or severe dysarthria.

NEUROPATHOLOGIC FEATURES OF CEREBRAL ANOXIA

Infarction in Cerebral and Spinal Boundary Zones

A period of circulatory arrest, preceded or followed by appreciable periods of hypotension, often leads to ischemic alterations concentrated in the boundary zones between ma-

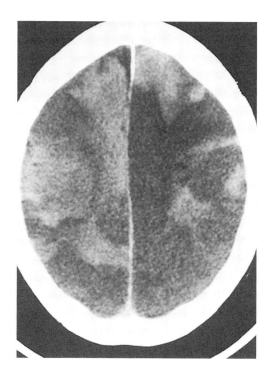

FIG. 17.1. Axial computed tomography scan 24 hours after cardiac arrest showing widespread infarction of convexities, including border zones between anterior cerebral and both middle and posterior cerebral arteries. There is also infarction within the anterior cerebral artery territory, demonstrating that cerebral ischemic damage does not always conform to watershed flow regions.

jor cerebral arteries in the cerebral cortex, basal ganglia, cerebellum, and spinal cord (35). In the cerebral cortex, ischemic necrosis after profound hypotension is most severe in the parieto-occipital regions, where the territories of the anterior, middle, and posterior cerebral arteries meet (Figs. 17.1 and 17.2). Necrosis is less prominent toward the frontal and temporal poles, and along the boundary zones of the anterior-middle and middle-posterior cerebral arteries. The cerebral cortex is commonly affected bilaterally but may occur unilaterally if there is carotid stenosis on one side. Cortical boundary zone infarcts often have petechial hemorrhages because of reperfusion when blood pressure is restored. Infarctions may coexist with focal injury to vulnerable neurons, as well as with diffuse cortical necrosis.

Within the spinal cord are border zones between the anterior spinal artery and the segmental arteries from the aorta. Severe hypotension or obstruction of the segmental arteries causes infarction of the spinal cord in the cervicothoracic and the thoracolumbar regions, as mentioned previously. The thoracic cord usually is involved at the boundary zone between the anterior spinal artery and the artery of Adamkiewicz (36).

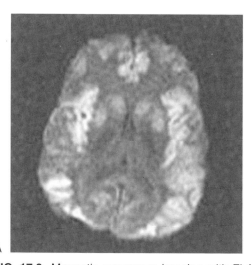

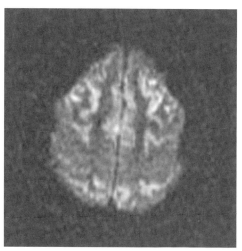

A   B

FIG. 17.2. Magnetic resonance imaging with FLAIR sequences demonstrates ischemic change in the border zone regions.

The relationship between vascular territories subjected to anoxia by microemboli, thrombi, or hypotension; and the location, size, and number of cerebral infarcts is often perplexing. Nevertheless, the boundary zone hypothesis best explains the focal neurological deficits observed in patients after profound hypotension. The predilection of infarcts for the boundary zones may reflect the fact that the tissue effects of reduced oxygen and glucose delivery are likely to be maximal in those regions most distant from the origin of a major artery, but neither the topography nor the severity of cerebral infarcts can be predicted from clinical estimates of the duration of hypotension or circulatory arrest. In addition, some clinical and experimental studies have not consistently found infarctions in boundary zones after hypotension. In primates subjected to cardiac arrest, Miller and Myers (37) observed that the brainstem was regularly affected, but cerebral infarcts did not occur as long as hypotension before and after circulatory arrest was prevented. Clinical and pathologic verification of infarction, predominantly of the brainstem, has been provided by Boisen and Siemkowicz (38), who observed the "locked-in" syndrome in three survivors of cardiac arrest, but such cases are rarely encountered.

Diffuse Central Nervous System Injury

Prolonged cardiac arrest causes widespread death of neurons. The following groups of neurons are vulnerable to even moderate degrees of anoxia: pyramidal cells in Sommer's sector of the hippocampus, Purkinje cells of the cerebellum, and pyramidal cells of the third and fifth layers of the cerebral cortex. In cases of the vegetative state, neuropathologic examination has revealed widespread necrosis of the cortex and thalamus, whereas the brainstem and spinal cord remained intact. Profound anoxia affects the cortex as well as the basal ganglia and brainstem nuclei and is not compatible with prolonged survival.

DIAGNOSTIC APPROACH TO ANOXIC COMA

Neurological Monitoring

Patients in coma initially require intensive care to support life and prevent complications. In most cases of coma, sequential observation of physical signs is paramount because they may indicate the degree of reversibility of CNS damage and predict likely outcome, or detect a loss of neurological function that precedes deterioration in cardiorespiratory function. The neurological examination of the comatose patient consists of an assessment of the level of consciousness as determined by eye opening, verbal responses, and reflex or purposive movements in response to noxious stimulation of the face, arms, and legs (39); neuroophthalmologic function as indicated by pupillary size and response to light, spontaneous eye movements, oculocephalic (doll's eyes) and oculovestibular (ice water caloric) responses; and vegetative function as reflected mainly by the respiratory pattern (39). Neurological signs can be correlated with specific anatomic sites to establish the severity and extent of CNS dysfunction (Table 17.2).

Levels of Consciousness

In post–cardiac arrest patients, like most other patients with unresponsiveness, the level of consciousness is best determined by the ease and degree of behavioral arousal, if any. Attempts should be made to elicit a behavioral motor response by verbal stimulation alone initially, then if no response, with a shout and gentle shake. Noxious stimulation can be applied to the face by cotton wisps in the nares or digital supraorbital pressure. Painful stimulation applied to individual arms and legs by compression of distal interphalangeal joints with a tongue blade or pen should be kept to a minimum, and pinching the skin or nipples is discouraged. Eye opening indicates activity of the reticular activating system; verbal responses indicate hemispheric function.

TABLE 17.2. *Correlation between levels of brain function and clinical signs*

Structure	Function	Clinical sign

Cerebral cortex	Conscious behavior	Speech (including any sounds)
		Purposeful movement
		  Spontaneous
		  To command
		  To pain

Brainstem sensory pathways (reticular activating system)	Sleep–wake cycle	Eye opening
		  Spontaneous
		  To command
		  To pain

Brainstem motor pathways	Reflex limb movements	Flexor posturing (decorticate) Extensor posturing (decerebrate)
Midbrain CN III	Innervation of ciliary muscle and certain extraocular muscles	Pupillary reactivity

Upper pons
  CN V
  CN VII
	
	Facial and corneal sensation
	Facial muscle innervation
		
		Corneal reflex–sensory
		Corneal reflex–motor response
		  Blink
		  Grimace

Lower pons CN VII (vestibular portion) connects by brainstem pathways with CN III, IV, VI	 Reflex eye movements	 Doll's eyes Caloric responses
Medulla	Spontaneous breathing maintains blood pressure	Breathing and blood pressure do not require mechanical or chemical support
Spinal cord	Primitive protective responses	Deep tendon reflexes Babinski response

Motor Response

In hypoxic–ischemic injury, the absence of motor response, especially with flaccidity and areflexia, indicates severe brainstem depression and frequently is found in terminal coma destined to become vegetative or reach brain death. Extensor posturing responses correlate with deep destructive lesions of the midbrain and upper pons but also may be present in reversible metabolic states such as anoxic encephalopathy. Flexor posturing responses occur after damage to the hemispheres, as well as in metabolic depression of brain function. Withdrawal and localizing responses imply purposive or voluntary behavior. Obeying commands is obviously the best response and marks the return of consciousness. Generalized or focal repetitive movements not affected by stimuli usually represent myoclonus or seizure activity. Focal seizures usually indicate a focal cortical lesion but can be seen in global hypoxic–ischemic insults because of prior focal lesions or vascular disease that predisposes some regions to ischemia preferentially.

Neuroophthalmologic Examination

The size, equality, and light reactivity of the pupils should be noted. In the acute post–cardiac arrest period, papilledema is not a reliable indicator of ICP. Deeply comatose patients may have no spontaneous eye movements. In such cases, "doll's eyes" (oculocephalic) responses and the ice water caloric test can be used to determine the integrity of the eighth, sixth, and third cranial nerves and their interconnecting brainstem pathways.

When the cortical influences are depressed with intact brainstem mechanisms, the head can be rotated horizontally to one side and the eyes deviate conjugately to the opposite side. Brisk back-and-forth eye movements, like those of a doll in response to rocking the head to and fro, are characteristic of metabolic coma. Doll's eyes indicate the integrity of proprioceptive fibers from the neck structures, vestibular nuclei, and nuclei of the third and sixth cranial nerves. Unilateral lesions of the brainstem eliminate the doll's eyes response to the side of the lesion. When the doll's eyes are absent, it becomes necessary to perform the ice water caloric test. In deep coma, the doll's eyes disappear before the ice water caloric responses because the latter are produced by a stronger stimulus. The caloric response is elicited in comatose patients by irrigating the tympanum with 30 to 50 mL of ice water. In the absence of cortical influences on the oculovestibular pathways, cold water produces tonic deviation of the eyes to the side of irrigation. Metabolic factors (e.g., sedative–hypnotic coma, phenytoin overdosage) and structural brainstem lesions eliminate the caloric response, as does labyrinthine disease, but the absence of elicited eye movements in anoxic coma is a grave sign.

Spontaneous, roving, horizontal eye movements in comatose subjects indicate only that the midbrain and pontine tegmentum are intact; they do not imply preservation of the frontal or occipital cerebral cortex. These movements, and those described in the following, appear to be release phenomena, namely, spontaneous movements generated by brainstem gaze mechanisms released from cortical or other suprasegmental control. Initially fixed eyes followed by the development of horizontal back and forth roving eye movements, are typical of the post–anoxic injury in our experience. Persistent downward deviation of the eyes, although characteristic of tectal compression by hydrocephalus, thalamic hemorrhage, or pineal tumor, also can occur in anoxic coma. Upward deviation may indicate nonconclusive epileptic activity. Two types of intermittent downward deviations of the eyes have been described in anoxic coma patients. Ocular bobbing, a movement disorder usually associated with damage to the lateral gaze centered in the pons, has been observed in post–cardiac arrest patients, some of whom recovered (40). Bob-

bing is characterized by spontaneous downward deviation of the eyes and less rapid upward movement. By contrast, ocular dipping, which is more common after global brain anoxia, consists of slow downward deviations followed by rapid upward movement (41).

Further Diagnostic Assessment

Neuroimaging

In acute anoxic coma, computed axial tomography usually fails to show any abnormalities unless the damage is catastrophic (Fig. 17.1). In the latter case, there initially is a blurring of the usual border between gray and white matter in the hemispheres. Approximately 48 hours after a prolonged anoxic episode, hypodensities in the cerebral and cerebellar cortices and in the caudate and lenticular nuclei appear as in Figure 17.1 (42). Days later, focal infarcts, edema, and diffuse and focal atrophy may be evident. Magnetic resonance imaging may be the most useful in revealing the typical border zone ischemic lesions, as well as the associated laminar necrosis. Hippocampal abnormalities have already been alluded to. In the early acute setting, the first 24 hours, MR diffusion-weighted images may demonstrate abnormalities in the basal ganglia, cerebellum, and cortex better than conventional MR imaging (43,44). Early abnormalities in white matter also have been reported using diffusion-weighted MR imaging (45). Conventional T2 and flip angle inversion recovery (FLAIR) sequences can demonstrate abnormalities in the 1- to 14-day interval (Fig. 17.2). Laminar necrosis becomes apparent on MR imaging in the 2- to 3-week interval followed by the evolution of diffuse atrophy (46). Even with optimal standard imaging, surprisingly little tissue injury is often appreciated in cases with persistent profound neurological dysfunction. In cases of persistent cerebral dysfunction, neuropsychological assessment combined with positron emission tomography (PET) scanning can further define the extent of damage (47).

Electroencephalography

The electroencephalogram (EEG) is a sensitive indicator of cerebral function (48). Compressed spectral array EEG can be used for continuous monitoring of comatose patients, as described in Chapter 8. With this method, hours of EEG activity are compressed into a pictorial representation that reveals time distribution and temporal characteristics of frequencies as well as the intensity of total electrical activity. These features may be helpful in the rapid assessment of the comatose state but have found their major use so far in long-term coma monitoring. In animal studies, EEG activity slows markedly when CBF falls below 16 mL/100 g per minute and becomes isoelectric below 12 mL/100 g per minute (48). Several groups have correlated the pattern and frequency spectra of the postresuscitation EEG with neurological outcome, but the absolute predictive value of the EEG has not been established (49). The EEG in metabolic–anoxic encephalopathy has been classified in terms of increasing severity in five categories: Grade I represents normal alpha with some theta-delta activity; grade II is theta-delta activity with some normal alpha activity; grade III is dominant theta-delta activity with no normal alpha activity; grade IV is low-voltage delta activity with alpha coma (nonreactive alpha activity); and grade V is isoelectric. Grade I is compatible with a good prognosis, grades II and III have no definitive predictive value, and grades IV and V are consistently associated with a poor prognosis and infrequent recovery (50,51). Alpha coma may occur after cardiac arrest and usually suggests a poor prognosis, but some groups have reported that this electrical pattern lacks prognostic significance (52). Electroencephalogram patterns with burst suppression and lack of reactivity have been associated with poor outcome (53). In general, the EEG can be useful in assessing the degree of cortical dysfunction and identifying the presence of epileptic activity.

Evoked Potentials

Evoked potentials provide information regarding the locus and severity of dysfunction in certain sensory systems and, unlike EEG, are not influenced by the level of consciousness (Chapter 8). If somatosensory cortical responses are bilaterally absent after global brain ischemia, mortality rate has been as high as 98% in most series (54–57). Patients who maintain normal responses throughout their illness have a better prognosis (58), but may suffer permanent neurological sequelae (59). In one study, normal somatosensory evoked potentials (SEPs) were associated with a survival rate of 74% (55). Others have emphasized that short latency somatosensory potentials (SSEPs) remain superior to motor evoked potentials in assessing outcome of comatose individuals (58). The ultra-early use of SSEPs has been reported in a series of 30 patients following successful cardiac resuscitation (60). When studied in the first 3 hours, 12 of the 30 demonstrated a cortical response. Eight of those 12 regained consciousness within 10 days, whereas none of those with absent cortical responses regained consciousness or survived.

For practical purposes, we occasionally use SSEPs in the 24- to 72-hour interval when additional prognostic evidence is needed in cases of anoxic coma, and the studies are most useful when the cortical responses are bilaterally absent supporting a uniformly dismal prognosis.

Brainstem auditory evoked potentials (BAEPs) can correlate with brainstem dysfunction during coma but are not as useful as somatosensory potentials in anoxic coma. Simultaneous latency increase of all components is consistent with progressive ischemia of the posterior fossa and a decrease in cerebral perfusion pressure. Mechanical distortion of the brainstem from hemispheral edema or a mass is usually reflected by loss of waves II, IV, and V, with preservation of wave I. Although BAEPs are not usually modified by exogenous factors (61), BAEPs can be falsely altered by hypothermia (62), anesthetics, and barbiturates, which can eventually abolish BAEPs (63).

MANAGEMENT OF POST–CARDIAC ARREST COMA

The clinical management of patients in coma after cardiac arrest involves the restoration of adequate cardiopulmonary function to prevent further cerebral injury, but no simple and effective delayed therapy yet exists that can reverse anoxic damage. Recent evidence suggests, however, that neuropathologic abnormalities continue to evolve for hours to days after ischemic anoxia has occurred (64). In addition, certain factors that determine the extent of cerebral injury have been identified. States of reduced cerebral energy requirement such as hypothermia prevent or reduce brain damage from anoxic insults, particularly if administered before the ictus (65,66). By contrast, hyperglycemia (67), cerebral lactic acidosis, loss of calcium homeostasis, raised ICP, and excessive release of excitatory neurotransmitters (as occurs with seizures) increase ischemic cerebral damage (68).

Hypothermia

Recent data from clinical trials of hypothermia following cardiac arrest have demonstrated benefit in both survival and neurological outcome. A multicenter trial randomized 273 patients successfully resuscitated following ventricular fibrillation arrest (69). Patients were given either standard care or hypothermia with a goal core temperature of 32°C to 34°C for 24 hours. Seventy-five of the 136 (55%) patients in the hypothermia group survived with good neurological recovery or moderate disability, compared to 54 of 137 (32%) in the control group. Another recent trial randomized survivors of out-of-hospital cardiac arrest to hypothermia with a goal core temperature of 33°C for 12 hours or to standard care (70). Twenty-one of 43 (49%) in the hypothermia

group survived with good outcome, compared to nine of 34 (26%) in the control group.

Both studies produced statistically significant results supporting hypothermia in this setting. Hypothermia was achieved with external cooling such as ice packs and cooling blankets. Patients routinely were sedated and paralyzed to block the shiver response. Many centers have now adopted hypothermia protocols for survivors of cardiac arrest based on these data. An example of a neurocritical care protocol for hypothermia is contained in Table 17.3. The imminent availability of intravascular cooling devices will allow much more accurate control of core temperature. This is the only treatment for the neurological aspect of cardiac arrest validated so far.

Hyperglycemia

The observation that animals made hyperglycemic before the onset of global ischemia have greater brain damage than do normoglycemic animals, suggests that the concentration of glucose in blood and brain may be an important determinant of ischemic cerebral injury (67). It has been postulated that severe cerebral lactic acidosis from anaerobic glycolysis during hyperglycemia contributes to irreversible damage of brain cells. Clinical studies also have correlated blood glucose concentrations with the severity of cerebral damage after cardiac arrest and stroke (71). Therefore, it seems prudent at this time to limit glucose-containing infusions in the immediate post–cardiac arrest period.

Raised Intracranial Pressure

The incidence of raised ICP after cardiac arrest is unknown but has been estimated to be as high as 30%. Brain swelling represents such a severe degree of anoxic damage that some have questioned the value of aggressive therapy when it occurs (Chapter 3). We have

TABLE 17.3. *Hypothermia after cardiac arrest protocol*

Inclusion criteria
1. Age 18 years or older
2. Women must be over 50 or have a negative pregnancy test
3. Cardiac arrest with return of normal rhythm (initial rhythm VF or pulseless VT; PEA can be considered if returned to normal rhythm and other criteria met)
4. Persistent coma as evidenced by no eye opening to pain after resuscitation (no waiting period required)
5. Blood pressure can be maintained at least 90 mm Hg systolic either spontaneously or with fluid and pressors (not aortic balloon pump)
6. Known time of cardiac arrest (excludes "found down" of unknown duration)

Exclusions
1. Another reason to be comatose (e.g., drug overdose, status epilepticus)
2. Pregnancy
3. A known terminal illness preceding the arrest
4. Known, preexisting coagulopathy or bleeding
5. No limit on duration of resuscitation effort; however, "down time" of <1 h most desirable
6. Preexisting *do not intubate* code status and patient not intubated as part of resuscitation efforts

Protocol (goal temperature 33°C to be achieved as soon as possible)
1. Patients should be enrolled as quickly as possible. For out-of-hospital arrests, emergency department attending will make decision to implement protocol. For in-hospital arrests, critical care unit resident in charge of completed code will make decision.
2. Neurological assessment prior to pharmacologic paralysis. *Do not delay initiation of hypothermia pending this assessment.*
3. Immediately place ice packs under the armpits, next to the neck, on the torso, and on the limbs.
4. Temperature-sensing Foley catheter should be placed if available; otherwise, rectal or tympanic temperatures should be used (in that order).
5. Two cooling blankets should be used, one under and one over the patient.
6. The ventilator heater should be turned off.
7. The room thermostat should be turned off.
8. Administer midazolam 2–6 mg/h and fentanyl 25–75 µg/h.
9. Once sedation is started, give vecuronium 0.1 mg/kg bolus, and then start a drip of 1 mg/h. Titrate the drip 0–5 mg/h to keep 1/4 twitches.
10. Patients should be on insulin drip if glucose >180 mg/dL, daily aspirin, on pressors and/or nitrates to maintain blood pressure, and any antiarrhythmic necessary.
11. Patients may receive other cardiac interventions, including systemic thrombolysis, anticoagulation, and urgent cardiac cath interventions as needed. Hypothermia should proceed concurrent with these interventions.
12. Once the patient reaches 33°C (bladder, rectal, or tympanic), keep patient at 33°C by removing ice packs and top cooling blanket if necessary.
13. Begin passive rewarming 24 hours after the beginning of cooling (not 24 hours after target temperature is reached):
    a. Turn room thermostat up to normal.
    b. Turn on ventilator heater.
    c. Turn off cooling blanket.
    d. May use regular blankets.
    e. Do not use warm air blanket unless temperature not 36°C after 12 hours of passive rewarming.

Paralysis, then sedation, may be discontinued during or after rewarming, based on shivering and other critical care issues.

PEA, pulseless electrical activity; VF, ventricular fibrillation; VT, ventricular tachycardia.
Adapted from Hypothermia after Cardiac Arrest Study Group. Mild therapeutic hypothermia to improve the neurological outcome after cardiac arrest. *N Engl J Med* 2002;346:549–556; and Bernard SA, et al. Treatment of comatose survivors of out-of-hospital cardiac arrest with induced hypothermia. *N Engl J Med,* 2002;346:557–563.

tended to agree with this concept, and proceed with ICP treatment only in occasional instances.

In practice, only a few young patients with swollen brains on CT scan and relatively good prognostic clinical signs are chosen for ICP monitoring. It is unclear if aggressive therapy to reduce ICP assists in recovery in these patients, but at a minimum it is advisable to avoid iatrogenic errors that raise ICP. Active treatment of raised ICP is best guided by direct ICP monitoring (Chapter 3), but postanoxic edema is typically resistant to conventional measures. Measurement of ICP, however, may be useful in highly selected cases, particularly, as mentioned, in young patients, or after drowning in children, when ICP is often greatly elevated but outcome may still be good. Most patients with intracranial pressure greater than 30 mm Hg are at risk for secondary damage and herniation (72,73).

Corticosteroids

Corticosteroids have not proved beneficial in post–cardiac arrest coma (74). In addition, steroids may elevate serum glucose and theoretically worsen cerebral ischemic damage. Steroids are not currently recommended after arrest, even if the CT scan shows cerebral swelling.

Barbiturates

Barbiturate anesthetics reduce cerebral metabolic requirements and have a protective effect on the brain when administered before or immediately after an ischemic insult in animals (12,75). In a benchmark clinical study of post–cardiac arrest patients, however, a single dose of thiopental after the arrest produced no improvement in outcome (76). In view of these negative results and the tendency of barbiturates to produce hypotension and arrhythmias, these agents cannot be recommended for the treatment of the post–cardiac arrest patient.

Calcium Channel Antagonists

The role of calcium channel blockers in the treatment of post–cardiac arrest patients has not been established (77). Nimodipine, in a rat model, has been shown to improve CBF and reduce brain edema after middle cerebral artery occlusion (78). A study evaluating the calcium-entry blocker lidoflazine in 520 comatose patients after cardiac arrest failed to demonstrate improvement in neurological recovery (79), and the use of calcium antagonists has not become routine.

Seizures

Excessive excitatory neurotransmitter release during brain ischemia can lead to paroxysmal discharges in the cerebrum, especially in the hippocampus, beginning within minutes and lasting several hours after arrest. Repetitive discharges may progress to clinically overt seizures, and suppression is then required to prevent further injury. Seizures, including status epilepticus and myoclonus, frequently follow cerebral anoxia. Approximately 40% of survivors of cardiac arrest in one study had residual seizures or myoclonus (80). Status epilepticus and myoclonic status epilepticus after anoxic encephalopathy have been found to be associated with poor outcome and persistent unconsciousness (81,80). In addition, electrographic status epilepticus without somatic motor manifestations also is suggestive of poor outcome (82).

Status epilepticus can result in permanent anoxic brain damage and requires immediate attention (Chapter 20). Generalized convulsions initially can be treated with diazepam intravenously, up to 10 mg total dose. Valproate can be useful in some cases of seizure and myoclonus, and can be loaded intravenously with 20 to 30 mg/kg at a maximum infusion rate of 3 to 6 mg/kg per minute. Precise loading doses are less clear for this agent, but this should provide therapeutic levels in most individuals. Other choices include phenytoin with a loading dose of 15 to 20 mg/kg infused at a rate not to exeed 50 mg/min. If status epilepticus continues, phenobarbital 20 mg/kg intravenously may be administered, but persistent convulsions may require general anesthesia with pentobarbital drip. In the case of generalized convulsions that are not consistent with status epilepticus, phenytoin may be administered, especially if there is EEG evidence of a persistent epileptic focus.

Myoclonus is generally recalcitrant to anticonvulsants, particularly if there is no organized paroxysmal EEG activity. We give intermittent doses of benzodiazepines in these circumstances.

PREDICTION OF OUTCOME FROM ANOXIC COMA

Clinical investigations have attempted to predict which cardiac arrest patients will do well and which will be left with severe cerebral damage. In early studies, Bell and Hodgson (83) reported that prolonged post–cardiac arrest coma was unfavorable and noted the rarity of full recovery if coma lasted for 3 days. Willoughby and Leach (84) reported that nonpurposive motor responses even 1 hour after cardiac arrest were incompatible with recovery of intellectual capacity. Snyder's group (85–88) found that comatose patients with seizures or myoclonus did not recover and that increased numbers of brainstem reflex abnormalities were associated with reduced chances for survival. All these studies, however, did not relate multiple signs to outcome, and they studied a relatively small number of patients. Earnest (89,90) reported on early and late outcomes from out-of-hospital cardiac arrest in more than 100 patients, and noted that the absence of pupillary light reactions, oculocephalic reflexes, and purposive movements to pain were each associated with reduced chances of recovery. Initial observations of only four signs were analyzed, and no comprehensive predictive technique was provided. Admission neurological signs did not correlate with late outcome. A retrospective analysis of patients in coma after out-of-hospital arrest (91) used information from charts collected over a 10-year period; consequently, approximately one-half of patients could not be evaluated for one of the five clinical variables. They concentrated almost entirely on whether a patient awakened after coma, rather than on the functional state. Retrospective design, missing data, and a relatively high error rate in identifying poor-prognosis patients limited the conclusions of this study.

Most of the current clinical prognostication is based on the work of Levy and Caronna (92,93). Clinical data were collected from 210 patients with nontraumatic coma lasting more than 6 hours, including 150 patients following cardiac arrest. Clinical examinations were performed 1, 3, 7, and 14 days after the insult. Functional recovery was assessed at 1, 3, 6, and 12 months and categorized as one of five grades: (a) no recovery (coma until death); (b) the vegetative state (wakefulness without awareness); (c) severe disability (conscious but dependent on others for aspects of daily living); (d) moderate disability (independent but with residual neurological deficits); and (e) good recovery; that is, able to resume prior level of function. The observations in this study confirm the clinical impression that the bulk of good recoveries occur within a short time. Within the first 3 days, 25 of the 210 patients had regained consciousness, whereas that number had increased only to 28 by 2 weeks. Forty-seven patients appeared vegetative on the first day, and only three of those ever improved to an independent state. Only 17 patients were in coma after 1 week, and only one of those ever regained consciousness. Of the 46 (22%) patients who regained consciousness, only 26 (13%) achieved a moderate or good recovery. Mortality was very high, with 64% of the patients dead at 1 week and 90% at 1 year.

Patient age, gender, or presence of postanoxic seizures failed to correlate with outcome. Specific neurological signs were linked to outcome, and provided the basis for predicting the potential for recovery (Fig. 17.3). The absence of specific brainstem activity was associated with poor prognosis. None of the 52 patients with absent pupillary light reflexes at initial examination ever recovered. Only three of the 71 patients with absent corneal responses at initial examination ever recovered, whereas none who lacked corneal response after the first day regained consciousness.

Important advances in assessing biochemical neuronal tissue injury may in the future be an adjunct to clinical data. Magnetic resonance spectroscopy can determine regional lactate and has been shown to correlate with outcome (94). Serum markers of tissue injury also can be measured, for example, neuron-specific enolase has been shown to correlate

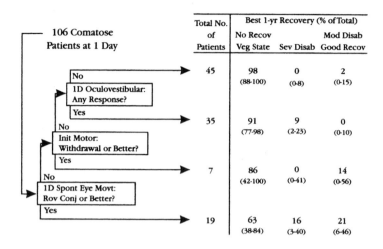

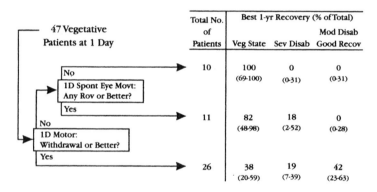

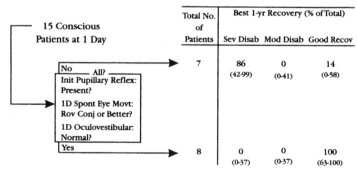

FIG. 17.3. Prognostic signs in hypoxic–ischemic encephalopathy. (From Levy DE, et al. Predicting outcome from hypoxic–ischemic coma. *JAMA* 1985;253:1420–1426, with permission.)

with injury, and high postresuscitation levels can predict persistent coma and death (95).

ACKNOWLEDGMENT

The authors thank Drs. Maise and Caronna for use of portions of the chapter from the previous edition.

REFERENCES

1. Bachman JW, McDonald GS, O'Brien PC. A study of out-of-hospital cardiac arrests in northeastern Minnesota. *JAMA* 1986;256:477–483.
2. Hallstrom AP, et al. Predictors of hospital mortality after out-of-hospital cardiopulmonary resuscitation. *Crit Care Med* 1985;13:927–929.
3. Weaver WD, et al. Considerations for improving survival from out-of-hospital cardiac arrest. *Ann Emerg Med* 1986;15:1181–1186.
4. Kaye W, et al. Can better basic and advanced cardiac life support improve outcome from cardiac arrest? *Crit Care Med* 1985;13:916–920.
5. Cummins RO, Eisenberg MS, Stults KR. Automatic external defibrillators: clinical issues for cardiology. *Circulation* 1986;73:381–385.
6. Weaver WD, et al. Cardiac arrest treated with a new automatic external defibrillator by out-of-hospital first responders. *Am J Cardiol* 1986;57:1017–1021.
7. Woollard M. Public access defibrillation: a shocking idea? *J Public Health Med* 2001;23:98–102.
8. Sanders AB, et al. Importance of the duration of inadequate coronary perfusion pressure on resuscitation from cardiac arrest. *J Am Coll Cardiol* 1985;6:113–118.
9. Brown CG, et al. Comparative effect of graded doses of epinephrine on regional brain blood flow during CPR in a swine model. *Ann Emerg Med* 1986;15:1138–1144.
10. Krause GS, et al. Ischemia, resuscitation, and reperfusion: mechanisms of tissue injury and prospects for protection. *Am Heart J* 1986;111:768–780.
11. Liberthson RR, et al. Prehospital ventricular defibrillation. Prognosis and follow-up course. *N Engl J Med* 1974;291:317–321.
12. Bass E. Cardiopulmonary arrest. Pathophysiology and neurological complications. *Ann Intern Med* 1985;103: 920–927.
13. Caronna JJ, Finklestein S. Neurological syndromes after cardiac arrest. *Stroke* 1978;9:517–520.
14. Finklestein S, Caronna JJ. Amnestic syndrome following cardiac arrest. *Neurology* 1978;28:389.
15. Volpe BT, Hirst W. The characterization of an amnesic syndrome following hypoxic ischemic injury. *Arch Neurol* 1983;40:436–440.
16. Plum F, Posner JB, Hain RF. Delayed neurological deterioration after anoxia. *Arch Intern Med* 1962;110:56.
17. Wainapel SF, Gupta PC, Matz R. Post-hypoxic leukoencephalopathy with late recovery. *Arch Phys Med Rehabil* 1984;65:201–212.
18. Ginsberg MD. Delayed neurological deterioration following hypoxia. In: Fahn S, Davis JN, Rowland LP, eds. *Advances in neurology.* New York: Raven, 1979:21–44.

19. Howard R, Trend P, Russell RW. Clinical features of ischemia in cerebral arterial border zones after periods of reduced cerebral blood flow. *Arch Neurol* 1987;44: 934–940.
20. Odeh M, Oliven A. Transient bilateral cortical blindness due to hypoxemia. *Anaesthesiol Int Care* 1996; 24:126.
21. Kam CA, Yoong FF, Ganendran A. Cortical blindness following hypoxia during cardiac arrest. *Anaesthesiol Int Care* 1978;6:143–145.
22. Lambert SR, et al. Visual recovery from hypoxic cortical blindness during childhood. Computed tomographic and magnetic resonance imaging predictors. *Arch Ophthalmol* 1987;105:1371–1377.
23. Sage JI, Van Uitert RL. Man-in-the-barrel syndrome. *Neurology* 1986;36:1102–1103.
24. Olejniczak PG, et al. Man-in-the-barrel syndrome in a noncomatose patient: a case report. *Arch Phys Med Rehabil* 1991;72:1021–1023.
25. Hurley JP, Wood AE. Isolated man-in-the-barrel syndrome following cardiac surgery. *Thorac Cardiovasc Surg* 1993;41:252–254.
26. Jennett B, Plum F. Persistent vegetative state after brain damage. A syndrome in search of a name. *Lancet* 1972; 1:734–737.
27. Ringel SP, Klawans HL. Carbon monoxide–induced parkinsonism. *J Neurol Sci* 1972;16:245–251.
28. Hallett M. Physiology of human posthypoxic myoclonus. *Mov Disord* 2000;15:8–13.
29. Wijdicks EF, Parisi JE, Sharbrough FW. Prognostic value of myoclonus status in comatose survivors of cardiac arrest. *Ann Neurol* 1994;35:239–243.
30. Lance JW, Adams RD. The syndrome of intention or action myoclonus as a sequel to hypoxic encephalopathy. *Brain* 1963;86:111–136.
31. Van Woert MH, et al. Long-term therapy of myoclonus and other neurological disorders with L-5-hydroxytryptophan and carbidopa. *N Engl J Med* 1977;296:70–75.
32. Goldberb MA, Dorman JD. Intention myoclonus: successful treatment with clonazepam. *Neurology* 1976;26: 24–26.
33. Fahn S. Post-anoxic action myoclonus: improvement with valproic acid. *N Engl J Med* 1978;299:313–314.
34. Welsh JP, et al. Why do Purkinje cells die so easily after global brain ischemia? Aldolase C, EAAT4, and the cerebellar contribution to posthypoxic myoclonus. *Adv Neurol* 2002;89:331–359.
35. Brierly JB, Graham DI. Hypoxia and vascular disorders of the central nervous system. In: Adams JH, Corsellis JAN, Duchen LW, eds. *Greenfield's neuropathology.* New York: Wiley, 1984:131–132.
36. Silver JR, Buxton PH. Spinal stroke. *Brain* 1974;97: 539–550.
37. Miller JR, Myers RE. Neuropathology of systemic circulatory arrest in adult monkeys. *Neurology* 1972;22: 888—904.
38. Boisen E, Siemkowicz E. Six cases of cerebromedullospinal disconnection after cardiac arrest. *Lancet* 1976; 1:1381–1383.
39. Teasdale G, Jennett B. Assessment of coma and impaired consciousness. A practical scale. *Lancet* 1974;2:81–84.
40. Hameroff SB, Garcia-Mullin R, Eckholdt J. Ocular bobbing. *Arch Ophthalmol* 1969;82:774–780.
41. Ropper AH. Ocular dipping in anoxic coma. *Arch Neurol* 1981;38:297–299.

42. Tippin J, Adams HP Jr, Smoker WR. Early computed tomographic abnormalities following profound cerebral hypoxia. *Arch Neurol* 1984;41:1098–1100.

43. Arbelaez A, Castillo M, Mukherji SK. Diffusion-weighted MR imaging of global cerebral anoxia. *AJNR Am J Neuroradiol* 1999;20:999–1007.

44. Liu AY, et al. Diffusion-weighted imaging in the evaluation of watershed hypoxic-ischemic brain injury in pediatric patients. *Neuroradiology* 2001;43:918–926.

45. Chalela JA, et al. MRI identification of early white matter injury in anoxic–ischemic encephalopathy. *Neurology* 2001;56:481–485.

46. Goto Y, et al. (Magnetic resonance imaging findings of postresuscitation encephalopathy: sequential change and correlation with clinical outcome). *No To Shinkei* 2001;53:535–540.

47. Alavi A, et al. Positron emission tomography imaging of regional cerebral glucose metabolism. *Semin Nucl Med* 1986;16:2–34.

48. Borel C, Hanley D. Neurological intensive care unit monitoring. *Crit Care Clin* 1985;1:223–239.

49. Joogensen EO, Malchow-Moller A. Natural history of global and critical brain ischaemia. Part III: cerebral prognostic signs after cardiopulmonary resuscitation. Cerebral recovery course and rate during the first year after global and critical ischaemia monitored and predicted by EEG and neurological signs. *Resuscitation* 1981;9:175–188.

50. Synek VM. Prognostically important EEG coma patterns in diffuse anoxic and traumatic encephalopathies in adults. *J Clin Neurophysiol* 1988;5:161–174.

51. Yamashita S, et al. Prognostic value of electroencephalogram (EEG) in anoxic encephalopathy after cardiopulmonary resuscitation: relationship among anoxic period, EEG grading and outcome. *Intern Med* 1995;34:71–76.

52. Austin EJ, Wilkus RJ, Longstreth WT Jr. Etiology and prognosis of alpha coma. *Neurology* 1988;38:773–777.

53. Young GB, et al. EEG and clinical associations with mortality in comatose patients in a general intensive care unit. *J Clin Neurophysiol* 1999;16:354–360.

54. Brunko E, Zegers de Beyl D. Prognostic value of early cortical somatosensory evoked potentials after resuscitation from cardiac arrest. *Electroencephalogr Clin Neurophysiol* 1987;66:15–24.

55. Firsching R, Frowein RA. Multimodality evoked potentials and early prognosis in comatose patients. *Neurosurg Rev* 1990;13:141–146.

56. Ganes T, Lundar T. EEG and evoked potentials in comatose patients with severe brain damage. *Electroencephalogr Clin Neurophysiol* 1988;69:6–13.

57. Haupt WF. (Prognostic value of multimodal evoked potentials in neurological intensive care patients). *Klin Wochenschr* 1988;66:53–61.

58. Zentner J, Ebner A. Prognostic value of somatosensory- and motor-evoked potentials in patients with a nontraumatic coma. *Eur Arch Psychiatry Neurol Sci* 1988; 237:184–187.

59. Ahmed I. Use of somatosensory evoked responses in the prediction of outcome from coma. *Clin Electroencephalogr* 1988;19:78–86.

60. Nakabayashi M, Kurokawa A, Yamamoto Y. Immediate prediction of recovery of consciousness after cardiac arrest. *Int Care Med* 2001;27:1210–1214.

61. Drummond JC, Todd MM, U HS. The effect of high dose sodium thiopental on brainstem auditory and median nerve somatosensory evoked responses in humans. *Anesthesiology* 1985;63:249–254.

62. Hall JW 3rd, Bull JM, Cronau LH. Hypo- and hyperthermia in clinical auditory brainstem response measurement: two case reports. *Ear Hear* 1988;9:137–143.

63. Garcia-Larrea L, et al. Transient drug-induced abolition of BAEPs in coma. *Neurology* 1988;38:1487–1489.

64. Pulsinelli WA, Brierley JB, Plum F. Temporal profile of neuronal damage in a model of transient forebrain ischemia. *Ann Neurol* 1982;11:491–498.

65. Michenfelder JD, Milde JH. Influence of anesthetics on metabolic, functional and pathological responses to regional cerebral ischemia. *Stroke* 1975;6:405–410.

66. Smith AL. Barbiturate protection in cerebral hypoxia. *Anesthesiology* 1977;47:285–293.

67. D'Alecy LG, et al. Dextrose containing intravenous fluid impairs outcome and increases death after eight minutes of cardiac arrest and resuscitation in dogs. *Surgery* 1986;100:505–511.

68. Siesjo BK, Wieloch T. Molecular mechanisms of ischemic brain damage Ca2+ related events. In: Rievich M, Hurtig H, eds. *Cerebrovascular diseases, 13th Research Conference.* New York: Raven, 1985:251–268.

69. Hypothermia after Cardiac Arrest Study Group. Mild therapeutic hypothermia to improve the neurological outcome after cardiac arrest. *N Engl J Med* 2002;346: 549–556.

70. Bernard SA, et al. Treatment of comatose survivors of out-of-hospital cardiac arrest with induced hypothermia. *N Engl J Med* 2002;346:557–563.

71. Longstreth WT Jr, et al. Neurological outcome and blood glucose levels during out-of-hospital cardiopulmonary resuscitation. *Neurology* 1986;36:1186–1191.

72. Moss E, et al. Intensive management of severe head injuries. A scheme of intensive management of severe head injuries. *Anaesthesia* 1983;38:214–225.

73. Nordby HK, Gunnerod N. Epidural monitoring of the intracranial pressure in severe head injury characterized by non-localizing motor response. *Acta Neurochir* 1985;74:21–26.

74. Grafton ST, Longstreth WT Jr. Steroids after cardiac arrest: a retrospective study with concurrent, nonrandomized controls. *Neurology* 1988;38:1315–1316.

75. Kirsch JR, Dean JM, Rogers MC. Current concepts in brain resuscitation. *Arch Intern Med* 1986;146:1413–1419.

76. Randomized clinical study of thiopental loading in comatose survivors of cardiac arrest. Brain Resuscitation Clinical Trial I Study Group. *N Engl J Med* 1986; 314:397–403.

77. Vibulsresth S, et al. Failure of nimodipine to prevent ischemic neuronal damage in rats. *Stroke* 1987;18:210–216.

78. Jacewicz M, et al. Nimodipine pretreatment improves cerebral blood flow and reduces brain edema in conscious rats subjected to focal cerebral ischemia. *J Cereb Blood Flow Metab* 1990;10:903–913.

79. A randomized clinical study of a calcium-entry blocker (lidoflazine) in the treatment of comatose survivors of cardiac arrest. Brain Resuscitation Clinical Trial II Study Group. *N Engl J Med* 1991;324:1225–1231.

80. Krumholz A, Stern BJ, Weiss HD. Outcome from coma after cardiopulmonary resuscitation: relation to seizures and myoclonus. *Neurology* 1988;38:401–415.

81. Jumao-as A, Brenner RP. Myoclonic status epilepticus: a clinical and electroencephalographic study. *Neurology* 1990;40:1199–1202.

82. Simon RP, Aminoff MJ. Electrographic status epilepticus in fatal anoxic coma. *Ann Neurol* 1986;20:351–355.

83. Bell JA, Hodgson HJ. Coma after cardiac arrest. *Brain* 1974;97:361–372.

84. Willoughby JO, Leach BG. Relation of neurological findings after cardiac arrest to outcome. *Br Med J* 1974;3:437–439.

85. Snyder BD, Ramirez-Lassepas M, Lippert DM. Neurological status and prognosis after cardiopulmonary arrest: I. A retrospective study. *Neurology* 1977;27:807–811.

86. Snyder BD, et al. Neurological prognosis after cardiopulmonary arrest: III. Seizure activity. *Neurology* 1980;30:1292–1297.

87. Snyder BD, et al. Neurological prognosis after cardiopulmonary arrest: IV. Brainstem reflexes. *Neurology* 1981;31:1092–1097.

88. Synder BD, et al. Neurological prognosis after cardiopulmonary arrest: II. Level of consciousness. *Neurology* 1980;30:52–58.

89. Earnest MP, et al. Quality of survival after out-of-hospital cardiac arrest: predictive value of early neurological evaluation. *Neurology* 1979;29:56–60.

90. Earnest MP, et al. Long-term survival and neurological status after resuscitation from out-of-hospital cardiac arrest. *Neurology* 1980;30:1298–1302.

91. Longstreth WT Jr, Diehr P, Inui TS. Prediction of awakening after out-of-hospital cardiac arrest. *N Engl J Med* 1983;308:1378–1382.

92. Levy DE, et al. Prognosis in nontraumatic coma. *Ann Intern Med* 1981;94:293–301.

93. Levy DE, et al. Predicting outcome from hypoxic–ischemic coma. *JAMA* 1985;253:1420–1426.

94. Berek K, et al. Early determination of neurological outcome after prehospital cardiopulmonary resuscitation. *Stroke* 1995;26:543–549.

95. Fogel W, et al. Serum neuron-specific enolase as early predictor of outcome after cardiac arrest. *Crit Care Med* 1997;25:1133–1138.

18

Critical Care of Guillain–Barré Syndrome

Guillain–Barré syndrome (GBS), as it is commonly known, or acute inflammatory polyneuropathy, is the most frequent cause of acute and subacute generalized paralysis now that polio has been largely eliminated. In the United States and elsewhere, it occurs at a rate of approximately 1.7 cases per 100,000 persons per year (1), and largely because of respiratory failure, it is among the most common neurological causes of admission to an intensive care unit (ICU). Reviews of the critical care aspects of GBS have appeared and may, in addition to this chapter, be useful to the reader (2,3). Weakness and sensory symptoms are the result of widespread immune-mediated damage to peripheral nerves; that is, it is a polyneuropathy. The central nervous system is very seldom affected. The polyneuropathy most often follows an acute infection, which may be of almost any type but with a proclivity for certain ones, particularly *Campylobacter jejuni* enteritis, Epstein–Barr virus, cytomegalovirus (CMV) and *Mycoplasma pneumoniae.*

The illness is not difficult to recognize based on acral paresthesias, bilateral limb weakness and sometimes cranial palsies and areflexia, all typically evolving over several days, without fever as described further in the following and in several monographs and reviews (4–6). Research criteria that have been established for the diagnosis of GBS provide reasonable guidelines in clinical practice (7). A classification based largely on electromyogram (EMG) findings and on presumed immunologic mechanisms sepa-rates several patterns: the common variety of GBS, acute inflammatory demyelinating polyneuropathy (AIDP); an acute motor-sensory neuropathy (AMSAN); and an acute motor axonal neuropathy (AMAN). The current authors find the clinical, pathologic, and antibody reactions associated with these categories to overlap and the incidence of the second two types in most practices to be low. Nonetheless, EMG plays a central role in confirming the diagnosis of GBS and in detecting severe axonal damage that leads to severe and prolonged paralysis. Examination of the spinal fluid for elevated protein and a paucity of white blood cells, considered the classic ancillary feature of the illness, continues to be useful but serves a subsidiary role in diagnosis.

Survival and gradual improvement is the rule in almost all patients. Recuperation is often lengthy and punctuated by major respiratory, autonomic, cardiovascular, and infectious problems that are the province of neurological intensive care. Several reviews of large series of GBS in the modern ICU era have reported approximately 5% mortality (4,8–12) and have suggested that outcome depends to a great extent on the quality of care received in the ICU. As discussed further on, corticosteroids have not proved effective in GBS, despite anecdotal exceptions, and several large randomized trials using either plasma exchange or intravenous infusions of gamma-globulin have demonstrated a reduction in the length of the acute illness and in the time on a ventilator.

PATHOPHYSIOLOGY OF GUILLAIN–BARRÉ SYNDROME

Immune Mechanisms

Several pathologic and pathophysiologic events account for the clinical signs and the course of GBS: (a) an immune-mediated destruction of the myelin surrounding the peripheral and cranial nerves, effected mostly, but not exclusively, by the cellular arm of the immune system (13); (b) an early, humorally mediated and complement dependent damage to myelin (14); (c) varying degrees of axonal damage that are most often secondary to very active inflammation but may also result from a primary immune attack on axonal elements in which there is poor and prolonged recovery (15) ("axonal GBS" or AS-MAN); and (d) a rapid and reversible electrophysiologic "conduction block" (16).

The immunologic nature of GBS seems undoubted, prompting studies of the cellular and humoral roles in experimental allergic neuritis (EAN), a model that closely resembles the disease in humans. The pathology in GBS and EAN consists mainly of lymphocytic infiltration of peripheral nerves, predominantly in perivascular regions, with adjacent demyelination of segmental type (loss of the myelin segments between adjacent nodes of Ranvier). Macrophages produce the stripping and destruction of myelin from the axonal surface. The lymphocytic infiltration occurs multifocally along the length of the nerve in both GBS and EAN and it may also affect dorsal root ganglia and the proximal portions of autonomic nerves. It has been proposed that extensive inflammation and myelin destruction can damage the underlying axons as they course through the zone. As mentioned, the distinction between demyelination and axonal disruption is often difficult but it assumes clinical importance because mild cases, with only demyelination, improve in weeks through a mechanism of remyelination, whereas those with axonal interruption require longer to recover, and are more likely to be left with residual weakness. As also mentioned, a primary axonal form of GBS occurs in which there is little inflammation and axonal disruption arises without primary destruction of myelin.

A considerable body of data suggests that plasma (humoral) factors participate in the pathogenesis of GBS. The earliest immunologic change that can be detected is deposition of complement on myelin surfaces. Cell-free serum from patients with GBS or animals with EAN can induce demyelination in cultured nerve tissue. Several histo pathologic reports indicate that some early cases may show a paucity of inflammation. Serum from animals with EAN and from patients with GBS also have been shown to induce electric conduction block and demyelination when injected into nerves in animals. Specific antibodies to peripheral nerve tissue have been isolated from a proportion of patients with GBS but not from control subjects.

The postinfectious nature of many, if not most, cases of GBS has been appreciated for many years and it has been presumed that the immune response to the infecting agent cross reacts with elements of normal neural tissue—a monophasic and self-limited autoimmune reaction. Direct evidence for this mechanism has been difficult to obtain, but it is supported by the singular relationship of preceding infection by the enteric bacterium, *Campylobacter jejuni* to acute GBS. Antibodies directed against this organism bind to specific ganglioside epitopes on peripheral nerve (in this case GM1) and are believed to generate the immune damage. There are certainly many cases of GBS that arise without an obvious prior infection and several case control series have attempted to show that there is no such relationship. It should be pointed out that in many instances there is only serologic evidence of recent infection without, for example, a febrile enteritis. The other infectious agents that have been regularly implicated in GBS are mainly EBV, CMV, and mycoplasma. Many cases of GBS following CMV are associated with antibodies to GM2, another neural ganglioside.

CLINICAL FEATURES

A summary of the clinical features of GBS in our patients from 1962 to 1979, before the use of plasma exchange and gamma-globulin had become routine, is presented in Table 18.1 and in the aforementioned texts on GBS (6,7). In most ways this parallels more recent experience with the exception that the institution of immune treatments has shortened the duration of hospitalization and introduced a number of related iatrogenic complications.

Preceding Infection

More than half of patients with GBS have a history of recent acute infection, usually a mild respiratory syndrome. A number of cases follow other well-defined illnesses such as mononucleosis, acute exanthemas, or surgery. When Epstein–Barr virus or CMV precede GBS, they often cause mildly abnormal liver function tests. These latter two infections are particularly likely to be seen in health care personnel. A preceding atypical or mild pneumonia suggests mycoplasma infection. As mentioned, *Campylobacter jejuni* enteritis is perhaps the most frequent identifiable pathogen that precedes GBS, accounting for up to 20% of cases in some series. An uncertain proportion of such cases occur without the typical enteritis and are detected only by serologic testing. It has been observed that *Campylobacter* may be associated with a severe axonal form of illness (AMSAN or AMAN), but there

seems little question that more typical and less severe cases, as well as variant illnesses such as Fisher syndrome, also may follow (17,18). In certain populations, symptomatic acute human immunodeficiency virus infection precedes GBS in up to 15% of cases (19). Postsurgical GBS is a less certain entity. Prior to the appreciation of what is now called critical illness polyneuropathy, postoperative GBS was said to occur 2 to 3 weeks after intracranial, abdominal, thoracic, and orthopedic operations as well as following epidural or spinal anesthesia; we have encountered several such cases (20,21). However, the incidence of this complication probably has been overestimated because many cases that follow postoperative sepsis are more likely to be of the "critical illness polyneuropathy" variety (Chapter 11).

Clinical Signs

In the most typical cases of GBS, the main clinical sign is weakness, usually appearing symmetrically in the legs, most often proximally. (The term *ascending paralysis* signifies weakness that begins in the legs and progresses to the arms, not weakness in the feet.) Bifacial paresis arises in about one half of patients and may be delayed in appearance, and oro-lingual-pharyngeal weakness is a feature in one third. The weakness in all parts evolves over 3 to 21 days (mean 2 weeks in untreated patients) and does not usually remit until a plateau of maximal weakness occurs.

TABLE 18.1. *Our experience with Guillain–Barré syndrome, 1962 to 1979 (Preplasma exchange and gamma-globulin era.)*

Number of cases	157
Average age	39 years
Age range	8–81 years
Prior illness	Upper respiratory infection (approximately 70%)
Onset to maximal deficit to plateau	Average 17 days
	40% by first week
	77% by second week
	89% by third week
Mortality	1.25%
Respiratory failure	29%
Average hospitalization	61 days
Average intubation	51 days
Residual deficits at 1 year	23% (severe in 8%)

Adapted from Truax BT. Autonomic disturbances in Guillain-Barré syndrome. *Semin Neurol* 1984;4:462–468.

Distal paresthesias with mild sensory loss are typical early in the illness; sensation is increasingly diminished in the distal limbs as the illness progresses, but it may be indistinct in the first several days. Patients with GBS exhibit few objective signs besides weakness and areflexia. Sensory signs early in the illness may be confined to mild or moderate glove and stocking loss of vibration and pain sensibility.

The deep tendon reflexes are usually lost in paretic limbs after several days of illness. In contrast, a brisk direct muscle percussion with a small hammer causes a local fascicular contraction.

Pain concentrated in the back or sciatica occurs in 10% to 25% of patients and is typically worse at night; it is described as a "charley horse" or deep aching pain similar to that experienced after exercise (22). The management of this pain is a major issue in the ICU and is addressed in the following. When it precedes weakness by several days, the diagnosis of lumbar spine disease or a painful muscle disorder may suggest itself. A separate acral dysesthetic pain may arise within days but is more often a delayed phenomenon and is managed differently.

One of the greatest problems in ICU practice is the identification and care of the approximately 5% of patients with a rapidly evolving and aggressive form of disease. They reach their worst clinical state in 1 to 3 days, resulting in quadriplegia and respiratory failure. In most other ways these cases resemble typical GBS. Feasby and colleagues showed that many of these patients have an acute axonal disruption with a paucity of inflammation of nerves, and coined the term "axonal GBS," which has come into wide use (15). In our experience and that of others, these patients have prolonged and incomplete recoveries (23); others have disagreed that the tempo of onset is related in this direct way to outcome (24); but there is no question that patients with signs of axonal degeneration on EMG have a more severe form of illness (see Treatment).

Dysautonomia of varying degrees occurs in approximately 20% of cases. Its various manifestations are more prominent in the most severely affected patients, including those with the axonal form of illness. For example, transient urinary sphincter dysfunction occurs in 15% of patients, particularly urinary retention that may occur early in the course of the disease and raise the possibility of spinal cord compression or myelitis. Respiratory muscle weakness, the main ICU issue in GBS (also discussed in greater detail in the following), occurs in one third of patients and is apparent within the first 2 weeks of illness with few exceptions.

Several variant illnesses of GBS are known; the most striking is a pattern of ophthalmoplegia and severe ataxia described by Fisher (25). Other unusual patterns or signs include cases of "descending" paralysis, beginning with ocular, facial, and pharyngeal paresis that simulates botulism or myasthenia gravis; ophthalmoplegia or ptosis; and predominantly or purely ataxic, motor, or sensory forms (26–28). About 3% of patients have abortive regional forms of the illness with preserved power and reflexes in either the arms or legs. The signs are relatively symmetric in all these variant cases. Failure of protective airway reflexes and the need for intubation are the main reasons these patients come to the attention of intensivists; diaphragmatic weakness is less common than in typical generalized GBS.

Electrophysiologic Tests

The electrophysiologic abnormalities associated with GBS provide confirmation of the diagnosis and are useful in distinguishing GBS from clinically similar diseases. They are more sensitive, and become abnormal earlier in the illness than does the classical laboratory abnormality of GBS, elevation of spinal fluid protein concentration. These tests also delineate a group of patients with early and severe axonal damage who typically require more intense and prolonged respiratory and ICU care.

Early in the illness, nerve conduction velocity is slightly slowed but it may be normal in mildly affected patients. Conduction block, the most specific EMG sign of demyelinating neuropathy, alluded to earlier, consists of a drop in the muscle action potential amplitude when proximal is compared to distal stimulation of the nerve. Abnormalities of the "late responses" are also sensitive indicators of early GBS. The main late responses (F-waves) are obtained by supramaximal stimulation of motor axons that propagates in a retrograde fashion toward the spinal cord and causes a discharge of motor neurons that can be recorded 25 to 35 msec later. In relation to axonal damage, inexcitable nerves or severely reduced motor action potential amplitudes, below 1 μV, or values that are less than 20% of the lower limit of normal, are predictive of prolonged illness and poor outcome (29). However, there are exceptions in which the inexcitability of nerves reflects severe focal demyelination with potential for recovery rather than indicating axonal disruption (30).

The electrical manifestation of the blink reflexes also can be recorded and are prolonged or absent in most patients with GBS. Somatosensory evoked potentials are typically abnormal in their peripheral nerve portions and rarely show central abnormalities. The severity of abnormalities in conventional electrophysiologic studies, except for early and widespread denervation on needle electromyography examination, only roughly parallels clinical weakness. Furthermore, there is usually a long interval between manifest clinical improvement and the normalization of electrophysiologic studies.

Other Laboratory Tests

Except for the examination of CSF and the discussed electrophysiologic testing, laboratory findings are of limited value in diagnosis. An increased level of CSF protein is helpful in confirming the diagnosis but may be detectable only after 5 to 10 days of illness. Occasionally, the CSF protein value is normal throughout the illness, including

some cases of severe or axonal type. The absence of cells in the CSF supports the diagnosis of GBS, but up to 5% of patients have 5 to 50 lymphocytes/mm^3; in all likelihood some of these cases represent other forms of polyneuropathy (e.g., Lyme, CMV, acquired immunodeficiency syndrome, etc.). Oligoclonal bands of CSF protein are present occasionally. Mild, asymptomatic abnormalities of liver function tests occur in about 5%, probably indicating a preceding viral hepatitis. In severe or particularly abrupt cases of GBS, it is interesting but not necessary for clinical work, to culture the patient's stool for *Campylobacter;* as mentioned, many of these cases also display circulating antibodies to GM1, a myelin glycolipid component. The sedimentation rate is normal.

Differential Diagnosis

The illnesses that simulate GBS are described in standard textbooks of neurology and in a monograph by one of the authors. The ones usually cited are: myasthenia gravis, transverse myelitis, and the rare entities of tick paralysis and porphyria. In the ICU setting, however, illnesses that cause acute areflexic quadriparesis include botulism, diphtheria, hyperalimentation-induced hypophosphatemia (31), and most importantly, the myopathy and polyneuropathy associated with sepsis and critical illness (Chapter 11). Several variants of GBS also may cause difficulty in diagnosis. Difficulty weaning from ventilation after general surgery is occasionally caused by GBS that develops postoperatively for unclear reasons, but the aforementioned critical illness myopathy and neuropathy as well as nutritional factors are more common causes of this problem.

INTENSIVE CARE UNIT COMPLICATIONS

The reasons for admitting a patient with GBS to an ICU are mostly self-evident but are summarized in Table 18.2. The clinical course can be expected to be weeks or

TABLE 18.2. *Criteria for admitting Guillain–Barré syndrome patients to an intensive care unit*

Vital capacity <12 mL/kg
Deteriorating vital capacity <18 to 20 mL/kg
Clinical signs of diaphragmatic fatigue including tachypnea, diaphoresis, and paradoxical breathing
Poor cough, difficulty swallowing, accumulating secretions, aspiration pneumonia
Major cardiovascular dysautonomic features (wide blood pressure and pulse fluctuations: arrhythmias, heart
  block, pulmonary edema, profound ileus with risk of visceral rupture)
Hypotension precipitated by plasma exchange, or plasma exchange planned in a ventilated or unstable patient
Sepsis
Pulmonary embolism or suspicion of same

months long in most patients who are ill enough to reach the ICU, but nonetheless the majority recover with little or no disability and a few require only days of ICU care. For this reason, attentive and anticipatory general medical care is the most important aspect of ICU treatment (32). In the modern ICU era the mortality rate for GBS in large series has been 1% to 8%, typically in the middle of this range. Hospital stays are complicated by intubation or tracheostomy (over 50% of ICU patients), pneumonia (25%), urinary infections (20%), phlebitis, gastrointestinal hemorrhage (5%), pulmonary embolus (approximately 2%), and psychologic depression. Hyponatremia arises as a consequence of mechanical ventilation but also independently as a result of either excess secretion of antidiuretic hormone or a salt-wasting syndrome. The special problems in GBS that are especially suited to ICU care are dysautonomia and respiratory failure. The rate of these complications in a series of 114 patients collected by Henderson and colleagues from the Mayo Clinic are similar to ours (33). They have reported an overall incidence of systemic infection of 20%, not surprisingly more frequently in patients who were more severely affected and on a ventilator.

Dysautonomia

Autonomic dysfunction, although potentially serious and relatively common in mild form (34–36), nonetheless may be a somewhat overrated clinical problem because most of its manifestations are inconsequential. We are dubious that autonomic dysfunction can represent the sole initial manifestation of generalized GBS, but putative cases have been reported (37). The status of "pure pandysautonomia" is likewise controversial, but we believe that many of its features conform to those of a postinfectious polyneuropathy.

The main concerns in GBS are cardiovascular changes ranging in seriousness from a fixed tachycardia (invariant R-R interval) usually in the range of 110 to 120 beats/min and reduced sweating, to more threatening manifestations such as profound hypotension or hypertension, as summarized in Table 18.3. Ileus, bladder dysfunction (particularly early urinary retention), various arrhythmias, electrocardiogram (ECG) changes, and paralysis of pupillary accommodation, are other components that arise in individual patients.

TABLE 18.3. *Autonomic dysfunction in a series of 169 patients with Guillain–Barré syndrome*

Dysautonomia	No. cases	Percent
Sinus tachycardia	62	37
Labile heart rate	14	8
Orthostatic hypotension	32	19
Sustained hypertension	5	3
Paroxysmal hypertension	40	24
"Vagal spells"	13	8
Other arrhythmias	8	5
Abnormal drug responses	2	1
Urinary retention	46	27
Urinary incontinence	4	2
Impotence (males)	2	2
Constipation	24	14
Ileus	15	9
Fecal incontinence	2	1

From Traux BT. Autonomic disturbances in Guillain-Barré syndrome. *Semin Neurol* 1984;4:462–468, with permission.

Among the less frequent changes, ileus should be emphasized because it impedes nasogastric feeding and may progress to the point of cecal rupture (Fig. 18.1). Its presenting features are abdominal discomfort and repeated "large residuals" following feeding. Often, in our experience, these patients have episodes of otherwise unexplained bradycardia. Interesting, but rare "parasympathetic discharges," or "vagal spells," are also known to occur, consisting of facial flushing, bradycardia, chest tightness, dermatographia, and a general sense of warmth, sometimes following a Valsalva maneuver. A number of patients, early in their course, have profound vasodepressor responses to the initiation of positive pressure ventilation. A probable manifestation of this same vagally induced abnormality is a high incidence of hypotension during elective intubation. These problems occur independently of dehydration.

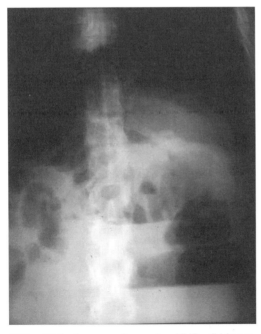

FIG. 18.1. Ileus radiograph. KUB (kidneys, ureters, bladder) radiograph of a severe ileus in a patient with Guillain–Barré syndrome during the second week of illness. There was a cecal rupture on the following day.

Electrocardiogram Changes and Arrhythmias

Morphologic changes of the ECG such as ST-T segment and T-wave abnormalities, occur in a small proportion of patients with GBS (6,38,39), and up to one third are reported to have mild elevation of serum creatine phosphokinase (CPK) concentrations early in the illness. When these ECG and enzyme findings coincide, concern arises regarding cardiac damage until the MB isoenzyme fraction is shown to be normal. The proportion of patients with elevations of CPK has been considerably lower in our experience than in many reported series; nonetheless, we exclude cardiac ischemia by echocardiography and other noninvasive means in appropriate clinical circumstances. Intramuscular injections of pain medications or other drugs are obviously a cause of enzyme elevation, but patients who have a great deal of deep muscular pain have had a higher rate of CK elevation in our series, independent of injections (40).

Diminished heart rate variation (RR interval) is ubiquitous in GBS, even in those without other feature of dysautonomia (41,42). Some of these patients have invariant tachycardia with pulse rates in the range of 106 to 126 beats/min, without other evident cause.

Arrhythmias that are more threatening than simply sinus tachycardia or bradycardia have occurred in approximately 4% of our patients, sometimes in the context of other signs of dysautonomia, but most instances can be traced to precipitants such as hypoxia, cardiac ischemia, or pulmonary embolus. A prospective study by Winer and Hughes (43) found that a reduced variation in the R-R interval and severe hypertension predicted for serious arrhythmias. Serious arrhythmias occurred in 11 of 100 of their patients on ventilators and were fatal in seven cases.

There are numerous reports of complete heart block or asystole requiring treatment with a pacemaker during acute GBS (44). Whether heart block or episodes of asystole can be anticipated in some way, such as by spectral analysis of ECG as elaborated by

Pfieffer (45) or provocative procedures such as pressure on the ocular globe, is uncertain. The approach to inserting a pacemaker has varied widely for this reason. Pfeiffer and colleagues also have indicated that serious bradycardia or sinus arrest usually is preceded for a period of time by increased daily variation in systolic blood pressure (46) or, paradoxically, by preservation of the normal respiratory induced heart rate variation (47). These are conclusions we cannot validate. Other types of trend monitoring or spectral analysis of heart rate variation have been similarly suggested as predictive of serious bradyarrhythmias (48), but these methods are best suited for investigation. The only guidance that can be given is to assume that a first episode of major bradyarrhythmia is a harbinger of further ones and that the threshold for insertion of a pacemaker should be correspondingly low.

Intravenous metoclopropamide caused repeated episodes of sinus arrest in one case (49), and we have seen it with narcotics. Myocarditis has been a very rare and usually fatal accompaniment of GBS that may be presaged by ventricular irritability.

Syndrome of Inappropriate Antidiuretic Hormone

The syndrome of inappropriate antidiuretic hormone (SIADH) secretion in GBS, described by Posner and colleagues (50), has since been reported numerous times (51). It is more frequent when positive pressure ventilation is used and it responds to fluid restriction. More recently, it has been appreciated that hyponatremia also may be the result of a natriuresis, probably related to elevations of atrial natriuretic factor (ANF) rather than to water retention (52). The appropriate treatment is the opposite of that for SIADH, namely, replenishment of sodium and intravascular volume, but the distinction between the two causes is difficult. Profound hyponatremia is more often caused by SIADH; however, if there is a question as to the cause, it is safest to measure the central venous pressure before embarking on aggressive fluid treatment. Rare instances of

pseudotumor cerebri with GBS have drawn much attention but remain unexplained (53).

Several other neuroendocrine abnormalities occur in GBS patients with cardiovascular dysautonomia, including elevated renin, atrial natriuretic factor, and catecholamines (54–56). These changes have been related in some instances to the hypertensive episodes that occur as a component of the dysautonomia of GBS (see the following).

Hypotension

Orthostatic hypotension is almost ubiquitous in GBS but is most often the result of prolonged bed rest, dehydration, and positive pressure ventilation. Autonomic failure may contribute in certain patients but little investigation has been done to differentiate these causes of hypotension.

Episodes of profound static hypotension are a more treacherous problem. These periods, lasting several minutes or less, often alternate with brief periods of hypertension, as discussed in the following (57–59). Some episodes of hypotension are precipitated by suctioning or other provocative vagal stimuli, but most seem to be spontaneous. Blood pressure may decrease profoundly enough to cause loss of consciousness even when the patient is in the supine position. In several such patients who have been studied physiologically, the pulse rate is seen to diminish slightly at the onset of each episode of hypotension (Fig. 18.2), whereas cardiac stroke volume remains constant. We concluded that reduced systemic vascular resistance was the cause, that is, a vasodepressor response. It appears paradoxical that most of these patients have lost vagal function (as reflected by a virtually invariant pulse), yet they are able to mount a profound vasodepressor response. However, the latter is mediated through medullary and sympathetic mechanisms, in contrast to the invariant pulse, which reflects a loss of efferent peripheral vagal function.

Treatment of the hypotension often is difficult, but fluid loading has ameliorated this component of the alternating hypoten-

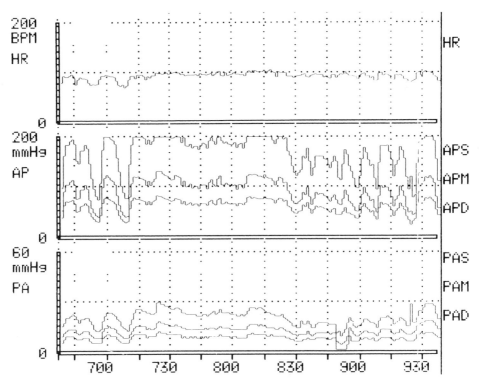

FIG. 18.2. Rapid and profound blood pressure swings in a patient with Guillain–Barré syndrome. During each episode of hypotension there is only a slight drop in pulse, suggesting a virtually pure vasodepressor episode. A drop in systemic vascular resistance was found to cause the hypotension, and loss of baroreceptor muting was theorized as the cause of hypertension. *AP*, arterial pressure; *PA*, pulmonary arterial pressure. (From Ropper AH, Wijdicks EFM. Blood pressure fluctuations in the dysautonomia of Guillain-Barré syndrome. *Arch Neurol* 1990;27:337–338, with permission.)

sion–hypertension episodes. Pressors such as phenylephrine may be used in limited amounts and with caution to stop the infusion as soon as the vasodepressor reaction ceases in order to avoid an exaggerated period of hypertension.

Pronounced and persistent hypotension (more than 1 or several minutes' duration) is invariably traced to an alternative cause other than dysautonomia, the most common ones being myocardial infarction, sepsis, pulmonary embolus, and a combination of narcotics or dehydration and the inception of positive pressure ventilation.

Hypertension

Hypertension is usually paroxysmal and sometimes severe enough to simulate pheochromocytoma. There has not been a consistent relationship between hypertension and heart block in our experience, but others differ on this point.

The associations of hypertension in exceptional instances with sudden death (60), subarachnoid hemorrhage (61–63), seizures (64), pulmonary edema, or hypertensive encephalopathy make anticipatory treatment advisable at higher levels of pressure. Episodes of severe hypertension (mean pressure greater than approximately 125 mm Hg) may be treated with intravenous labetalol, esmolol, or nitroprusside infusions. However, β-adrenergic or calcium channel blockers should be used cautiously if episodes of hypertension alternate with hypotension because they may exaggerate the degree of hypotension. More typical are lesser blood pressure elevations, in the range of 100 mm Hg mean, that do not generally cause clinical problems or require therapy. If there is considerable pain from the GBS itself, distention of a viscus or other source, analgesic medications may be enough to reduce the blood pressure.

Further discussion and citations regarding dysautonomia in GBS may be found in a monograph by one of the authors (6).

Respiratory Failure

Guillain–Barré syndrome is the prototype of neuromuscular respiratory failure owing to weakness of the diaphragm. Prior to the inception of immune treatments for GBS, approximately one third of patients required ventilators at some time in their course (65,66). More recent series have had a slightly lower number (Table 18.4). Detailed

discussions of the pathophysiology of neuromuscular respiratory failure can be found in the pulmonary literature (67–70) and in Chapter 4, but several features bear emphasis here. The phrenic nerve is affected as a component of the polyneuropathy in most cases of GBS, the shorter nerves to the accessory muscles apparently being spared until advanced stages of disease. The latter muscles provide an increasing proportion of respiratory effort as the diaphragm weakens. There is a relatively predictable progression of the clinical signs of respiratory failure, the reduction in pulmonary mechanical volumes, and certain pathophysiologic abnormalities, represented schematically in Figure 18.3. The main point to be made is that carbon dioxide retention, the traditional indicator of mechanical ventilatory failure, is a late sign in this subacute process and indicates that diaphragmatic weakness has progressed well beyond a safe point.

TABLE 18.4. *Respiratory failure in two large series of Guillain–Barré syndrome patients, before and after the routine use of plasma exchange*

	Mayo Clinic[a]	Personal series
Years of study	1974–1979	1981–1984
No. patients	13	18
Age	55 ± 22	53 ± 14 years
Days to intubation		9 ± 8
VC on admission		2.5 ± 0.91 mL/kg (38 mL/kg)
VC before intubation		0.9 ± 0.37 mL/kg (14 mL/kg)
VC at weaning	1.6 ± 0.461 ($n = 11$; 2 died)	1.8 ± 0.71 mL/kg (28 mL/kg)
IF (inspiratory force) at weaning	−48 ± 21 cm H_2O	−43 ± 15 cm H_2O ($n = 10$)
Po_2 before intubation		72 ± 14 mm Hg ($n = 12$)
Pco_2 before intubation		40 ± 4 mm Hg ($n = 12$)
Pco_2 at weaning		43 ± 4 mm Hg
Days on ventilator (including IMV)	45 (6–93)	49 ± 53 (6–220)
Days intubated (including EET)	54 (10–104)	51 ± 53 (8–220)
Tracheostomy	100%	63%
Tracheostomy day after EET	4 ± 4	11 ± 3
Hospital; intensive care unit days	82 ± 30; 58 + 26	105 ± 83; 50 ± 43
Complications (second data include patients without respiratory failure)		
Pneumonia	5/13 (38%)	15/18 (83%)
Pulmonary embolus	0/13; 1/21 (5%)	1/18 (5%); 2/38 (5%)
Tracheal stenosis/erosion	1/13 (7%)	1/18 (5%)
Death	2/13 (15%); 3/79 (4%)	0/18; 1/38 (3%)

[a]Data from Gracey DR, McMichan JC, Divertie M, et al. Respiratory failure in Guillain–Barré syndrome. A 6-year experience. *Mayo Clin Proc* 1982;57:742–746.
EET, endotracheal tube; IF, inspiratory force; IMV, intermittent mechanical ventilation; VC, vital capacity.
Adapted from Ropper AH, Kehne SM. Guillain-Barré syndrome: management of respiratory failure. *Neurology* 1985;35:1662–1665.

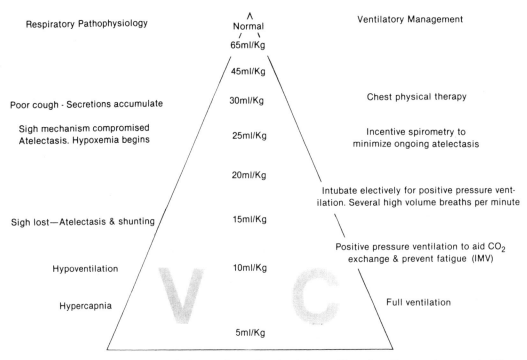

FIG. 18.3. Relationship among vital capacity, pathophysiology of lung function, and suggested therapy in mechanical ventilatory failure. This applies equally well to the respiratory failure of Guillain–Barré syndrome, myasthenia, botulism, paralyzing drugs, and high spinal cord lesions.

Physiology of Acute and Subacute Neuromuscular Respiratory Failure

As the vital capacity (VC) diminishes, the expiratory flow rate decreases and the cough becomes weak, causing difficulty in clearing pulmonary secretions. Mild hypoxia at this point is the result of ventilation–perfusion mismatching. With a further reduction, the spontaneous sigh mechanism is reduced; without this periodic hyperexpansion of the lungs, peripheral alveoli collapse for increasingly longer portions of the respiratory cycle. At some point the affected alveoli lose their surfactant coating and remain collapsed, creating unventilated but perfused areas. The resulting pulmonary vascular "shunting" is a progressive phenomenon, and results in a diminished PaO_2. Tidal volume, in contrast to forced vital capacity, decreases only slightly in the early stages of mechanical respiratory failure. It is worth emphasizing that dyspnea occurs at various times in different patients, depending on age and preexisting lung conditions, but generally it is not a complaint until VC is reduced to less than half of the predicted normal. It has been proposed that, as a result of vagal dysfunction, some patients are insensitive to the afferent impulses from the lung that induce dyspnea but there is no confirmation of this notion.

A controversial feature of mechanical respiratory failure in GBS is the role of physiologic fatigue of the intercostal muscles and diaphragm. These muscles normally function in a rather narrow window of energy metabolism that is quickly exceeded when moderate weakness demands more of the motor units (motor neuron and innervated muscles) than they can provide (28,71) (Fig. 18.4). Borel and colleagues studied GBS respiratory failure from the point of view of traditional notions of diaphragmatic fatigue (72). They found that patients with GBS and myasthenia gravis were

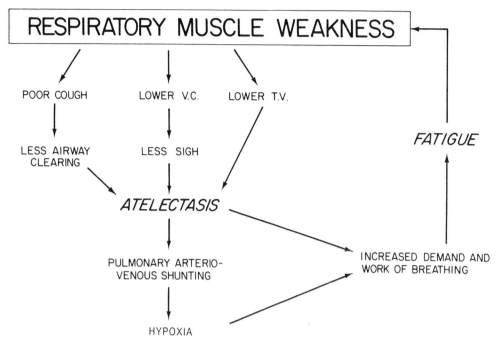

FIG. 18.4. Schematic summary of the proposed effects of fatigue and decreased vital capacity on progressive atelectasis, in patients with mechanical respiratory weakness. (From Ropper AH, Shahani BT. Diagnosis and management of acute areflexic paralysis with emphasis on Guillain-Barré syndrome. In: Asbury AK, Gilliat RW, eds. *Peripheral nerve disorders.* London: Butterworth, 1984:21–45, with permission.)

unable to wean from the ventilator despite a time–tension integral (TTdi) from the diaphragm that did not exceed the expected fatigue threshold of 0.15 (as judged from work on chronic obstructive pulmonary disease where fatigue is a topic of great interest). The TTdi concept was developed for application in patients with parenchymal lung disease (73) and may not apply to neuromuscular ventilatory failure. Or, it may be necessary to prorate indices such as TTdi to the proportion of functioning motor units in the diaphragm in order to make the measurement relevant to respiratory failure in neuromuscular disease.

Similar uncertainty pertains to the role of central respiratory drive in the respiratory failure of GBS and myasthenia. Some evidence supports a failure of central drive prior to the cessation of diaphragmatic action. The main evidence is a retained ability to generate diaphragmatic contraction by stimulation of the phrenic nerve or transcortical magnetic stimulation immediately after respiratory arrest (74,75). These issues have been better studied in chronic neuromuscular failure, such as muscular dystrophy.

Respiratory Measurements

The issue of the ideal measurement of respiratory strength also remains controversial because there is no clinical standard by which to judge the efficacy of various methods. An accurate but impractical measurement is transdiaphragmatic pressure, a cumbersome and effort-dependent test best suited for research. Traditional notions in pulmonary physiology suggest that midexpiratory (or inspiratory) flow rates are the most accurate indicators of diaphragmatic contraction. Griggs and colleagues and others have suggested that maximum expiratory pressure is the most sensitive indicator of weakness in chronic neuromuscular disease (76,77). However, these and related dynamic measurements are difficult to use in an ICU. The simpler forced vital capacity (VC) and the useful but more variable inspiratory force (NIF) are indirectly reflective of diaphragmatic function, and therefore adequate for routine use. It should be kept in mind that these volumetric measurements are surrogates for diaphragmatic strength and are compromised by the use of small hand-held devices that have two drawbacks: They do not truly collect gas in order to quantitate volume and they are sensitive to flow rates and therefore may underestimate volume in weak patients.

In any case, it should be emphasized that the trend of these measurements over hours or days and the clinical signs of respiratory failure as described in the following are as indicative as any single measurement of the need for intubation and mechanical ventilation.

Detecting Respiratory Failure

In a deteriorating patient, it is advisable to measure VC (by an experienced nurse, therapist, or physician) approximately once every 2 to 4 hours during the day and every 4 to 6 hours at night until the patient is stable and the measurements are no longer declining. In patients with facial weakness, care should be taken to seal the nose and lips over the mouthpiece in order to prevent air leakage. As a rough rule, the ability to count rapidly from 1 to 25 on one breath reflects a VC above 2L, to 10, a VC of 1L. Awakening a stable patient at night to check VC generally is not necessary; if there is a concern that a patient will rapidly deteriorate in the middle of the night, it is probably appropriate to intubate that patient electively. Because the usual measurement of VC by forced exhalation promotes atelectasis, inspiratory exercises are recommended afterward; alternatively, inspiratory VC or inspiratory force, somewhat more variable measurements than expiratory VC, may be used to test respiratory effort.

Patients with GBS should be prepared early in their illness for the possibility of intuba-

tion. Elective intubation is probably indicated when VC reaches approximately 10 to 12 mL/kg or is rapidly decreasing above these levels (12,78). Clinical signs of fatigue, brow sweating, tachycardia, and slight distractibility are important factors in deciding on the precise time of intubation and mechanical ventilation. Protection of the airway also must be considered in timing the decision to intubate a patient with oropharyngeal weakness. This approach has produced the results shown in Table 18.4 (12).

It is common for patients whose respiration is marginally compensated to become rapidly dyspneic, diaphoretic, and moderately hypoxic without obvious worsening of their generalized weakness. This tends to occur when the VC is in the range of 10 to 12 mL/kg. The majority of such patients have difficulty swallowing or clearing their secretions from the airways, for reasons already mentioned. For these reasons, we and others have empirically encouraged conservative, early intubation in order to minimize the chance of pneumonia and prevent precipitous respiratory failure that requires emergency intubation. The substantial risk of aspiration related to emergent intubation is avoided thereby.

Once intubation has taken place, daily determinations with the patient in the same body position are useful in gauging the likelihood of recovery (79). Such measurements may also be useful in determining the timing of tracheostomy but general guidelines can be given that usually prove effective.

Mechanical Ventilation and Tracheostomy

The optimal system of respiratory support in these awake patients is positive pressure volume cycled mechanical ventilation. Most attempts to use negative pressure, cuirass devices, even for nocturnal ventilation early in the course of the illness, have been ineffective and cumbersome; this was our experience in the 1980s. Occasional cases, especially in children, nevertheless have been managed in this way (80). Early in the course of mechanical respiratory failure, two to four high-volume breaths

(12 to 15 mL/kg each) per minute suffice to minimize further atelectasis and usually to reduce dyspnea if it is present. Peak inspiratory pressures (PIP) are usually low in GBS because of weakness and flaccidity of the diaphragm and chest muscles. As VC decreases further, a respirator rate between 4 and 10 beats/min is used that is comfortable for the patient and gives a normal $PaCO_2$. Of course, there is no reason to hyperventilate these patients.

Intermittent mandatory ventilation (IMV) is generally used and the waveform of the ventilator breath seems to make little difference, which is why it should be adjusted for the patient's comfort. The technique of pressure support ventilation may be an alternative to IMV in patients with vital capacities of near 10 mL/kg, and it has been used frequently to supplement IMV, ostensibly to make patients more comfortable; its value in GBS, as in most other circumstances, is untested.

Anxiety that leads to breathlessness is often difficult to differentiate from an inadequate ventilator volume. Tachypnea from this cause (that is not the result of cardiopulmonary disease) can be managed with sedatives. Sometimes the sense of inadequate positive pressure volume can be allayed by prolonging the machine inspiration or by several seconds of a large volume sigh, best accomplished with a large anesthesia bag.

The proper timing of tracheostomy has long been a topic of discussion, with some groups preferring to perform the procedure as soon as mechanical ventilation becomes necessary. Because up to one third of patients with modern immune treatments may improve greatly within 2 or 3 weeks, most units delay tracheostomy until that period has passed (81). In a series from the Mayo Clinic, of 60 patients in an ICU, only 13 could be weaned within 3 weeks and those who were older or who had preexisting pulmonary disease, were least likely to succeed (82). That group of patients who become rapidly paralyzed and appear clinically and electrophysiologically to have the axonal type of disease are probably better served by early tracheostomy because their chances for rapid recovery are quite small. The risks of soft cuffed low-pressure endotracheal tubes in these immobilized patients are minimal even after weeks of use; however, patient comfort and ease of clearing secretions make tracheostomy preferable (83). We can only offer limited personal comment on the "mini-trach" in patients with GBS where it has proved cumbersome and often restricts airflow and access for the suction catheter.

Regarding weaning, the observation of rapid shallow breathing, and various indices of respiratory effort, have been found to predict a failure of weaning; however, it is not known if this applies to GBS and other forms of neuromuscular respiratory failure (84,85). The ability to voluntarily double minute ventilation also usually predicts successful weaning and this is the measure we use most frequently. Weaning is accomplished by slowly reducing the intermittent mandatory ventilation rate as VC increases. The process is begun when VC reaches 8 to 10 mL/kg, and is usually successful when VC is approximately 18 mL/kg and inspiratory force is −35 to −45 cm H_2O. This method is usually less stressful to the patient than increasingly long intervals on a T-piece (off the respirator) (86,87). Factors such as hypokalemia, malnutrition, or alkalosis should be considered if difficulty is encountered in weaning.

It has been our experience that acute episodes of dyspnea that occur in the first 2 or 3 weeks of illness are most often caused by airway plugging by secretions, endotracheal cuff leaks, or anxiety; whereas those episodes that occur later are associated with pulmonary embolism or other serious cardiorespiratory diseases. Only a few of our patients have had respiratory dyscoordination, a syndrome more commonly associated with isolated phrenic nerve or cervical spinal cord damage. The problem was resolved with repeated slow attempts at weaning.

Guillain–Barré Syndrome Mimicking Brain Death

This striking state, reported regularly because of its novelty, is only commented on here because it is likely to arise in the ICU setting. Experienced clinicians are rarely misled into mistaking the complete de-efferented state of severe GBS for brain death, if for no other reason than it arises over time from a typical, usually axonal, type of generalized paralysis. There may be understandable confusion in the diagnosis if the early progression is not observed or an unheralded respiratory arrest is the first sign of GBS (88). Unexplained areflexia should then tip one off to the correct diagnosis. The pupils may indeed be unreactive and large or mid-position in severe GBS and all other brainstem function can be obliterated. In such a case, an electroencephalogram may be performed if there is a question of whether the patient has retained brain function.

GENERAL INTENSIVE CARE UNIT APPROACH

As already emphasized, attention to the small details of daily care is of equal importance to treatments directed specifically at the underlying immune neuropathy. Particular emphasis should be placed on positioning patients to avoid nerve pressure palsies. Ravn has shown that some residual disabilities are associated with the secondary effects of pressure of nerves, particularly the peroneal nerves (89), and inflamed nerves are believed (with little confirmation) to be prone to this type of damage.

The use of "mini-heparin" (5,000 U subcutaneously every 12 hours) seems to be effective (a randomized trial has not been performed) in reducing leg vein thrombosis and pulmonary embolism with GBS, a problem that continues to cause morbidity in bed-bound patients (90). After several weeks of intermittent subcutaneous heparin, some patients no longer have a small rise in the partial thromboplastin time, risking an embolus, and a higher dose of heparin may be required. If a prolonged bedridden period is anticipated and a tracheostomy already has been performed, we institute warfarin anticoagulation instead of heparin. An alternative for prevention of venous thromboembolism are long-leg inter-

mittent pneumatic calf compression boots that are cut out at the knees to prevent peroneal nerve compression. We have seen two patients with mild hypercalcemia, not caused by hyperparathyroidism, after immobilization for 6 months from GBS.

Nasogastric or gastric tube feeding (we prefer the former) should be instituted early but slowly. These patients are generally catabolic and high-energy (40 to 45 nonprotein kcal/kg) and high-protein (2 to 2.5 g/kg) feedings have been recommended. Presumably this approach reduces muscle wasting and assists respiratory weaning (91). The potential for developing adynamic ileus, as emphasized in the preceding, always should be kept in mind if there is abdominal pain or high residual volume of feeding. Continuous enteral feeding seems to be tolerated better than bolus feeding in these patients.

Surveillance for infections with weekly or more frequent sputum and urine cultures in debilitated and bed-bound patients may be useful but the use of these tests should be guided by clinical circumstances.

Pain is an underrated ICU problem in GBS (28,92). Because it is often worse at night, it disrupts sleep and contributes to physical and respiratory fatigue. Gabapentin or carbamazepine (93) may be effective in suppressing the discomfort but they are not often completely effective. The most effective treatment in severe cases has been epidural analgesia; we resort to this regularly. Narcotics are effective but sedation and bowel hypomotility become problematic. In severe cases, a single large dose of corticosteroids may be helpful for several days. Warm packs and massage offer temporary relief at night. Some patients prefer a water mattress; others prefer a foam mattress contoured with small pyramids. We have not had success relieving pain with quinine or nonsteroidal antiinflammatory drugs. As with other conditions associated with prolonged immobilization and disuse atrophy, the use of suxamethonium for intubation or other procedures is hazardous and may cause hyperkalemic cardiac arrest (94).

The "de-efferented" state that occurs in severe GBS requires considerable psychologic support. Explanation that the illness is usually self-limited and has a good outcome in most instances seems to have a beneficial effect on patients. We regularly arrange visits by patients who have recovered. Orientation to surroundings and adequate sleep improve the patient's overall motor and respiratory performance and psychologic outlook.

Communication is facilitated by a signboard; the type we have found most useful is a piece of Plexiglas on which is written the letters of the alphabet and commonly desired phrases such as, "I am in pain," "Turn me," "I am short of breath," etc. The board is held between the patient and nurse or physician and the patient's gaze can be used quite efficiently and rapidly to glean the message. Use of newly available electronic keyboard devices with touch-triggered buttons has greatly eased the burden of communication for these and other intubated and paretic patients. For those without eye movement, devices that move a cursor on a screen by means of a chin- or lip-operated lever may be useful. In cases simulating brain death (see the preceding) some small flicker of lid or ocular movement sometimes can be used as a signal; otherwise, sedation may be advisable.

The timing and benefits of physical therapy in the ICU for GBS are somewhat controversial, although it is certainly not suggested that it should be omitted. We generally allow patient comfort to dictate how aggressive a program is instituted in the first 2 weeks. Often, nighttime pain is worsened by even passive motion; at other times patients are more comfortable after physical therapy or massage. A good general rule is to limit early active therapy because occasional patients develop profound weakness in a limb that has been used excessively on the days after the onset of illness (e.g., a carpenter whose right arm becomes most severely affected). Of course, there is benefit in establishing an early relationship between patient and physical therapist so that treatments after the acute stage seem like a natural progression from early

therapy. The early application of plastic foot splints or high-topped sneakers prevents shortening of the Achilles tendons.

SPECIFIC THERAPY

Plasma Exchange

Since the original report by Brettle and coworkers (95) in 1978, a number of studies have achieved favorable results with plasma exchange in acute GBS. A large collaborative randomized North American trial (The Guillain–Barré Syndrome Study Group) (96), as well as French (97) and Swedish (98) randomized studies have all demonstrated its efficacy. Several results from these reports deserve emphasis (Table 18.5):

1. The time required to improve one clinical grade on a five-point scale (e.g., wean from ventilation, walk after being bedbound) was reduced by 50% in the treated group.
2. The length of time required before patients could walk independently was reduced by 40% (85 versus 53 days median).
3. The differences between groups were even greater in ventilated patients.
4. The treated and untreated groups differed only if plasma exchange was instituted more than 2 weeks from the onset of the illness.
5. Treated patients were better off after 1 year.

It should be emphasized that these results were achieved in centers with experienced plasma exchange and ICU staffs and depend on similarly low complication rates outside the auspices of a large trial.

It seems reasonable to conclude that the usual plasma exchange regimen used in these trials (total volume exchanged approximately 200 mL/kg over 7 to 14 days, or four to five exchanges of 3.5 to 4 L in a typical patient) improves outcome in acute GBS. There is no apparent value in rushing the series of treatments, but starting them early probably is beneficial. One study has suggested that six exchanges are

TABLE 18.5. *Results of North American Guillain–Barré Syndrome Plasma Exchange Trial: Status of Guillain–Barré syndrome patients 4 weeks after randomization*

Group	Plasmapheresis	Conventional	P value
All patients			
Improved at least one grade	64/108 (59%)	47/120 (39%)	<0.01
Mean grade change	1.1 grade	0.4 grade	<0.001
Respirator patient subgroup			
Improved at least one grade	26/52 (50%)	18/52 (35%)	0.08
Mean grade change	0.8 grade	0.1 grade	<0.001
Time required for all patients to improve one grade			
All patients—median days	19	40	<0.001
Respirator patients—median days	24	48	<0.01
Time for patients to reach grade 2 (able to walk unassisted)			
All patients			
Median days	53	85	<0.001
Respirator patients			
Median days	97	169	<0.01

From Guillain-Barré Syndrome Study Group. Plasmapheresis and acute Guillain-Barré syndrome. *Neurology* 1985;35:1096–1104, with permission.

no better than four in severely affected patients (99). The replacement fluid has varied between centers (100), but is usually a solution of 850 mL saline with 150 mL of 25% albumin per liter; solutions with more albumin may be associated with mild hypotension toward the end of the procedure. The issue of retreatment or sequential treatment with intravenous immune globulin (IVIG) in cases that do not improve is addressed in the following.

The type and incidence of complications, including infections, do not differ between groups. The risks of treatment are small and vascular catheter insertion, usually in the subclavian vein, is justified if adequate flow cannot be established from the arm.

Approximately 10% of patients who improve after a course of several plasma exchanges deteriorate again in the week or two following the end of the course of treatment (at times, up to 40 days later). A small number of these instances owe to purely respiratory decompensation in fatigued patients with marginal pulmonary reserve or to pulmonary embolism, sepsis, or pneumonia; however, most are the result of a limited relapse of the neuropathy, presumably because of a return of immune activity directed against nerves. As with relapses following IVIG, most such patients have improved with a second course of

several exchanges and generally do not go on to have a chronically relapsing course.

Plasma exchange does not appear to involve excessive risks for patients with minor autonomic dysfunction. Hypotension and minor arrhythmias occur more often in these patients, but they can be minimized by using adequate fluid replacement and cardiac rhythm monitoring if necessary. We have avoided exchanging patients with myocardial infarctions in the previous 6 months, those with new arrhythmias, or episodes of profound hypotension discussed in the preceding. It should be kept in mind that plasma exchanges produce a mild coagulopathy as a result of the depletion of fibrinogen and other clotting factors, for which reason procedures such as lumbar puncture and tracheostomy should be performed only after delay or after assuring adequate clotting mechanisms.

Gamma-Globulin (IVIG)

The intravenous administration of pooled gamma-globulin has been as effective as plasma exchange in treating acute GBS and its relative ease of use has made it the more popular immune treatment. A Dutch randomized study concluded that 0.4 g/kg per day immunoglobulin intravenously for 5 days is effective (101) and several subsequent reports confirm this. The cost of the two treatments in the United States is comparable. Adverse effects are infrequent but may include anaphylaxis, local vascular immune responses in the veins, myocardial infarction, and congestive heart failure. Renal failure is rare (102). A few patients have an aseptic meningitis and severe headache that virtually precludes further treatment.

Corticosteroids

Because of their lympholytic effect, high-dose steroids have been used for GBS even though there is no satisfactory evidence that they alter the course of the acute disease. Hughes and colleagues have shown in two randomized trials that there is no overall benefit (103,104). Some neurologists (some of the authors included), on the strength of personal cases that showed impressive improvement, still use large doses of corticosteroids occasionally when other treatments are precluded in rapidly deteriorating patients (e.g., intravenous methylprednisolone 125 mg every 6 hours for 1 to 3 days followed by slowly tapering oral steroids) (20); however, in view of the available data, this therapy cannot be recommended for routine use.

Failure to Respond to Treatment and Combined Treatments

It should be stated that improvement in the clinical state is evident only when large populations of patients are examined, not in an individual patient under observation. Two issues derived from this are likely to arise in severely affected ICU patients. First is the problem of a patient who deteriorates despite treatment with IVIG or plasma exchange and who becomes quadriplegic and ventilator dependent. Cases such as these that evolve rapidly, over days or less, are usually caused by the axonal type of GBS and, in our experience, benefit little from any immune treatment; large trials indicate minimal improvement when com-

pared to no treatment. The understandable inclination to continue treatment or switch to the alternative (IVIG after exchanges or vice versa or even to resort to corticosteroids) probably should be resisted in these cases, but no definitive data can be brought to bear on the subject. One study has suggested that retreatment with IVIG may salvage some severely affected patients but this requires confirmation (105). Retrospective analyses have suggested that certain immune profiles may be associated with better outcomes with IVIG but the applicability and practicality of these data are difficult to judge.

Regarding sequential treatment with IVIG after plasma exchange, the only large randomized trial so far has failed to detect a definite benefit, although there may have been a trend in that direction (106). Using plasma exchange after the apparent failure of IVIG has not been studied, ostensibly because the second therapy removes the first. Studies in small groups of patients have suggested that the addition of corticosteroids to one of the conventional therapies may be efficacious, but this also must be considered a tentative conclusion and not the standard approach.

REFERENCES

1. Kennedy RH, Danielson MA, Mulder DW, et al. Guillain-Barré syndrome: a 42-year epidemiologic and clinical study. *Mayo Clin Proc* 1980;53:93–99.
2. Ropper AH. Intensive care of acute Guillain-Barré syndrome. *Can J Neurol Sci* 1994;21:S23.
3. Fulgham JR, Wijdicks EF. Guillain-Barré syndrome. *Crit Care Clin* 1997;52:635–638.
4. Ropper AH. The Guillain-Barré syndrome. *N Engl J Med* 1992;326:1130–1136.
5. Ropper AH, Wijdicks EFM, Truax BT. *Guillain-Barré syndrome.* Philadelphia: FA Davis, 1991.
6. Hughes RAC. *Guillain-Barré syndrome.* London: Springer-Verlag, 1990.
7. Asbury AK. Diagnostic considerations in Guillain-Barré syndrome. *Ann Neurol* 1981;9:1–5.
8. McLeave DJ, Fletcher J, Cruden LC. The Guillain-Barré syndrome in intensive care. *Anaesthesiol Int Care* 1976;4:46–52.
9. Moore P, James O. Management of Guillain-Barré syndrome: incidence management and outcome of major complications. *Crit Care Med* 1981;9:549–555.
10. O'Donohue W, Baker J, Bell G, et al. Respiratory failure in neuromuscular disease: management in a respiratory intensive care unit. *JAMA* 1976;235:733–735.
11. Ropper AH, Kehne SM. Guillain-Barré syndrome:

management of respiratory failure. *Neurology* 1985; 35:1662–1665.

12. Lawn ND, Wijdicks EF. Fatal Guillain-Barré syndrome. *Neurology* 1999;52:635–638.

13. Asbury AK, Arnason BG, Adams RD. The inflammatory lesion in idiopathic polyneuritis. Its role in pathogenesis. *Medicine* 1969;48:173–215.

14. Hafer-Macko CE, Sheikh KA, Li CY, et al. Immune attack on the Schwann cell surface in acute inflammatory demyelinating polyneuropathy. *Ann Neurol* 1996; 39:625–635.

15. Feasby TE, Gilbert JJ, Brown WF, et al. An acute axonal form of Guillain-Barré polyneuropathy. *Brain* 1986;109:1115–1126.

16. Brown WF, Feasby TE. Conduction block and denervation in Guillain-Barré polyneuropathy. *Brain* 1984; 107:219–239.

17. Kaldor J, Speed BR. Guillain-Barré syndrome and *Campylobacter jejuni:* a serological study. *BMJ* 1984;288:1867–1870.

18. Rhodes KM, Tattersfield AE. Guillain-Barré syndrome associated with *Campylobacter jejuni* infection. *BMJ* 1982;285:172.

19. Cornblath DR, McArthur JC, Kennedy PGE, et al. Inflammatory demyelinating peripheral neuropathies associated with human T-cell lymphotropic virus type III infection. *Ann Neurol* 1987;21:320.

20. Arnason BG, Asbury AK. Idiopathic polyneuritis after surgery. *Arch Neurol* 1968;18:500–507.

21. Steiner I, Argov Z, Cahan C, et al. Guillain-Barré syndrome after epidural anesthesia: direct nerve root damage may trigger disease. *Neurology* 1985;35:1473–1475.

22. Ropper AH, Shahani BT. Pain in Guillain-Barré syndrome. *Arch Neurol* 1984;41:511–514.

23. Ropper AH. Severe acute Guillain-Barré syndrome. *Neurology* 1986;36:429–432.

24. Pleasure DE, Lovelace RE, Duvoisin RC. The prognosis of acute polyradiculoneuritis. *Neurology* 1968;18: 1143–1148.

25. Fisher CM. An unusual variant of acute idiopathic polyneuritis (syndrome of ophthalmoplegia, ataxia, and areflexia). *N Engl J Med* 1956;255:57–65.

26. Ropper AH. Unusual clinical variants of and signs of Guillain-Barré syndrome. *Arch Neurol* 1986;43: 1150–1152.

27. Ropper AH. Further regional variants of acute immune polyneuropathology. Biofacial weakness or sixth nerve paresis with paresthesias and lumbar polyradiculopathy, and ataxia with pharngeal-cervical-brachial weakness. *Arch Neurol* 1994;51:671–675.

28. Ropper AH, Shahani BT. Diagnosis and management of acute areflexic paralysis with emphasis on Guillain-Barré syndrome. In: Asbury AK, Gilliat RW, eels. *Peripheral nerve disorders.* London: Butterworth, 1984: 21–45.

29. Winer JB, Hughes RAC, Greenwood RJ, et al. Prognosis in Guillain-Barré syndrome. *Lancet* 1985;1: 1202–1203.

30. Triggs, WJ, Cros D, Gorminak SC, et al. Motor nerve inexcitability in Guillain–Barré syndrome. The spectrum of distal conduction block and axonal degeneration. *Brain* 1992;115:1291–1302.

31. Furlan A, Hanson M, Copperman A, et al. Acute areflexic paralysis. Association with hyperalimentation and hypophosphatemia. *Arch Neurol* 1975;32:706–707.

32. Loeffel N, Rossi L, Mumenthaler M, et al. The Landry-Guillain-Barré syndrome. Complications, prognosis and natural history in 123 cases. *J Neurol Sci* 1977;33:71–79.

33. Henderson RD, Lawn ND, Fletcher DD, et al. The morbidity of Guillain-Barré syndrome admitted to the intensive care unit. *Neurology* 2003;60:17–21.

34. Appenzeller O, Marshall J. Vasomotor disturbance in Landry-Guillain-Barré syndrome. *Arch Neurol* 1963; 9:368–372.

35. Lichtenfield P. Autonomic dysfunction in the Guillain-Barré syndrome. *Am J Med* 1971;50:772–780.

36. Traux BT. Autonomic disturbances in Guillain-Barré syndrome. *Semin Neurol* 1984;4:462–468.

37. Ferraro-Herrera AS, Kern HB, Ngler W. Autonomic dysfunction as the presenting feature of Guillain-Barré syndrome. *Arch Phys Med Rehabil* 1997;78:777–779.

38. Davies AG, Dingle HR. Observations on cardiovascular and neuroendocrine disturbance in the Guillain-Barré syndrome. *J Neurol Neurosurg Psychiatry* 1972; 35:176–179.

39. Greenland P, Griggs RC. Arrhythmic complications in the Guillain-Barré syndrome. *Arch Intern Med* 1980; 140:1053–1055.

40. Ropper AH, Shahani B. Pain in Guillain-Barré syndrome. *Arch Neurol* 1984;41:511–514.

41. Frison J, Sanchez L, Garnacho A, et al. Heart rate variations in the Guillain-Barré syndrome. *BMJ* 1980;281: 694.

42. Smith SA, Smith SE. Heart rate variations in the Guillain-Barré syndrome. *BMJ* 1980;281:1009.

43. Winer JB, Hughes RAC. Identification of patients at risk of arrhythmias in the Guillain-Barré syndrome. *Q J Med* 1988;68:735–739.

44. Pace NL. Cardiac monitoring and demand pacemaker in Guillain-Barré syndrome. *Arch Neurol* 1976;33: 374.

45. Pfeiffer G. Dysautonomia in Guillain-Barré syndrome. *Nervenartz* 1999;70:136–148.

46. Pfeiffer G, Schiller B, Kruse J, et al. Indicators of dysautonomia in severe Guillain-Barré syndrome. *J Neurol* 1999;246:1015–1022.

47. Pfeiffer G, Netzer J. Spectral analysis of heart rate and blood pressure in Guillain-Barré patients with respiratory failure. *J Neurol Sci* 1997;150:39–48.

48. Flachenecker P, Reiners K. Twenty-four-hour heart rate power spectrum for evaluation of autonomic dysfunction in Guillain-Barré syndrome. *J Neurol Sci* 1999;165:144–153.

49. Malkoff MD, Ponzillo JJ, Myles GL, et al. Sinus arrest after administration of intravenous metoclopramide. *Ann Pharmacother* 1995;29:381–383.

50. Posner JB, Ertel NH, Kossmann RJ, et al. Hyponatremia in acute polyneuropathy. *Arch Neurol* 1967;17: 530–541.

51. Penney MD, Murphy D, Walters G. Resetting of osmoreceptor response as a cause of hyponatremia in acute idiopathic polyneuritis. *BMJ* 1979;2:1474–1476.

52. Wijdicks EFM, Ropper AH. Elevated atrial natriuretic factor and blood pressure fluctuations in Guillain-Barré syndrome. *Ann Neurol* 1990;27:337–338.

53. Ropper AH, Marmarou A. Mechanism of pseudotumor in Guillain-Barré syndrome. *Arch Neurol* 1984;41: 259–261.

54. Durocher A, Servias B, Cardroix M, et al. Autonomic

dysfunction in the Guillain-Barré syndrome. Hemodynamic and neurobiochemical features. *Int Care Med* 1980;6:3–6.

55. Lauffer J, Passwell J, Kern G, et al. Raised renin activity in the hypertension of the Guillain-Barré syndrome. *BMJ* 1981;282:1272–1273.

56. Mitchell PL, Meilman E. The mechanism of hypertension in the Guillain-Barré syndrome. *Am J Med* 1967;42:986–995.

57. Dalos NP, Borel C, Hanley DF. Cardiovascular autonomic dysfunction in Guillain-Barré syndrome. Therapeutic implications of Swan-Ganz monitoring. *Arch Neurol* 1988;45:115–117.

58. Ropper AH, Wijdicks EFM. Blood pressure fluctuations in the dysautonomia of Guillain-Barré syndrome. *Arch Neurol* 1990;27:337–338.

59. Weintraub MI. Autonomic failure in Guillain-Barré syndrome-value of Swan-Ganz catheterization. *JAMA* 1979;242:513–514.

60. Eiben RM, Gersony WM. Recognition, prognosis, and treatment of Guillain-Barré syndrome. *Med Clin North Am.* 1963;47:1371–1380.

61. Bredin DP. GBS: the unresolved cardiac problems. *Irish J Med Sci* 1977;146:273.

62. Richards AM, Nicholls MG, Beard MEJ, et al. Severe hypertension and raised hematocrit: unusual presentation of Guillain-Barré syndrome. *Postgrad Med J* 1985;61:53–55.

63. Gande AR, Taylor Nolan KN. Autonomic instability and hypertension resulting in subarachnoid hemorrhage in the Guillain-Barré syndrome. *Int Care Med* 1999;25:1432–1434.

64. McQuillan JJ, Bullock RF. Extreme labile blood pressure in Guillain-Barré syndrome. *Lancet* 1988;2: 172–173.

65. Gracey DR, McMichan JC, Divertie M, et al. Respiratory failure in Guillain-Barré syndrome. A 6 year experience. *Mayo Clin Proc* 1982;57:742–746.

66. Hewer RL, Hilton PJ, Smith AC, et al. Acute polyneuritis requiring artificial respiration. *QJ Med* 1968;147: 479–491.

67. Hedley-White J, Burgess G, Fealey T, et al, eds. *Applied physiology of respiratory care.* Boston: Little, Brown, 1976:245–268.

68. Pontoppidan H, Geffin B, Lowenstein E. Acute respiratory failure in the adult (second of three parts). *N Engl J Med* 1972;287:743–752.

69. Pontoppidan H, Geffin B, Lowenstein E. Acute respiratory failure in the adult (third of three parts). *N Engl J Med* 1972;287:799–806.

70. Ringel SP, Carroll JE. Respiratory complications of neuromuscular disease. In: Weinger WJ, ed. *Respiratory dysfunction in neurological disease.* Mt. Kisco, NY: Futura, 1980:113–115.

71. Roussos C, Macklem PT. The respiratory muscles. *N Engl J Med* 1982;307:786–797.

72. Borel CO, Tilford C, Nichols DG, et al. Diaphragmatic performance during recovery from acute ventilatory failure in Guillain-Barré syndrome and myasthenia gravis. *Chest* 1991;99:444–451.

73. Bellemare F, Grassino A. Force reserve of the diaphragm in patients with chronic obstructive pulmonary disease. *J Appl Physiol* 1983;53:1190–1195.

74. Zifko UA. Electrophysiological respiratory studies in the critical care unit. *Can J Neurol Sci* 1998;25:S21–26.

75. Johnson DC, Kazemi H. Central control of ventilation in neuromuscular disease. *Clin Chest Med* 1994;15: 607–617.

76. Black LF, Hyatt RE. Maximal static respiratory pressures in generalized neuromuscular disease. *Am Rev Respir Dis* 1969;99:696–702.

77. Griggs R, Donohue M, Utell M, et al. Evaluation of pulmonary function in neuromuscular disease. *Arch Neurol* 1981;38:9–12.

78. Ropper AH. Tips for neurologists who care for patients with mechanical respiratory failure. *Semin Neurol* 1984;4:497–498.

79. Lawn N, Wijdicks EF. Post-intubation pulmonary function test in Guillain-Barré syndrome. *Muscle Nerve* 2000;23:613–616.

80. Lands L, Zinman R. Maximal static pressures and lung volumes in a child with Guillain-Barre syndrome ventilated by a cuirass respirator. *Chest* 1986;89:757–760.

81. Newsum JK, Smith RM, Croker D. Intubation for acute respiratory failure in Guillain-Barré syndrome. *JAMA* 1979;242:1650–1651.

82. Lawn ND, Wijdicks EF. Tracheostomy in Guillain-Barré syndrome. *Muscle Nerve* 1999;22:1058–1062.

83. Stauffer JL, Olson DE, Petty TL. Complications and consequences of endotracheal intubation and tracheotomy: a prospective study of 150 critically ill adult patients. *Am J Med* 1981;70:65–76.

84. Yang KL, Tobin MJ. A prospective trial of indexes predicting the outcome of trials of weaning from mechanical ventilation. *N Engl J Med* 1991;324:1445–1450.

85. Tobin MJ. Advances in mechanical ventilation. *N Engl J Med* 2001;344:1986–1996.

86. Downs JB, Klein EF Jr, DeSautels D, et al. Intermittent mandatory ventilation: a new approach to weaning patients from mechanical ventilators. *Chest* 1973;64: 331–335.

87. Kennedy SK, Weintraub RM, Skillman JJ. Cardiorespiratory and sympathoadrenal responses during weaning from controlled ventilation. *Surgery* 1977;82: 233–240.

88. Vargas F, Hilbert G, Gruson D, et al. Fulminant Guillain-Barré syndrome mimicking cerebral death: case report and literature review. *Int Care Med* 2000;26: 623–627.

89. Ravn H. The Landry-Guillain-Barré syndrome. A survey and report of 127 cases. *Acta Neurol Scand* 1967; 43:1–64.

90. Raman TK, Blake JA, Harris TM. Pulmonary embolism in Landry-Guillain-Barré-Strohl syndrome. *Chest* 1971;60:555–557.

91. Roubenoff RA, Borel CO, Hanley DF. Hypermetabolism and hypercatabolism in Guillain-Barré syndrome. *JPEN J Parent Enter Nutr* 1992;16:464–472.

92. Moulin DE, Hagen N, Feasibly TE, et al. Pain in Guillain-Barré syndrome. *Neurology* 1997;48:328–331.

93. Tripathi M, Kaushik S. Carbamazepine for pain management in Guillain-Barré syndrome patients in intensive care units. *Crit Care Med* 2000;28:655–658.

94. Fergusson RJ, Wright DJ, Willey RF, et al. Suxamethonium is dangerous in polyneuropathy. *BMJ* 1981; 282:298–299.

95. Brettle RP, Gross M, Legg NJ, et al. Treatment of acute polyneuropathy by plasma exchange. *Lancet* 1978;2: 1100.

96. Guillain-Barré Syndrome Study Group. Plasmaphere-

sis and acute Guillain-Barré syndrome. *Neurology* 1985;35:1096–1104.

97. Raphael JC, Chastang Cl, Masson C, et al. Guillain-Barré syndrome and plasma exchange. *Lancet* 1985; 2:45.

98. Osterman PO, Lundemo G, Pirskanen R, et al. Controlled trial of plasma exchange in acute inflammatory polyradiculoneuropathy. *Lancet* 1984;1:877–879.

99. The French Cooperative Group on Plasma Exchange in Guillain-Barré Syndrome. Appropriate number of plasma exchanges in Guillain-Barré syndrome. *Ann Neurol* 1997;41:287–288.

100. Shumak HH, Humphrey JG, Chin JY, et al. The effect of replacement solution (plasma or albumin) on the response of acute Guillain-Barré syndrome to plasma exchange. *Plasma Ther Transfus Techno* 1985;6: 427–431.

101. van der Meché FGA, Schmitz PIM. Dutch Guillain-Barré Study Group. A randomized trial comparing intravenous gamma-globulin and plasma exchange in acute Guillain-Barré syndrome. *N Engl J Med* 1992; 326:1123–1129.

102. Levy JB, Pusey CD. Nephrotoxicity of intravenous immunoglobulin. *QJM* 2000;93:751–756.

103. Hughes RA, Newsom-Davis JM, Perkins GD, et al. Controlled trial prednisolone in acute polyneuropathy. *Lancet* 1978;2:750–753.

104. Hughes RAC. Ineffectiveness of high-dose methyl prednisolone in Guillain-Barré syndrome. *Lancet* 1991;338:1142.

105. Farcas P, Avnun L, Frisher S, et al. Efficacy of repeated intravenous immunoglobulin in severe unresponsive Guillain-Barré syndrome. *Lancet* 1997;350:1747.

106. Plasma exchange/Sandoglobulin Guillain-Barré Syndrome Trial Group. Randomised trial of plasma exchange, intravenous immunoglobulin, and combined treatments in Guillain-Barré syndrome. *Lancet* 1997;349:225–230.

19

Treatment of the Critically Ill Patient with Myasthenia Gravis

Myasthenia gravis (MG) is an uncommon disorder of immune pathogenesis that affects neuromuscular transmission and causes regional and generalized fatigable weakness. Its prevalence is 0.5 to five per 100,000 population (1). The effectiveness of anticholinesterase medications in ameliorating the symptoms was discovered in the 1930s by Walker, and the relationship of thymectomy to clinical improvement was first noted in 1939 by Blalock. Simpson proposed the role of the immune system in 1960, and antibodies to the acetylcholine receptor were discovered in 1973 by Patrick and Lindstrom.

The event that initiates the production of autoimmune acetylcholine receptor antibodies is unknown, but the increased incidence of autoimmune thyroid disease (10%), systemic lupus erythematosus, rheumatoid arthritis, pernicious anemia, and idiopathic thrombocytopenia in patients with myasthenia and their relatives suggests a more pervasive problem in the immune system. Furthermore, a genetic predisposition exists in young women with human leukocyte antigen types A1, B8, DRW3, and B12 (2). There are no important geographic factors, and curiously, few familial cases have been reported (3). The disease most commonly occurs in two age groups: young women (15 to 30 years old) and older men (60 to 75 years old) (4,5). About 10% of patients manifest a thymoma; most other patients have thymic enlargement owing to hyperplasia. Thymomas tend to occur in the older age group, and the long-term prognosis for these patients is far worse because of the severity of their myasthenia regardless of type of treatment or the extent of spread of the thymoma (6).

The relative importance of the roles of cell- and antibody-mediated damage to the acetylcholine receptor have not yet been determined, but it is clear that the main clinical feature of the disease, fluctuating skeletal muscle weakness, is related largely to binding of IgG antibodies to the postsynaptic acetylcholine receptor. There is destruction of the receptors and a reduction in the surface area of the postsynaptic membrane (7). In myasthenia, the normal process of receptor degradation is reduced from 7 days to less than 48 hours by a complement-mediated destruction and phagocytosis.

In the last two decades, treatment with corticosteroids, immunosuppressive medications, plasma exchange, and intravenous immunoglobulin has been added to the standard approach with anticholinesterase drugs, thymectomy, and advanced respiratory care to improve greatly the prognosis of patients with MG (8). At Columbia–Presbyterian Medical Center during the 1940s and 1950s, the mortality in patients with MG was greater than 30% (9). This declined to 12% during the 1960s, 3.3% during the 1970s, and even lower in the 1980s and 1990s (10).

CLINICAL FEATURES

The fluctuating nature of myasthenic weakness, truly a work-related fatigue, makes it a unique clinical disorder. Patients complain less of fatigue than of weakness

TABLE 19.1. *Modified Osserman classification of myasthenia gravis*

Class 1	Patients with ocular involvement alone
Class 2	Mild weakness, not incapacitating, without oropharyngeal or respiratory muscle involvement
Class 3	Moderate weakness, not incapacitating, including oropharyngeal and respiratory muscle weakness
Class 4	Incapacitating weakness of any muscle system, including oropharyngeal and respiratory muscle weakness
Class 5	Life-threatening respiratory insufficiency requiring ventilatory assistance (crisis)

and this weakness is regional in the early stages of illness. In the majority, ocular muscles are affected first, resulting in ptosis and diplopia in about 40%; these muscles are ultimately affected in 90% of patients. The facial and oropharyngeal muscles are also commonly affected, resulting in dysarthria, dysphagia, and facial diplegia. On occasion, swallowing is impaired before the ocular signs appear. Virtually all patients with MG have some involvement of oropharyngeal and ocular muscles at some time during the course of illness. Isolated limb or diaphragm weakness is rare. An exacerbation with generalized weakness that includes respiratory muscles to the point of ventilatory failure is termed "myasthenic crisis." Thirty percent of patients with MG develop some degree of respiratory muscle weakness, and 15% to 20% experience at least one episode of "crisis." Numerous series of such patients with acute worsening have been reported, all emphasizing a high rate of morbidity and mortality (see the following for treatment of myasthenic crisis) (11–14).

A practical clinical classification for the severity of MG was devised by Osserman in 1958 and is still used with modifications by most centers that specialize in the treatment of MG (Table 19.1) (15,16).

The specialist in critical care can expect to treat severely ill patients in class 4 or 5. Only rarely does such a patient enter the hospital without a previously known diagnosis of MG. Most patients have been symptomatic for at least several months before developing respiratory compromise (Table 19.2). On occasion, a patient with unsuspected MG who has acute respiratory failure of unknown cause (17–19) is admitted from the emergency room or transferred from another hospital. Rare instances of myasthenia presenting as stridor or isolated respiratory failure have been reported and may come to the attention of the intensivist (20). Another such idiosyncrasy occurs during obstetric delivery or general surgery, in which a previously undiagnosed myasthenic patient may develop respiratory failure as a result of the administration of neuromuscular blocking drugs,

TABLE 19.2. *Characteristics of myasthenic crisis*

	1960–1980[a]	1983–1994[b]
No. patients	61	53
Average age	38 yr F; 62 y M	55 yr; 2:1 F:M
Duration before crisis (range)	21 mo, median; (2 mo–8 y)	8 mo, mean (20–82 wk)
Crisis within 1 year of onset of myasthenia gravis	36%	53%
Duration of mechanical ventilation (range)	2 wk median	13 d; (1 d–5 mo)
Mortality	42%	4% before extubation; 6% after extubation

[a]Data from Cohen MS, Younger D. Aspects of the natural history of myasthenia gravis: crisis and death. *Ann NY Acad Sci* 1981;377:670–677.
[b]Data from Thomas CS, Mayer SA, Gungor Y, et al. Myasthenic crisis: clinical features, mortality, complications and risk factors for prolonged mechanical ventilation. *Neurology* 1997;48:1253–1260.

agents known to greatly exaggerate the neuromuscular failure of MG (21).

Many other medications are known to worsen the symptoms of MG (22,23) but their propensity to uncover a previously unsuspected case is low in comparison to the neuromuscular blocking drugs. In this regard, the risk of the use of aminoglycoside and related antibiotics is often raised in the treatment in urinary or pulmonary infections. There is an undoubted effect on strength in marginally compensated individuals but most such patients are already intubated and the drugs can be used freely. In others less affected, surveillance for respiratory failure should be enhanced. Other medications, particularly β-blockers, present a similar but lesser risk.

Diagnosis

The diagnosis of MG depends on the presence of the appropriate clinical syndrome combined with electrodiagnostic features of impaired neuromuscular transmission (decremental response with repetitive nerve stimulation or increased "jitter" and blocking of impulses with single-fiber electromyography), a clinical response to cholinergic drugs [edrophonium (Tensilon)] or neostigmine test, and the presence in the serum of antibodies against the acetylcholine receptor. The sensitivity of these tests varies with the severity of the disease and the level of experience of the laboratory. The most frequently employed technique is repetitive stimulation of a muscle to elicit a decremental contraction. An increase in the variability of the timing of firing of linked muscle fibers within a motor unit, called "jitter," can be demonstrated in 90% of weak muscles by the use of single-fiber electromyography. This reflects intermittent blocking of impulses at individual neuromuscular junctions. Acetylcholine receptor antibodies are present in high titer in 90% of patients with generalized or longstanding myasthenia, but in only 50% of patients with ocular signs alone (24). Restated, at least 10% of patients with typical MG are "seronegative" (25,26). The intravenous edrophonium

test most clearly, but only briefly, ameliorates weakness (i.e., is positive) in patients with ocular signs (ptosis and strabismus) but the results are more difficult to assess in patients with limb weakness or respiratory failure alone. An alternative test using neostigmine, 2 mg intramuscularly is generally preferable in patients with respiratory failure or unusual patterns of limb weakness. The action of intramuscular neostigmine reaches a peak at 15 to 30 minutes, allowing for repeated clinical examination and measurements of vital capacity (VC) and maximal expiratory pressure in order to detect a definite increment.

In the critical care setting, the differential diagnosis of myasthenic crisis is limited mainly to other neuromuscular diseases that cause oropharyngeal and respiratory muscle weakness, namely Lambert–Eaton myasthenic syndrome, periodic paralysis, Guillain–Barré syndrome—particularly the oropharyngeal variant (Chapter 18), mitochondrial myopathies, muscular dystrophy, polymyositis, motor neuron diseases, botulism, organophosphate poisoning, and poison snake or spider bites (27,28). Central nervous system diseases with prominent brainstem features and processes that affect multiple cranial nerves may mimic the oculopharyngeal features of MG. Two such examples are a 35-year-old woman who underwent thymectomy for presumed myasthenic bilateral ptosis and ophthalmoparesis and was later found to have bilateral giant cavernous-carotid aneurysms; and a 68-year-old man who developed dysphagia and dysarthria followed by respiratory failure. He required intubation and mechanical ventilation, was treated with intensive plasma exchange, and improved over a 2-week period. After extubation, magnetic resonance imaging (MRI) of the brainstem revealed a cavernous angioma with recent hemorrhage in the medulla.

Myasthenic Crisis

This aspect of the disease is most likely to involve the neurointensivist. Two of the most extensive and useful clinical analyses of myasthenic crisis are from the Columbia–Presbyterian Medical Center and in most ways reflect our general experience. Most points regarding the problem can be gleaned from a record review of 447 myasthenic patients between 1960 and 1980 (29), and a more recent survey comprising 53 patients with crisis (30). Of patients seen during the earlier 20-year period, 16% (61 patients) had at least one episode of crisis. Among 36 women, crisis occurred at a mean age of 38 years; the first crisis in men occurred later at a mean age of 62 years; the average age was 55 years in the later series. The interval between onset of myasthenia and the first crisis is shown in Table 19.2. The often-stated dictum, concordant with our own experience, that most crises occur within the first year of illness, was found in the more recent series of Thomas and colleagues (8 months average duration of illness before crisis) (30). One third of their patients had more than one episode of crisis, again usually within a year of the first. In up to one half of the episodes, there was no obvious cause for the exacerbation other than progressive myasthenic weakness. However, many patients had severe dysarthria and dysphagia at the time. In others, overt pneumonia or other respiratory infection precipitated respiratory failure but not always severe generalized weakness. Four patients in the older series had sudden cardiorespiratory arrest, two had respiratory depression secondary to sedative drugs, two had pulmonary embolism, and two patients, not known previously to have MG, were given curare during elective surgery and had prolonged ventilatory failure. Therefore, many of these cases did not conform to the usual definition of myasthenic crisis but were operationally equivalent because they resulted in admission to the intensive care unit (ICU).

In the later series, the mean VC just prior to intubation was high, 27 mL/kg, presumably reflecting the need to intubate some patients for protection of the airway rather than for ventilatory failure. Positive-pressure ventilation was required for varying periods, ranging from several hours to 1 year. In the more modern series, half of patients were extubated by 13 days, and 75% by 31 days. It is notable that three patients died from cardiac arrest during tracheostomy, presently a rare occurence.

Steroid therapy was being administered to 16 patients at the onset of crisis. These agents, used as treatment for crisis, were started for the first time in 11 patients who had been on a respirator for more than 2 weeks. In a retrospective analysis, it was impossible to ascertain if steroids had a beneficial effect in weaning the patient off the respirator.

The mortality rate of crisis has declined in recent years; presumably this reflects modern critical care techniques and possibly the introduction of plasma exchange and immunoglobulin therapy (see the following). In a review of patients by Chang and Fink from 1983 to 1991 (31), there had been no deaths from crisis, but in subsequent years there certainly have been several. In the later Columbia series the mortality rate was 10% overall, half of those dying after extubation. It is reemphasized that although plasma exchange and immune globulin are routinely used in the treatment of crisis, their efficacy remains uncertain, as discussed more extensively in the following.

Cholinergic Crisis

The frequency of cholinergic crisis in MG is somewhat uncertain. These crises indisputably occur with overdosage of cholinesterase-binding organophosphate toxins. Whereas much was made of the problem in the older literature, recent experience suggests their importance is overrated (32) in all likelihood because of the more cautious use of anticholinesterase drugs. The types and equivalent dosages of the cholinesterase inhibitors in clinical use are listed in Table 19.3.

Osserman and Genkins (15,16) described the syndrome as a worsening of myasthenic weakness caused by depolarization blockade of certain muscle groups from excessive anticholinesterase administration. To optimize the dosage of medications, they advocated an

TABLE 19.3. *Cholinergic drug dosage equivalents and duration of action*

	Equivalent dose	Onset	Maximum response
Pyridostigmine (Mestinon)	60 mg (p.o.)	40 min	1 h
Neostigmine (p.o.)	15 mg (p.o.)	1 h	1.5 h
Neostigmine (i.m.)	1.5 mg (i.m.)	30 min	1 h
Neostigmine	0.5 mg (i.v.)	Immediate	20 min

i.m., intramuscular; i.v., intravenous; p.o., oral.

edrophonium test. As originally described, 1 or 2 mg of edrophonium is injected intravenously. If weakness improved, true "myasthenic" crisis was assumed to be the problem, and the dosage of cholinesterase inhibitor was increased. If there was no improvement or if weakness worsened, "cholinergic" crisis was assumed, and the dosage of cholinesterase inhibitor was decreased. This technique is now little used in the management of patients with MG who have an exacerbation but it may have some utility in selected cases where the distinction is unclear. More often, patients are so weakened that they require intubation in any case, and the drugs are temporarily withdrawn.

At most institutions, it has become standard practice to discontinue all cholinergic medication whenever a patient requires mechanical respiratory support. We have only rarely observed a patient to improve immediately after discontinuing cholinergic medication; usually, the weakness becomes worse. If cholinergic crisis occurs, some patients should improve immediately with medication withdrawal. In their review of myasthenic crisis, Cohen and Younger (29) noted cessation of cholinergic medication in 50 of 94 attacks. Cholinergic crises could not be confidently diagnosed in any of these patients because improvement did not occur in the following 72 hours.

EVALUATION OF THE CRITICALLY ILL MYASTHENIC PATIENT

Readers are referred to several authoritative sources for the routine evaluation of a patient with suspected myasthenia gravis (33–35). This chapter focuses on patients with severe exacerbations and impending ventilatory failure.

The clinical manifestations of respiratory failure in a patient with MG are similar to other acute neuromuscular diseases. Patients may display the following symptoms or signs: early on, restlessness, insomnia, anxiety, tachycardia, diaphoresis, and tachypnea; and much later, headache, central cyanosis, hypotension, confusion and asterixis. It is impossible to predict accurately the arterial oxygen tension (PaO_2) and arterial carbon dioxide tension ($PaCO_2$) by clinical observation alone, and the diagnosis of respiratory failure requires arterial blood gas analysis. PaO_2 less than 60 mm Hg or $PaCO_2$ greater than 50 mm Hg unequivocally demonstrates respiratory failure. However, as emphasized in Chapter 18 regarding Guillain–Barré syndrome, it is more important to detect deteriorating function before overt respiratory failure develops (36). Rieder and colleagues have suggested that repeated measurement of VC is a poor guide to the need for intubation in MG (37). Their series was small, retrospective, and compared VC less than 20 mL/kg to less than 13 mL/kg or to a derived index as predictors of the need for mechanical ventilation. Our experience does not accord with theirs but their main point, that the course of the illness is unpredictable, is well taken. By the time hypoxemia occurs, the patient may be near respiratory arrest. As VC falls and the cough and sigh mechanisms deteriorate, basal atelectasis develops. This results in mild hypoxemia because of shunting of blood through the poorly ventilated lung (as described in Chapters 4 and 18). In neuromuscular ventilatory failure, the earliest indication ancillary sign of critical impending respiratory failure is usually mild hypoxemia. Weakness of the oropharyngeal muscles represents a separate but often coexisting risk. Elective endotracheal intubation at the appropriate time can prevent aspiration pneumonia and respiratory arrest.

The simplest and most reliable way to determine impending ventilatory failure is by the use of frequent bedside measurements of VC with a hand-held spirometer. A normal VC is approximately 55 mL/kg depending on body size, age, and preexisting respiratory disease; a reduction to 30 mL/kg is associated with a poor cough and accumulation of oropharyngeal secretions. At a level of 25 mL/kg, the sigh mechanism is impaired, atelectasis develops, and mild hypoxemia may result. If the VC falls below 15 mL/kg, elective intubation is usually necessary to provide positive pressure ventilation (Fig. 18.3).

Because of the high incidence of respiratory infection associated with myasthenic crisis, a high-quality chest x-ray should be obtained, and appropriate culture specimens should be taken. Other causes of respiratory failure unrelated to myasthenia must be excluded in certain circumstances (pulmonary embolism, pneumothorax, cardiac failure). Even if all objective measurements indicate adequate spontaneous ventilation, a patient with myasthenic crisis should be considered very unstable and monitored in an intensive care or close-observation unit. Abrupt deterioration from muscle fatigue is common.

Treatment of Myasthenic Crisis

Mechanical Ventilation

Nasotracheal intubation may be preferred in a patient with neuromuscular disease who is fully awake (38–40). It is more comfortable for the patient and has less chance of tube displacement during movement. Many anesthesiologists dispute this and prefer oral intubation to prevent nasal bleeding. Following the usual respiratory ICU practices, a low-pressure cuff is inflated to just barely seal the trachea during inspiration. Each shift, the nurse should deflate and reinflate the cuff, noting the volume required to make a seal. An initial inspired oxygen concentrations of 50% is used until arterial blood gases are determined. The FIO_2, is gradually reduced to provide a PaO_2 of 85 to 100 mm Hg. Typical respirator settings are positive end-expiratory pressure of 3 to 5 mm Hg, tidal volume of 12 mL/kg, initial respiratory rate of 12 per minute, inspiratory flow rate of 30 to 40 L/minute. The addition, or in mild cases, the exclusive use of "pressure-support" is advocated; however, eventually most such patients require large volume cycles. Cuirass negative-pressure techniques and novel respiratory patterns such as low-volume jet ventilation have not been studied systematically in neuromuscular disease, but our experience suggests they have limited utility.

Cholinergic medications are generally discontinued after the initiation of mechanical ventilation (see discussion further on). These drugs are not necessary after the patient is intubated, and they cause excessive bronchial secretions and diarrhea when used in conjunction with nasogastric tube feedings. Most patients have cholinergic medications restarted when the acute episode has resolved. The optimal timing for reintroducing these medications is uncertain, but our experience suggests that there is no benefit in starting them in the presence of fever, pulmonary infection, or severe respiratory failure. The best results are obtained when medication is restarted during spontaneous improvement in respiratory function and the patient is ready to wean from mechanical ventilation. Others continue them in low doses before recovery from crisis.

Tracheostomy is considered if the patient requires airway protection or mechanical ventilation for more than 2 weeks. Other reasons for tracheostomy include poor patient tolerance of the endotracheal tube because of pain, inadequate access for suctioning through the endotracheal tube, or unsuccessful tracheal intubation. Tracheostomy should be performed in a stable elective situation to prevent long-term complications such as tracheal stenosis. If possible, there should be an interval of 1 day or more after plasma exchange in order to avoid excessive bleeding; in any case, coagulation parameters guide this timing. Emergency airway protection can be performed by cricothyroid membrane puncture if endotracheal intubation is impossible.

After several days of rest on a mechanical ventilator without any other treatment, a proportion of patients with MG (about one third in our experience) improve spontaneously and can tolerate extubation. At 2 weeks, about one half of patients with myasthenic crisis can be extubated. Bedside pulmonary function tests are used to determine readiness for weaning and extubation: guidelines are a VC greater than 15 mL/kg, inspiratory pressure greater than 25 cm H_2O, expiratory pressure greater than 40 cm H_2O, Pao_2 greater than 80 mm Hg with FIo_2 of 40%, Pco_2 less than 42, and a spontaneous respiratory rate less than 20 allow weaning (see Chapter 18). The ability to voluntarily double the resting minute volume is a popular threshold for extubation but few of our myasthenic patients have been able to achieve it and are nonetheless weaned. As mentioned in Chapter 18, the use of the pressure support mode of ventilation may assist in gradually weaning the patient but many alternative methods are equivalent.

As in other critically ill patients, adverse medical conditions delay weaning and extubation—fluid overload, anemia, diminished consciousness, fever, acidosis, alkalosis, gastric distention, drug-induced respiratory depression, cardiac arrhythmias, renal failure, and hypovolemia. Hyperthyroidism is common in patients with MG and may precipitate respiratory failure or delay the weaning process (41). Aggressive nutritional therapy should be initiated as early as possible lest inadequate nutrition impair spontaneous respiratory strength and weaning.

Cholinergic Drugs

Some aspects of the use of these medications in myasthenic crisis have already been mentioned, namely their discontinuation once mechanical ventilation has been established

and their slow reintroduction as the patient improves. The maximal effective dose of pyridostigmine (Mestinon) is about 120 mg every 3 hours; some patients tolerate slightly more when they are well. There are fewer gastrointestinal side effects with pyridostigmine than with neostigmine. If the patient is unable to swallow because of severe oropharyngeal muscle weakness, we usually resort to a nasogastric feeding tube to administer medications. Some authorities have suggested using parenteral forms of pyridostigmine for patients who are unable to swallow. In our experience, the response to this form is unpredictable, and it may induce extreme bronchorrhea and airway obstruction.

Our practice has been to restart cholinergic medications at one half the previous dosage when the patient has reached the criteria for weaning from the ventilator. Some patients show a marked response to a neostigmine test with a significant increase in VC and expiratory pressures. In those situations, cholinergic drugs may be started sooner.

An alternative used in some centers is continuous infusion of pyridostigmine, beginning at 2 mg/hour and slowly increasing the dose until a benefit occurs in respiratory function (42,43). We have scant experience with this technique but have had difficulty as a result of bronchial secretions and the need for frequent atropine administration.

Corticosteroids and Immunosuppressive Drugs

Adrenocorticotrophic hormone was used for the treatment of MG as far back as 1951, but it was not until 1971, when oral prednisone became popular, that the use of corticosteroids in the treatment of MG became widespread. Although corticosteroids are widely used and accepted as appropriate treatment for MG, their efficacy has never been studied in randomized placebo-controlled clinical trials. It has long been recognized that these agents may have a direct adverse effect on neuromuscular transmission when they are first introduced; indeed, they may precipitate a crisis. There is also controversy about the merits of various dosage schedules (44,45). Some investigators have recommended high-dose intravenous "pulse" therapy, some recommend high-dose oral therapy, and others recommend both high- and low-dose alternate-day schedules (46–49). In one of the largest uncontrolled clinical series from the University of Virginia, 116 patients were treated with prednisone, 60 to 80 mg daily until improvement and then were changed to lower-dose alternate-day therapy for up to several years (50). With this regimen, 80% achieved either remission or marked improvement. Patients older than 60 years had a higher response rate (95%) and the time to the onset of improvement was about 2 weeks. Within the first 6 months of treatment, rapid reduction of dosage often was associated with a relapse, as has been our unfortunate experience. Almost 50% of patients experienced temporary worsening of their myasthenia within a few days of starting treatment.

We use corticosteroids for patients who are not already on immunosuppressive drugs, are in crisis, and remain ventilator-dependent for 2 weeks despite intensive plasma exchange or immunoglobulin. In severe crisis, an appropriate regimen is 1 mg/kg of prednisone in a single daily dose continued for at least 1 month. If there is improvement, the patient is generally committed to at least 6 months of treatment. After several weeks the daily dosage can be changed to alternate-day therapy (2 mg/kg) and then gradually reduced by 2.5 mg every 2 weeks as long as the disease is stable. During crisis, significant improvement infrequently occurs until 10 to 14 days. In lesser-affected patients and those improving rapidly after plasma exchange or immunoglobulin, slightly lower doses can be used. Those who have been on steroids prior to the onset of crisis have the drugs continued or the dose raised. Patients with severe disease who undergo thymectomy may already be treated with steroids preoperatively, and the medication is continued intraoperatively and postoperatively.

Azathioprine (Imuran) has not enjoyed the widespread use that corticosteroids have attained but clinical studies have shown an 80% remission or improvement rate in patients treated with azathioprine for more than 6 months (51,52). Some patients who have not responded to steroids have shown an excellent response to azathioprine, but unfortunately often have significant side effects (53). In the critical care setting, however, the necessity to begin azathioprine is reduced because of a delay of 3 to 6 months before benefits are observed. Nevertheless, it can be started in anticipation of longer-term therapy, as a steroid-sparing drug.

In recalcitrant patients who cannot be weaned from the ventilator or remain bedbound as a result of weakness, other immunosuppressive agents, such as methotrexate, mercaptopurine, and cyclosporine, have been shown to be effective in small clinical trials. Cyclosporine was more effective than placebo in a small double-blind, randomized trial, and larger trials comparing it with placebo and other immunosuppressive agents have given conflicting but generally positive results (54–56).

Plasma Exchange, Immunoglobulin Infusion, and Immunoadsorption

Since its first use to treat MG in the 1970s, plasma exchange has been reported in numerous uncontrolled clinical series of varying sizes to have a beneficial effect on myasthenic weakness (57,58). The mechanism of action is uncertain, and there is only a rough correspondence between clinical improvement and reduction in acetylcholine receptor antibody titers. As noted below, plasma exchange for MG has been subjected to study in few controlled trials, yet most clinicians consider it to be effective (59–61). There is general agreement that plasma exchange has short-term benefit only, and it is generally recommended for situations where temporary improvement is sought until more definitive therapy is effective (62).

Three to five daily plasma exchanges are performed, and sometimes more (1.5 to 2 L per exchange), until pulmonary function reaches 80% of its predicted normal value. Plasma is replaced with saline and 5% normal serum albumin. A 2-L plasma exchange theoretically removes 88% of the antiacetylcholine receptor antibody from blood, and equilibration with the extracellular compartment reduces tissue antibody levels in 3 to 5 days. This corresponds with the timing of clinical improvement but it is not clear that the two are linked. If plasma exchange is performed first, the worsening that is sometimes associated with corticosteroid therapy is not often observed.

Most centers use plasma exchange only to treat patients with severe generalized MG, for crisis, or for those with such severe oropharyngeal weakness that they are at risk of aspiration. The most frequent justification is to shorten the time on mechanical ventilation and prevent the morbidity associated with respiratory failure (63). There are dozens of small anecdotal series supporting its use in these situations, but this approach has not been evaluated in a randomized clinical trial. In a retrospective review of patients treated with plasma exchange for crisis from 1983 to 1990 at Columbia Presbyterian Hospital, there was no difference in the time spent on a ventilator compared with an historic control group from the 1970s (Mathew Fink, personal communication). The complications of plasma exchange are well known and have been reviewed elsewhere (64). The most treacherous ones in our experience have derived from insertion of a subclavian or jugular venous double or triple lumen catheter for venous access, including one fatality from a hemothorax.

The only prospective randomized comparison of plasma exchange versus immunoglobulin (comprising 87 patients) in the treatment of exacerbation of myasthenia of varying severity found no differences in outcome (65). In a retrospective study of 54 instances of crisis, exchanges were felt to be superior to immunoglobulin with regard to ventilatory status 2 weeks later but the complication rate was higher (66). Two small groups (four and 12 patients) have been reported in which plasma exchange was apparently beneficial

after immunoglobulin had failed (67,68). There are no clear reasons to choose one treatment over the other but it has been our impression that exchanges are more often successful.

Plasma exchange is also used to prepare patients for thymectomy if they have evidence of respiratory muscle weakness (see the following), but most do not require this treatment because they have the operation at an earlier stage of the illness. The regimen is the same as for crisis.

During the past several years, intravenous infusion of pooled human immunoglobulin has been tried, again, with numerous anecdotal reports of benefit (69–72). The dose has generally reflected practice in acute Guillain–Barré syndrome (400 mg/kg per day for 4 or 5 consecutive days). The mechanism of action is not known but is thought to be effective by binding of the receptor antibodies by the infused immunoglobulin or blockade of phagocytes that destroy the receptors. Some investigators have suggested infusion of immunoglobulin after plasma exchange, as mentioned.

Immunoadsorption of acetylcholine receptor antibodies is an alternative newer technique that has been used to supplant plasma exchange in the treatment of MG (73–76). It is safe and feasible for long-term use in patients with chronic refractory disease. There are fewer complications than with the use of repeated plasma exchange but the procedure has not been extensively studied and is not widely available; therefore, its role in comparison to plasma exchange during crisis is not clear.

ROLE OF THYMECTOMY AND PERIOPERATIVE MANAGEMENT FOR OTHER SURGERIES

Between 1939 and 1941, Blalock published results of thymectomies in the treatment of MG. At the time, the morbidity and mortality of the operation was high but so was the untreated disease. Initially, thymectomy was reserved for patients with thymomas. After pathologic confirmation of thymic hyperplasia in most patients with MG, thymectomy became the accepted standard therapy for most patients with generalized MG (77). Exceptions are made in elderly patients with severe medical problems or thymomas, all of whom tend to have a complicated surgical course and poor outcome after thymectomy. Here again, there has not been a randomized clinical trial to evaluate the benefits of thymectomy or compare its efficacy to immunosuppressive medications, and we must rely on natural history studies.

One of the most helpful of such series from the Netherlands reported the long-term outcome in 73 patients diagnosed between 1926 and 1965 and followed until 1985 (78). The only treatment was anticholinesterase medication. The maximum severity of disease occurred during the first 7 years after onset in 87% of patients. Eighteen (29%) patients died, of whom eight had a thymoma. At the end of the study, 16 (22%) patients were in complete remission, 13 (18%) improved considerably, 12 (16%) improved moderately, 12 (16%) remained the same, and two patients deteriorated. If the patients who died are excluded from analysis, the spontaneous improvement rate is 75% (41 of 55). For comparison, one of the best published series regarding thymectomy reported 95 patients with generalized myasthenia undergoing "maximal" thymectomy and followed for up to 89 months (79). In the 72 patients without thymoma, 46% (33) were in complete remission, and 33% (24) were symptom-free on minimal doses of anticholinesterase medication, for a total improvement rate of 79%. Although thymectomy is considered standard treatment (we do not doubt that it is), it is difficult to prove that it improves the natural history. One alternative explanation for the reduced mortality of the disease in recent years is that improvements in overall medical care allow patients to survive long enough to have a spontaneous remission.

The surgical technique (median sternotomy with "maximal" thymectomy versus transcervical thymectomy) is a somewhat controversial issue and beyond the scope of this chapter. The transcervical approach has less morbidity and greater patient acceptance. However, there are many cases of incomplete removal of the thymus with the transcervical approach, resulting in disease relapse and need for reoperation through the transsternal approach (80). Nevertheless, most large series of transcervical thymectomies report similar rates of remission and improvement as transsternal operations.

Just prior to the procedure, anticholinesterase medications are withheld and large doses of corticosteroids are administered approximately 6 hours before, just prior to, and after the procedure, but only if these drugs had been used previously.

Postoperative problems after thymectomy are usually few because the procedure is done at early stages of the disease. If the myasthenic patient has normal pulmonary function tests preoperatively, the postoperative course is uneventful and most patients are extubated immediately or on the next postoperative day (81,82).

In severely affected patients, thymic removal is usually delayed until the patient has improved; occasionally it is undertaken if younger patients, especially women, remain ventilator-bound after months of medical treatment. Preoperative pulmonary function tests, including vital capacity, forced expiratory volume, maximum minute ventilation, maximum inspiratory force, and maximum expiratory force, are recommended to determine if there is respiratory muscle weakness (83). Measurements of expiratory force correlate well with respiratory muscle strength and the ability to cough in MG. It may be the single best predictor of rapid, uncomplicated extubation after thymectomy. These tests may be performed before and after a 2-mg intramuscular injection of neostigmine. If VC and maximum expiratory force are better than 80% of predicted values for age, height, and weight, no preoperative treatment is required. If the pulmonary function tests indicate significant muscle weakness, patients undergo preoperative plasma exchange until their respiratory measurements reach the 80% mark.

If plasma exchange is unsuccessful at improving respiratory function, treatment with corticosteroids is considered, and a tracheostomy may be performed at the time of thymectomy in anticipation of prolonged mechanical ventilation. If there is a significant response to the neostigmine test, cholinergic drugs are instituted before weaning and extubation.

PROGNOSIS

With modern immunosuppressive medications, thymectomy, and advanced critical care techniques, death from MG is infrequent. Most deaths have occurred in older patients who require prolonged ventilation. The causes of death in our experience have been pneumonia, pulmonary embolism, gastrointestinal bleeding in relation to steroid treatment, and problems of venous catheter placement. However, as already alluded to, the natural history of the disease is difficult to define, making it impossible to assess the overall impact of various treatments. Current therapy has apparently reduced mortality in the early years of disease activity when most complications occur. Unfortunately, we are now beginning to see the late complications of immunosuppressive therapies, such as malignancies and opportunistic infections. It is uncertain if our current treatments have increased the rate of long-term remission or have just traded early mortality from myasthenic weakness for late morbidity and mortality related to the complications of therapy. Evaluation of the various immune treatments must continue, particularly in reference to their most effective use during myasthenic crisis.

ACKNOWLEDGMENT

The authors thank Dr. Mathew Fink for use of material from his chapter in the third edition of this book.

REFERENCES

1. Vincent A, Palace J, Hilton-Jones D. Myasthenia gravis. *J Neurol Neurosurg Psychiatr* 2001;357:2122–2128.
2. Compston DAS, Vincent A, Newsom-Davis J, et al. Clinical, pathological, HLA antigen and immunological evidence for disease heterogeneity in myasthenia gravis. *Brain* 1980;103:579–601.
3. Kerzin-Storrar L, et al. Genetic factors in myasthenia gravis: a family study. *Neurology* 1988;38:38–42.
4. Donaldson DH, Ansher M, Horan S, et al. The relationship of age to outcome in myasthenia gravis. *Neurology* 1990;40:786–790.
5. Perlo VP, Poskanzer DC, Schwab RS, et al. Myasthenia gravis: evaluation of treatment in 1355 patients. *Neurology* 1966;16:431–439.
6. Somnier FE, Keiding N, Paulson OB. Epidemiology of myasthenia gravis in Denmark. A longitudinal and comprehensive population survey. *Arch Neurol* 1991;48:733–739.
7. Drachman DB, Adams RN, Josifek LF, et al. Functional activities of autoantibodies to acetylcholine receptors and the clinical severity of myasthenia gravis. *N Engl J Med* 1982;307:769–775.
8. Drachman DB, ed. *Myasthenia gravis: biology and treatment,* vol. 505. New York: The New York Academy of Sciences, 1987:914.
9. Rowland LP, Hoefer PF, Aranow H, et al. Fatalities in myasthenia gravis. A review of 39 cases with 26 autopsies. *Neurology* 1958;6:307–326.
10. Chang I, Fink ME. Plasmapheresis in the treatment of myasthenic crisis. *Neurology* 1992;42:242.
11. Ferguson IT, et al. Ventilatory failure in myasthenia gravis. *J Neurol Neurosurg Psychiatry* 1982;45:217–222.
12. Mantegazza R, Beghi E, Pareyson D, et al. A multicentre follow-up study of 1152 patients with myasthenia gravis in Italy. *J Neurol* 1990;237:339–344.
13. Schmidt-Nowara WW, et al. Respiratory failure in myasthenia gravis due to vocal cord paresis. *Arch Neurol* 1984;41:567–568.
14. Gracey DR, Divertie MB, Howard FM. Mechanical ventilation for respiratory failure in myasthenia gravis: two year experience with 22 patients. *Mayo Clin Proc* 1983;58:597–602.
15. Osserman K, Genkins G. Studies in myasthenia gravis: reduction in mortality rate after crisis. *JAMA* 1963;183:97.
16. Osserman KE. *Myasthenia gravis.* New York: Grune & Stratton, 1958.
17. Dushay KM, Zibrak JD, Jensen WA. Myasthenia gravis presenting as isolated respiratory failure. *Chest* 1990;97:232–234.
18. Mier A, Laroche C, Green M. Unsuspected myasthenia gravis presenting as respiratory failure. *Thorax* 199;45:422–423.
19. Nagappan R, Kletchko S. Myasthenia gravis presenting as respiratory failure. *NZ Med J* 1992;105:152.
20. Hanson JA, Lueck CJ, Thomas DJ. Myasthenia gravis presenting with stridor. *Thorax* 1996;51:108–109.
21. Plauche WC. Myasthenia gravis in mothers and their newborns. *Clin Obstet Gynecol* 1991;34:82–99.
22. Argov Z, Mastaglia FL. Disorders of neuromuscular transmission caused by drugs. *N Engl J Med* 1979;301:409–413.
23. Wittbrodt ET. Drugs and myasthenia gravis: an update. *Arch Int Med* 1997;157:399–408.
24. Vincent A, Newsom-Davis J. Anti-acetylcholine receptor antibodies. *J Neurol Neurosurg Psychiatry* 1980;43:590–600.
25. Birmanns B, Brenner T, Abramsky O, et al. Seronega-

tive myasthenia gravis: Clinical features, response to therapy and synthesis of acetylcholine receptor antibodies *in vitro. J Neurol Sci* 1991;102:184–189.

26. Soliven BC, et al. Seronegative myasthenia gravis. *Neurology* 1988;38:514–517.

27. Engle AG. Myasthenia gravis and myasthenic syndromes. *Ann Neurol* 1984;16:519–534.

28. Swift TR. Disorders of neuromuscular transmission other than myasthenia gravis. *Muscle Nerve* 1981;4: 334–353.

29. Cohen MS, Younger D. Aspects of the natural history of myasthenia gravis: crisis and death. *Ann NY Acad Sci* 1981;377:670–677.

30. Thomas CS, Mayer SA, Gungor Y, et al. Myasthenic crisis: clinical features, mortality, complications and risk factors for prolonged mechanical ventilation. *Neurology* 1997;48:1253–1260.

31. Chang I, Fink ME. Plasmapheresis in the treatment of myasthenic crisis. *Neurology* 1992;42:242A.

32. Rowland LP. Controversies about the treatment of myasthenia gravis. *J Neurol Neurosurg Psychiatry* 1980;43:644–659.

33. Lisak RP, Barchi RL. *Myasthenia gravis.* Philadelphia: WB Saunders, 1982.

34. Drachman DB. Myasthenia gravis. *N Engl J Med* 1994;330:1797–1801.

35. Engel AG, ed. *Myasthenic gravis and myasthenic disorders.* New York: Oxford University Press, 1999.

36. Griggs RC, Donohoe KM, Utell MJ, et al. Evaluation of pulmonary function in neuromuscular disease. *Arch Neurol* 1981;38:9–12.

37. Rieder P, Louis M, Jolliet P, et al. The repeated measurement of VC is a poor predictor of the need for mechanical ventilation in myasthenia gravis. *Int Care Med* 1995;21:663–668.

38. Pontoppidan H, Geffin B, Lowenstein E. Acute respiratory failure in the adult. *N Engl J Med* 1972;287:690.

39. West JB. *Pulmonary pathophysiology. The essentials,* 2nd ed. Baltimore: Williams & Wilkins, 1982.

40. Weiner WJ, ed. *Respiratory dysfunction in neurological disease.* Mt. Kisco, NY: Futura, 1980.

41. Teoh R, Chow CC, Kay R, et al. Response to control of hyperthyroidism in patients with myasthenia gravis and thyrotoxicosis. *Br J Clin Pract* 1990;44:742–744.

42. Saltis LM, Martin RB, Traeger XM, et al. Continuous infusion of pyridostigmine in the management of myasthenic crisis. *Crit Care Med* 1993;21:938–940.

43. Borel CO. Management of myasthenic crisis: continuous anticholinesterase infusions (editorial). *Crit Care Med* 1993;21:821–822.

44. Miano MA, Bosley TM, Heiman-Patterson TD, et al. Factors influencing outcome of prednisone dose reduction in myasthenia gravis. *Neurology* 1991;41: 919–921.

45. Miller RG, et al. Prednisone-induced worsening of neuromuscular function in myasthenia gravis. *Neurology* 1986;36:729–732.

46. Arsura E, Brunner NG, Namba T, et al. High-dose intravenous methylprednisolone in myasthenia gravis. *Arch Neurol* 1985;42:1149–1153.

47. Seybold ME, Drachman DB. Gradually increasing doses of prednisone in myasthenia gravis. Reducing the hazards of treatment. *N Engl J Med* 1974;290:81–84.

48. Wakata N, Kawamura Y, Kobayashi M, et al. Intermit-

tent long-term adrenocorticosteroid treatment of myasthenia gravis. *J Neurol* 1991;238:16–18.

49. Warmolts JR, Engel WK. Benefit from alternate-day prednisone in myasthenia gravis. *N Engl J Med* 1972;286:17–20.

50. Pascuzzi RM, Coslett HB, Johns TR. Long-term corticosteroid treatment of myasthenia gravis: report of 116 patients. *Ann Neurol* 1984;15:291–298.

51. Niakan E, et al. Immunosuppressive drug therapy in myasthenia gravis. *Arch Neurol* 1986;43:155–156.

52. Witte AS, Cornblath DR, Parry GJ, et al. Azathioprine in the treatment of myasthenia gravis. *Ann Neurol* 1984; 15:602–605.

53. Hohlfeld R, et al. Azathioprine toxicity during long term immunosuppression of generalized myasthenia gravis. *Neurology* 1988;38:258–261.

54. Antonini G, Bove R, Filippini C, et al. Results of an open trial of cyclosporine in a group of steroid-dependent myasthenic subjects. *Clin Neurol Neurosurg* 1990; 92:317–321.

55. Tindall RS, Phillips JT, Rollins JA, et al. Cyclosporin in the treatment of myasthenia gravis. *Monogr Allergy* 1988;25:135–147.

56. Tindall RSA, et al. Preliminary results of a double-blind randomized, placebo-controlled trial of cyclosporine in myasthenia gravis. *N Engl J Med* 1987;316: 719–724.

57. Kornfeld P, Ambinder EP, Mittag T, et al. Plasmapheresis in refractory myasthenia gravis. *Arch Neurol* 1981; 38:478–481.

58. Perlo VP, Shahani BT, Huggins CE, et al. Effect of plasmapheresis in myasthenia gravis. *Ann NY Acad Sci* 1981;377:709–724.

59. Antozzi C, Gemma M, Regi B, et al. A short plasma exchange protocol is effective in severe myasthenia gravis. *J Neurol* 1991;238:103–107.

60. National Institutes of Health. The utility of plasmapheresis for neurological disorders. *JAMA* 1986;256: 1333–1337.

61. Tindall RSA. Plasmapheresis for neurological disorders. In: Appel SH, ed. *Current neurology,* vol 10. Chicago: Year Book, 1990:177–193.

62. Newsom-Davis J, Vincent A, Wilson SG, et al. Long-term effects of repeated plasma exchange in myasthenia gravis. *Lancet* 1979;1:464–468.

63. Gracey DR, Howard FM, Divertie MB. Plasmapheresis in the treatment of ventilator-dependent myasthenia gravis patients. Report of four cases. *Chest* 1984;85: 739–743.

64. Henze T, Prange HW, Talartschik J, et al. Complications of plasma exchange in patients with neurological diseases. *Klin Wochenschr* 1990;68:1183–1188.

65. Gajdos P, Chevret S, Clair B, et al. Clinical trial of plasma exchange and high-dose intravenous immunoglobulin in myasthenia gravis. Myasthenia Gravis Clinical Study Group. *Ann Neurol* 1997;41:789–796.

66. Qureshi AI, Choudhry MA, Akbar MS, et al. Plasma exchange versus intravenous immunoglobulin treatment in myasthenic crisis. *Neurology* 1999;52:629–632.

67. Stricker RB, Kwiatkowski BJ, Habis JA, et al. Myasthenic crisis: response to plasmapheresis following failure of intravenous immune globulin. *Arch Neurol* 1993; 50:837–840.

68. Kornfeld P, Ambinder E, Papatestas AE, et al. Plasma-

pheresis in myasthenia gravis: controlled study. *Lancet* 1979;2:629.

69. Arsura E. Experience with intravenous immunoglobulin in myasthenia gravis. *Clin Immunol Immunopathol* 1989;53:S170–179.

70. Arsura EL, Bick A, Brunner NG, et al. High-dose intravenous immunoglobulin in the management of myasthenia gravis. *Arch Intern Med* 1986;146:1365–1368.

71. Liblau R, Gajdos P, Bustarret FA, et al. Intravenous gamma-globulin in myasthenia gravis: Interaction with anti-acetylcholine receptor autoantibodies. *J Clin Immunol* 1991;11:128–131.

72. Achiron A, Barak V, Miron S, et al. Immunoglobulin treatment in refractory myasthenia gravis. *Muscle Nerve* 2000;23:551–555.

73. Shibuya N, Sato T, Osame M, et al. Immunoadsorption therapy for myasthenia gravis. *J Neurol Neusorsug Psychiatr* 1994;57:578–581.

74. Sato T, Ishigaki Y, Komiya T, et al. Therapeutic immunoadsorption of acetylcholine receptor antibodies in myasthenia gravis. *Ann NY Acad Sci* 1988;540:554–556.

75. Haupt WF, Rosenow F, van der Ven C, et al. Immunoadsorption in Guillain-Barré syndrome and myasthenia gravis. *Ther Apher* 2000;4:195–197.

76. Grob D, Simpson D, Mitsumoto H, et al. Treatment of myasthenia gravis by immunoadsorption of plasma. *Neurology* 1995;45:338–344.

77. Durelli L, Maggi G, Casadio C, et al. Actuarial analysis of the occurrence of remission following thymectomy for myasthenia gravis in 400 patients. *J Neurol Neurosurg Psychiatry* 1991;54:406–411.

78. Oosterhuis HJG. The natural course of myasthenia gravis: a long term follow up study. *J Neurol Neurosurg Psychiatry* 1989;52:1121–1127.

79. Jaretzki A, Penn AS, Younger DS, et al. "Maximal" thymectomy for myasthenia gravis: results. *J Thorac Cardiovasc Surg* 1988;95:747–757.

80. Miller RG, Filler-Katz A, Kiprov D, et al. Repeat thymectomy in chronic refractory myasthenia gravis. *Neurology* 1991;41:923–924.

81. Gorback MS, Moon RE, Massey JM. Extubation after transsternal thymectomy for myasthenia gravis: A prospective analysis. *South Med J* 1991;84:701–706.

82. Chevalley C, Spiliopoulos A, de Perrot M, et al. Perioperative medical management and outcome following thymectomy in myasthenia gravis.*Can J Anaesthesiol* 2001;48:446–451.

83. Younger DS, Braun NMT, Jaretzki A, et al. Myasthenia gravis: determinants for independent ventilation after transsternal thymectomy. *Neurology* 1984;34:336–340.

20

Status Epilepticus

Status epilepticus (called "status" throughout this chapter) is a life-threatening neurological emergency with a high mortality and morbidity. In several series it accounts for 1% to 8% of all hospital admissions for epilepsy (1), and in the United States is estimated to affect between 50,000 and 152,000 patients per year (2); furthermore, as many as 50,000 deaths per year may be associated with this condition. Nonconvulsive status epilepticus (NCSE) is an allied condition that is reportedly rare, although probably underrecognized, with an incidence of perhaps one per million for an absence variety and 35 per million of complex partial status. About 44% of adults admitted to an urban San Francisco hospital with status had no prior history of seizures (3). Between one tenth to one third of adults with new onset seizures present with status (4). Status shows two age-related peaks, one during infancy and one in late adulthood (2).

CLASSIFICATION AND DEFINITIONS

Recurrent or continuous seizures occur with all seizure type. Commonly used categories of status include generalized convulsive status (GCSE); simple partial status; myoclonic SE; and NCSE. Nonconvulsive status encompasses absence, complex partial, and atonic seizures. Kaplan suggests classifying NCSE into three types: NCSE of generalized epilepsies; NCSE of localization-related epilepsies [subclassified by electroencephalographic (EEG) features]; and an indeterminate form of NCSE not fitting the prior categories (5).

Debate persists regarding the duration of seizure activity constituting status. At the 1962 Marseilles conference, status was defined as an "enduring epileptic state" (6). The International League against Epilepsy defined it as a seizure persisting for sufficient length of time to produce such an enduring state, or repeated seizures occurring frequently without recovery between attacks (7). Subsequent attempts to define status as 30 minutes of continuous or recurrent seizure activity reflected experimental and epidemiologic evidence of the approximate time needed to produce cerebral injury (8). However, this definition interferes with management, because aggressive treatment to status should not be delayed to achieve success and prevent brain injury. A typical secondarily generalized tonic–clonic seizure generally stops by 3 minutes and almost always by 5 min (6,9). Seizures may last somewhat longer in children and still remit spontaneously, but a seizure in a child that has lasted 12 minutes is unlikely to do so within the next 30 minutes (10). Whether one chooses to define status based on such operational definitions (11), or maintains the older definition but begins treatment earlier in order to stop seizure activity before it lasts 30 minutes is a point of intellectual but not clinical relevance.

PATHOPHYSIOLOGY

The brain has intrinsic inhibitory mechanisms that serve to prevent seizures, and to terminate those that do occur. However, these mechanisms fail in status, either because of increased neuronal excitability or loss of normal inhibitory pathways (12). Receptors for the major inhibitory transmitter, γ-amino butyric acid (GABA), are the site of most effective antistatus agents (e.g., the benzodiazepines). Conversely, proconvulsant agents such as penicillin can precipitate status by antagonizing the inhibitory neurotransmitter. However, the GABA agonists lose efficacy over many minutes, perhaps because GABA receptors undergo rapid changes in subunit composition, which decreases their affinity for these substances (13). Excitatory neurotransmitters are considered to be important in the maintenance of status, including glutamate, aspartate, and acetylcholine. *N*-methyl-*D*-aspartate (NMDA)–linked calcium channels appear to be particularly involved in the pathogenesis of status (14), and NMDA antagonists are promising agents for the control of refractory status (15).

Cerebral injury occurs from status independent of the systemic metabolic disturbances it produces (16), although the latter undoubtedly contribute to neuronal damage in many cases (17). Primary neuronal injury appears to be a consequence of calcium-mediated excitotoxicity and increased metabolic demands from excessive neuronal activity. The upregulation of glial metabotropic glutamate receptors has been proposed as a mechanism in the epileptogenesis induced by status (18). Recently, nerve growth factor and other neurotrophins were suggested to have specific protective roles against excitotoxic cell stress (19), but many of these notions currently are speculative.

During the first several minutes of GCSE, recurrent isolated or continuous clinical convulsions are manifestations of discrete electrographically recordable seizures. There is sympathetic overactivity with hypertension and tachycardia. Blood lactate and glucose levels increase, with reduced pH secondary to metabolic acidosis, and respiratory acidosis as well when there is airway compromise. Cerebral glucose metabolism, oxygen use, and blood flow increase acutely, and brain lactate levels are also increased.

With persistence of status beyond 30 to 60 minutes, visible seizures become more subtle, seen only as focal myoclonic twitches, followed by complete disappearance of motor manifestations despite persistence of ongoing electrographic seizures. Discrete seizures are initially seen on the EEG, corresponding to the clinical events. Subsequently, waxing and waning electrographic seizures develop, followed by continuous ictal activity. With time, the pattern degenerates into continuous epileptiform activity interrupted by flat periods, and eventually into periodic lateralizing epileptiform discharges (PLEDs) (20). Hypotension develops, along with persistently increased lactate, hypoglycemia, hyperthermia, and respiratory compromise. Cerebral autoregulation is impaired with decreased cerebral blood flow related to systemic hypotension. Cerebral glucose and oxygenation are also reduced (18). Vasogenic cerebral edema occurs with prolonged seizures.

ETIOLOGY

Status occurs either because of an overwhelming acute insult to the brain or in situations in which acute processes are superimposed on prior brain injury. It may be precipitated *de novo* in patients with no prior history of seizures owing to acute metabolic or structural injury to the brain. Anticonvulsant noncompliance or withdrawal from other hypnosedative agents, including ethanol, is the commonest precipitating cause of status in our practices. Acute electrolyte disturbances (especially acute hypoosmolar states), renal failure, sepsis, nervous system infections, stroke, toxicity from medications, hypoxia, and head trauma are also among the common causes of status (3). These latter acute derangements are associated with poorer outcome and are more refractory to treatment (21). Conversely, status in patients with preexisting epilepsy usually follows poor compliance or tapering of medications. There is frequently good response to treatment in this situation and other etiologies (including ethanol abuse, cerebral tumors, and late epilepsy following prior strokes).

MANAGEMENT

The following discussion of management applies to status of generalized tonic–clonic seizure type and is based on our general experience, drawn in part from the experiences of others of course. The management of complex partial NCSE is similar; however, absence NCSE is usually approached less aggressively than the generalized variety because there are no data suggesting that simple partial status causes significant injury. Less vigorous efforts are also recommended because these seizures are remarkably resistant to treatment and efforts to completely abolish them generally result in medication-induced side effects.

There are five aspects to the management of status: *general supportive care, termination of status, prevention of seizure recurrence, correction of precipitating causes, and prevention and treatment of complications.* The aggressiveness of treatment reflects the likelihood of brain injury and systemic complications with prolonged convulsive status. Early initiation of treatment appears to be critical to a favorable outcome.

Initial therapy follows the general principles of any emergency medical condition regarding the basics of airway, breathing, and circulation. However, there are some precautions and difficulties specific to status. Airway management is critical to avoid exacerbating status through hypoxia. In those patients with spontaneous adequate breathing, airway patency should be maintained by either oral or nasopharyngeal devices supplemented by 100% oxygen. Intubation with mechanical ventilation is required in those with evidence of respiratory compromise. This should be considered prior to respiratory compromise once the decision is made to treat with agents that tend to cause respiratory suppression. Patients with status frequently need neuromuscular blocking agents to facilitate intubation. It is important to use short-acting

neuromuscular blocker (e.g., vecuronium, 0.1 mg/kg), because the cessation of muscle activity makes diagnosing seizure activity clinically difficult. Neostigmine (50 to 70 µg/kg) reverses the neuromuscular blockade once it begins to wear off. Use of succinylcholine should be discouraged because of the potential for severe hyperkalemia associated with this drug in neurological patients.

Secure intravenous access is essential for blood samples, management of fluid and electrolytes, and administration of medications. Cardiac monitoring allows recognition and treatment of potentially life-threatening arrhythmias, which occasionally develop in these patients. If a patient is hypotensive, one should begin volume replacement and consider the use of vasoactive agents. Conversely, if a patient is hypertensive, delay treating the blood pressure primarily, because the drugs used to terminate status tend to cause hypotension. With prolonged status, intensive care unit (ICU) admission is essential. If the blood glucose concentration is low, 50 mL of 50% dextrose (or 1 mL/kg) along with 100 mg thiamine should be administered intravenously, because hypoglycemia commonly presents with seizures, which may be partial. Hypoglycemia also can occur as a complication of prolonged status. If one contemplates the use of phenytoin, at least one line containing normal saline as the infusion fluid is required.

Routine laboratory analysis should include complete blood count, serum glucose, electrolytes, liver enzymes, and renal function tests; arterial blood gas, anticonvulsant levels, urinalysis, and blood and urine screening for psychotropic agents as appropriate.

The role of the EEG in the management of status cannot be overestimated. Patients without improving responsiveness, in whom neuromuscular blocking has been used, or patients with refractory status, require some form of EEG monitoring. Persistent electrographic seizures after control of visible seizures were seen in 20% of the patients in the Department of Veterans Affairs (DVA) cooperative study (22) and in about 15% in the study by DeLorenzo and coworkers (23).

Early initiation of treatment is crucial in these patients. Animal and human experiments indicate that status becomes progressively refractory to anticonvulsants with increasing duration (24). In experimental status induced by lithium and pilocarpine, the total dose of diazepam required to control seizures more than doubled if therapy was delayed until the second seizure compared to the dose required following the first (25). Lowenstein and Alldredge (3) showed that status was terminated in 80% of patients when treated within 30 minutes of onset, but was less than 40% successful if delayed for 2 hours or more.

Various anticonvulsants and anesthetic agents are effective in the management of status (Table 20.1).

Lorazepam has smaller volume of distribution and longer duration of action than *diazepam,* which are somewhat advantageous when treating status; the slightly slower brain uptake appears not to be clinically significant. There is also no important difference in the degree of respiratory depression between the two drugs (26). *Midazolam* is also highly lipophilic and rapidly metabolized by liver. However, it has a very short half-life and requires continuous infusion; indeed, continuous intravenous administration frequently is successful in refractory status (27). Tachyphy-

laxis to midazolam develops, sometimes quickly, requiring upward titration of the dose. We have used up to 22 mg/hour with success. Cardiovascular depression seems less prominent than that seen with barbiturates. The well-known side effects related to benzodiazepines include impaired consciousness (20% to 60%), hypotension (less than 2%), and respiratory depression (3% to 10%) (28).

Phenytoin, which continues to be a mainstay of the treatment of status, is lipid soluble but insoluble in aqueous solutions. Parenteral forms contain 40% propylene glycol, 10% ethanol, and sodium hydroxide at a pH of 12. Peak brain levels occur about 6 minutes after infusion is complete (29). Infusion of a loading dose (20 mg/kg) at the maximal safe rate of 50 mg/minute takes over 20 minutes, and the clinical effect may not be seen until after the completion of the infusion. It is metabolized in the liver by hydroxylation. The cardiovascular risks associated with a loading dose of phenytoin are mainly hypotension and cardiac arrhythmias (particularly bradyarrhythmias and heart block) (30). These adverse effects result from both phenytoin itself and to a lesser extent, the diluent; slowing or stopping the infusion generally diminishes these complications (31). Phenytoin infusion also carries some risk of subcutaneous ex-

TABLE 20.1. *Antiseizure medications used in the management of status epilepticus*

Drug	Route	Loading dose (mg/kg)	Maintenance dose
Diazepam	i.v., e.t.	0.2–0.5 at 2–4 mg/min	None
Lorazepam	i.v., e.t.	0.1 at 2 mg/min	9 mg/h
Midazolam	i.v.	0.05–2 at <4 mg/min	0.75–10 µg/kg/min
Phenytoin	i.v.	20 at 50 mg/min or 1 mg/kg/min	5 mg/kg
Fosphenytoin	i.v.	20 at 150 mg/min or 3 mg/kg/min	5 mg/kg
Phenobarbital	i.v.	15–20 at 2 mg/kg/min or 50–75 mg/min	1–4 mg/kg/h
Thiopental	i.v.	12 over seconds	250 mg/min
Pentobarbital	i.v.	5–12 at 0.2–0.4 mg/kg/min or over 1 h	0.5–5 mg/kg/h
Etomidate	i.v.	0.3	30 mg/sec
Propofol	i.v.	2–3	1–15 mg/kg/h
Paraldehyde	i.m., p.r.	60–150 mg/kg or 0.07–0.35 mL/kg (1 g/mL)	1 mg/min
Lidocaine	i.v., e.t.	2–3 at <50 mg/min	1–3 mg/kg/h or 100 mg/min
Valproate	i.v.	20–40 at 3–6 mg/kg/min	
Isoflurane	Inhalant	—	—
Ketamine	i.v.	1–4.5	10–50 µg/kg/min

e.t., endotracheal; i.m., intramuscular; i.v., intravenous; p.r., rectally.

travasation, especially with poor intravenous access, which can lead to thrombophlebitis and soft-tissue necrosis. Known serious reactions to the drug probably contraindicate its use but exceptions can be made in dire situations.

Fosphenytoin is water-soluble prodrug of phenytoin, the phosphate ester group of which is rapidly removed by phosphatases once it is in the bloodstream. It is supplied at a pH of 8. Fosphenytoin can be given at a faster maximal rate (150 mg/minute) than phenytoin. The advantages of fosphenytoin as an alternative to phenytoin include faster maximal rate infusion, no restriction of the vehicle of infusion, and the near absence of infusion-site reactions. The incidence of hypotension requiring intervention is uncommon (1% for fosphenytoin and 9% for phenytoin) at the recommended rates of administration (32). Infusion site reactions are significantly reduced with fosphenytoin except for pruritus, which may be generalized also, but is not an issue in status patients. We generally employ phenytoin because of its ease of use and availability.

Phenobarbital is lipophilic, with therapeutic brain levels reached in 3 minutes and much faster during seizure activity (33). Its half-life ranges from 50 to 150 hours after a loading dose and a wide range of levels are obtained after a loading dose. Sedation, hypotension, and respiratory depression are common following a loading dose. Maintenance dosage adjustments are required in patients with hepatic dysfunction, and the loading dose may be lower in patients with renal failure because of diminished protein binding. The usual dose of phenobarbital is 20 mg/kg given at 50 to 75 mg/minute.

Thiopental is a very rapidly acting barbiturate, with peak brain levels obtained within 30 seconds. Extravasation into subcutaneous tissues can cause tissue necrosis. Due to its high lipophilicity, it accumulates in fat when given for long periods, resulting in delayed clearance. It is metabolized to pentobarbital, which is an active anticonvulsant and has a half-time of up to 90 hours. Rare hypersensitivity reactions can occur once in 30,000 people.

Thiopental can cause significant hypotension and respiratory suppression and must be used only in intubated and carefully monitored patients.

Propofol is very short-acting, highly lipid soluble, and metabolized by the liver; its use in status requires a continuous infusion. It is a GABA-A receptor agonist with additional possible mechanisms of action. Prolonged administration can result in hyperlipidemia and metabolic acidosis. Although an effective treatment for refractory status (34), its use has declined with the recognition of several potential adverse effects (35).

Ketamine, commonly used throughout the world for general anesthesia, also appears to be effective in the treatment of status. The optimum dose in refractory status is uncertain. The anesthetic dose is 1 to 4.5 mg/kg with supplements of 0.5 to 2.5 mg/kg every 30 to 45 minutes or 10 to 50 µg/kg per minute.

Parenteral *valproate,* made available more recently than the previously discussed drugs, may have efficacy in several types of status. Given its broad antiepileptic activity, ease of administration, lack of significant cardiorespiratory depression, less sedation, it can be a very useful alternative in the treatment of status. Doses of 20 to 40 mg/kg given at 3 to 6 mg/kg per minute may achieve levels effectively controlling status without the respiratory and cardiovascular depression of most other antiseizure agents (36). Our limited experience suggests it may not be as effective as phenytoin but it has utility and further experience will be interesting to follow.

The DVA Status Epilepticus Cooperative Study addressed essential elements of drug selection in the *initial* treatment of status and serves in part as a guide for the short-term treatment of status (28,39). Patients were divided into overt and subtle status based on their clinical and electrographic manifestations. The overt status (convulsing) group was randomized to lorazepam (0.1 mg/kg); diazepam (0.15 mg/kg) followed by phenytoin (18 mg/kg); phenytoin alone; and, phenobarbital (15 mg/kg) alone. Successful treatment was defined as complete cessation of clinical and electrographic seizures within 20 minutes of therapy. Patients failing the first drug were given a second drug, and if necessary, a third one. Lorazepam was effective in terminating status 65% of the time, which was statistically significantly better than phenytoin alone. In another study, lorazepam was effective in 85% of status patients (26). However, in this study only clinical cessation of seizures were taken into consideration. As mentioned, this study indicated that about 20% of patients with clinical control of seizures have ongoing electrographic seizures (22).

Perhaps more importantly from a tactical point of view, preliminary data from the VA trial show that if one drug fails, successful termination of status becomes unlikely with the subsequent use of conventional antiseizure drugs. Many neurologists try phenytoin or fosphenytoin as a second-line drug, but these data suggest that this approach is unlikely to succeed. Others have had similar findings, and although probably correct in most cases, this has not always accorded with our own experience, in part because it refers again to the initial control of seizures (37).

Refractory Status Epilepticus

Status not responding to the initial two or more anticonvulsants should be considered refractory, and a more aggressive approach pursued (37). These patients generally have respiratory and cardiovascular compromise and associated systemic complications. Patients should be intubated and placed on mechanical ventilation. Hypotension should be corrected, and some patients need central venous or pulmonary artery catheter placement for hemodynamic monitoring and management. Once a patient reaches a stage of refractory status, following the seizures clinically become nearly impossible, and continuous EEG monitoring is required both to identify ongoing electrographic seizures as well as for adjusting anticonvulsant dosing (38).

Agents available in the treatment of refractory status include high-dose barbiturates (pentobarbital, thiopental, and phenobarbital),

high-dose benzodiazepines (midazolam, lorazepam), propofol, ketamine, and other anesthetics. There are few comparisons of these drugs in refractory status. Midazolam and propofol have emerged as useful medications in refractory status. Midazolam is administered as 0.2 mg/kg bolus followed by 0.1 to 2 mg/kg per hour (2 to 40 µg/kg per minute) (39). Advantages of midazolam include its rapid onset and its water solubility, avoiding the metabolic acidosis of propylene glycol seen with high doses of other benzodiazepines and barbiturates. All of these drugs are potentially immunosuppressant as well as being negative inotropes and vasodilators.

Propofol has gained popularity recently in the treatment of refractory status. It can be given as a 2- to 5-mg/kg bolus followed by 1 to 15 mg/kg per hour infusion (34). The onset of action is within 3 minutes, and activity persists only for 5 to 10 minutes after the drug has been stopped, even though the plasma half-time is much longer. Potential side effects are respiratory suppression, hypotension, and particularly, infections with prolonged infusions; the latter has tempered enthusiasm for it but we still find it useful. A notable issue, not shared with other infused drugs, is the need to adjust dietary caloric intake to prevent overfeeding from the lipid vehicle. Rapid discontinuation should be avoided, because it may precipitate withdrawal seizures (40). The advantages of propofol include less tachyphylaxis than midazolam and less hypotension than phenobarbital. However, recent concerns over the potential toxicity of prolonged infusions at high doses suggest that midazolam be tried before propofol (35).

When high-dose midazolam and propofol fail or must be discontinued because of toxicity, high-dose barbiturates remain useful. Recent shortages of the substrate for intravenous pentobarbital and phenobarbital production have fueled a return to thiopental as the barbiturate of choice for this indication, even though this drug may produce more autonomic instability than the other barbiturates. The rapid central nervous system entry of thiopental facilitates dosing, as the EEG effect is apparent within minutes of a loading dose. The possible doses and combinations of previously administered drugs makes it difficult to predict the initial dose of thiopental necessary for the control of refractory status; hence, administration of 300-mg increments every few minutes to terminate seizure activity is a reasonable approach. The initially rapid redistribution of thiopental requires a constant intravenous infusion of the drug, with the rate titrated to maintain seizure control. Vasopressor and inotrope support is almost always necessary, and is facilitated by data from a pulmonary artery catheter or the newer, less invasive methods for determining cardiac output and the adequacy of intravascular volume.

Abundant experimental evidence characterizes refractory status as a state with diminished sensitivity to GABA agonists (41), and suggests that NMDA antagonists may be more useful (42). Initial clinical experience with ketamine suggests that it is effective for the control of refractory status (4,15), but a randomized trial is needed. Loading with topiramate via an orogastric tube may be useful also.

Isoflurane may be a useful agent for the rare patient who cannot tolerate adequate doses of intravenous agents (19).

The EEG goal of treatment for refractory status remains a subject of debate. Older suggestions that a suppression-burst background is necessary and sufficient for the control of status are not supported by newer information (43). In the absence of a randomized trial, we recommend that continuous EEG monitoring be employed, with the dose of antiseizure agent titrated to prevent seizure activity regardless of whether the EEG background activity so produced is slow, suppression-burst, or isoelectric.

Once seizures have been suppressed for some period of time (e.g., 12 to 24 hours), one can decrease the dose of the agent by 25% to 50% and observe for seizure recurrence. Many prefer to have the patient loaded with sufficient phenytoin to produce a plasma level of 20 to 25 μg/mL before attempting to withdraw the other agents; this is a reasonable but unstudied approach. Many refractory patients also need loading with phenobarbital to allow withdrawal of the continuous infusion of other drugs. If the seizures do not recur, then a comparable percentage of drug is again withdrawn.

Patients who develop refractory status owing to withdrawal from anticonvulsants or ethanol usually can be kept out of status with GABA agonists, or restitution of their original antiseizure regimen, once their status has been broken. However, many patients who reach the stage of refractory status have an ongoing stimulus for epileptogenicity such as encephalitis, and may require high-dose therapy for weeks or months (44). In this circumstance one is often faced with staff and family members who become despondent over the patient's potential for recovery. However, desires to withdraw therapy should be tempered by the fairly frequent occurrence of functional recovery, and even return to normal function, among patients with encephalitis or cryptogenic status despite very long periods of treatment. Unless there is radiographic evidence of cortical atrophy or necrosis, one should be reticent to withdraw aggressive support until seizure control has been achieved and the patient's level of function assessed in the absence of sedating drugs. One should also keep in mind that functional recovery may continue for months after resolution of active encephalitis or seizure activity.

INTENSIVE CARE UNIT APPROACH TO STATUS

In general, we try to determine if: (a) a patient in status has been on anticonvulsants, and if so which ones; and (b) if there is an endogenous metabolic disturbance, intoxication, infection, or a new structural lesion. In most cases, we use a benzodiazepine to control convulsions and electrographic seizures first, followed by a loading dose of phenytoin. Although the data from the DVA cooperative study do not suggest utility for phenytoin in the control of status, it remains a useful agent to prevent seizure recurrence. In recent years, we have stopped the practice of adding phenobarbital in adults who fail to cease seizing after the administration of these first two drugs.

If convulsive seizures persist and the patient has been intubated, we have generally instituted neuromuscular paralysis and a continuous infusion or midazolam. (Propofol may be an alternative if used for less than several consecutive days.) The role of neuromuscular junction blockers in this setting is an expedient for temperature control, but adds the difficulty of loss of the neurological examination and thus requires the concomitant use of electroencephalographic monitoring. Note that neuromuscular junction blocking agents do nothing to prevent cerebral damage other than control temperature.

Failing this approach, there is no certain course and the addition of valproate may be tried but is not likely to succeed. Instead, some form of general anesthesia is called for; thiopental, exceedingly high doses of a benzodiazepine, or the inhalation agent isoflurane may be tried. Most such patients have a poor prognosis, but we have had numerous survivors with good neurological recovery over the years, and suggest caution in abandoning an aggressive program too early. Of course, an underlying structural brain lesion should be sought by imaging, and spinal fluid examination when safe; decisions regarding the degree of aggressiveness in treatment are guided by these findings as well.

Nonconvulsive status epilepticus presents similar problems but does not add the risks of neuromuscular paralysis and intubation in most patients. However, as stated, a consensus is developing that NCSE is so often refractory that an overly ambitious approach may not be justified. This leaves the physician with an ambiguous plan because only a modest proportion of cases in our experience burn themselves out. We have tried the sequential use of two or three conventional anticonvulsants, usually given by nasogastric tube and again seek the underlying cause.

In both these cases, treatment often is thwarted by medical problems such as ileus, chest or other infection and fever, loss of intravenous access because of local tissue reactions to infusions, undernutrition, and difficulty with ventilation (most dire). A special issue pertains to the production of hypotension as a result of high-dose anticonvulsant infusion. Here we usually use small doses of vasopressors, particularly phenylephrine, after assuring adequate hydration. If larger doses are required, we usually abandon the anticonvulsant (most often phenytoin is responsible) and institute an alternative. Ketamine becomes particularly attractive in this setting as its intrinsic sympathomimetic effects serve to raise blood pressure. When other general anesthetic agents are required, vascular monitoring to insure adequate volume expansion and vasopressor agents typically are required.

All of these suggestions are tempered by particular circumstances and require the astute implementation of several intensive care skills.

REFERENCES

1. Hauser WA. Status epilepticus: epidemiologic considerations. *Neurology* 1990;40:9–13.
2. DeLorenzo RJ, Pellock JM, Towne AR, et al. Epidemiology of status epilepticus. *J Clin Neurophysiol* 1995; 12:316–325.
3. Lowenstein DH, Alldredge BK. Status epilepticus at an urban public hospital in the 1980s. *Neurology* 1993; 43:483–488.
4. Sung CY, Chu NS. Status epilepticus in the elderly: etiology, seizure type and outcome. *Acta Neurol Scand* 1989;80:51–56.
5. Kaplan PW. Nonconvulsive status epilepticus. *Semin Neurol* 1996;16:33–40.
6. Gastaut H. Classification of status epilepticus. *Adv Neurol* 1983;34:15–35.
7. Proposal for revised clinical and electroencephalographic classification of epileptic seizures: from the Commission on Classification and Terminology of the International League Against Epilepsy. *Epilepsia* 1981; 22:489–501.
8. Bleck TP. Convulsive disorders: status epilepticus. *Clin Neuropharmacol* 1991;14:191–198.
9. Theodore WH, Porter RJ, Albert P, et al. The secondarily generalized tonic–clonic seizure: a videotape analysis. *Neurology* 1994;44:1403–1407.
10. Shinnar S, Berg AT, Moshe SL, et al. How long do newonset seizures in children last? *Ann Neurol* 2001;49: 659–664.

11. Lowenstein DH, Bleck T, Macdonald RL. It's time to revise the definition of status epilepticus. *Epilepsia* 1999;40:120–122.

12. Fountain NB, Lothman EW. Pathophysiology of status epilepticus. *J Clin Neurophysiol* 1995;12:326–342.

13. Kapur J, Macdonald RL. Rapid seizure-induced reduction of benzodiazepine and Zn2+ sensitivity of hippocampal dentate granule cell GABA^A receptors. *J Neurosci* 1997;17:7532–7540.

14. Lothman E. The biochemical basis and pathophysiology of status epilepticus. *Neurology* 1990;40:13–23.

15. Bleck TP. Refractory status epilepticus in 2001. *Arch Neurol* 2002;59:188–189.

16. Meldrum BS, Vigouroux RA, Brierley JB. Systemic factors and epileptic brain damage. Prolonged seizures in paralyzed, artificially ventilated baboons. *Arch Neurol* 1973;29:82–87.

17. Meldrum BS. Metabolic factors during prolonged seizures and their relation to nerve cell death. *Adv Neurol* 1983;34:261–275.

18. Kreisman NR, Rosenthal M, Sick TJ, et al. Oxidative metabolic responses during recurrent seizures are independent of convulsant, anesthetic, or species. *Neurology* 1983;33:861–867.

19. Kofke WA, Bloom MJ, Van Cott A, et al. Electrographic tachyphylaxis to etomidate and ketamine used for refractory status epilepticus controlled with isoflurane. *J Neurosurg Anesthesiol* 1997;9:269–272.

20. Treiman DM, Walton NY, Kendrick C. A progressive sequence of electroencephalographic changes during generalized convulsive status epilepticus. *Epilepsy Res* 1990;5:49–60.

21. Towne AR, Pellock JM, Ko D, et al. Determinants of mortality in status epilepticus. *Epilepsia* 1994;35:27–34.

22. Craven W, Faught E, Kuzniecky R, et al. Residual electrographic status epilepticus after control of overt clinical seizures. *Epilepsia* 1995;36:46.

23. DeLorenzo RJ, Waterhouse EJ, Towne AR, et al. Persistent nonconvulsive status epilepticus after the control of convulsive status epilepticus. *Epilepsia* 1998;39:833–840.

24. Walton NY, Treiman DM. Rational polytherapy in the treatment of status epilepticus. *Epilepsy Res Suppl* 1996;11:123–139.

25. Walton NY, Treiman DM. Response of status epilepticus induced by lithium and pilocarpine to treatment with diazepam. *Exp Neurol* 1988;101:267–275.

26. Leppik IE, Derivan AT, Homan RW, et al. Double-blind study of lorazepam and diazepam in status epilepticus. *JAMA* 1983;249:1452–1454.

27. Kumar A, Bleck TP. Intravenous midazolam for the treatment of refractory status epilepticus. *Crit Care Med* 1992;20:483–488.

28. Treiman DM, Meyers PD, Walton NY, et al. A comparison of four treatments for generalized convulsive status epilepticus. Veterans Affairs Status Epilepticus Cooperative Study Group. *N Engl J Med* 1998;339:792–798.

29. Ramsay RE. Pharmacokinetics and clinical use of parenteral phenytoin, phenobarbital, and paraldehyde. *Epilepsia* 1989;30:S1–3.

30. Wilder BJ. Efficacy of phenytoin in treatment of status epilepticus. *Adv Neurol* 1983;34:441–446.

31. Cranford RE, Leppik IE, Patrick B, et al. Intravenous phenytoin in acute treatment of seizures. *Neurology* 1979;29:1474–1479.

32. Ramsay RE, DeToledo J. Intravenous administration of fosphenytoin: options for the management of seizures. *Neurology* 1996;46:S17–19.

33. Walton NY, Treiman DM. Phenobarbital treatment of status epilepticus in a rodent model. *Epilepsy Res* 1989;4:216–221.

34. Stecker MM, Kramer TH, Raps EC, et al. Treatment of refractory status epilepticus with propofol: clinical and pharmacokinetic findings. *Epilepsia* 1998;39:18–26.

35. Prasad A, Worrall BB, Bertram EH, et al. Propofol and midazolam in the treatment of refractory status epilepticus. *Epilepsia* 2001;42:380–386.

36. Sinha S, Naritoku DK. Intravenous valproate is well tolerated in unstable patients with status epilepticus. *Neurology* 2000;55:722–724.

37. Mayer SA, Claassen J, Lokin J, et al. Refractory status epilepticus: frequency, risk factors, and impact on outcome. *Arch Neurol* 2002;59:205–210.

38. Claassen J, Hirsch LJ, Emerson RG, et al. Continuous EEG monitoring and midazolam infusion for refractory nonconvulsive status epilepticus. *Neurology* 2001;57:1036–1042.

39. Bleck TP. Management approaches to prolonged seizures and status epilepticus. *Epilepsia* 1999;40 (Suppl 1):S59–S63; discussion S64–S66.

40. Finley GA, MacManus B, Sampson SE, et al. Delayed seizures following sedation with propofol. *Can J Anaesthesiol* 1993;40:863–865.

41. Kapur J, Coulter DA. Experimental status epilepticus alters gamma-aminobutyric acid type A receptor function in CA1 pyramidal neurons. *Ann Neurol* 1995;38:893–900.

42. Borris DJ, Bertram EH, Kapur J. Ketamine controls prolonged status epilepticus. *Epilepsy Res* 2000;42:117–122.

43. Krishnamurthy KB, Drislane FW. Depth of EEG suppression and outcome in barbiturate anesthetic treatment for refractory status epilepticus. *Epilepsia* 1999;40:759–762.

44. Mirski MA, Williams MA, Hanley DF. Prolonged pentobarbital and phenobarbital coma for refractory generalized status epilepticus. *Crit Care Med* 1995;23:400–404.

21

Viral Encephalitis and Bacterial Meningitis

In the past 20 years the complexity of caring for patients with acute encephalitis and meningitis in the critical care setting has increased. This is the result of the emergence of new pathogens, advances in diagnostic technology, the development of new forms of antiviral and antibacterial chemotherapy, and the increasing sophistication of supportive care and monitoring techniques used in the neurological intensive care unit (neuro-ICU) setting. Defined in their simplest terms, encephalitis is inflammation of the brain, and meningitis is inflammation of the leptomeninges. In establishing the diagnosis, noninfectious inflammatory disorders need to be excluded. The archetypal presentation of infectious encephalitis or meningitis is the clinical triad of fever, headache, and altered mental status. Patients with encephalitis are more prone to develop seizures, mental status changes, and focal neurological deficits, which signify direct brain infection; whereas those with meningitis have more prominent signs of meningeal irritation. Both encephalitis and meningitis may present as isolated infections, or as a component of a systemic infection in which nervous system involvement is but one feature. This chapter focuses on the diagnosis and ICU management of severe acute viral encephalitis and bacterial meningitis.

VIRAL ENCEPHALITIS: GENERAL CONSIDERATIONS

Pathogenesis

Viruses may gain access to the central nervous system either by hematogenous of neuronal routes (1,2), the former being more common. Systemic viral infections arise from inoculation via a mosquito bite (arthropod-borne infection), animal bite, contaminated needle stick, or blood transfusion, or through direct infection of the mucous membranes lining the respiratory, gastroenteric, or genitourinary tracts (Table 21.1). After the initial infection of local tissues, continued viral replication results in transient viremia, diffuse seeding of the reticuloendothelial system, and secondary infection of other organs including the nervous system. Alternatively, a number of special viruses access the nervous system by intraneuronal routes, probably via retrograde transport through the peripheral or olfactory nerves, as occurs with herpes simplex, varicella-zoster, and rabies viruses.

Whether the virus reaches the central nervous system (CNS) via neural or hematogenous routes, widespread infection of the brain occurs only if the virus can attach to and penetrate susceptible cells (neurotropism), and continue to spread and replicate (2,3). Specific cell populations—including the leptomeningeal epithelial tissues, neurons, vascular endothelium, and glia—may have varying degrees of susceptibility to infection, which explains in part why the primary locus of viral infection of the nervous system is so variable. Clinical syndromes related to direct viral infection include encephalitis, meningitis, myelitis, and polyradiculitis, or combinations of these entities.

In viral encephalitis, inflammation occurs primarily in the gray matter and there is a pre-

TABLE 21.1. *Causes of acute viral encephalitis in humans*

Virus	Mode of transmission
Herpes group viruses	
Herpes simplex virus 1	Saliva
Herpes simplex virus 2	Venereal
Epstein–Barr virus	Saliva
Cytomegalovirus	Saliva, blood transfusion, venereal
Varicella–zoster virus	Respiratory droplet
Human herpesvirus 6 and 7	Saliva, respiratory droplet
Herpesvirus simiae	Animal bite
Arboviruses (see Table 22.11)	
Flaviviruses (e.g., St. Louis, dengue)	Arthropod bite
Togaviruses (e.g., eastern and western equine)	Arthropod bite
Reoviruses (e.g., Colorado tick fever)	Arthropod bite
Bunyaviruses (e.g., California, La Crosse)	Arthropod bite
Enteroviruses	
Coxsackievirus	Enteric
Echovirus	Enteric
Poliovirus	Enteric
Enterovirus 70 and 71	Enteric
Hepatitis A virus	Enteric
Paramyxoviruses	
Mumps	Respiratory droplet
Measles	Respiratory droplet
Nipah virus	Respiratory droplet
Arenaviruses	
Lymphocytic choriomeningitis	Respiratory droplet
Rhabdoviruses	
Rabies	Animal bite, transplantation
Adenoviruses	
Adenovirus	Respiratory droplets, enteric
Parvoviruses	
Parvovirus B19	Respiratory droplets
Togavirus/Rubivirus genus	
Rubella	Transplacental
Orthomyxoviruses	
Influenza A and B	Respiratory droplet
Parainfluenza virus	Respiratory droplet
Retroviruses	
HIV-1 and HIV-2	Blood transfusion, venereal, transplacental

Adapted from Johnson RT. Pathogenesis of CNS infections. In: *Viral infections of the nervous system,* 2nd ed. New York: Lippincott–Raven, 1998:35–60.

dominance of perivascular lymphocytic infiltrates. Disruption of the blood–brain barrier (BBB) is a component of all these viral invasions and results from the local expression of chemokines and nitric oxide synthetase, which incite vasogenic cerebral edema (4,5). As the infection progresses, reactive astrocytosis and gliosis become more prominent. Certain unique histopathologic features in encephalitis, such as Cowdry type A intranuclear inclusions with herpesvirus and Negri bodies with rabies virus infection, facilitate the pathologic diagnosis.

Epidemiology

The incidence of clinically diagnosed acute encephalitis is between 3.5 and 7.4 per 100,000 patient-years; in children, the incidence is far higher, exceeding 16 cases per 100,000 patient-years (6). Approximately 20,000 new cases are diagnosed in the United States each year, making this entity slightly less common than aneurysmal subarachnoid hemorrhage. The illness appears in epidemic or sporadic forms. Most epidemics occur in the summer or early fall, and result from arboviruses or enteroviruses.

Establishing the specific causative agent often is difficult, and the likely pathogen depends on geography, the time epoch studied, and the method of diagnosis. In the United States, the most common causes of acute viral encephalitis are herpesviruses, arboviruses, and enteroviruses. In 1977, of all cases of infectious encephalitis reported to the U.S. Centers for Disease Control, 73% were of undetermined etiology, 11% were associated with arboviruses, 6% with exanthem viruses, 3% with mumps, and 7% with other viruses (7). Other studies attempting to identify the most common causes of viral encephalitis have yielded highly variable results. In a classic study conducted from 1953 to 1963 at the Walter Reade Army Institute of Research, which relied on serologic confirmation of the diagnosis, mumps virus was the leading cause of viral encephalitis (Table 21.2) (8). With the advent of modern vaccination, mumps encephalitis is now rare. In two more recent European studies relying on polymerase chain reaction (PCR) technology to detect viral DNA in the cerebrospinal fluid (CSF), enteroviruses (9) and varicella–zoster

(10) were the most common causes of CNS infection, whereas arboviral infections were uncommon (Table 21.2). In the United States, mundane encephalitic enteroviruses such as Epstein–Barr virus (EBV) and cytomegalovirus (CMV) probably account for a large group of cases and among the enteroviruses, LaCrosse is currently the commonest but others, particularly West Nile, have evinced great interest because it is novel and may cause a poliomyelitis. In our experience, CSF PCR testing has greatly increased the frequency with which a specific cause of viral encephalitis is identified; however, a large number of cases still remain undiagnosed.

Clinical Manifestations

The hallmark of viral encephalitis, well known to neurologists, is the clinical triad of fever, headache, and alteration of consciousness. Other neurological manifestations may include disorientation, delirium and other behavioral and language disturbances, memory impairment, hallucinations, hemiparesis, and (perhaps most characteristically) seizures. These illnesses usually reach their

TABLE 21.2. *Relative frequency of viral causes of central nervous system infection among patients referred for diagnostic testing*

Location	Walter Reade Hospital, Washington, DC, U.S.A.	Oxford, U.K.	Helsinki, Finland
Years	1953–1963	1994–1996	1995–1996
Method of diagnosis	Serologic	PCR	PCR and serologic
Enteroviruses	15[a]	53	8
Mumps virus	26	0	0
Lymphocytic choriomeningitis virus	16	0	0
Arboviruses	19	0	6
Herpes simplex virus 1 or 2	16	23	14
Human herpesvirus 6	0	0	7
Varicella–zoster	0	11	32
Epstein–Barr	0	8	3
Adenovirus	0	0	4
Influenza A	0	0	8
Others	9	5	18
TOTAL diagnosed, *n* (% of total studied)	129 (57)	144 (7)	336 (33)
TOTAL studied, *n*	227	2,162	1,014

Values are percent of all diagnosed cases, except where indicated. PCR, polymerase chain reaction.
[a]Poliovirus (8%), Echovirus (3%), Coxsackievirus A (2%), Coxsackievirus B (2%).

full extent within 10 days (11), but severe cases may progresses rapidly to coma with motor posturing. Deterioration is most often owing to extension of the virus through the cerebrum, but cerebral edema with mass effect and elevated intracranial pressure (ICP) are as often responsible. Approximately 40% of severe cases are complicated by seizures. Convulsive or nonconvulsive status epilepticus tends to be highly refractory to treatment when it occurs.

Diagnosis

History and Examination

Noninfectious processes simulate viral encephalitis; among these, acute disseminated encephalomyelitis, CNS vasculitis, Behçet's disease, or mitochondrial encephalopathy, lactic acidosis and stroke-like episodes (MELAS) should be considered (Table 21.3). Noninfectious processes frequently masquerade as viral encephalitis: In one prospective study (perhaps not representative of the modern era), 22% of brain biopsies for suspected herpes simplex encephalitis (HSE) yielded a noninfectious diagnosis (12). Many of these conditions are recognized by paying particular attention to extracranial manifestations of the disease, such as a rash, renal or cardiac involvement, or hematologic abnormalities. A large number of nonviral

TABLE 21.3. *Noninfectious processes that can mimic viral encephalitis*

Vascultis
Behçet disease
Acute disseminated encephalomyelitis
Multiple sclerosis
Systemic lupus erythematosus
Mitochondrial encephalopathy, lactic acidosis, and stroke-like episodes (MELAS)
Sarcoidosis
Thrombotic thrombocytopenia purpura
Cerebral neoplasm
Adrenoleukodystrophy
Reye syndrome
Cerebral infarction
Paraneoplastic limbic encephalitis

TABLE 21.4. *Nonviral causes of infectious encephalitis*

Mycoplasma pneumonia
Brucellosis
Meningovascular syphilis
Lyme disease
Rocky Mountain spotted fever
Q fever
Leptospirosis
Toxoplasma gondii
Tuberculosis
Whipple disease
Plasmodium falciparum
Cryptococcus neoformans
Histoplasma capsulatum
Naegleria
Acanthamoeba and Balamuthia
Cat scratch fever
Listeriosis
Bacterial endocarditis
Cysticercosis

causes of infectious encephalitis must be considered also, particularly because the majority of these infections are treatable (Table 21.4).

As mentioned, efforts to achieve a specific etiologic diagnosis rely on careful attention to the epidemiologic setting, clinical manifestations of the process, and the appropriate use of the laboratory tests. Important historical elements include recent travel and recreational activities, contact with animals, and occupational exposures (Table 21.5) (13). It has been noted by others that the features of the neurological syndrome itself generally are not helpful for differentiating between specific viral etiologies. For instance, when signs and symptoms of viral encephalitis were compared between patients with and without biopsy-proven HSE, no distinguishing characteristics could be identified (Table 21.6) (12). We are not in full agreement because language and memory difficulties early in the illness are suggestive of herpes infection and certain viruses cause basal ganglionic features. An important exception also is West Nile virus encephalitis, which is often associated with neuromuscular abnormalities, specifically the aforementioned poliomyelitis (14).

TABLE 21.5. *Historical data and physical findings that suggest the cause of viral encephalitis*

Variable	Virus(es)
Historical data	
Season	Arboviruses in tick and mosquito season; mumps in spring; enteroviruses in late summer and fall
Travel	Other arboviruses, exotic viruses (e.g., Nipah virus)
Family illnesses	Enteroviruses cause family outbreaks of varied disease
Recreational activity	California encephalitis in woodlands
Animal exposures	Lymphocytic choriomeningitis carried by mice or hamsters; rabies by bat, wild carnivore, dog or cat bites; herpes Simiae virus with monkey bites
Immunization and transfusions	Hepatitis B and human immunodeficiency virus (HIV) via transfusion
Physical findings	
Rash	Viruses causing childhood exanthems (i.e., measles, rubella), enteroviruses, human herpesvirus 6
Herpangina	Coxsackie viruses
Adenopathy	HIV, Epstein–Barr, cytomegalovirus.
Parotitis and/or orchitis	Mumps virus, lymphocytic choriomeningitis virus
Pneumonitis	Adenoviruses, lymphocytic choriomeningitis virus

Adapted from Johnson RT. Meningitis, encephalitis, and poliomyelitis. In: *Viral infections of the nervous system*, 2nd ed. New York: Lippincott–Raven, 1998:87–132.

TABLE 21.6. *Presenting symptoms and signs in patients with biopsy-proven herpes simplex encephalitis (HSE)*

	HSE+	HSE–
Historic findings		
Alteration of consciousness	109/112 (97%)	82/84 (98%)
Fever	101/112 (90%)	66/85 (78%)
Headache	89/110 (81%)	56/73 (77%)
Personality change	62/87 (71%)	44/65 (68%)
Seizures	73/109 (67%)	48/81 (59%)
Vomiting	51/111 (46%)	38/82 (46%)
Hemiparesis	33/100 (33%)	19/72 (26%)
Memory loss	14/59 (24%)	9/47 (19%)
Clinical findings at presentation		
Fever	101/110 (92%)	64/79 (81%)
Personality change	69/81 (85%)	43/58 (74%)
Dysphasia	58/76 (76%)	36/54 (67%)
Autonomic dysfunction	53/88 (60%)	40/71 (56%)
Ataxia	23/55 (40%)	18/45 (40%)
Hemiparesis	41/107 (38%)	24/81 (30%)
Seizures	43/112 (38%)	40/85 (47%)
Cranial nerve defects	34/105 (22%)	27/81 (33%)
Visual field loss	8/58 (14%)	4/33 (12%)
Papilledema	16/111 (14%)	9/84 (11%)

Data are those with finding/total number evaluable (%).
From Whitley RJ, Soong SJ, Linneman C, et al. Herpes simplex encephalitis. Clinical assessment. *JAMA* 1982;247:317–320, with permission.

Cerebrospinal Fluid Examination

CSF examination is essential for establishing the diagnosis and identifying the cause of viral encephalitis. CSF abnormalities generally include pleocytosis (usually lymphocytic) and elevation of protein; glucose levels usually are normal. A small proportion of patients (3% to 5%) with severe viral infections of the CNS, including HSE, may have completely normal CSF, particularly early in the illness (15). We have twice in the last year given the erroneous opinion that a patient with headache, confusion, and fever did not have a meningoencephalitis because the spinal fluid on the first day was normal. Elevated intrathecal IgG production is a nonspecific finding that occurs with many CNS inflammatory or infectious processes and cannot be depended on to aid in diagnosis. An increase in CSF lactate levels has been associated with a poor prognosis, mainly in meningitis (16). Although cultures of CSF are of limited value for isolating virus, the detection of viral DNA with PCR technology has revolutionized the way in which viral encephalitis is identified, and it has become almost a necessity in modern diagnosis (9,10). In the National Institute of Allergy and Infectious Diseases (NIAID) collaborative study, CSF PCR was 98% sensitive and 94% specific when compared to brain biopsy as the standard for certain agents (17). Multiplex PCR assays that simultaneously test a single CSF sample for the most common and important causes of viral encephalitis are particularly useful and efficient (18).

Neuroimaging and Electroencephalogram

Magnetic resonance brain imaging is more sensitive than CT for evaluating cerebral pathology in viral encephalitis (19,20). Diffusion-weighted imaging (DWI), reflecting cytotoxic edema, is useful for identifying focal pathology when vague abnormalities are seen on T2-weighted and FLAIR sequences (Fig. 21.1) (21). Electroencephalography is of value for demonstrating periodic lateralized epileptiform discharges (PLEDs), a physiologic marker of structural temporal lobe damage, or electrographic seizure activity in comatose patients (22). Periodic lateralized epileptiform discharges are seen most commonly with HSE, which has a predilection for involvement of the temporal lobes, but are not sensitive or specific for this entity (15).

Ancillary Testing

Successful serologic or PCR confirmation of the cause of viral encephalitis usually occurs several weeks into the illness, and thus is not helpful for guiding therapy, which should be empiric. Nonetheless, it is of some value to establish a specific diagnosis if possible in order to identify epidemic forms of viral encephalitis, and for determining the prognosis. Serologic diagnosis depends on demonstrating the production of organism-specific IgM antibodies in the CSF or plasma, or seroconversion or seroboosting (a fourfold rise) of IgG titers between the acute and convalescent (3 to 4 weeks) phase of the illness. Even with PCR technology, it remains important to perform acute and convalescent serologic testing in patients with viral encephalitis, because CSF PCR is not 100% sensitive or specific. To facilitate diagnosis, viral cultures of throat (influenza, enterovirus), rectal (enterovirus), urine (adenovirus, CMV), saliva (rabies), and skin exudate (herpes) specimens also should be obtained (11).

Brain Biopsy

Tissue biopsy remains the gold standard for establishing the diagnosis of viral encephalitis but is unnecessary in most circumstances. Nonetheless, in experienced hands, the procedure has a low rate of complications (23). The morbidity consists primarily of bleeding or hematoma at the biopsy site and occurs in less than 3% of patients. The specificity of a positive brain biopsy approaches 100% (24). The sensitivity of brain biopsy for viral encephalitis is approximately 95%; a false-negative biopsy can result when an uninvolved area of brain is analyzed, or from errors in pathologic

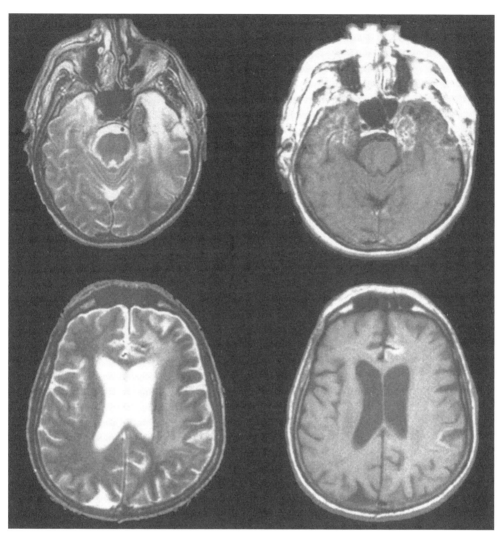

FIG. 21.1. Chronic magnetic resonance imaging abnormalities (*left,* T2; *right,* T1 with gadolinium) in a 56-year-old man with viral encephalitis who developed behavioral abnormalities consistent with the Klüver–Bucy syndrome (hyperphagia, hypersexuality, amnesia, visual agnosia). The causative viral agent was not identified by cerebral spinal fluid polymerase chain reaction studies or brain biopsy. The images reveal hemorrhagic necrosis with dystrophic calcification of the left medial temporal lobe, and laminar necrosis (increased T1 signal) of the left medial frontal and parietal lobes.

specimen processing or interpretation. Immunohistochemical stains have recently made rapid diagnosis possible from brain biopsies, and confocal microscopy can facilitate these analyses by identifying specific regions of abnormal staining that then can be processed for more detailed ultrastructural and electron microscopy studies (25). Magnetic resonance imaging should be used for guidance in se-

lecting an involved area for biopsy: Open leptomeningeal and tissue biopsies from cortical regions with contrast enhancement yield the best diagnostic results. Although specific histopathologic findings such as intranuclear inclusions may be present in only one third of brain biopsies from patients with HSE, a negative culture carries more diagnostic weight if it is obtained from an abnormal area of brain.

Brain biopsy is generally indicated only when a patient is responding poorly to treatment and the precise diagnosis remains in question after noninvasive testing. The exception is that biopsy should be performed with a lower threshold in immunocompromised patients, in whom opportunistic infections frequently mimic HSE.

Treatment

General Treatment Measures

As is the case for all serious neurological conditions managed in the ICU, treatment begins with meticulous attention to general supportive measures that can minimize complications. Comatose patients who are unable to protect their airway should be intubated. Unintubated patients who are agitated or delirious should be treated with general orienting measures at the bedside and haloperidol 1 to 10 mg every 2 to 6 hours or a similar agent. Intubated patients can be sedated with propofol or midazolam infusions, with frequent "wake-ups" to allow serial assessment of neurological status. In both cases, an opioid such as morphine or fentanyl or nonsteroidal analgesia such as ketorolac should be given if pain is felt to be a contributing factor. Only isotonic intravenous fluids such as 0.9% saline solution should be administered, to avoid the exacerbation of cerebral edema that can result from hypotonic fluids. Early and aggressive enteral feeding should be provided to combat the protein catabolism that is characteristic of most serious neurological illnesses.

With regard to seizures, phenytoin (15 to 20 mg/kg followed by 5 mg/kg per day) is recommended by some authorities to prevent seizures, and frequent drug levels should be obtained to ensure that serum concentrations are in the therapeutic range. However, we have not used anticonvulsants prophylactically and instead waited for an indication that seizures will be a problem. Surveillance EEG monitoring is advisable in patients whose level of consciousness is fluctuating or in those who are persistently comatose, to rule out nonconvulsive status epilepticus (Chapter 8). Aggressive intervention with acetaminophen and cooling blankets to control fever should be pursued, although these measures are often ineffective (26).

Intracranial Pressure Management

Clinical deterioration in patients with viral encephalitis may be associated with cerebral edema and increased ICP. In the NIAID collaborative antiviral study of herpes encephalitis, two thirds of patients had progression after the diagnosis was confirmed by brain biopsy, and one third of the patients lapsed into coma (27). As in other diseases, the indication for placement of an ICP monitor includes: (a) coma; (b) a CT or MR scan demonstrating significant intracranial mass effect (e.g., global edema with effacement of the basal cisterns); and (c) a prognosis that merits aggressive ICU intervention (28). In our small series of comatose encephalitis patients, intracranial monitoring revealed the progressive development of increased ICP during the first 2 weeks, and control of ICP was associated with better outcomes (29). The proportion of patients with encephalitis who may be expected to develop raised ICP is not known but is certainly highest among those with HSE.

The role of corticosteroids in treating brain edema associated with viral encephalitis is controversial. One small trial failed to demonstrate a benefit from dexamethasone in Japanese encephalitis (30). However, case reports have described dramatic clinical improvement after the initiation of steroid therapy for varied forms of encephalitis (31–33). In our opinion, a brief course of dexamethasone (4 to 10 mg every 6 hours) is a reasonable treatment option for stuporous or comatose encephalitis patients with severe brain edema on neuroimaging. Mild to moderate hypothermia may be a promising treatment for these patients as well (34–36). In febrile infants with influenza encephalitis and low CPP (less than 70 mm Hg), brain temperature can exceed core body temperature by greater than 2°C, a phenomenon termed "brain thermo-pooling" (34). Therapeutic hypothermia has been associated with clinical and radiographic improvement and reduced ICP in case reports (35,36); however, well-designed studies of temperature modulation on the course of viral encephalitis have yet to be performed. As a last resort, decompressive hemicraniectomy may be life-saving for young patients with severe necrotizing viral encephalitis resulting in focal mass effect and transtentorial herniation; good recoveries after this procedure have been described (37,38).

Antiviral Therapy

Specific therapy is available for only a few of the viruses that cause acute encephalitis (Table 21.7). If there is any possibility of herpes simplex infection, intravenous acyclovir should be started immediately. Clinical trials indicate that acyclovir, when started early, reduces mortality from approximately 70% to 25%, and that almost 40% of those who survive make a good recovery with minimal long-term disability (27,39). Serious varicella–zoster infections, including encephalitis and polyradiculitis, can be treated with acyclovir in combination with other agents (Table 21.7). In patients with CMV encephalitis, ganciclovir is the preferred agent, with or without concurrent foscarnet. Though these agents have demonstrated efficacy against CMV retinitis in HIV infected patients, the clinical response of CMV encephalitis patients treated with a single agent is usually poor, which has prompted the recommendation for combination therapy (40). Pleconaril is a novel agent with activity against picornavirus enteroviral infections (e.g., polio, Coxsackie, enterovirus 71), which is currently in clinical trials and is available for compassionate use (41). Quantitative CSF PCR testing, which measures the burden of viral DNA (number of DNA copies per μL CSF), is becoming increasingly used to assess the response to treatment. Almost all patients with HSE have a negative CSF PCR after 14 days of treatment with acyclovir; persistence is associated with resistant strains and poor prognosis, and probably is an indication for prolonged therapy with additional agents (42).

Outcome

Outcome after encephalitis depends primarily on the virulence of the infecting agent. Rabies (mortality greater than 90%) and Eastern equine encephalitis (mortality greater than 30%) are generally regarded as the most lethal forms of viral encephalitis in the United States. Other determinants of poor outcome include increasing age, absent or late (greater than 4 days) initiation of antiviral therapy, coma, status epilepticus, and elevated ICP (11). Approximately half of those who survive

TABLE 21.7. Antiviral agents for serious acute central nervous system viral infections

Agent	Targets	Dosage	Comments
Acyclovir (Zovirax)	HSV, VZV	10 mg/kg q8 h i.v. for 14–21 d	First-line therapy for HSV
Gancyclovir (Cytovene)	CMV	10 mg/kg q12 h i.v. for 14–21 d	First-line therapy for CMV, often combined with foscarnet
Foscarnet (Foscavir)	CMV, VZV	180 mg/kg i.v. q8 h for 14–21 d	Often combined with gancyclovir for CMV infection
Pleconaril (Picovir)	Picornaoviruses	5 mg/kg p.o. t.i.d. for 7 d	Pending FDA approval; available for compassion use at www.viropharma.com
Valacyclovir (Valtrex)	HSV, VZV	1,000 mg p.o. b.i.d.	Being tested as follow-up therapy after I.V. acyclovir for HSV encephalitis
Famciclovir (Famvir)	HSV, VZV	500 mg t.i.d. for 7–14 d	Used primarily for genital herpes and Zoster infections

b.i.d., twice per day; CMV, cytomegalovirus; FDA, U.S. Food and Drug Administration; HSV, herpes simplex virus; i.v., intravenous; p.o., orally; t.i.d., three times per day; VZV, varicella–zoster virus.

an episode of viral encephalitis are disabled by cognitive or motor impairment, which can be profound (43). Focal damage of the hippocampi, medial temporal lobes, and frontal and cingulate cortex from HSE and other infections can result in dramatic amnestic and behavioral abnormalities, including the Klüver–Bucy syndrome (hyperphagia, hypersexuality, amnesia, and visual agnosia, Fig. 21.1) (44,45). Although functional independence can improve with intensive rehabilitation, the rate of recovery varies and is generally less than that for traumatic brain injury (46). Late epilepsy develops in up to 20% of encephalitis patients (47). The majority of this latter group has survived severe infections complicated by coma and seizures, experience complex-partial seizures related to multiple seizure foci, and are highly refractory to anticonvulsant therapy (48).

SPECIFIC CAUSES OF ACUTE VIRAL ENCEPHALITIS

Herpes Simplex Encephalitis

Clinical Presentation

Herpes simplex virus comprises approximately 10% of cases of viral encephalitis in the United States, and is the most frequently cause of fatal sporadic encephalitis (49). Occurring throughout the year, about one half of cases develop in patients older than 50 (1). The majority of HSE is caused by HSV-1. It has been proposed that approximately half of HSE cases are related to primary infection, and half are the result of viral reactivation (1,50). Experimental evidence suggests that latent HSV-1 infection may result from reactivation of the virus in the trigeminal ganglia, with transport of the virus from the nasal mucosal to the olfactory tract to the brain (1). The medical history with respect to prior labial or genital herpes simplex infection is not helpful in establishing the diagnosis. A history of herpes simplex labialis or genitalis is elicited in approximately 25% of patients with HSE, and in the same percentage of patients with other forms of encephalitis.

The stereotypical presentation of a patient with HSE includes 24 to 48 hours of gradually increasing headache, fever, and confusion, which may be preceded by olfactory hallucinations (15). In addition, patients may experience memory loss, personality changes, aphasia, and focal or generalized seizures, and may or may not have focal motor findings (Table 21.6). Although this clinical constellation should raise the suspicion of HSE, few patients present in such a straightforward fashion, and no single finding or combination of findings rules in or out the diagnosis. The more recent use CSF PCR instead of brain biopsy to establish the diagnosis of HSE has expanded awareness of milder or atypical forms of presentation, such as brainstem encephalitis (51), which comprise approximately 20% of all cases (52). This subset of patients has a higher than expected number of individuals infected with HSV-2 rather than HSV-1, suggesting that HSV-2 is more likely to cause milder or atypical disease.

Diagnosis

Most but not all HSE patients have abnormal CSF. The initial lumbar puncture usually exhibits a moderate pleocytosis (50 to 500 lymphocytes/mm^3), which is usually primarily lymphocytic. Even though HSE is often thought of as a hemorrhagic, only 20% of patients have more than 500 red blood cells/mm^3. The CSF glucose may be normal or decreased, but is only rarely extremely low. The CSF protein is usually mildly elevated, but it is normal at clinical presentation in approximately 20% of patients. Herpes simplex virus is only rarely cultured from the spinal fluid of adults with HSE.

Much emphasis has been placed on noninvasive neurodiagnostic studies as a useful approach to separate patients with HSE from those with other forms of encephalitis. Patients with HSE are more likely than patients with other forms of encephalitis to have localized abnormalities on EEG, technetium-99 (^{99}Tc) perfusion scans, or CT than are patients with other forms of encephalitis (15). However, localized abnormalities are seen frequently enough in patients with other forms of encephalitis that these studies cannot be used to make an etiologic diagnosis. The EEG is abnormal in 80% of patients with HSE; diffuse slowing, spike and slow waves localized to the area of involved brain, and PLEDS are the most frequently encountered EEG findings.

Many studies have explored the value of CSF examination in establishing the diagnosis of HSE (53–55). Although serum and CSF antibodies to herpes simplex rise in many patients with HSE, this is neither universal nor specific, and important changes are rarely present early enough in the course of illness to be clinically useful. More recently PCR technology has been applied to the diagnosis of HSE (56,57). One study that evaluated 43 patients with HSE and 60 patients with acute nonherpetic encephalitis revealed a positive PCR signal in 42 patients with HSE and in none of the control subjects (56). In this study, CSF samples were positive for herpes simplex virus DNA as early as the first day of illness.

With the advent of acyclovir as the drug of choice for treatment of HSE and the wide availability of CSF PCR testing, there has been much less enthusiasm in many centers for brain biopsy to establish the diagnosis. Although it is clear that acyclovir has relatively little toxicity, it bears repeating that physicians remain aware of the fact that other diagnoses were established in 22% of patients undergoing brain biopsy with the presumptive diagnosis of HSE in the NIAID studies; 40% of these cases had entities for which specific therapy is available, including pyogenic brain abscess, cryptococcal meningitis, toxoplasma encephalitis, CNS lymphoma, and tuberculosis (12). Mitochondrial encephalopathy, lactic acidosis and stroke-like episodes, enteroviruses, parainfluenza virus, or human herpesviruses (HHV)-6 may also present in a fashion that mimics HSE (58–61). Although it can no longer be argued that most patients with suspected HSE should undergo brain biopsy (62), the threshold for obtaining tissue for biopsy confirmation in cases of suspected HSE should remain low, particularly if the patient fails to respond well to treatment. Several elaborate decision-making analysis paradigms have been applied to the question as to whether to perform brain biopsies on all, some, or no patients with suspected herpes simplex encephalitis (63–65). Although these analyses are elegant exercises, they are rarely of substantive use in approaching individual patients.

Treatment

After initial favorable reports of idoxuridine in uncontrolled trials in the early 1970s were shown to be flawed by the absence of controls (66), a randomized placebo-controlled study of adenine arabinoside was conducted by the NIAID Collaborative Antiviral Study Group. This study documented a reduction in mortality of patients with HSE from 70% to 30% (27). A subsequent study that compared adenine arabinoside with acyclovir established acyclovir as the drug of choice for treating patients with HSE (39). Side effects of acyclovir include renal insufficiency, which can be minimized with aggressive hydration, thrombocytopenia, transaminase elevation, fever, leukopenia, and metabolic encephalopathy with prominent myoclonus and tremor (67). An entity of early relapse after completion of short-term acyclovir also has been recognized (68). Although this phenomenon generally should prompt the reinstitution of therapy, it has more recently been proposed that this form of late deterioration may represent a postinfectious immune-mediated phenomenon.

Outcome

Despite the decreased mortality associated with acyclovir therapy, morbidity remains high, especially in patients older than 30 years of age, when therapy is delayed, and in those who are stuporous or comatose. Early treatment is critical: If acyclovir is started within 4 days or less, mortality falls from approximately 35% to almost zero (1). Quantitative CSF PCR may provide valuable information about prognosis. In one study, survival with a good outcome occurred in all patients with less than

100 HSV DNA copies/μL CSF, whereas mortality was 22% and residual impairment was the rule in those with more copies (69). Outcomes are generally more favorable in children; in one series, mortality was only 7%, and more than one half of the survivors had no neurological sequelae (70). Clear-cut neurocognitive abnormalities are often present in long-term survivors of HSE, even in individuals who exhibit normal performance in bedside clinical mental status tests (71).

Epstein–Barr Virus

Clinical Presentation

Primary infection with EBV may be subclinical or it may be associated with the syndrome of infectious mononucleosis (72). In adolescents and adults the classic triad of fever, pharyngitis, and lymphadenopathy may be present in as few as 10% or as many as 70% of patients with primary EBV infection, depending on the setting (73–75). Laboratory features of the illness include an atypical lymphocytosis and the appearance of heterophile antibodies in the peripheral blood (72). However, these laboratory findings are far from universal (76).

In a subset of patients with primary EBV infection, dramatic neurological complications can occur (77–80). Neurological manifestations of EBV infection include focal abnormalities such as Bell's palsy, and more global abnormalities such as encephalitis or Guillain–Barré syndrome (Table 21.8). Al-

TABLE 21.8. *Neurological complications of primary Epstein–Barr virus infection*

Encephalitis
Meningitis
Transverse myelitis
Guillain–Barré syndrome
Optic neuritis
Cranial nerve palsies
Mononeuritis multiplex
Seizures
Psychosis
Hallucinations and illusions ("Alice-in-Wonderland" syndrome)

though direct infection of the CNS can occur, in some situations such as Guillain–Barré syndrome, it has been postulated that the clinical manifestations are the result of a secondary autoimmune response induced by the virus. The onset of EBV encephalitis can be dramatic, with a rapid progression from headache to coma. In some patients, cerebellitis is present as one of the earliest manifestations of a global encephalitis (81).

Diagnosis

Cerebrospinal fluid PCR analysis is the diagnostic modality of choice for diagnosing EBV infection of the CNS. Semiquantitative analysis of EBV DNA suggests that copy numbers are substantially higher in those with active infection than in latently infected patients who are seropositive for EBV (82). Primary CNS lymphoma in HIV-infected patients is also highly associated with positive EBV PCR in the CSF (42). Epstein–Barr virus–specific serologic testing also can be helpful in establishing the diagnosis: IgM antibody directed against the viral capsid antigen indicates primary infection (83).

Treatment

In patients with EBV-induced encephalitis, management consists primarily of supportive care. There is no indication for corticosteroid use. Although EBV is sensitive *in vitro* to acyclovir and it has been studied in acute infectious mononucleosis (84), there have been no controlled trials of acyclovir in patients with EBV encephalitis. Treatment with acyclovir is a reasonable option for patients with severe disease, but there is no evidence to support its efficacy.

Outcome

In patients with EBV-induced neurological complications, full recovery should be expected in 85% of patients without specific therapeutic intervention (72).

Varicella–Zoster Virus

Clinical Presentation

Disseminated primary infection with varicella–zoster virus (VZV) is associated with chickenpox. In most children, chickenpox is a self-limiting illness unassociated with neurological manifestations. In some, and more frequently in adults, however, chickenpox may be associated with encephalitis (Table 21.9) (85). In addition, the use of aspirin in children with varicella may be associated with the now rare Reye syndrome (86). As in the case of EBV, varicella encephalitis often presents with cerebellar signs; this complication usually occurs 5 to 10 days after the onset of the rash, but it may, on rare occasions, precede the onset of the rash (87,88).

Encephalitis may accompany recurrent herpes zoster infection of the spinal ganglia ("shingles"), in both immunocompetent and immunocompromised patients (89). Aseptic meningitis is a more common accompanying feature of herpes zoster, and is usually minimally symptomatic. Aseptic meningitis, polyneuritis, myelitis, or encephalitis related to VZV infection also can occur in the absence of cutaneous findings (90). In the setting of HIV infection, VZV can cause an acute necrotizing encephalitis or a more chronic progressive form of encephalitis (91,92).

Infection of cerebral arteries by VZV can produce unifocal or multifocal vasculopathy. Unifocal large-vessel vasculopathy (granulomatous arteritis) usually affects elderly immunocompetent persons, whereas multifocal vasculopathy occurs in persons who are immunocompromised (93). In the most common scenario, ophthalmic zoster is followed after several weeks by ipsilateral middle cerebral artery territory infarction related to vasculitis, which is the result of retrograde spread of VZV via the trigeminal system. Less typical presentations include cerebral vasculopathy following a remote site of Zoster infection (i.e., sacral), a progressive leukoencephalopathy, and ischemic optic neuropathy (93).

Diagnosis

Cerebrospinal fluid PCR analysis is the test of choice for diagnosis CNS VZV infection (94), but is not 100% sensitive, particularly in patients with delayed vasculopathy. In these cases the demonstration of intrathecal anti-VZV IgG production (CSF greater than serum titers) can establish the diagnosis.

Treatment

Central nervous system VZV infections should be treated with intravenous acyclovir (Table 21.7). The limited gastrointestinal absorption of acyclovir, coupled with its relatively lower activity against VZV compared with simplex viruses, renders oral therapy in-

TABLE 21.9. *Neurological complications of varicella–zoster virus infection*

Type of infection	Comments
Primary infection	
Encephalitis	Increases in frequency with age; cerebellar involvement common
Cranial mononeuropathy or polyneuropathy	Rare
Reye syndrome	Accompanying administration of aspirin to children with varicella
Guillain–Barré syndrome	Virus triggers an autoimmune response
Reactivation (herpes zoster)	
Aseptic meningitis	Common accompaniment of uncomplicated zoster; usually self-limiting
Encephalitis	More frequent in association with systemic dissemination in immunocompromised individuals
Delayed cerebral vasculopathy	Ophthalmic zoster with MCA involvement most common; viral transport along trigeminal system is thought to trigger giant cell arteritis

MCA, middle cerebral artery.

adequate for CNS manifestations of VZV infection. Foscarnet can be added for severe or resistant infections. There is good evidence that early antiviral therapy can prevent secondary dissemination of VZV infection in immunocompromised patients with herpes zoster (95). Although controlled trials have not yet addressed the issue of treatment for VZV-associated vasculopathy, treatment with acyclovir is probably advisable (93).

Prognosis

In patients with the cerebellar form of varicella encephalitis the spinal fluid is usually normal, and prospects for recovery are excellent. With frank encephalitis the prognosis is not as good as with the cerebellitis, but still most patients recover without sequelae. Most of our nonimmunocompromised patients who have CNS complications of herpes zoster also do well.

Other Herpesviruses

Cytomegalovirus

Cytomegalovirus rarely causes encephalitis in immunocompetent patients (96). One case of simultaneous CNS infection with herpes simplex virus and CMV has been reported (97). In the setting of HIV, chorioretinitis is the most common manifestation of CMV infection; its frequency has fallen dramatically with the advent of highly active antiretroviral therapy (HAART) (42). Central nervous system infection in immunocompromised patients may also be accompanied by systemic evidence of CMV infection, such as hepatitis or colitis (98). In AIDS, acute ependymitis with prominent oculomotor signs mimicking Wernicke encephalopathy can occur (99). The ubiquity of CMV and the neurotropism of the HIV virus make it difficult to ascribe a cause-and-effect relationship between CMV infection and HIV-related dementia (100). Like the other herpesviruses, CMV infection has also been associated with Guillain–Barré syndrome

(101). The diagnosis of CMV encephalitis is best established by CSF PCR analysis (102). Ganciclovir and foscarnet alone or in combination are used for treatment; chronic maintenance therapy is required to prevent relapses in immunosuppressed patients (Table 21.7) (103).

Herpesvirus simiae

Herpesvirus simiae also known as simian B virus, is enzootic in rhesus and other Old World monkeys (104). Analogous to herpes simplex virus in humans, the agent is shed intermittently from the oropharynx of infected monkeys. Symptomatic disease caused by this agent resulting from an animal bite is rare in humans but is devastating when it occurs (105). Several days to several weeks after the exposure, vesicles or pain and paresthesias may appear at the site of the inoculation. Aseptic meningitis and encephalitis then develop over the course of the next several days. A subgroup may present with the central nervous manifestations without antecedent peripheral manifestations. Death occurs in 70% to 85% of humans with symptomatic disease. Although the agent is not exquisitely sensitive to acyclovir *in vitro,* intravenous acyclovir (10 mg/kg every 8 hours) should be used in individuals with signs or symptoms suggestive of *Herpesvirus simiae* infection (106).

Human Herpesviruses 6 and 7

HHV-6 and HHV-7 cause exanthema subitum (also known as roseola infantum or sixth disease), childhood febrile illnesses with a spreading maculopapular rash (42). Review of CSF specimens of patients initially suspected to have HSE infection found HHV-6 DNA in 7% of specimens, suggesting that this virus may be a more common cause of sporadic focal encephalitis than was previously suspected (107). Their sensitivity to antiviral agents parallels that of CMV, with most isolates resistant to acyclovir, but sensitive to ganciclovir and foscarnet (42).

Arboviral Encephalitis

The term *arbovirus* (*ar*thropod-*bo*rne) is derived from older taxonomic criteria in which viruses were classified by mode of spread. *Arboviral encephalitis,* however, is a useful term to describe encephalitis caused by any one of several agents that may be transmitted by mosquitoes or ticks. In the United States eight agents account for the vast majority of cases of arboviral encephalitis (Table 21.10). These agents are single- or double-stranded RNA viruses that belong to the Togavirus, Flavivirus, or Bunyavirus families. They share the features of being transmitted primarily by mosquitoes or ticks and of being geographically or seasonally clustered to one degree or another. Although geographically named, it is important to recognize that the terminology reflects the site of initial description more accurately than it does the distribution of the agent. In recent years, most U.S. arboviral infections have been caused by the LaCrosse and St. Louis viruses (42). Following a dramatic outbreak in New York City in 1999, however, West Nile virus (WNV) has now emerged as the most important cause of arboviral encephalitis in the United States.

Japanese Encephalitis

Japanese encephalitis, transmitted by Culex mosquitoes, causes more cases of encephalitis worldwide than the other arthropod-borne viruses combined (1). During the past 75 years, Japanese encephalitis has expanded from China and southeast Asia to include India and Pakistan, eastern Russia, the Philippines, and Australia. In China alone, at least 20,000 cases are reported annually, most commonly in children (108). Only a minority of infections lead to encephalitis. After a few days of nonspecific symptoms, patients with Japanese encephalitis develop headache, altered mental status, and vomiting; seizures occur in 10% of adults and 85% of children. Other characteristic signs include tremor, dystonia, rigidity, and a masklike facies (1). Magnetic resonance imaging shows a characteristic pattern of mixed intensity lesions, especially in the thalamus and basal ganglia (109). Diagnosis is facilitated by the detection of IgM antibodies in the CSF. The mortality rate is 30%, and 50% of survivors are permanently disabled. Although there is no established treatment, a clinical trial of interferon alpha is currently underway.

TABLE 21.10. *Characteristics of selected mosquito-borne arbovirus encephalitides in the United States*

Virus	Geographical distribution	Age-group affected	Mortality	Symptoms
Western equine	West, midwest U.S.	Infants and adults (>50 years old)	Moderate in infants; 5%–10% in other ages	Headache, altered consciousness, seizures
Eastern equine	East, Gulf Coast, southern U.S.	Children and adults	>30%	Headache, altered consciousness, seizures
Venezuelan	South America, southern U.S.	Adults	1%	Headache, myalgias, pharyngitis, leukopenia
St. Louis	Central, west, southern U.S.	Adults (>50 years old)	20%	Headache, nausea, vomiting, disorientation, stupor, irritability
California	Northcentral U.S.	Children	2%	Fever, headache, leukocytosis
La Crosse	Central, eastern U.S.	Children	5%–15%	Seizures, paralysis, focal weakness
Colorado tick fever	Western U.S.	Children and adults	<1%	Transmitted by tickbite; fever and chills precede encephalitis
West Nile	East Coast U.S., Africa, Middle East, Europe	Adults	Low	Seizures, myelitis, polyradiculitis, optic neuritis

Adapted from Ebel H, Kuchta J, Balogh A, et al. Operative treatment of tentorial herniation in herpes encephalitis. *Child Nerv System* 1999;15:84–86.

Eastern Equine Encephalitis

Eastern equine encephalitis (EEE) is associated with a mortality rate exceeding 30% (110). Nonetheless, subclinical infection or an influenza-like illness is 20 to 30 times more common with EEE infection than is classical encephalitis. Symptomatic disease is experienced most frequently by infants and adults older than the age of 55. Eastern equine encephalitis occurs principally along the eastern and gulf coasts of the United States between June and September, but cases have been reported as far west as South Dakota. Outbreaks in humans in a given area are usually preceded by epizootics in horses. The clinical illness is usually abrupt in onset, with confusion, somnolence, headache, and fever developing over 24 to 48 hours. Seizures are present in 25% of patients on admission (110). Cerebrospinal fluid findings include a lymphocyte pleocytosis that may be as high as 1,000 cells/mm^3; protein is usually elevated and glucose is usually normal. Magnetic resonance imaging most often reveals focal lesions in the basal ganglia, thalami, and brainstem (110). The diagnosis is established by detecting IgM antibodies in the CSF, demonstrating a fourfold rise in serum anti-EEE antibodies, or by isolating virus from the CSF or brain tissue. Poor outcome is predicted by a CSF WBC count exceeding 500 cells/mm^3 or the presence of hyponatremia (less than 130 mEq/L) (110).

Treatment is primarily supportive; antiviral therapy is not yet available for EEE.

Western Equine Encephalitis

Western equine encephalitis (WEE), initially described in California, is found throughout the United States. Although the clinical manifestations in a given patient are indistinguishable from EEE, the illness in general is much less severe, with a mortality rate of less than 5% (111). Cerebrospinal fluid findings usually include a lymphocytic pleocytosis, although polymorphonuclear cells may predominate early in the illness. Treatment is supportive.

Mortality and major sequelae are much more frequently encountered in infants and individuals older than 55 years of age (111, 112).

St. Louis Encephalitis

With its nationwide distribution, St. Louis encephalitis (SLE) is in some older series the most common arboviral disease in the United States (113,114). St. Louis encephalitis is less restricted than most other arboviruses in its choice of vectors, being spread by at least three different mosquitoes. In the urban United States, the virus is spread by a mosquito that breeds in stagnant sewer water. In the West, the mosquito vector breeds in primarily irrigated fields, thus explaining the rural distribution and greater frequency among men with occupational exposure. The typical patient presents with a flulike illness followed by meningoencephalitis. In general, both the severity of disease and propensity of the virus to infect the CNS increases with age (113). The disease often occurs in outbreaks, and the clinical manifestations, CSF findings, and method of diagnosis are similar to those encountered in EEE or WEE. Treatment is primarily supportive; mortality ranges from 2% to 20% (113). Neurological sequelae are present in about 5% of surviving patients and consist primarily of speech defects, ataxia, and visual disturbances.

Venezuelan Equine Encephalitis

Venezuelan equine encephalitis (VEE) is primarily distributed in South and Central America, but also occurs in the southern United States (115). Venezuelan equine encephalitis can be spread by a number of different mosquito vectors during an epizootic. In most patients VEE causes a mild acute febrile illness with no neurological complications. In some individuals, however, headache, confusion, seizures, or tremors may occur. Cerebrospinal fluid findings are nonspecific, consisting of a lymphocytic pleocytosis and a normal or slightly elevated protein concentration. Treatment is supportive. Uncomplicated recovery occurs over a week with few sequelae in most patients. The mortality rate is less than 1% in most series.

West Nile Virus

In August of 1999, an epidemic of viral encephalitis occurred in and around New York City, which ultimately resulted in 62 cases and seven deaths (14). The initial assumption, based on IgM positivity in some patients, was that SLE was the causative agent. After it was noticed that birds in the region were dying at an alarming rate, DNA sequencing and antigenic analysis of specimens obtained from birds and humans implicated WNV, a virus previously restricted to North Africa and the Mediterranean, as the causative agent (116).

Over the past several years, epidemic WNV infection during the summertime months has spread to the mid-Atlantic, midwestern, and southern United States. The most common neurological syndromes caused by WNV infection in the New York City epidemic included encephalitis with muscle weakness (39%), aseptic meningitis (32%), encephalitis without muscle weakness (22%), and a milder illness with headache and fever only (7%) (116). Neuromuscular manifestations of WNV infection include polyradiculitis, axonal polyneuropathy, and a striking poliomyelitis; on occasion, a syndrome indistinguishable from Guillain–Barré syndrome can occur (117). The diagnosis can be established with CSF PCR analysis, by detecting anti-WNV IgM antibodies in the CSF, or by demonstrating a fourfold increase in serum titers. There is no treatment, although ribavirin has been reported to inhibit WNV replication in cell culture (42).

Mumps

Mumps virus is a paramyxovirus that usually causes a self-limiting febrile illness associated with fever and inflammation of the salivary glands. On occasion, however, neurological complications of mumps may dominate the clinical presentation (118,119). A subclinical CSF pleocytosis is not uncommon in mumps, having been recognized in 50% of patients with uncomplicated mumps who underwent lumbar puncture (119). Mumps-associated aseptic meningitis is usually self-limiting, although the CSF abnormalities may persist for as long as a month.

Before the widespread application of mumps vaccine, mumps accounted for 20% to 30% of cases of viral encephalitis in the United States (120). When encephalitis occurs, CNS manifestations usually follow the onset of meningeal symptoms by several days, and the onset of parotitis by 1 to 2 weeks (118). The clinical presentation is usually that of a nonfocal encephalitis, with changes in mental status and fever being the most frequent manifestations. Patients may also have seizures, aphasia, paralysis, or involuntary movements. The encephalitis resolves over a 1- to 2-week period in most patients. Neurological sequelae may include seizure disorders or psychomotor retardation (118,119). Death occurs in 1% to 2% of cases. Diagnosis of mumps encephalitis is facilitated by the recognition of other manifestations of mumps (e.g., parotitis, orchitis, hyperamylasemia), but it may occur in the absence of these findings. Serologic studies for viral isolation from saliva, urine, or CSF may be used to confirm the diagnosis. Treatment is supportive.

Measles and Rubella

Measles (rubeola) is infrequently associated with encephalitis, although subclinical involvement of the CNS as documented by EEG abnormalities is present in up to 50% of cases of uncomplicated measles (121). Measles encephalitis is usually nonfocal in presentation and often presents during convalescence from the typical rash and systemic viral syndrome. Patients present with recurrent fever, seizures, or alteration of mental status. The pathogenesis of measles encephalitis is not known with certainty; the delayed timing of onset and difficulty in isolating virus from brain suggests that it may result from an immune response to the virus in brain tissue (122). The demonstration that levels of neopterin in the CSF are elevated in children with measles-associated encephalitis supports the concept that immune activation in the CNS plays an important role in the pathogenesis of measles encephalitis (123). Although most patients survive, neurological sequelae are common. Diagnosis is usually possible on clinical grounds but may be confirmed serologically. Although the pathogenesis may be immune mediated, there are no convincing data to support the use of immunosuppressive drugs or corticosteroids in the treatment of measles encephalitis. Besides causing acute encephalitis, measles can also cause: (a) a relentlessly progressive subacute encephalitis in immunosuppressed patients; (b) postinfectious immune-mediated demyelinating encephalomyelitis; and (c) subacute sclerosing panencephalitis (SSPE), a "slow" viral infection characterized by progressive dementia, ataxia, myoclonus, periodic sharp and slow wave complexes on EEG, elevated titers of antimeasles antibodies in the CSF, and pathologic intracellular viral inclusion bodies. Rubella (German measles) is very infrequently associated with encephalitis, but the mortality rate is significant (20% to 50%) in patients in whom this complication occurs (124).

Enteroviruses

Enteroviruses cause 40% to 60% of all cases of viral meningitis, most cases of paralytic poliomyelitis, and a small number of cases of encephalitis (13). Most enteroviral infections occur in children and are caused by fecal–oral transmission. With successful eradication owing to vaccines, epidemic paralytic poliomyelitis—which presents as fever, flaccid paralysis, and meningismus with a polymorphonuclear CSF pleocytosis—has not been reported in the United States since 1980 (13). However, rare imported cases still occur. Coxsackievirus and echovirus infections usually are asymptomatic; when they occur, systemic manifestations of infection may include

rash, respiratory symptoms, pleurodynia, carditis, and diarrhea. Group A Coxsackieviruses also cause herpangina, characterized by grayish vesicular lesions on the tonsillar fauces, soft palate, and uvula. Coxsackievirus and echovirus are common causes of aseptic meningitis, and occasionally can cause encephalitis. Usually the encephalitis is mild, and permanent sequelae are rare. Less common CNS manifestations of Coxsackievirus and echovirus infection include cerebellitis, opsoclonus-myoclonus, polyradiculitis, and focal encephalitis with hemiplegia (13). Enteroviral infection detected by PCR has been reported in association with bilateral hippocampal lesions on MR, mimicking HSE (59). Enterovirus (71) can cause a severe form of epidemic spinal and brainstem encephalitis in children, presenting as myoclonus, vomiting, and ataxia; fatal cases have been associated with neurogenic shock and pulmonary edema resulting from medullary involvement (125). Pleconaril is currently being evaluated as a specific antiviral treatment for enteroviral meningoencephalitis; it is not currently FDA approved (41).

Influenza Virus

Encephalitis is a rare complication of influenza virus infection. Some recent strains of influenza A virus in the Far East have been markedly neurovirulent. In Japan, a recent epidemic of influenza A encephalitis was associated with a 25% mortality rate; death was associated with systemic abnormalities such as coagulopathy and hepatic dysfunction (126). Influenza B encephalitis has been associated with seizures, PLEDs, and focal temporal lobe abnormalities on MRI, mimicking HSE (127). In addition to routine serologic testing, CSF PCR analysis can now be used to establish the diagnosis (127,128).

Nipah Virus

This newly recognized paramyxovirus caused a massive outbreak of encephalitis among pig farmers in Malaysia in 1999; 100

people died during the epidemic (116). It is named after the village where the infectious agent was initially isolated, and is similar to Hendra virus, which was first isolated from horses and human beings in Australia in 1995 (42). Clinical signs include fever, headache, altered mental status, areflexia, cerebellar and brainstem signs, segmental myoclonus, and cardiovascular autonomic instability (116). Magnetic resonance imaging demonstrates multiple scattered white matter lesions, which are felt to represent microinfarctions from underlying vasculitis of the cerebral small vessels (129). The mortality rate is 32%, and treatment is supportive. In some cases, a delayed relapse 4 to 6 weeks after the original infection may result from ongoing inflammatory vasculitis (129).

BACTERIAL MENINGITIS

Bacterial infection of the leptomeninges and subarachnoid space that develops over hours or days is referred to as *acute bacterial meningitis.* Leptomeningeal infection that develops indolently over a period of at least 2 weeks is known as *chronic meningitis;* examples include CNS Lyme infection and syphilis. This chapter focuses on acute bacterial meningitis, which is usually life threatening and treated in an ICU. Nosocomial bacterial CNS infections are discussed in Chapter 7.

Pathogenesis

The events leading to neurological damage in meningitis are complex. The majority of the injury appears to be mediated by the immunological response to infection, rather than the infection itself. The development of bacterial meningitis progresses through four stages that are sequential but also interconnected: (a) bacterial penetration of the meninges or BBB and infection of the CNS; (b) bacterial multiplication and induction of inflammation in the subarachnoid space; (c) progression of inflammation owing to the host immune response; and (d) the development of neuronal damage (130,131).

Once bacteria gain access to the CSF, they multiply rapidly because leukocytes, immunoglobulin, and complement are largely excluded from the CNS by the BBB. However, bacterial cell wall components (lipopolysaccharides and peptidoglycans) are potent inducers of inflammation; they stimulate an initial surge of cytokine expression from CNS glial and endothelial cells, which in turn incite a much larger secondary host inflammatory response. Besides being directly toxic, interleukin-1 and tumor necrosis factor released during the initial phase of infection stimulate secondary neutrophil chemoattraction and inflammation (132). Other important mediators of the inflammatory cascade in meningitis include other interleukins and chemokines, complement, prostaglandins, matrix-metalloproteases, reactive oxygen radicals, and the urokinase plasminogen activator system (131,133–135).

The preceding events can lead to diffuse BBB breakdown and vasogenic cerebral edema, intracranial hypertension, focal cerebritis or abscess formation, vasculitic arterial thrombosis leading to secondary infarction, acute or chronic hydrocephalus, cranial nerve injury, dural sinus thrombosis, or the development of subdural effusions or empyema (131,132). Bacterial meningitis is also associated with marked changes in cerebral blood flow (CBF). In the early phases of the disease, an increase in CBF occurs, which is related to overexpression of nitric oxide (136). Blood–brain barrier breakdown during this early hyperemic phase is an important pathophysiologic event, because it allows for increased extravasation of cytokines and other neurotoxic factors into the CNS. Severe generalized brain swelling during the early phase of infection, if left unchecked, can lead to herniation and death.

Cerebral blood flow is reduced in advanced meningitis. This may result from global depression of cerebral metabolism, low cerebral perfusion pressure associated with elevated ICP, diffuse small-vessel arterial vasoconstriction related to reactive oxygen species and endothelin release, and large-vessel thromboocclusive disease related to inflammation of arteries or veins that traverse the subarachnoid space (131). Excitatory amino acids such as glutamate, in the presence or absence of ischemia, appear to be the most important mediators of direct neuronal toxicity in bacterial meningitis (131).

Epidemiology

With the advent of *H. influenzae*, vaccination programs and more effective antimicrobial therapy, bacterial meningitis has gradually transformed from a disease of very young children to a condition that affects individuals of all ages. The average patient with meningitis is 25 years of age, and *S. pneumoniae* is the most common pathogen, accounting for 50% of cases overall and the majority of cases in adults. *Neisseria meningitidis* is the second leading pathogen, accounting for 25% of cases, and is the most common cause in children aged 2 to 18. *Streptococcus agalactiae* and *Listeria monocytogenes* account for 12% and 8% of cases, respectively, whereas *Haemophilus influenza* is now responsible for 7% of cases (130).

Clinical Manifestations

Fever, headache, meningismus, and signs of cerebral dysfunction such as confusion, delirium, or depressed level of consciousness are well-known classic signs and occur in 85% of patients. Neonates and the elderly are somewhat less likely to present with these classic symptoms. The meningismus may be subtle or obvious, and are accompanied by Kernig (inability to extend the knee with the hip flexed) or Brudzinski (flexion at the hip and knee with passive flexion of the neck) signs in approximately 50% of cases. Other findings may include cranial nerve palsies (20% of cases), focal cerebral signs (25%), seizures (10% to 15%), vomiting (35%), and dysautonomia (10%) (132,137).

A specific cause of community-acquired meningitis may be suggested by certain symptoms or signs. For example, approximately 50% of patients with meningococcal infection present with a distinctive rash on the extremities that evolves from a maculopapular to petechial to purpuric form as the infection progresses. *Listeria* infection may present with ataxia, nystagmus, and other features of rhombencephalitis. Meningitis associated with otitis media, sinusitis, or pneumonia is usually caused by *S. pneumoniae* infection, but can also occur in patients with *H. influenzae* (137).

Diagnosis

The diagnosis of bacterial meningitis is based on examination of the CSF. The CSF white cell count is usually in the range of 1,000 to 5,000 cells/μL, with a polymorphonuclear predominance. Predominance of lymphocytes or mononuclear cells suggests *Listeria monocytogenes* infection, or Gram-negative bacillary meningitis. A relatively low CSF white cell count in the presence of high CSF bacterial concentrations portends a poor prognosis. A decreased CSF glucose level (below 40 mg/dL) and CSF:serum glucose ratio (below 30%) occurs in two thirds of cases. CSF protein elevation (greater than 100 mg/dL) occurs in almost all cases (138).

The CSF Gram stain is positive in 60% to 90% of cases, and has a specificity of nearly 100%. However, the probability of detecting the organism by Gram stain or culture decreases in patients who have already been given an antibiotic. Cultures become sterile in 90% to 100% of patients after 24 to 36 hours of treatment with appropriate antibiotics, despite the absence of concomitant improvement in the CSF profile (139). In patients with negative cultures, latex agglutination can detect the presence of bacterial antigen for *S pneumoniae, H. influenzae* type B, *N. meningitidis, E. coli,* K1, *L. monocytogenes,* and *S. agalactiae* with reasonable specificity. However, because the sensitivity of latex agglutination ranges from 50% to 100%, a negative test cannot rule out the diagnosis. Polymerase chain reaction technology is now available for diagnosing the presence of DNA for most of these organisms as well (140,141). The merits of PCR as opposed to latex agglutination testing for evaluating culture-negative meningitis remain unclear.

An algorithm for the emergency evaluation and management of patients with suspected bacterial meningitis is presented in Figure 21.2. Whenever possible, a lumbar puncture should be performed and empiric antimicro-bial therapy initiated within 30 minutes of presentation (132). In patients with pa-pilledema or focal neurological signs, a CT scan of the head with contrast should be performed to rule out a mass lesion, because lumbar puncture in this situation can precipitate cerebral herniation (141–142). The risk of herniation from a diagnostic lumbar puncture in patients with bacterial meningitis is small

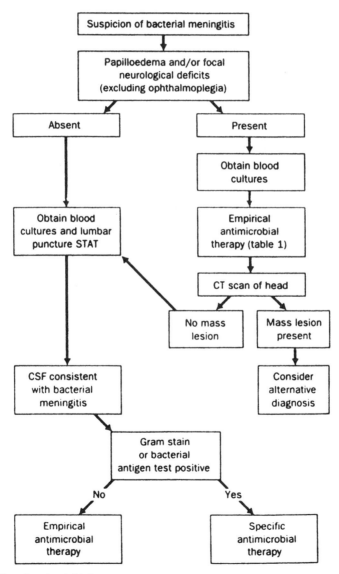

FIG. 21.2. Algorithm for the initial management of patients with acute bacterial meningitis. *CSF,* cerebrospinal fluid; *CT,* computed tomography; *STAT,* at once. (From Tunkel AR, Scheid WM. Acute bacterial meningitis. *Lancet* 1995;346:1675–1680, with permission.)

but real, and a normal head CT cannot entirely exclude this possibility. In one of the few studies to systematically address this issue, 4.3% of 445 children with bacterial meningitis experienced herniation at some point during their illness (142). Sixty-three percent of these episodes occurred during the first 12 hours after the initial lumbar puncture, making the risk of herniation 32 times more likely during this period than other time intervals. Of particular importance is the fact that the CT scan was normal in 36% of these cases. We have witnessed fatal herniation immediately following lumbar puncture in patients with AIDS-related cryptococcal meningitis. Herniation in these and other CT-negative cases is presumably caused by a thick inflammatory exudate that packs the basal cisterns and impairs the normal flow of CSF, resulting in a compartmentalized ICP gradient once fluid is removed from the lumbar space.

Treatment

Antimicrobial Therapy

If the causative agent cannot be identified by Gram stain within 30 minutes of presentation, empiric antibiotic therapy for community-acquired bacterial meningitis should be initiated based on the patient's age (Table 21.11). Most adults should be treated with ampicillin and ceftriaxone pending the results of CSF cultures; cefotaxime is a reasonable alternative for ceftriaxone in this setting. The use of empiric third-generation cephalosporins has become increasingly emphasized as penicillin-resistant strains of pneumococcus have become more prevalent. Once the specific bacterial isolate has been identified, subsequent antibiotic therapy should be based on sensitivity testing. The total duration of antibiotic therapy should be 14 to 21 days.

Steroid Therapy

Despite numerous small trials that gave conflicting results in adult meningitis, a recent randomized study has shown that early treatment with dexamethasone improves the outcome of acute bacterial meningitis. Glucocorticoids such as dexamethasone have powerful antiinflammatory and immunomodulatory effects, particularly on cell-mediated immune mechanisms, and may lower ICP related to vasogenic cerebral edema. To be ef-

TABLE 21.11. *Common pathogens and empiric antibiotic regimens in patients with suspected bacterial meningitis*

Age or risk group	Etiologies	Antibiotic coverage
0–12 weeks	1. *S. agalactiae* 2. *E. coli* 3. *L. monocytogenes* 4. *K. pneumoniae* 5. *H. influenzae*	Cefotaxime 150 mg/kg/d q4–6 h + ampicillin 50–100 mg/kg/d q12 h
3 months to 18 years	1. *N. meningitidis* 2. *H. influenzae* 3. *S. pneumoniae*	Ceftriaxone 100 mg/kg/d q12 h ± ampicillin 50–100 mg/kg/d q12 h
18–50 years	1. *S. pneumoniae* 2. *N. meningitidis*	Ceftriaxone 2 g i.v. q12 h ± ampicillin 2 g i.v. q4 h
>50 years	1. *S. pneumoniae* 2. *N. meningitidis* 3. *L. monocytogenes* 4. Aerobic Gram-negative bacilli	Ceftriaxone 2 g i.v. q12 h + ampicillin 2 g i.v. q4 h
Postneurosurgical procedure or head trauma	1. *S. aureus* 2. Aerobic Gram-negative bacilli 3. *S. pneumoniae*	Ceftazidime 1–2 g i.v. q8 h + vancomycin 1 g i.v. q12 h

i.v., intravenous.

fective, it appears that the steroid therapy must be instituted prior to initiating antibiotics, probably in order to blunt the severe inflammatory response that accompanies lysis of large amounts of bacteria.

In children, dexamethasone 0.15 mg/kg every 6 hours for 4 days reduces long-term sensorineural hearing loss from *H. influenzae* infection, and mortality from pneumococcal infection (130,144,145). A more recent study of 301 adults found that 10 mg of dexamethasone given 15 minutes before the first dose of antibiotic, followed by 6 mg every 6 hours for 4 days, was associated with a 52% reduction in mortality and a 13% increase in the likelihood of survival without disability (146). These beneficial effects were most apparent in patients with pneumococcal meningitis. In addition, both seizures and coma were less frequent in steroid-treated patients.

Intracranial Pressure Management

The general approach for treating elevated ICP in bacterial meningitis is the same as for other conditions, beginning with CSF drainage (if feasible), sedation, CPP optimization, osmotherapy, and hyperventilation (28). Few studies have systematically studied ICP patterns in bacterial meningitis. In one study of 12 patients, all experienced elevations exceeding 20 mm Hg, although only five had radiological signs of brain swelling (143). A small study in children found that oral glycerol administration reduced the frequency of neurological sequelae from 19% to 7%, but this result was of marginal statistical significance (147). There is a paucity of clinical research directly examining the effects of glucocorticoids, CPP manipulation, osmotherapy, hyperventilation, or barbiturates on ICP and outcome in bacterial meningitis. Promising experimental work suggests that hypothermia (32°C to 34°C) started shortly after the administration of antibiotics lowers ICP, raises CPP, reduces brain edema, and has beneficial effects on the CSF profile and a variety of inflammatory mediators in animals with meningitis (148,149). Translational studies in humans are needed.

Anticoagulation

Heparin-induced anticoagulation has been suggested to have beneficial effects in terms of minimizing the frequency of vasculitic infarction in bacterial meningitis (150). In an observational study of 86 patients, 28% had focal neurological signs, 15% had angiographically documented arterial or venous occlusive disease, and 7% had delayed cerebral infarction (151,152). The prognosis of patients with cerebrovascular complications was extremely poor. Approximately 50% of meningitis patients develop transcranial Doppler velocity accelerations related to large vessel narrowing, which peak between days 3 and 5 (150,153). In an experimental model of pneumococcal meningitis, heparin was shown to interfere with leukocyte endothelial interactions, and to ameliorate early hyperemia, ICP elevation, brain edema, and leukocyte influx (154). Additional studies investigating the impact of neurovascular monitoring and anticoagulation on cerebrovascular complications from meningitis are needed.

Outcome

With appropriate therapy, mortality rates for bacterial meningitis range between 5% and 30%, with most studies showing a hospital mortality rate of 20% (132). Mortality is chiefly determined by: (a) the virulence of the infecting organism; (b) the age and underlying medical condition of the patient; and (c) the speed with which effective antibiotic therapy is initiated. The highest mortality rate (greater than 40%) is associated with meningococcal meningitis and septic shock (155). Mortality and neurological sequelae have been linked to high concentrations of bacteria and bacterial antigen in the CSF and serum TNF levels (156,157).

REFERENCES

1. Whitley RJ, Gnann JW. Viral encephalitis: familiar infections and emerging pathogens. *Lancet* 2002;359: 507–513.
2. Johnson RT. Pathogenesis of CNS infections. In: *Viral infections of the nervous system,* 2nd ed. New York: Lippincott–Raven, 1998:35–60.
3. Schweighardt B, Atwood WJ. Virus receptors in the human central nervous system. *J Neurovirol* 2001;7: 187–195.
4. Asensio VC, Campbell IL. Chemokines and viral diseases of the central nervous system. *Adv Viral Res* 2001;56:127–173.
5. Komatsu T, Ireland DDC, Chung N, et al. Regulation of the BBB during viral encephalitis: roles of IL-12 and NOS. *Nitric Oxide* 1999;3:327–339.
6. Johnson RT. Acute encephalitis. *Clin Infect Dis* 1996; 23:219–226.
7. Downs AG. Arboviruses. In: Evans AS, ed. *Viral infections of humans: epidemiology and control.* New York: Plenum, 1989:105–132.
8. Buescher EL, Artenstein MS, Olsen LC. Central nervous system infections of viral etiology: the changing patterns. *Res Publ Assoc Nerv Ment Dis* 1968;44; 147–163.
9. Jeffery KJM, Read SJ, Peto TEA, et al. Diagnosis of viral infections of the central nervous system: clinical interpretation of PCR results. *Lancet* 1997;349: 313–317.
10. Koskiniemi M, Rantalaiho T, Piiparinen H, et al. Infections of the central nervous system of suspected viral origin: a collaborative study from Finland. *J Neurovirol* 2001;7:400–408.
11. Wijdicks EFM. Acute viral encephalitis. In: Wijdicks EFM. *The clinical practice of critical care neurology.* New York: Lippincott–Raven, 1998:252–261.
12. Whitley RJ, Cobbs CG, Alford CA Jr, et al. Diseases that mimic herpes simplex encephalitis. Diagnosis, presentation, and outcome. NIAID Collaborative Antiviral Study Group. *JAMA* 1989;262:234–239.
13. Johnson RT. Meningitis, encephalitis, and poliomyelitis. In: *Viral infections of the nervous system,* 2nd ed. New York: Lippincott–Raven, 1998:87–132.
14. Nash D, Mostashari F, Fine A, et al. The outbreak of West Nile virus infection in the New York City area in 1999. *N Engl J Med* 1999;344:1807–1814.
15. Whitley RJ, Soong SJ, Linneman C, et al. Herpes simplex encephalitis. Clinical assessment. *JAMA* 1982; 247:317–320.
16. Read SJ, Kurtz JB. Laboratory diagnosis of common viral infections of the central nervous system by using a single multiplex PCR screening assay. *J Clin Microbiol* 1999;37:1352–1355.
17. Büttner T, Dorndorf W. Prognostic value of computed tomography and cerebrospinal fluid analysis in viral encephalitis. *J Immunol* 1988;20:163–164.
18. Lakeman FD, Whitley RJ, and the national institute of Allergy and Infectious Diseases Collaborative Antiviral Study group. Diagnosis of herpes simplex encephalitis: application of polymerase chain reaction to cerebrospinal fluid from brain-biopsied patients and correlation with disease. *J Infect Dis* 1995;171: 857–863.
19. Domingues RB, Fink MC, Tsanaclis SM, et al. Diagnosis of herpes simplex encephalitis by magnetic resonance imaging and polymerase chain reaction in assay of cerebrospinal fluid. *J Neurol Sci* 1998;157:148–153.
20. Deck MD, Drayer BP, Anderson RE, et al. Imaging of intracranial infections. *Radiology* 2000;215:535–545.
21. Tokunaga Y, Kira R, Takemoto M, et al. Diagnostic usefulness of diffusion-weighted magnetic resonance imaging in influenza-associated acute encephalopathy or encephalitis. *Brain Development* 2000;22;451–453.
22. Krumholz A, Sung GY, Fisher RS, et al. Complex partial status epilepticus accompanied by serious morbidity and mortality. *Neurology* 1995;45:1499–1504.
23. Morawetz RB, Whitley RJ, Murphy DM. Experience with brain biopsy for suspected herpes encephalitis: a review of forty consecutive cases. *Neurosurgery* 1983;12:654–657.
24. Nahmias AJ, Whitley RJ, Visintine AN, et al. Herpes simplex virus encephalitis: laboratory evaluations and their diagnostic significance. *J Infect Dis* 1982;145: 829–836.
25. Howell DN, Miller SE. Identification of viral infection by confocal microscopy. *Meth Enzymol* 1999;307: 573–591.
26. O'Donnell J, Axelrod P, Fisher C, et al. Use and effectiveness of hypothermia blankets for febrile patients in the intensive care unit. *Clin Infect Dis* 1997;24: 1208–1213.
27. Whitley RJ, Soong SJ, Dolin RD, et al. Adenine arabinoside therapy of biopsy-proved herpes simplex encephalitis. *N Engl J Med* 1977;297:289–294.
28. Mayer SA, Chong J. Critical care management of increased intracranial pressure. *J Int Care Med* 2002;17: 55–67.
29. Barnett GH, Ropper AH, Romeo J. Intracranial pressure and outcome in adult encephalitis. *J Neurosurg* 1988;68:585–588.
30. Hoke CH Jr, Vaugn DW, Nisalak A, et al. Effect of high-dose dexamethasone on the outcome of acute encephalitis due to Japanese encephalitis virus. *J Infect Dis* 1992;165:631–637.
31. Kovama S, Morita K, Yamaguchi S, et al. An adult case of mumps brainstem encephalitis. *Int Med* 2000;39: 499–502.
32. Matsui M. Infection in the central nervous system and corticosteroid therapy. *Rinsho Shinkeigaku* 1999;39: 26–28.
33. Sommer JB, Heckmann JG, Kraus J, et al. Generalized brain edema in non-purulent meningoencephalitis. The anti-edema effect with dexamethasone. *Nervarzt* 2000; 71:112–115.
34. Hayashi N. Brain thermo-pooling is the major problem in pediatric influenza encephalitis. *No to Hattatsu* 2000;32:156–162.
35. Yokota S, Imagawa T, Miyamae T, et al. Hypothetical pathophysiology of acute encephalopathy and encephalitis related to influenza virus infection and hypothermia therapy. *Ped Int* 2000;42:197–203.
36. Ohtsuki N, Kimura S, Nezu A, et al. Effects of mild hypothermia and steroid pulse combination therapy on acute encephalopathy associated with influenza virus infection: report of two cases. *No to Hattatsu* 2000; 32:318–322.
37. Ebel H, Kuchta J, Balogh A, et al. Operative treatment of tentorial herniation in herpes encephalitis. *Child Nerv Syst* 1999;15:84–86.

38. Taferner E, Pfausler B, Kofler A. et al. Craniectomy in severe, life-threatening encephalitis: a report on outcome and long-term prognosis of four cases. *Int Care Med* 2001;27:1426–1428.

39. Whitley RJ, Alford CA, Hirsch MS, et al. Vidarabine versus acyclovir therapy in herpes simplex encephalitis. *N Engl J Med* 1986;314: 144–149.

40. Cinque P, Cleator GM, Weber T. Diagnosis and clinical management of neurological disorders caused by cytomegalovirus in AIDS patients. European Union Concerted Action on Virus Meningitis and Encephalitis. *J Neurovirol* 1998;4:120–132.

41. Rotbart HA. Webster AD. Pleconaril Treatment Registry Group. Treatment of potentially life-threatening enterovirus infections with pleconaril. *Clin Infect Dis* 2001;32:228–235.

42. Redington J, Tyler KL. Viral infections of the nervous system, 2002. *Arch Neurol* 2002;59:712–718.

43. Aygun A, Kabakus N, Celik I, et al. Long-term neurological outcome of acute encephalitis. *J Trop Pediatr* 2001;47:243–247.

44. Bonno S, Raschilas F, Mari I, et al. Klüver-Bucy syndrome in herpetic meningoencephalitis. *Presse Med* 2001;30:115–118.

45. Kennedy PG, Adams JH, Graham DI, et al. A clinicopathologic study of herpes simplex encephalitis. *Neuropathol Appl Neurobiol* 1988;14:395–415.

46. Moorthi S, Schneider WN, Dombovy ML. Rehabilitation outcomes in encephalitis: a retrospective study. *Brain Inj* 1999;13:139–146.

47. Annegers JF, Hauser WA, Beghi E, et al. The risk of unprovoked seizures after encephalitis and meningitis. *Neurology* 1988;38:1407–1410.

48. Trinka E, Dubeau F, Andermann F, et al. Clinical findings, imaging characteristics and outcome in catastrophic post-encephalitic epilepsy. *Epileptic Disord* 2000;2:153–162.

49. Olson LC, Buescher EL, Artenstein MS, et al. Herpesvirus infection of the human central nervous system. *N Engl J Med* 1967;277:1271–1272.

50. Nahmias AJ, Whitley RJ, Visintine AN, et al. Herpes simplex virus encephalitis: Laboratory evaluations and their diagnostic significance. *J Infect Dis* 1982;145: 829–836.

51. Chu K, Kang DW, Lee JJ, et al. Atypical brainstem encephalitis caused by herpes simplex virus 2. *Arch Neurol* 2002;59:460–463.

52. Domingues RB, Tsanaclis AM, Pannuti CS, et al. Evaluation of the range of clinical presentations of herpes simplex encephalitis by using polymerase chain reaction assay of cerebral spinal fluid samples. *Clin Infect Dis* 1997;25:86–91.

53. Revello MG, Gualandri R, Manservigi R, et al. Development and evaluation of an ELISA using secreted antibody to herpes simplex virus. *J Virol Meth* 1991; 34:57–70.

54. Kahlon J, Chatterjee S, Lakeman FD, et al. Detection of antibodies to herpes simplex virus in the cerebrospinal fluid of patients with herpes simplex encephalitis. *J Infect Dis* 1986;155:38–44.

55. Vandvik B, Vartdal F, Norrby E. Herpes simplex virus encephalitis: intrathecal synthesis of oligoclonal virus-specific IgG, IgA, and IgM antibodies. *J Neurol* 1982; 228:25–38.

56. Aurelius E, Johansson B, Skoldenberg B, et al. Rapid diagnosis of herpes simplex encephalitis by nested polymerase chain reaction assay of cerebrospinal fluid. *Lancet* 1991;1:189–192.

57. Rowley AH, Whitley RJ, Lakeman FD, et al. Rapid detection of herpes-simplex-virus DNA in cerebrospinal fluid of patients with herpes simplex encephalitis. *Lancet* 1990;335:440–441.

58. Sharfstein SR, Gorden ME, Libman RB, et al. Adult-onset MELAS presenting as herpes encephalitis. *Arch Neurol* 1999;56:241–243.

59. Liow K, Spanaki MV, Bover RS, et al. Bilateral hippocampal encephalitis caused by enteroviral infection. *Ped Neurol* 1999;21:836–838.

60. McCarthy VP, Zimmerman AW, Miller CA. Central nervous system manifestations of parainfluenza virus type 3 infections in childhood. *Pediatr Neurol* 1990;6: 197–201.

61. Ishiguro N, Yamada S, Takahashi T, et al. Meningo-encephalitis associated with HHV-6 related exanthem subitum. *Acta Paediatr Scand* 1990;79:987–989.

62. Hanley DF, Johnson RT, Whitley RJ. Yes, brain biopsy should be a prerequisite for herpes simplex encephalitis treatment. *Arch Neurol* 1987;44:1289–1290.

63. Barza M, Pauker SG. The decision to biopsy, treat, or wait in suspected herpes encephalitis. *Ann Intern Med* 1980;92:641–649.

64. Braun P. The clinical management of suspected herpes virus encephalitis: a decision-analytic view. *Am J Med* 1980;69:845–902.

65. Soong SJ, Watson NE, Caddell GR, et al. Use of brain biopsy for diagnostic evaluation of patients with suspected herpes simplex encephalitis: a statistical model and its clinical implications. NIAID Collaborative Antiviral Study Group. *J Infect Dis* 1991;163:17–22.

66. Nolan DC, Lauter CB, Lerner AM. Idoxuridine in herpes simplex virus (type I) encephalitis: experience with 29 cases in Michigan, 1966 to 1971. *Ann Intern Med* 1973;78:243–246.

67. Haefli WE, Schoenenberger RAZ, Weiss P. Acyclovir-induced neurotoxicity: concentration side-effect relationship in acyclovir overdose. *Am J Int Med* 1993; 94:212–215.

68. Barthez MA, Billard C, Santini JJ, et al. Relapse of herpes simplex encephalitis. *Neuropediatrics* 1987;18:3–7.

69. Domingues RB, Lakeman FD, Mayo MS, et al. Application of competitive PCR to cerebrospinal fluid samples from patients with herpes simplex encephalitis. *J Clin Microbiol* 1998;36:2229–2234.

70. Lahat E, Barr J, Barkai G, et al. Long term neurological outcome of herpes encephalitis. *Arch Dis Child* 1999;80:69–71.

71. Gordon B, Selnes DA, Hart J Jr, et al. Longterm cognitive sequelae of acyclovir-treated herpes simplex encephalitis. *Arch Neurol* 1990;47:646–647.

72. Schooley RT, Dolin R. Epstein Barr virus. In: Mandell GE, Douglas RG, Bennett JE, eds. *Principles and practice of infectious diseases.* New York: Wiley, 1985: 971–982.

73. Hallee TJ, Evans AS, Niederman JC, et al. Infectious mononucleosis at the United States Military Academy. *Yale J Biol Med* 1974;3:182–195.

74. Sawyer RN, Evans AS, Niederman JC, et al. Prospective studies of a group of Yale freshmen. I. Occurrence of infectious mononucleosis. *J Infect Dis* 1971;123: 263–270.

75. Lehane DE. A seroepidemiological study of infectious mononucleosis. *JAMA* 1970;212:2240–2242.
76. Fleisher G, Lennette ET, Henle G, et al. Incidence of heterophil antibody responses in children with infectious mononucleosis. *J Pediatr* 1979;94:723–728.
77. Bernstein TC, Wolff HG. Involvement of the nervous system in infectious mononucleosis. *Ann Intern Med* 1948;33:1120–1138.
78. Silverstein A, Steinberg G, Nathanson M. Nervous system involvement in infectious mononucleosis. *Arch Neurol* 1972;26:353–358.
79. Gautier-Smith PC. Neurological complications of glandular fever (infectious mononucleosis). *Brain* 1965;88:323–334.
80. Grow C, Henle W, Henle G, et al. Primary Epstein-Barr virus infections in acute neurological diseases. *N Engl J Med* 1975;292:392–395.
81. Bajada S. Cerebellitis in glandular fever. *Med J Aust* 1976;1:153–156.
82. Meerbach A, Gruhn B, Egerer R, et al. Semiquantitative PCR analysis of Epstein-Barr virus DNA in clinical samples of patients with EBV-associated diseases. *J Med Virol* 2001;65:348–357.
83. Schmitz H, Scherer M. IgM antibodies to Epstein-Barr virus in infectious mononucleosis. *Arch Gesamte Virusforsch* 1972;37:332–339.
84. Andersson J, Britton S, Ernberg I, et al. Effect of acyclovir on infectious mononucleosis: a double blind, placebo-controlled study. *J Infect Dis* 1986;153: 283–290.
85. Underwood EA. The neurological complications of varicella: a clinical and epidemiological study. *Br J Child Dis* 1935;32:83–107.
86. Hierwitz ES, Nelson DB, Davis C, et al. National surveillance for Reye's syndrome: a five year review. *Pediatrics* 1982;70:895–897.
87. Peters ACB, Versteeg J, Lindeman J, et al. Varicella and acute cerebellar ataxia. *Arch Neurol* 1978;35: 769–771.
88. Goldston AS, Millichap JA, Miller RH. Cerebellar ataxia with preeruptive varicella. *Am J Dis Child* 1963;106:197–200.
89. Jemsek J, Greenberg SB, Taber L, et al. Herpes zoster-associated encephalitis: clinicopathologic report of 12 cases and review of the literature. *Medicine* 1983; 62:81–97.
90. Mayo DR, Booss J. Varicella-associated neurological disease without skin lesion. *Arch Neurol* 1989;46: 313–315.
91. Gilden DH, Murray RS, Wellish M, et al. Chronic progressive varicella-zoster virus encephalitis in an AIDS patient. *Neurology* 1988;38:1150–1153.
92. Weaver S, Rosenblum MK, DeAngelis LM. Herpes varicella zoster encephalitis in immunocompromised patients. *Neurology* 1999;52:193–195.
92. Gilden DH. Varicella zoster virus vasculopathy and disseminated encephalomyelitis. *J Neurol Sci* 2002; 195:99–101.
93. Gilden DH, Lipton HL, Wolf JS, et al. Patients with unusual forms of varicella–zoster virus vasculopathy. *N Engl J Med* 2002;347:1500–1503.
94. Puchhammer-Stockl E, Popow-Kraupp T, Heinz FX, et al. Detection of varicella-zoster virus DNA by polymerase chain reaction in the cerebrospinal fluid of patients suffering from neurological complications associated with chicken pox or herpes zoster. *J Clin Microbiol* 1991;29:1513–1516.
95. Whitley RJ, Soong SJ, Dolin R, et al. Vidarabine therapy to control the complications of herpes zoster in immunosuppressed patients. *N Engl J Med* 1982;307: 971–975.
96. Duchowny M, Caplan L, Siber G. Cytomegalovirus infection of the adult nervous system. *Ann Neurol* 1979; 5:458–461.
97. Larsen JK, Melgaard B. Simultaneous neuroinfection with herpes simplex virus and cytomegalovirus in an immunocompetent adult. *J Intern Med* 1989;226: 59–61.
98. Witte T, Werwitzke S, Schmidt RE. CMV complications in variable immune deficiency. *Immunobiology* 2000;202:194–198.
99. Torgovnick J, Arsura EL, Lala D. Cytomegalovirus ventriculoencephalitis presenting as Wernicke's encephalopathy. *Neurology* 2000;55:1910–1913.
100. Wiley CA, Nelson JA. Role of human immunodeficiency virus and cytomegalovirus in AIDS encephalitis. *Am J Pathol* 1988;133:73–81.
101. Schmitz H, Enders G. Cytomegalovirus as a frequent cause of Guillain-Barré syndrome. *J Med Virol* 1977; 1:21–27.
102. Burke DG, Leonard DG, Imperiale TF, et al. The utility of clinical and radiographic features in the diagnosis of cytomegalovirus central nervous system disease in AIDS patients. *Mol Diagn* 1999;4:37–43.
103. Anduze-Faris BM, Filet AM, Gozlan J, et al. Induction and maintenance therapy of cytomegalovirus central nervous system infection in HIV-infected patients. *AIDS* 2000;14:517–524. ·
104. Benson PM, Malane SL, Banks R, et al. B virus (Herpesvirus simiae) and human infection. *Arch Dermatol* 1989;125:1247–1248.
105. Hummeler K, Davidson WL, Henle W, et al. Encephalomyelitis due to infection with Herpesvirus simiae (herpes B virus). *N Engl J Med* 1959;261: 64–68.
106. Boulter EA, Thornton B, Bauer DJ, et al. Successful treatment of experimental B virus (Herpesvirus simiae) infection with acyclovir. *Br Med J* 1980;280: 681–683.
107. McCullers JA, Lakeman FD, Whitley RJ. Human herpesvirus 6 is associated with focal encephalitis. *Clin Infect Dis* 1995;21:571–576.
108. Vaughn DW, Hoke CH Jr. The epidemiology of Japanese encephalitis: prospects for prevention. *Epidemiol Rev* 1992;14:197–221.
109. Kalita J, Mista UK. Comparison of CT scan and MRI findings in Japanese encephalitis. *J Neurol Sci* 2000; 174:3–8.
110. Deresiewicz RL, Thaler SJ, Hsu L, et al. Clinical and neuroradiographic manifestations of Eastern Equine encephalitis. *N Engl J Med* 1997;336:1867–1874.
111. Earnest MP, Goolishian HA, Calverley JR, et al. Neurological, intellectual, and psychological sequelae following western encephalitis. *Neurology* 1971;21: 969–974.
112. Annette EH, Longshore WA. Western equine and St. Louis encephalitis in man. California 1945–1950. *Cal Med* 1951;75:189–195.
113. Powell KE, Blakey DL. St. Louis encephalitis. *JAMA* 1977;237:2294–2298.

114. Southern PM, Smith JW, Luby JP, et al. Clinical and laboratory features of epidemic St. Louis encephalitis. *Ann Intern Med* 1969;71:681.

115. Ventura AK, Buff EE, Ehrenkranz NJ. Human Venezuelan equine encephalitis virus infection in Florida. *Am J Trop Med Hyg* 1974;23:507–512.

116. Hinson VK, Tyor WR. Update on viral encephalitis. *Curr Opin Neurol* 2001;14:369–374.

117. Ahmed S, Libman R, Wesson K, et al. Guillain–Barré syndrome: an unusual presentation of West Nile virus infection. *Neurology* 2000;55:144–146.

118. Levitt LP, Rich TA, Kinde SW, et al. Central nervous system mumps. *Neurology* 1970;20:829–834.

119. Bang HO, Bang J. Involvement of the central nervous system in mumps. *Acta Med Scand* 1943;113:487–490.

120. Russell RR, Donald JC. The neurological complications of mumps. *Br Med J* 1958;2:27–30.

121. Gibbs FA, Gibbs EL, Carpenter PR, et al. Electroencephalographic changes in "uncomplicated" childhood diseases. *JAMA* 1959;171:1050–1055.

122. Meulen VT, Muller D, Kackell Y, et al. Isolation of infectious measles virus in measles encephalitis. *Lancet* 1972;2:1172–1174.

123. Griffin DE, Ward BJ, Jaurequi E, et al. Immune activation during measles: interferon-gamma and neopterin in plasma and cerebrospinal fluid in complicated and uncomplicated disease. *J Infect Dis* 1990;79:987–989.

124. Sherman FE, Michaels RH, Kenny FM. Acute encephalopathy (encephalitis) complicating rubella. *JAMA* 1965;192:675–681.

125. Huang C-C, Liu C-C, Chang Y-C, et al. Neurological complications in children with enterovirus 71 infection. *N Engl J Med* 1999;341:936–942.

126. Yoshikawa H, Yamazaki S, Watanabe T, et al. Study of influenza virus associated encephalitis/encephalopathy in children during the 1997 to 2001 influenza seasons. *J Child Neurol* 2001;16:885–890.

127. Kurita A, Furushima H, Yamada H, et al. Periodic lateralized epileptiform discharges in influenza B-associated encephalopathy. *Int Med* 2001;40:13–16.

128. McCullers JA, Facchini S, Chesney PJ, et al. Influenza B encephalitis. *Clin Infect Dis* 1999;28:898–900.

129. Sarji SA, Abdullah BJ, Goh KJ, et al. MR imaging features of Nipah encephalitis. *AJR* 2000;175:437–442.

130. Coyle PK. Glucocorticoids in central nervous system bacterial infection. *Arch Neurol* 1999;56:796–801.

131. Leib SL, Tauber MG. Pathogenesis of bacterial meningitis. *Infect Dis Clin N Am* 1999;13:527–548.

132. Tunkel AR, Scheid WM. Acute bacterial meningitis. *Lancet* 1995;346:1675–1680.

133. Tauber MG, Kim YS, Lieb SL. Neuronal injury in meningitis. In: Peterson PK, Remington JS, eds. *In defense of the brain*. Malden, MA: Blackwell Science, 1997:124.

134. Winkler F, Kastenbauer S, Koedel U, et al. Role of the urokinase plasminogen activator system in patients with bacterial meningitis. *Neurology* 2002;59:1350–1355.

135. Leppert D, Leib SL, Grygar C, et al. Matrix metalloproteinase (MMP)-8 and MMP-9 in cerebrospinal fluid during bacterial meningitis: association with blood-brain barrier damage and neurological sequelae. *Clin Infect Dis* 2000;31:80–84.

136. Koedel U, Bernatowicz A, Paul R, et al:. Experimental pneumococcal meningitis: cerebrovascular alterations, brain edema, and meningeal inflammation are linked to the production of nitric oxide. *Ann Neurol* 1995;37:313.

137. Miller JR, Jubelt B. Bacterial infections. In: Rowland LP, ed. *Merritt's textbook of neurology,* 10th ed. Philadelphia: Lippincott Williams & Wilkins, 2000:103–127.

138. Spanos A, Harrell FE Jr, Durack DT. Differential diagnosis of acute meningitis: an analysis of the predictive value of initial observation. *JAMA* 1989;262;2700–2707.

139. Bonadio WA. The cerebrospinal fluid: physiologic aspects and alterations associated with bacterial meningitis. *Pediatr Infect Dis J* 1992;11:423–432.

140. Margall CN, Majo MM, Latorre OC, et al. Use of universal PCR on cerebrospinal fluid to diagnose bacterial meningitis in culture-negative patients. *Eur J Clin Microbiol Infect Dis* 2002;21:67–69.

140. Lu JJ, Perng CL, Lee SY, et al. Use of PCR with universal primers and restriction endonuclease digestions for detection and identification of common bacterial pathogens in cerebrospinal fluid. *J Clin Microbiol* 2000;38:2076–2080.

141. Marton KI, Gaen AD. The spinal tap: a new look at an old test. *Ann Int Med* 1986;104:840–848.

142. Rennick G, Shann F, de Campo J. Cerebral herniation during bacterial meningitis in children. *BMJ* 1993;306:953–955.

143. Grande PO, Myhre EB, Nordstrom CH, et al. Treatment of intracranial hypertension and aspects on lumbar dural puncture in severe bacterial meningitis. *Acta Anaesthesiol Scand* 2002;46:264–270.

144. Lebel MH, Freij BJ, Syrogiannopoulos GA, et al. Dexamethasone therapy for bacterial meningitis; results of two double-blind, placebo controlled trials. *N Engl J Med* 1988;319:964–971.

145. Girgis NI, Farid Z, Mikhail IA, et al. Dexamethasone treatment for bacterial meningitis in children and adults. *Am J Dis Child* 1989;8:848–851.

146. de Gans J, van de Beek D, for the European Dexamethasone in Adulthood Bacterial Meningitis Study Investigators. Dexamethasone in adults with bacterial meningitis. *N Engl J Med* 2002;347:1549–1556.

147. Kilpi T, Peltola H, Jaunhiainen T, et al. Oral glycerol and intravenous dexamethasone in preventing neurological and audiologic sequelae of childhood bacterial meningitis. *Pediatr Infect Dis J* 1995;14:270–278.

148. Irazuzta JE, Pretzlaff RK, Zingarelli B, et al. Modulation of nuclear factor-kappa B activation and decreased markers of neurological injury associated with hypothermic therapy in experimental bacterial meningitis. *Crit Care Med* 2002;30:2553–2559.

149. Irazuzta JE, Pretzlaff R, Rowin M, et al. Hypothermia as an adjunctive treatment for severe bacterial meningitis. *Brain Res* 2000;881:88–97.

150. Haring HP, Rötzer HK, Reindl H, et al. Time course of cerebral blood flow velocity in central nervous system infections: a transcranial Doppler sonography study. *Arch Neurol* 1993;50:98–101.

151. Pfister HW, Feiden W, Einhäupl KM. Spectrum of complications during bacterial meningitis in adults. Results of a prospective clinical study. *Arch Neurol* 1993;50:575–581.

152. Pfister H-W, Borasio GD, Dirnagl U, et al. Cerebrovascular complications of bacterial meningitis in adults. *Neurology* 1992;42:1497–1504.

153. Müller M, Merkelbach S, Huss GP, et al. Clinical relevance and frequency of transient stenoses of the middle and anterior cerebral arteries in bacterial meningitis. *Stroke* 1995;26:1399–1403.

154. Weber JR. Angstwurm K, Rosenkranz T, et al. Heparin inhibits leukocyte rolling in pial vessels and attenuates inflammatory changes in a rat model of experimental bacterial meningitis. *J Cereb Blood Flow Metab* 1997;17:1221–1229.

155. Gedde-Dahl TW, Bjark P, Hoiby EA, et al. Severity of meningococcal disease: assessment by factors and scores and implications for management. *Rev Infect Dis* 1990;12;973–992.

156. Feldman WE. Relation of concentrations of bacteria and bacterial antigen in cerebrospinal fluid to prognosis in patients with bacterial meningitis. *N Engl J Med* 1977;296:433–435.

157. Waage A, Halstensen A, Espevik T. Association between tumour necrosis factor in serum and fatal outcome in patients with meningococcal disease. *Lancet* 1987;I:355.

22

Spinal Cord Injury

Approximately 10,000 patients a year in the United States are rendered paraplegic or quadriplegic as a result or injuries to the spinal cord. There are an estimated 200,000 quadriplegics in this country. Although prevention programs have been initiated, there is no evidence that the incidence is declining. Even though the life expectancy of these mostly young and healthy patients is slightly reduced, most patients now survive the acute period and may live for many years or many decades with their handicap. The great psychological impact of these accidents of the patient and family as well as the socioeconomic significance have been repeatedly emphasized in various writings. Most such patients are cared for initially in an intensive care unit (ICU) and demand the attention of a neurosurgeon. Here we review the main considerations that should be known to neurointensivists and list the main types of spinal fractures with some details of their management in order to give a fuller account of the problem.

PATHOPHYSIOLOGY OF CORD COMPRESSION

Experimental investigation of the mechanisms and pathology of spinal cord injury began early this century when Allen developed a standardized low-force model of injury to the spinal cord (1). He recognized that secondary damage develops progressively during the first few hours after the injury. These changes have been attributed to vascular mechanisms that ultimately lead to spinal cord infarction (2). The earliest changes occur within minutes of an experimental injury; they consist of hyperemia and small hemorrhages in the central gray matter of the cord. Microscopic pericapillary hemorrhages coalesce, and by 1 hour, grossly visible hemorrhagic areas appear in the central gray matter. Tissue oxygen saturation is decreased in the injured segments during these early stages (3). Osterholm and Mathews (4) observed that there is an accumulation of vasoactive amines in the injured segments of the cord during this initial period, suggesting that vasoconstrictive substances in the injured area might be responsible for vasospasm and decreased blood flow, which potentiate damage. Since that time there has been considerable controversy regarding the nature and significance of these changes and their role has not been emphasized (5,6). Within 4 hours of injury, the gray matter is infarcted and spreading white matter edema is noted that progresses at 8 hours to infarction of the white matter (7,8). The delay in the appearance of white matter necrosis has raised the hope of preventing irreversible damage to long tracts by therapeutic intervention during the first few hours. These attempts, for the most part unsuccessful, have included laminectomies and myelotomies to decompress the central edema and hemorrhage; early spinal cord cooling to prevent secondary damage to the white matter (9,10); and hyperbaric oxygenation during the early stages of experimental cord injury. A variety of pharmacologic agents, including corticosteroids, diuretics, plasma expanders (including low-molecular-weight dextran), dimethyl sulfoxide, α-methyltyrosine (a monamine synthesis blocker), and endogenous opiate antagonists, have been found to have a beneficial effect in experimental cord injury (11,12). However, none of these surgical or pharmacologic interventions have been proven to alter the prognosis of human spinal cord injury.

The one exception, albeit now controversial, has been the often-cited randomized controlled trial that reported beneficial effects of high-dose methylprednisolone administered soon after the injury (13). This study was driven by experimental models in which corticosteroids were found to be beneficial in a rather restricted range of mechanical force applied to the spinal column (typically between 300 and 500 g/cm^2). Injuries produced by lower forces did not result in paraplegia, and higher forces caused irreversible damage regardless of treatment. It is only an occasional clinical injury that conforms to forces within this narrow window. At present, of all these forms of therapeutic intervention, only corticosteroids are sufficiently safe to be recommended for wide clinical use; however, the validity of the conclusions of this study has been questioned from a number of perspectives. Soon after the results of the study were published, treatment with high-dose corticosteroids was considered obligatory but subsequent criticisms have emerged based largely on the study design and the analysis of results (14,15). There now seems to be a consensus that corticosteroids may offer only a slight benefit. Nevertheless, many centers continue to utilize a loading dose of 30 mg/kg methylprednisolone over 15 minutes followed by 5.4 mg/kg per hour for 23 hours. Others have recommended that the medication be continued for only 4 hours.

INITIAL EVALUATION AND TREATMENT

It cannot be overemphasized that the care of the patient with spinal cord injury begins at the scene of the accident. The significance of this early phase of treatment is underscored in a study by Rogers (16), who, a half decade ago, found that one of ten patients with spinal cord injury deteriorated between the time of the accident and the time of arrival at a medical facility. Because most of these patients do not lose consciousness, simple questioning reveals that the patient is paralyzed or has the cardinal signs of spinal injury, namely, numbness or severe neck or back pain. It has become well-established practice that in the presence of any of these symptoms or if the patient is unresponsive after a severe injury, a spinal injury is suspected and the patient is handled in such a way as to avoid any further dislocation of the spinal segments (17). Cardiopulmonary resuscitation when appropriate, insurance of a proper airway, control of obvious hemorrhage, and immobilization of evident long bone fractures are the other integral parts of initial care. If spinal cord injury is confirmed, the option of using intravenous methylprednisolone is available at the dose described in the preceding.

Many authorities have emphasized the utility of standardized protocols that cue physicians and nurses to various aspects of treatment and, more importantly, the avoidance of further injury at each stage (18).

Once the patient arrives at the emergency room, continued immobilization of the suspected spinal injury must be ensured until definitive radiologic studies are obtained. The first priority is an adequate airway. Tracheal intubation is indicated if the patient is hypoventilating, unable to handle secretions, or comatose. Most patients can be intubated nasotracheally or by direct laryngoscopy without extending the head on the neck. The recent development of a fiberoptic laryngoscope has greatly facilitated intubation while eliminating the need to alter the position of the head and neck. With the flexible laryngoscope passed through a nasotracheal tube, the tube may be manipulated and its placement in the trachea determined under direct vision.

Most patients with high thoracic and cervical injuries have mild *hypotension* and bradycardia that is caused by sympathetic failure and peripheral vascular vasodilation that accompanies the state of "spinal shock." These patients appear well perfused; their skin is warm; they do not appear in any way hypovolemic but nonetheless they respond to rapid infusions of crystalloid solutions or plasma expanders. Only infrequently is it necessary to use vasopressors to support blood pressure. Pressor use should be dictated by signs of hypoperfusion of the brain, heart, or kidneys and not solely by the failure of fluid infusions to bring the systemic pressure to normal. Atropine also can be used to restore blood pressure briefly if the hypotension is associated with bradycardia.

Recognition of *other life-threatening injuries* is of vital importance and sometimes can be quite difficult in the paralyzed patient. With spinal gunshot wounds a second small bullet entry in the back may be missed while concentrating on the more obvious neck wound. Signs of hypovolemic shock may be absent in a patient with even profuse visceral bleeding because sympathetic tone is absent; therefore, the expected vasoconstriction and pallor may not be present; instead of the expected tachycardia, the patient may be bradycardic. It is then possible to misinterpret hypotension as caused by spinal shock while the patient continues to bleed. It should be emphasized that spinal shock is usually not responsible for profound hypotension, and it is not associated with a continuing drop in systemic blood pressure while the patient is receiving fluids. Furthermore, an acute abdominal injury, even when resulting in massive spillage of blood or gastrointestinal contents, may not be associated with any signs of peritoneal irritation in the patient with a complete spinal lesion. Therefore, when in doubt, it is appropriate to look for free air by performing a careful abdominal tap and abdominal plain films or computed tomography (CT) scan.

Head injuries frequently accompany and complicate spinal injuries, and their proper recognition is, of course, vital. As an extension of preceding comments, it is almost always incorrect to attribute a deteriorating state of consciousness to cerebral hypoperfusion related to spinal shock. Conversely, a spinal cord injury must be suspected in the comatose, head-injured patient who exhibits muscular flaccidity rather than reflex posturing. Only in the agonal stages of deterioration from a brain injury does flaccidity arise. Obvious long bone fractures should be properly immobilized to assist in the prevention of fat embolism and skin erosions.

During the acute stages of spinal cord injury, as also noted in the following, the *bladder and gastrointestinal* tract are atonic. An indwelling urinary catheter must be inserted except in institutions where a special team of trained personnel is available continuously for intermittent catheterization. If the latter is available, the patient should be committed to this form of treatment from the beginning. Otherwise, an indwelling catheter, placed with careful sterile technique, may be preferable (19). Gastric atony can result in significant gastric dilatation that compounds respiratory failure by causing upward pressure on the diaphragm, or it may promote aspiration. These patients are understandably anxious and as a result swallow a considerable amount of air. Because they do not feel pain, gastric dilatation can reach massive proportions rapidly and, if untreated, result in gastric rupture, a frequent cause of early death in past eras. These problems can be prevented by early insertion of a nasogastric tube.

NEUROLOGICAL ASSESSMENT AND SPINAL CORD SYNDROMES

Following these initial steps, a careful neurological assessment must be undertaken to determine the level and severity of the spinal cord injury. In cervical injuries the *motor examination* usually establishes the level. Patients with cervical and high thoracic lesions will have lost intercostal movement and their respirations are fully diaphragmatic. With injuries in the upper cord above C5, the phrenic motor neuronal pools are damaged and respiration is impaired. With complete injuries at the T1 level, there is paraplegia and some impairment of intrinsic hand function. At the C7-T1 level, there is also impairment of finger and wrist flexors (C8 nerve root). At the C6-C7 level, the triceps, wrist extensors, and forearm pronators (C7 root) also are lost. At C5-C6, in addition to the preceding, the biceps and forearm supinators are weak (C6 root), and at C4-C5 the deltoid and supraspinatus and infraspinatus muscles are impaired (C5 root). Thoracic injuries result in paraplegia, and the level can be determined by correlating the radiographic findings and the sensory examination. Lower thoracic and thoracolumbar injuries often result in complex neurological syndromes with mixtures of upper and lower motor neuron (conus), and peripheral nerve (cauda equina) deficits. Lumbar injuries, of course, result in cauda equina deficits, which are usually incomplete, and as noted in the following, reversible for a considerable period.

The *sensory examination* also is of utility in determining the level, type, and severity of the neurological injury. Careful testing of pain sensation must be carried out to identify areas of spared sensation, especially in the sacral and perineal regions, which are of considerable prognostic significance. In determining the level of injury by pinprick examination, recalling that cutaneous branches of the cervical plexus, corresponding mostly to C3 and C4, innervate the skin over the lower collar and upper chest areas, sometimes as far down as the nipples, avoids the error of calling a cervical lesion incomplete because sensation is preserved in the upper chest. Careful sensory examination of the upper extremities (C5 through T1) and the axilla (T1 and T2) usually demonstrates a correspondence between the sensory and motor functions. It is also of value to identify cases of complete loss of motor function and pain sensation but with preserved proprioception (posterior column) function.

Deep tendon reflexes initially usually are absent below the level of a complete spinal cord lesion; however, they may return within a few hours of the injury, and their presence should not be taken as an indication of an incomplete lesion. In thoracolumbar injuries, the presence of an anal or bulbocavernosus reflex in the absence of motor power or sensation indicates that spinal shock has subsided and there is an upper motor neuron lesion as opposed to a cauda equina lesion. The latter,

as discussed, has a much better prognosis. During the initial evaluation, appropriate films can be obtained, as discussed, and it is advisable to also obtain routine blood tests and arterial blood gases.

Partial spinal cord injuries generally fall into one of the following neurological syndromes. The *Brown–Sequard syndrome* of hemiparesis with ipsilateral loss of proprioception and contralateral impairment in pain perception can occur in relatively pure form from penetrating injuries such as stab wounds. The prognosis is good when caused by closed injuries, and nearly 90% of these patients make a functional recovery.

The *central cord syndrome of Schneider* is characterized by loss of strength of the upper extremities out of proportion to the weakness of the lower extremities. The sensory deficits and impairment of bladder and bowel function are variable and unpredictable (20,21). The prognosis is good, and close to 60% of patients regain the ability to ambulate, although they may be left with some impairment of hand function. Usually, function of the legs returns first, followed by bladder function and ultimately function of the upper extremities.

The *anterior cord syndrome* consists of loss of motor function and pain sensibility below the level of the lesion, with preservation of posterior column function. The prognosis here is poor, but occasionally a patient improves after decompression of the cord by removal of an anterior disc or bone fragment. The rare instances of relatively pure impairment of posterior column function carry a good prognosis. As discussed, lesions of the conus medullaris are associated with a poor prognosis for return of bladder and rectal function, but the prognosis is good when the deficit is due to root dysfunction, which is sometimes hard to distinguish from conus lesions in cases of thoracolumbar injuries.

When there is spinal malalignment with obvious or possible compression of the spinal cord, we and the neurosurgeons who advise us have felt that rapid reduction of the dislocation is preferable in all patients and is essential in those patients with only a partial neurological injury. There is less urgency in reducing lumbar fractures that compress only the cauda equina.

Thoracic fractures usually present with either no neurological deficit or with a complete neurological syndrome. These fractures are usually stable and reduction is rarely necessary unless marked kyphosis is present. *Thoracolumbar fractures* frequently require open reduction to decompress the cornus medullaris and to ensure stability. In these cases, reduction should be accomplished as early as feasible once the patient is stable from the hemodynamic point of view and other urgent injuries have been attended to.

With rare exceptions, displaced *cervical fractures* should be treated initially by skeletal traction. The halo ring is preferred in our institutions, but other methods of skeletal traction are also satisfactory. There is no clear rational or scientific justification for the traditional method of reducing these dislocations by slow increases in weights over periods of many hours or days (22). In cases of high cervical dislocations, reduction usually can be easily accomplished with weights of no more than 10 to 15 pounds. For lower cervical dislocations, traction can be initiated with 20 pounds under careful radiographic control, preferably with an image-intensifying fluoroscopic unit, to detect early distraction. The weights can be increased by increments of 5 to 10 pounds every few minutes, with radiographic observation between each increase, until reduction is accomplished. This may take as much as 70 to 80 pounds, which is safe for a short period of time, provided that excessive distraction at any level is not detected radiographically. Only an exceptional dislocation (usually associated with a unilateral jumped facet) fails to be reduced within 1 or 2 hours with 80 pounds of traction and careful administration of parenteral muscle relaxants. Once reduction is achieved, the weight can be reduced to approximately 20 pounds, which is usually sufficient to maintain proper alignment until a definitive form of immobilization is chosen.

It should be noted that a multicenter study has documented delayed deterioration in approximately 5% of patients with spinal cord injuries (23). Others indicate the rate is closer to 1% if considering only irreversible syndromes of "ascending cord necrosis." Usually, these are younger patients with cervical cord injuries and there is substantial swelling of the cord on magnetic resonance imaging scan. In most of these patients, the decline in function was associated with a specific event (e.g., surgery, moving the patient, or application of traction, etc.). In the case of cervical cord injury and delayed ascension of the deficit, there has been an association with mortality. Furthermore, deterioration within 24 hours was associated with traction, between 24 and 72 hours with hypotension, and later deterioration, with vertebral artery injury (24).

RADIOLOGIC ASSESSMENT

In all patients who are unconscious from a head injury, or who complain of neck or back pain, or in whom a spinal injury is suspected for any reason, initial anteroposterior and lateral plain films of the area in question should be obtained with the patient properly immobilized. In cases of suspected cervical spine injuries, an open-mouth view of the odontoid is also essential. Careful, systematic review of plain spine films should be performed to exclude injury at each spinal level (25). It is advisable to obtain a chest film during this initial period.

The availability of emergency CT scanning greatly facilitates the early evaluation of cervical injuries. This has become a major mode of diagnostic evaluation after plain films. In patients with a short neck or large shoulders, CT scanning may be the only way to properly evaluate the lower cervical area. The cervical spine must be studied at least down to the C7-T1 junction in cases of suspected cervical injury. Computed tomography studies may also be necessary to detect a unilateral jumped facet or bone fragments that have been displaced into the spinal canal or root foramen. They are valuable in confirming that complete reduction of a dislocation has been achieved when an anterior fusion is contemplated. Between 15% and 20% of patients who have cervical spinal injuries have no overt radiographic abnormality on plain films, but two thirds of these have abnormalities on CT scan. More extensive fractures than appreciated with plain radiographs have been visualized in more than 50% of patients who had CT scans (26). Flexion and extension films of the neck in the acute stage of a spinal injury are not recommended except in patients with a normal neurological examination who complain of neck pain and have no obvious evidence of dislocation or fracture on plain radiography. We have had no experience with discography which was used in the past (27). Magnetic resonance imaging (MRI) has proved to be of benefit in evaluating the chronically injured spinal cord (28). This modality of imaging can be used after bony alignment has been achieved.

Despite the relative ease of CT, MRI affords a far superior view of cord compression and is used if there is a neurological deficit; it also demonstrates soft-tissue injury, such as ligamentous rupture, that is not apparent on CT. Myelography in acute spinal injury has largely been replaced by MRI (29). The dye can be injected through a C1-C2 puncture with the patient supine and in the reverse Trendelenburg position to demonstrate a block, which is the main finding of immediate clinical relevance in this setting.

EARLY COMPLICATIONS

During the first week of intensive care, several problems related to the spinal cord injury patient merit discussion. Those with high cervical cord injuries frequently develop worsening of their respiratory status during the initial few days, and for this reason these patients must be nursed in an ICU environment. In a few, the neurologic level of injury ascends, even to the medulla. More frequently, clinical deterioration is related to associated lung contusions, aspiration or bacterial pneumonitis, tracheobronchitis, inspissated secretions with bronchial plugs, fat embolisms or other causes. These problems can be prevented with meticulous pulmonary toilet, adequate hydration, and aerosols. It is, of course, preferable to avoid prophylactic antibiotics and to treat only radiologically established pulmonary infection rather than positive sputum cultures alone.

Some form of rotation or repositioning is critical in avoiding skin breakdown and is imperative once the spine has been mechanically stabilized. Prevention of *decubitus ulcers* is a major goal of the early care of these patients. Turning is appropriate approximately every 2 hours, and pressure areas must be padded carefully. A Stryker-type bed facilitates turning, but when enough trained personnel are available to turn the patient properly, a regular bed is adequate. Recently developed beds that provide gradual, continued alteration in body position while maintaining traction have been useful.

With high cervical injuries there can be significant *variations in blood pressure and heart rate* during tracheal suctioning or changes in position. A cardiac monitor and arterial line are therefore useful but some authoritative sources differ on their proper use.

Particularly pertinent in ICU cases is the *syndrome of hypoventilation* and, in its extreme, sleep apnea. This may begin with a vague subjective sensation of air hunger. The patient may sigh frequently and seem to be anxious and confused. The unwary physician may interpret these symptoms as anxiety and gravely exacerbate the problem by sedating the patient. Patients who display progressive hypoventilation may have very prolonged episodes of apnea or even cease breathing during sleep. If awakened, normal breathing resumes. The syndrome seems to be caused by a decreased sensitivity of the respiratory drive to carbon dioxide and is compounded by mechanical factors such as immobilization and a diminished oropharyngeal space causing obstructive apnea. Oxygen should be administered carefully in these patients who may be dependent on hypoxic drive. The arterial blood gas measurements are usually satisfactory when the patient is awake. Upon recognizing this syndrome nocturnal mechanical ventilation must be provided. The condition usually subsides in 5 to 10 days.

Acute *neurogenic pulmonary edema* (discussed in Chapter 5) has been reported rarely in patients with acute spinal cord injuries but is more common after acute head injury (although still infrequent). *Pulmonary embolism* occurs in immobilized spinal injury patients, usually after the second week and remains a constant threat to the paraplegic. Unless there is bleeding from associated injuries, we use "miniheparin" prophylaxis (5,000 U subcutaneously twice daily), pneumatic air boots, or both. Low molecular weight heparin may be equivalently or more effective (30).

Gastrointestinal atony may persist for several days, and patients with thoracolumbar fractures can have a reflex paralytic ileus for as long as 2 weeks. In addition, patients with spinal cord injuries invariably develop a negative nitrogen balance caused by an exaggerated catabolic state and by immobilization. This may lead to hypoproteinemia and hypocalcemia. Furthermore, some form of *prophylaxis for gastric erosion and bleeding* should be instituted, usually an H-2 histamine blocker, given initially intravenously and later, orally.

Electrolyte disturbances, most frequently hyponatremia, is sometimes related to inappropriate secretion of antidiuretic hormone. Anemia may develop in these patients because of blood loss from the initial injury, marrow depression, sequestration, and prominently from phlebotomy for tests. These problems can be prevented to some extent with early, intelligent nutritional replacement and continued attention to appropriate laboratory values.

Autonomic dysfunction occurs, particularly so-called "cholinergic crises," that consist of reflex bradycardia, sweating, pilomotor erection, and headache. These may arise early or, more often, after recovery from spinal shock. Cardiac arrest has been reported in extreme cases. Bladder fullness, tracheal suctioning, and other painful stimuli below the level of cord transection can precipitate these crises.

Anticholinergic drugs can block them; however, these drugs may exacerbate bladder and gastrointestinal atony and therefore must be used cautiously. At times, placement of a temporary cardiac pacemaker has been required to prevent recurrent severe bradycardic episodes associated with hypotension and loss of consciousness. Before inserting a pacemaker, an associated bradyarrhythmia (often missed because patients are seen moments afterward) must be demonstrated rather than assuming that loss of consciousness was caused by dysautonomia.

Spontaneous *temperature fluctuations* are common and can make the recognition and proper treatment of serious infections difficult. In addition, vasodilatation below the level of the lesion increases heat loss such that rectal temperature may be several degrees lower than oral.

Meticulous *urinary care* is known to be essential. Continuing use of an indwelling catheter beyond the first 2 or 3 weeks should be avoided and, depending on the type of neurological injury and the state of recovery of the sacral autonomic centers, a definitive program of bladder care should be established as early as possible. Early urologic consultation is helpful in this respect. This complex aspect of the treatment of spinal cord injuries has been discussed in detail in reviews of the subject (31). *Sepsis* probably accounts for the majority of deaths after the first week of injury and the commonest source is the urinary tract, followed by pulmonary infection. To this end, we have encouraged the acquisition of cultures from these areas once or twice weekly for the first week or two and the avoidance of antibiotic treatment except with well documented infections (i.e., not bacteruria). Whether this preemptive approach, and the comparable practice of obtaining routine chest radiographs is helpful, is not known.

Succinylcholine and other depolarizing agents should probably not be used during the first 2 or 3 months after severe spinal cord injuries (and perhaps even afterward if the patient has been immobile) to avoid hyperkalemia from muscle potassium release with attendant ventricular fibrillation. This susceptibility is related to the response of denervated or atrophic–immobile muscle cell membranes to depolarization, similar to what occurs in other paralytic states. Acute and unpredictable hypertensive responses to a variety of anesthetic techniques have been observed in these patients and must be treated vigorously, preferably with direct smooth muscle relaxants such as nitroprusside as opposed to ganglionic blockers.

RECOGNITION AND TREATMENT OF SPECIFIC SPINAL INJURIES

The two most important surgical goals in the management of spinal injuries are decompression of neural structures and assuring the stability of the spine. Immediate stability as well as potential for late instability must be considered after an initial period of treatment. It is also important to keep in mind that osseous lesions, especially through cancellous bone, heal well when immobilized, but ligamentous injuries are slow to heal if they heal at all. Holdsworth has emphasized the importance of considering two basic soft-tissue support units for each segment of the spine (32). The anterior support complex is formed by the anterior and posterior longitudinal ligaments, the disc, and the annulus. The posterior complex is comprised of the supraspinous and interspinous ligaments, the ligamentum flavum, and the facet capsules. When the posterior complex of ligaments is disrupted, the spine becomes unstable and operative fusion is frequently necessary to ensure immediate as well as eventual stability of the spine. Disruptions of the anterior complex heal better and are more stable, especially when extension is prevented by immobilization in a slightly flexed position with a rigid brace.

It is difficult to consider the two goals of decompression and stability in general terms; therefore they are considered in reference to each of the common types of spinal injuries. Table 22.1 summarizes the mechanism of injury and the probability of immediate and late stability for each of the most important specific types of spinal injury.

Atlantooccipital Dislocations

These dislocations are almost invariably fatal when severe. They are most common in children. The clue to their radiologic recognition is the finding of an abnormal relationship between the occipital condyles and the lateral masses of the atlas. Survivors should not be

TABLE 22.1. *Fractures and dislocations of the spine: mechanisms and stability*

Type	Mechanism	Stability[a]	
		Immediate	Late
Atlanto-occipital dislocation	Twisting force to the head	Poor	Poor
Atlantoaxial dislocation	Flexion	Poor	Poor
Fractures of the waist or base of the odontoid	Flexion or (rarely) extension	Poor	Fair
Jefferson fracture	Axial load to the head	Good	Good
Hangman fracture	Hyperextension and distraction	Poor	Good
C3–T1 anterior dislocation with bilateral jumped facets	Flexion	Poor	Fair
Unilateral jumped facets	Flexion and rotation	Good	Fair
Simple wedge fractures	Flexion and axial compression	Good	Good
Bursting fractures	Flexion and axial compression	Fair	Good
Teardrop fractures with anterior subluxation	Flexion and axial compression	Poor	Poor
Hyperextension fractures	Extension	Good in flexion	Good
Thoracic fractures	Direct trauma or flexion	Good	Good
Thoracolumbar fractures	Flexion	Poor	Poor
Open fractures	Penetrating injuries	Good	Good

[a]"Immediate" refers to stability at the time of injury; "late" refers to potential for future stability after an appropriate period of nonoperative immobilization.

placed in traction, which increases distraction. These injuries are highly unstable, and their potential for late stability is poor because the injury is mostly ligamentous. Therefore, a posterior fusion of the occiput to the atlas and the axis followed by a period of 2 to 3 months of immobilization in a halo apparatus is indicated.

Atlantoaxial Dislocations

Atlantoaxial dislocations can result from incompetence of the ligamentous complex holding the dens to the anterior ring of the atlas or from fractures of the dens. Rheumatoid arthritis occasionally causes weakening of the ligaments and predisposes to this injury (33). Atlantoaxial dislocations caused by traumatic fractures of the dens can result in immediate death from respiratory arrest but quite frequently result in no neurological damage. When acute, they are often unstable and the patient must be immobilized. If there is significant dislocation, it should be reduced with no more than 10 to 15 pounds of traction. When the fracture involves the base of the odontoid through the cancellous bone of C2 (actually this is a fracture of the body of C2), it heals well after a period of 2 to 3 months of immobilization in tongs or a halo apparatus (34). Chip fractures through the tip of the odontoid are of no consequence and heal well. Fractures through the neck (waist) of the odontoid are problematic because of nonunion in 40% to 50% of cases. Early posterior fusion has been recommended with displaced fractures, especially if the patient is older than 40 years or if the fracture is displaced more than 4 mm (5). A conservative approach with halo apparatus immobilization may be preferable for patients with undisplaced fractures and for children (35). The problem with the displacement criteria is that a fracture that may have been markedly displaced could reduce itself spontaneously, and when initially recognized radiographically, it may appear undisplaced. A rational approach is to offer adult patients with these fractures the choice between at least 3 to 6 months (de-

pending on the amount of callus seen radiographically) of immobilization with the halo apparatus, with a small chance of nonunion and need for subsequent surgery, or early operative fusion followed by a period of 2 to 3 months wearing a stiff cervical collar.

Jefferson's Fractures

Jefferson's fractures are burst fractures of the ring of the atlas produced by an axial force through the vertex; they are usually asymptomatic. Only when markedly displaced do they require reduction by gentle traction. They heal well after a period of 6 to 8 weeks of immobilization in a halo apparatus because the injury is osseous rather than ligamentous.

Hangman's Fractures

These are fractures through the pedicles of C2 with avulsion and anterior displacement of the body of C2 onto C3. They are produced by hyperextension–distraction injuries such as occur in penal hangings or in a head-on collision when the driver's head is propelled forward and the chin is caught in the steering wheel. Although usually associated with devastating neurological damage, they may present with no deficit at all. The injury is highly unstable initially, but because the injury is mostly bony, it heals well after a period of 2 to 3 months of immobilization in a halo apparatus or traction. Initial reduction must be accomplished with gentle traction (usually 15 to 20 pounds) when the fracture is displaced.

Hyperflexion Dislocations of C3 to T1

Hyperflexion dislocations of any of the levels between C3 to T1 are probably the most common cause of traumatic paraplegia and quadriplegia. Occasionally, however, a patient with a markedly displaced fracture presents only with neck pain and has no neurological deficit. Any degree of subluxation has to be treated as a potentially unstable injury if it is associated with any indication of posterior ligamentous disruption, such as an exaggerated interspinous gap on the anteroposterior film. This precaution is necessary because it is not possible to know how much displacement had been present before the initial films were obtained. In patients presenting with serious neurological deficit, it must be assumed that at one time the displacement was marked enough to have caused significant cord compression. These injuries must be realigned promptly by traction, especially when the injury is associated with a partial neurological deficit. Usually the dislocation is reduced with 30 to 40 pounds of traction, but occasionally 70 pounds are necessary. If the dislocation cannot be reduced, open reduction by a posterior approach is indicated soon in any case but as an emergency in cases of partial neurological deficits.

To mobilize patients early, many surgeons in the United States favor early operative fusion (36,37). In Europe and Australia, a conservative approach has been preferred, particularly in specialized spinal cord injury centers (38). Most agree that the indiscriminate use of wide decompressive laminectomies in acute spinal injuries is to be condemned (39). However, in patients with partial neurological deficit and demonstrated cord compression, the careful removal of any offending material is felt to be not only desirable, but urgent. The approach in our institutions has been to reduce the dislocation rapidly. If the patient has a complete neurological deficit below the level of injury that does not improve with reduction or if the patient is neurologically intact, traction with 15 to 20 pounds is continued for a few days. The decision is then made, after considering the patient's age and medical condition, to recommend either a period of 3 to 6 months of halo immobilization or an early posterior fusion with wire and bone. The posterior fusion offers immediate stability and deals with the pathology that allows potential redislocation (i.e., disruption of the posterior support complex). Posterior fusion without laminectomy has less chance of worsening the neurological deficit than does anterior fusion (40). When a partial neurological deficit is present and not improving rapidly after complete reduction, we recommend a imaging of the spine. If compression is demonstrated, it usually is anteriorly by an extruded disc that can be removed from the anterior route. An alternative is to follow the anterior fusion with internal fixation with instrumentation such as that designed by Caspar and coworkers (41). Even when the dislocation appears well reduced on plain films, CT may reveal that one facet is still jumped. Under these circumstances, an anterior fusion is unlikely to succeed and redislocation is expected.

Flexion–Rotation Injuries of C3 to T1

Flexion–rotation injuries of C3 to T1 characteristically result in anterior subluxation with a unilaterally jumped facet. On the lateral cervical film, all that may be seen is mild anterior subluxation with some narrowing of the disc space. With careful observation, it may be noted that the alignment of the spine shifts suddenly from a lateral to a more oblique position at the area in question. The alignment of the facets, as seen in profile, is disturbed at the level involved. In the anteroposterior projection, the main finding is a steplike shift of alignment in the spine as manifested by abrupt discontinuity of the normal straight line or gentle continuous curve (when the patient's neck is slightly rotated) formed by an imaginary line through the center of the spinous processes (42). Oblique views of the spine demonstrating the neural foramen at each level often help demonstrate a jumped facet.

Most surgeons agree that an effort should be made to reduce these dislocations with traction, because if unreduced they can lead to persistent neck and radicular pain and deficits from root impingement by the jumped inferior facet of the upper vertebrae. The same approach is used as for reduction in the section on hyperflexion dislocations. Before surgery an MRI or CT myelogram is obtained to assess the possibility of a herniated disc, which can be removed at the time of surgery.

Compression Fractures of C3 to TI

Compression fractures of C3 to T1 occur as a result of a flexion with significant axial loading. They form a spectrum from simple wedge compression fractures to teardrop and bursting fractures. Simple wedge compression fractures with intact posterior elements are stable and heal well with simple immobilization in a stiff collar for a few weeks. Burst injuries are caused by a more severe axial force and are frequently accompanied by serious neurological damage. When the deficit is partial and not improving rapidly, an anterior surgical approach with removal of at least the central portion of the shattered vertebral body followed by fusion is indicated. When the posterior elements are intact, these fractures heal well and operative fusion is indicated only if decompression is necessary.

Teardrop fractures are produced by an extreme flexion injury with axial loading. One vertebral body is crushed by the vertebral body superior to it, causing the anterior portion of the compressed body to break away. They are usually accompanied by some disruption of the posterior ligamentous complex, which allows forward dislocation and great instability. When a partial neurological deficit persists, an anterior decompression followed by fusion with either internal fixation or a period of postoperative halo immobilization is indicated.

Hyperextension Fractures

Hyperextension injuries to the spine involve only ligamentous and muscular injuries and, with some exceptions (notably when there is preexisting spondylosis), are well tolerated. Simple cervical collar immobilization until the pain subsides is sufficient. More severe forces result in variable degrees of fracture to the posterior elements but are stable when the anterior support complex is intact. The most severe hyperextension injuries result in disruption of the anterior ligaments and occasionally posterior displacement. These fractures are stable in flexion, and a stiff cervical collar that will prevent extension for a period of 10 to 12 weeks usually results in good stability.

Hyperextension injuries of the spine are frequently associated with the central cord syndrome of Schneider, which was discussed in the preceding. This syndrome occurs frequently in elderly patients with spondylosis but also can occur in the young, especially as a result of football injuries. A conservative approach is preferred for as long as these patients show some improvement.

Fractures of T2 Through T10

These fractures, in most instances, are stable because the thoracic cage acts as a rigid unit that supplies sufficient stability to obviate the need for operative fusion in all but the most severe dislocations. Severe kyphosis requires stabilization with rods. In cases of progressive neurological deficit secondary to anterior cord compression, an anterior transthoracic approach may be necessary. Acute anterior operations in the thoracic (as well as lumbar) regions tend to be very bloody and carry significant morbidity. It may be preferable to avoid such an operation in an acutely traumatized patient, especially if there are associated thoracic or abdominal injuries. An alternative that avoids thoracotomy are the costo-transversectomy approach or a bilateral transpedicular approach. These approaches are less satisfactory from the point of view of achieving complete anterior decompression but have the advantages of minimizing postoperative respiratory difficulties.

Thoracolumbar Fractures

Common thoracolumbar fractures occur as a result of acute flexion of the thoracic on the lumbar spine such as a weight falling on the back while in a bent position (43). neurological deficits resulting from these injuries can be complex, with a mixture of upper motor neuron, lower motor neuron (conus), and root (cauda equina) deficits. In addition, the potential for instability is considerable in this region. The use of anterior, anterolateral, or posterolateral (transpedicular) approaches to displaced thoracolumbar fractures with neurological deficit has gained considerable popularity because extensive laminectomies in this region exacerbate instability and carry some danger of further cord damage when the pathology is located anteriorly. When there is significant dislocation, the approach has been to reduce these fractures as early as the patient's condition permits. If the fracture is not reduced by simple positional maneuvers (lying supine on padded support under the fracture), operative reduction is carried out. Evoked potentials recorded intraoperatively are helpful (Chapter 8). Either anterior or posterolateral decompression and fusion, depending on the CT delineation of the compressing elements, may be performed if a partial neurological deficit persists (44).

Lumbar Fractures

Lumbar fractures can be unstable when there is massive disruption of the posterior ligaments. In these cases, a posterior fusion with instrumentation is indicated. If a neurological deficit is present, Magnetic resonance imaging or CT-myelography should be performed. When a block is present, a posterior decompression through a limited laminectomy is almost always indicated even when the deficit appears complete, because roots in the lumbar area (cauda equina) have a great potential for recovery when decompressed even days and weeks after an injury.

Open (Penetrating) Injuries of the Spine

It has traditionally been recommended that all these injuries be explored to decompress the spinal canal, remove foreign bodies, and repair dural lacerations and potential CSF leaks. This principle still holds for military high-velocity missile injuries, which produce extensive tissue damage and necrosis with a great potential for infection. However, a more conservative approach may be reasonable in civilian low-velocity bullet or knife wounds.

Norrell recommended exploration of these wounds only under the following circumstances: (a) when the entrance wound is directly over the injured cord, in which case there is a short tract with easy access for microorganisms; (b) when fecal contamination is likely, such as when a bullet transverses the colon on its way to the spine; (c) when there is significant bony comminution or an obvious missile within the spinal canal; (d) when there is progressive neurological deficit; (e) in injuries to the cauda equina; and (e) in the rare instances of pleural–CSF fistulas (7).

PROGNOSIS

It is widely acknowledged that there is virtually no chance of recovery when a spinal cord injury results in total loss of neurological function and no recovery has taken place during the first 24 hours. Any evidence of neural transmission through the injured level of the cord, such as a slight voluntary movement or some sensory sparing, indicates that the cord is not totally disrupted and that the injury has been of the threshold type with a potential for recovery.

The repeated recording of somatosensory evoked potentials has been advocated as a useful technique in prognosticating spinal cord injuries. These techniques are considered in Chapter 8. In general, the ability to record cortical evoked potentials from stimulation below the injury seems to indicate that the lesion is incomplete and carries the same prognostic significance as detecting minimal but definite residual neurological function below the level of injury. The reverse, of course, does not hold; that is, the absence of recordable cortical evoked potentials does not imply a complete cord lesion, although the prognosis in these cases is obviously poor if indeed no neurological function can be detected. The loss or deterioration of once-present cortical evoked responses is a good early indicator of subtle deterioration of cord function. The value of using this technique intraoperatively during reduction of thoracolumbar fractures already has been mentioned. In the patient who is unconscious, whether from anesthesia or from associated head injury, the measurement of evoked potentials is one of the most useful techniques for assessing cord function.

An effective and vigorous rehabilitation program is essential in ensuring that the patient with spinal cord injury eventually functions at the highest level possible. Discussion of this aspect of care of spinal cord injuries is beyond the scope of this chapter, but its planning must begin during this early phase of treatment.

PSYCHOLOGICAL FACTORS

Rigoni (45) wrote a concise report over 20 years ago dealing with the psychological aspects of the care of these patients that is still relevant today. The long-term psychological impact of severe spinal cord injuries has been a matter of a number of more recent reviews (46). Dealing with patients with acute catastrophic spinal cord injuries can be most difficult for the physician as well as for the nursing personnel. Frequently, simple greeting statements such as, "How are you today?" or "How do you feel today?" are difficult for the physician to articulate for fear that the patient may respond, "How would you feel if you were in my shoes?" These fears must be overcome. In general, during the acute stages, these patients are too busy dealing with immediate survival matters to concern themselves with long-term philosophic considerations. It is preferable to let the patient ask about what he or she wants to know. Generally, the patient asks questions such as, "Will I ever be able to walk again?" only when he or she is ready to hear the answer. In fact, the patient generally knows already before being told. When questioned by the patient, and at all times with the family, the physician must be honest and forthright, offering no false hopes where no hope exists but also carefully avoiding withdrawing even the slightest hope where there is some or when the patient desperately wants to hold on to some. During the early stages, there is no need to emphatically deny the question, "But, doctors, miracles do happen, don't they?"

A coordinated and unified approach to these patients and their families is necessary for the physicians, nurses, physical therapists, social workers, and others involved in their early care. This approach must be positive. The quadriplegic patient is not helped by the daily requests from nurses and physicians to "Lift your legs off the bed" or "Hold both arms up in front of you." Instead, the patient should be positively reinforced for what he or she can do. The patient indicates soon enough when he or she can move the legs, and there is no advantage to finding out at the earliest hour. Another important aspect of the early approach to these patients is to devise and emphasize a realistic short-goal–oriented schedule to be understood and reinforced by all personnel dealing with the patient. In the intubated patient one may talk daily about the day when the tube may be removed if he or she continues to do well. Then one may look forward to the day when the patient can be moved out of the ICU if everything remains stable. Next, one can start talking about physical therapy, then transfer to a rehabilitation facility, and so on.

ACKNOWLEGMENT

The authors thank Drs. Christopher Ogilvy and Roberto Heros for use of material from their chapter in the third edition of this book.

REFERENCES

1. Allen AR. Surgery of experimental lesion of the spinal cord equivalent to crush injury of fracture dislocation of spinal column. *JAMA* 1911;57:878–880.
2. Tator CH, Fehlings MG. Review of secondary injury theory of acute spinal cord trauma with emphasis on vascular mechanisms. *J Neurosurg* 1991;75:15–26.
3. Kelly DL, Lassiter KRL, Calogero LA, et al. Effects of local hypothermia and tissue oxygen studies in experimental paraplegia. *J Neurosurg* 1970;33:554–563.
4. Osterholm JL, Mathews GJ. Altered norepinephrine metabolism following experimental spinal cord injury. Part 1. Relation to hemorrhagic necrosis and post-wound neurological deficits. *J Neurosurg* 1972;36:386–394.
5. Kobrinde AI, Doyle F, Martins AN. Local spinal cord blood flow in experimental traumatic myelopathy. *J Neurosurg* 1975;42:144–149.
6. Naftchi NE, Demeny M, Decreschito V, et al. Biogenic amine concentrations in traumatized spinal cords of cats. *J Neurosurg* 1974;40:52–57.

7. Norrell HA. Fractures and dislocations of the spine. In: Rothman RH, Simeone FA, eds. *The spine,* vol 2. Philadelphia: WB Saunders, 1975:529–566.

8. White RJ. Pathology of spinal cord injury in experimental lesions. In: Urist MR, ed. *Clinical orthopaedics and related research.* Philadelphia: JB Lippincott, 1975:16–26.

9. Albin MS, White RJ, Acosta-Rua G, et al. Study of functional recovery produced by delayed localized cooling after spinal cord injury in primates. *J Neurosurg* 1968;29:113–120.

10. White RJ. Current status of spinal cord cooling. *Clin Neurosurg* 1972;20:400–408.

11. Tator CH. Acute spinal cord injury: a review of recent studies of treatment and pathophysiology. *Can Med Assoc J* 1972;107:143–150.

12. Yashon D. *Spinal injury.* New York: Appleton-Century-Crofts, 1978.

13. Bracken MB, Shepard MJ, Collins WF, et al. A randomized controlled trial of methylprednisolone or naloxone in the treatment of acute spinal-cord injury. *N Engl J Med.* 1990;322:1405–1411.

14. Hurlbert RJ. Methylprednisolone for acute spinal cord injury: an inappropriate standard of care. *J Neurosurg* 2000;93:175–179.

15. Coleman WP, Benzel D, Cahill DW, et al. A critical appraisal of the reporting of the National Acute Spinal Cord Injury Studies (I and II) of methylprednisolone in acute spinal cord injury. *J Spinal Disord* 2000;13: 185–189.

16. Rogers WA. Fractures and dislocation of the cervical spine and end results study. *J Bone Joint Surg Am* 1957; 39A:341–376.

17. Pierce DS. Acute treatment of spinal cord injuries. In: Pierce DS, Nickel VH, eds. *The total care of spinal cord injuries.* Boston: Little, Brown, 1977:1–51.

18. Green BA, David C, Falcone S, et al. Spinal cord injury in adults. In: Youmans JR, ed. *Neurological surgery,* 4th ed. Philadelphia: WB Saunders, 1996:1969–1990.

19. Comarr AE. The neurogenic bladder. In: Pierce DS, Nickel VH, eds. *The total care of spinal cord injuries.* Boston: Little, Brown, 1977:165–169.

20. Schneider R, Crosby E, Russo H, et al. Traumatic spinal cord syndromes and their management. *Clin Neurosurg* 1972;20:424–492.

21. Schneider RC. Trauma to the spine and spinal cord. In: Kahn EA, Crosby EC, Schneider RC, et al, eds. *Correlative neurosurgery,* 2nd ed. Springfield, IL: Charles C Thomas, 1969:597–684.

22. Dickson JH, Harrington PR, Erwin WD. Results of reduction and stabilization of the severely fractured thoracic and lumbar spine. *J Bone Joint Surg Am* 1978; 60A:799–805.

23. Marshall LF, Knowlton S, Garfin SR, et al. Deterioration following spinal cord injury: A multicenter study. *J Neurosurg* 1987;66:400–404.

24. Harrop JS, Sharan AD, Vaccaro AR, et al. The cause of neurologic deterioration after acute cervical spine cord injury. *Spine* 2001;26:340–346.

25. Hudgins PA, Hudgins RJ. Radiology of cervical spine trauma. *Clin Neurosurg* 1991;37:571–595.

26. Heiden JS, Weiss MH. Cervical spine injuries with and without neurological deficit, Part 2. *Contemp Neurosurg* 1980;2:1–8.

27. Raynor RB. Discography and myelography in acute injuries of the cervical spine. *J Neurosurg* 1971;35: 529–535.

28. Quenger RM, Sheldon JJ, Post MJD, et al. MRI of the chronically injured spinal cord. *Am J Radiol* 1986; 147:125–132.

29. Heiden JS, Weiss MH. Cervical spine injuries with and without neurological deficit, Part 1. *Contemp Neurosurg* 1980;2:1–6.

30. Attia J, Ray JG, Cook DJ, et al. Deep vein thrombosis and its prevention in critically ill adults. *Arch Int Med* 2001;161:1268–1279.

31. Wyndaele JJ, Madersbacher H, Kovindha A. Conservative treatment of the neuropathic bladder in spinal cord injured patients. *Spinal Cord* 2001;39:294–300.

32. Holdsworth F. Fractures, dislocations, and fracture-dislocations of the spine. *J Bone Joint Surg Am* 1970; 52A:1534–1551.

33. Alexander E Jr, Davis CH Jr. Reduction and fusion of fractures of the odontoid process. *J Neurosurg* 1969; 31:580–582.

34. Anderson LD, D'Alonzo RT. Fractures of the odontoid process of the axis. *J Bone Joint Surg Am* 1974;56A: 1663–1674.

35. Apuzzo MLJ, Heiden JS, Weiss MH, et al. Acute fractures of the odontoid process. *J Neurosurg* 1978;48:85–91.

36. Clark K. Use of anterior operative approach in the treatment of cervical spine injuries. In: Youmans JR, ed. *Neurological surgery,* vol 2. Philadelphia: WB Saunders, 1973:1067–1074.

37. Cloward RB. Acute cervical spine injuries. *Clin Symp* 1980;32:2–32.

38. Bedbrook GM. Spinal injuries with tetraplegia and paraplegia. *J Bone Joint Surg Br* 1979;61B:267–284.

39. Morgan TH, Wharton GW, Austin GN. The results of laminectomy in patients with incomplete spinal cord injuries. *Paraplegia* 1971;9:14–23.

40. Kraus DR, Stauffer ES. Spinal cord injury as a complication of elective anterior cervical fusion. In: Urist MR, ed. *Clinical orthopaedics and related research.* Philadelphia: JB Lippincott, 1975:130–141.

41. Caspar W, Barbier DD, Klara PM. Anterior cervical fusion and Caspar plate stabilization for cervical trauma. *Neurosurgery* 1989;25:491–502.

42. Harris JH Jr. *The radiology of acute cervical spine trauma.* Baltimore: Williams & Wilkins, 1978.

43. Durward QJ, Schwiegel JF, Harrison P. Management of fractures of the thoracolumbar and lumbar spine. *Neurosurgery* 1981;8:555–561.

44. Schmidek HH, Gomes FB, Seligson D, et al. Management of acute unstable thoracolumbar (T-11–L-1) fractures with and without neurological deficit. *Neurosurgery* 1980;7:30–35.

45. Rigoni HC. Psychological coping in the patient with spinal cord injury. In: Pierce DS, Nickel VH, eds. *The total care of spinal cord injuries.* Boston: Little, Brown, 1977:299–307.

46. Craig AR, Hancock KM, Dickson M, et al. Psychological consequences of spinal injury: a review of the literature. *Aust NZ J Psychiatry* 1990;24:418–425.

23

Ethical and Legal Aspects Applicable to the Neurological Intensive Care Unit

Neurologists and neurosurgeons in the neurological intensive care unit (neuro-ICU) frequently must decide on the level of care to be provided for certain patients with severe and irreversible brain damage. When confronted with the ostensible meaninglessness of life for such patients, the suffering felt by their families, the risk of survival without neurological recovery, and the duty to fulfill the prior wishes of the patient, the physician might be in a position that recommends a level of treatment that predictably shortens the patient's survival. Physicians faced with such literally life-and-death decisions must be knowledgeable about the medical, ethical, and legal bases for such decision making. Most patients for whom these decisions to terminate treatment are considered are permanently comatose or vegetative. The starting point for discussion is the assumption of individual self-determination, rather than societal or religious judgment. Much of the current ethical and legal debate arises because such patients lack decision-making capacity (are incompetent) to decide about their own care. Consequently, others (families, proxies, physicians) must, in essence, decide for them. This chapter reviews the ethical and legal aspects of end-of-life decision making, particularly for incompetent, severely brain-damaged patients, and provides some guidelines for physicians responsible for their care. This chapter is intended only to be an overview, because laws regarding informed decision making and medical malpractice might vary; therefore, it is at times important to consult

with experts in a particular state or jurisdiction regarding specific issues. It might be pointed out that medical ethics does not always equate with ethical behavior on the part of the individual physician, the latter having more to do with settling in one's own mind the personal role one plays in guidance of patients and families in difficult situations. Some of these dilemmas are referred to further on.

All decision making regarding the extent of treatment begins with a clear definition of the patient's diagnosis and prognosis. Restated, the issue is to determine how prognostic information should be factored into ethical clinical decision making regarding the level of care to be provided to patients who have had severe neurological damage. In the most common situation, the neurologist is asked to state the likelihood that the patient's brain functioning will recover more or less to normal. Examples of such determinations include coma and vegetative states after cardiac arrest, head trauma, and stroke. Before any decision regarding withdrawal of life-prolonging treatment, the physician should strive to reach a prognosis with the highest possible level of certainty. (See Chapters 9 and 17 for discussions of prognostication and its limitations.) When using prognostic indicators, there is always a degree of uncertainty that should be considered before making decisions, but the precise level of certainty required for ethically sound decision making remains uncertain. Of course, the most grievous error is an incorrect prediction of poor outcome in which patients may die from withdrawal of care when they might have survived with a good outcome. They may also suffer, however, if there is an inappropriate prediction of good outcome that leads to survival in a persistent vegetative or completely dependent state, which may not have been their wish. It is inappropriate for the physician to initiate steps to limit treatment if the prognosis remains altogether uncertain. Instead, the clinician should provide support and postpone decision making until the prognosis for return of consciousness becomes more certain. Although physicians are expected to supply information about prognosis to their patients, the Supreme Court of California in *Arato v. Avedon* held that physicians do not legally have to provide specific survival or mortality percentages to their patients, recognizing the leeway needed in giving individual recommendations (1). Ethical clinical decisions are based on both medical facts and individual values where the physician has expertise only about the former and the patient or patient's surrogate has expertise only about the latter, and the decisions emerge from this joint expertise rather than from unilateral physician recommendations (2).

WITHDRAWAL OF LIFE SUPPORT: THE COMPETENT PATIENT

Four principal bioethical concepts form the foundation for decisions to terminate treatment: respect for autonomy, nonmaleficence, beneficence, and justice (3).

U.S. Supreme Court Justice Benjamin Cardozo described respect for autonomy in the medical context when he wrote, "Every human being of adult years and sound mind has a right to determine what shall be done with his own body" (4). The practice of informed consent is based on this concept of respect for autonomy (5). Physicians consider the duties of nonmaleficence and beneficence whenever they balance the burdens and benefits of a particular therapy. Justice embodies rules for the societal distribution of resources. Under the ethical principle of autonomy, patients have the right to refuse life-prolonging treatment, including artificial nutrition and hydration (6).

Competent, terminally ill patients sometimes ask their physicians to discontinue their life support systems to permit them to die. A relatively common scenario of this type in a neuro-ICU is that of a patient with amyotrophic lateral sclerosis who is dependent on a ventilator. Faced with a relatively short life expectancy and dependence on mechanical ventilation, some patients opt to be withdrawn from the ventilator even though this action results in almost certain death. From a purely ethical perspective in Western society, the physician's role in such decision making is relatively easy. The rational wishes of competent patients are followed. Choosing a rapid death from respiratory failure over a protracted death from the other complications of motor neuron disease is generally considered to be a rational decision. It is emotionally difficult for the physician to witness and participate in such a death, but when the patient is competent and is completely informed of the alternatives, his or her wishes should be followed (7). The legal requirement for physicians to extubate such patients is grounded in the doctrine of informed consent, as ruled in *Satz v. Perlmutter* (8). The Florida court in *Satz v. Perlmutter* affirmed the right of a competent individual (Mr. Satz, a man totally paralyzed as a result of amyotrophic lateral sclerosis), to have life-support measures discontinued if the family agrees and there are no dependents.

Physicians have several well-defined duties in the care of dying patients who refuse respiratory support. First, the patient must be carefully and compassionately counseled about his or her prognosis, with and without treatment. The appropriateness and efficacy of various types of ventilatory support should be discussed in detail (7,9). A series of discussions, specifically more than one, should be held to ascertain that the patient's wish to forgo ventilatory support is not an impulsive reaction to his or her illness, but rather is a carefully considered and consistently held choice based on a full knowledge of the consequences and treatment alternatives. The ambiguity here, in our view, is in regard to the issue of reactive depression. Some view any desire to die as a reflection of an unnatural depression. Input from the patient's family is valuable in determining the constancy and rationality of the patient's decision. Another perspective, based on conservative religious doctrine, is that only God has the power to terminate life. Over the past few decades even the latter view has been modified by mainstream pronouncements that allow, but do not necessarily endorse, the withdrawal of care in certain circumstances. If the physician has a moral objection to carrying out the patient's decision, he or she should transfer the care of the patient to another physician.

From a practical perspective, physicians should assure the patient and family that they would attempt to maintain comfort throughout the extubation and death. Morphine (or other narcotics or benzodiazepines) may be prescribed in doses (from 2 to 10 mg per hour of morphine as boluses or continuous infusion) that minimize suffering and lessen the pain and anxiety of air hunger in the recently extubated patient, even if this contributes, as a secondary effect, to respiratory depression, coma, or death (6,s10–13). The ethical principle of double effect supports the use of pain medication in doses that may risk respiratory depression because the primary intention is pain relief, although the foreseen but unintended result may be a hastening of death (12).

WITHDRAWAL OF LIFE SUPPORT: THE INCOMPETENT PATIENT

Ethical Aspects

The more frequent context for decisions to terminate treatment arise with the incompetent patient. Physicians can continue to respect patients' autonomy by attempting to identify and follow their previously stated wishes. *Advance directives* are formal or informal instructions, executed by competent individuals that pertain to their medical care in the event they become incompetent. Physicians who follow patients' advance directives permit their patients to consent to or refuse their treatment, despite their present incompetence. Informal advance directives refer to verbal statements made by patients to family members or friends that reveal their attitudes about maintaining life support in the setting of hopeless illness. Formal advance directives are of two types: (a) written instructional directives in the form of the legally nonbinding *living will* or in those states with statutory provisions, in the form of a legally binding *terminal care document* or *natural death act;* and (2) proxy appointments that designate a person to make surrogate decisions, which in those states with statutory provisions, can be made in the form of a legally binding *Durable Power of Attorney for Health Care* (DPAHC). The instructional directives have the advantage of providing a statement of the patient's exact wishes, whereas the proxy appointments have the advantage of providing greater flexibility to adapt the patient's wishes to each particular clinical situation (14).

Written advance directives do have inherent limitations. The patient's medical situation can change significantly from the time of execution of an advance directive to the moment of treatment choices so that circumstances that may have been anticipated are not the circumstances present during the patient's incompetence. Directives of the living will type often state that the patient refuses "life-prolonging" therapy and other "extraordinary measures" if he or she is in a hopeless "terminal condition." The ambiguity arises in the interpretation of these vague phrases. Does the persistent vegetative state count as a terminal condition, given that patients have been recorded to survive for many years in such states? Furthermore, does continued artificial hydration and nutrition by gastrostomy tube count as life-prolonging therapy or an extraordinary measure? Patients and physicians may differ on their interpretation of these terms, and physicians may be thrust into the difficult position of being asked to make life-and-death decisions based on ambiguous directives. The DPAHC provision enacted by many states in the United States provides flexibility to overcome many of these ambiguities. The agent named as DPAHC should know the values and preferences of the individual he or she represents. The DPAHC can then interpret these wishes and make judgments in specific clinical contexts. Patients can protect themselves to the greatest extent by executing both a terminal care document and a DPAHC.

In those more frequent situations in which advance directives do not exist, it is still of great value to have a proxy decision maker appointed. This may be done formally, as in states with Health Care Proxy laws, or informally by the physician appointing either one close relative or all the close family members and even all interested parties (e.g., the patient's fiancé or closest friend) to participate in the decision making. Using the values of the patient, the proxy should be guided to attempt to reproduce the decision that the patient would have made in the particular situation. This type of decision making is called the standard of *substituted judgment.* Proxies must be told that their prediction of the patient's preference may not be the same as the decision that the surrogate would choose for himself or herself. The realistic limit of the ideal of substituted judgment was shown in a survey of spouses who were asked to predict elderly patients' preferences for cardiopulmonary resuscitation (CPR) (15). In more than one third of instances, spouses predicted that the patients would desire CPR when they would not. Interestingly, physicians erred frequently in predicting that elderly patients would not want CPR when, in fact, they did. Although imperfect, substituted judgment is the decision-making standard that best permits respect for a patient's autonomy. In our view, the physician has an appropriate role in judging whether the proxy understands the mandate to make a substituted judgment.

In some situations, the proxy decision maker is thrust into the difficult position of not knowing which choice the patient would have made. In this circumstance, he or she should be asked to assess the relative benefits and burdens to the patient with or without treatment. This type of decision making is

called the standard of *best interest.* The best interest standard is ethically less powerful than the substituted judgment standard because it requires the decision maker to use his or her own values to balance the benefits and burdens of treatment. The proxy's values, hence his or her judgment, may or may not correspond to the decision that the patient would have made.

It is not uncommon, in our experience, for the proxy to solicit the advice of the physician on the correct course of action, beyond asking for prognostic information. We have taken the point of view that the physician should develop the personal discipline to avoid directly interposing personal belief systems, even to the extent of using expressions such as "if it were me or my family member." This requires that guidance, rather than even subtle paternalism, be used as a method of support. More helpful in giving guidance are: (a) reassurance that the proxy is making the correct decision if his or her instinct is that the patient's wishes would lie in one direction or the other; and (b) the physician's experience with various prior cases. Even the reassurance that most patients who are severely injured will die in some short or intermediate period of time of medical complications, if not offered disingenuously, can be very helpful to families in realizing that some uncertainty must be a part of the process but can be put in perspective. Some families hang on a comment, often appropriate on the part of the physician, that there is no absolute certainty regarding a poor outcome; comments such as these should be couched in broad terms that indicate the chances are very small indeed. And, again in our view, the physician should not be the agent of efficiency or the subtly expressed desire of a hospital or insurance company to free up space or limit resources. One solution to this problem is to attempt to move the patient to a less intensive care environment, if possible, while decisions are being made.

In the severely brain-damaged patient for whom it can be determined with a high level of certainty that recovery of consciousness will not occur, continued treatment only prolongs his or her dying and confers no benefit to the patient. It is morally permissible to withdraw treatment provided that the prognosis for recovery of consciousness is hopeless and that there is evidence that, while competent, the patient wished to be permitted to die in this situation. In the absence of any such evidence, it is morally permissible for the physician to withdraw therapies if the prognosis for recovery of consciousness is hopeless and the proxy chooses no treatment. In the absence of proxy involvement, it is morally acceptable to discontinue care if the physician and family agree that the burdens of continued treatment outweigh the benefits (5,16–20). Treatment without benefit to the patient is considered futile.

Although the medical community may have reached consensus that there is no moral obligation to continue treatment deemed futile (21), there is still no legal consensus on the issue (22). In general, it is very telling that when there is a prospective disagreement about whether or not a treatment is futile, the courts have ruled in favor of the party wishing to initiate or continue treatment (1,23,24). In our own experience, even with a living will stating the patient's wish not to have his or her life artificially prolonged, the court has ruled in favor of the one dissenting family member wishing to prolong aggressive treatment. It should be kept in mind also that some parts of society, particularly some non–Western societies, hold the belief that regardless of how dismal the prognosis, even if the patient is vegetative, the person should be kept alive at all costs. In terms of risk management, physicians should be aware of any policies addressing futile situations and continuing care that are in place at the hospitals where they practice. Following hospital policies demonstrates that the physician met the professional standard of behavior.

If the patient or surrogate disagrees with a medical decision, many hospitals have an ethics committee that can help improve communication and be of assistance from a risk management perspective. The President's Commission recommended that *hospital ethics committees* provide oversight for physicians' orders to terminate treatment on patients who are hopelessly but not terminally ill (5). The ethics committee has a strictly defined role in such proceedings. It is not their prerogative to decide whether the termination of treatment order is appropriate; that responsibility lies with the attending physician. The committee functions to protect the patient by guaranteeing that a proper decision-making process was followed. They ascertain that a firm diagnosis and prognosis have been made, that the previous wishes of the patient have been sought, and that the current wishes of the family are known. This oversight role obviates the need for judicial review of the decision in most cases. However, it should be acknowledged that a physician who countermands the opinion of such a committee is in a difficult position. Our experience with ethics committees has been that they are most helpful when a family takes an extreme position of prolonging care in cases of brain death or a severely brain-damaged state.

Legal Aspects

Several legal cases in the United States have served as benchmarks for the evolution of thinking on medical ethics in neurological care. The sequence of decisions is instructive in understanding the current state of affairs but cannot be used to surmise future directions. It may reasonably be assumed that these cases were decided on the basis of prevailing societal opinion, which may change with the evolution of society, as noted in the next section.

A legal precedent was set for the right of the incompetent patient to discontinue life-support measures in the *Karen Quinlan* case. Karen Quinlan was a young woman who had suffered unexplained periods of apnea during which she received no adequate ventilatory support (25). When she arrived at the hospital she was comatose and, despite ventilator support, persisted in a vegetative state. The family believed that the ventilator should be discontinued and that Karen ought to be allowed to die, but physicians on the hospital staff disagreed. The New Jersey court granted permission to the father, who had been appointed legal guardian, to discontinue the life-supporting ventilator, acknowledging that there was no reasonable chance of recovery and that Karen, before becoming incompetent, had indicated that she would not want to be supported by a ventilator. The court indicated that the patient had a right to privacy and a right to die that could be exercised on her behalf by her legal guardian. The ventilator was discontinued but Karen continued to breathe on her own. (This case is of some interest to neurologists in that the neuropathology explaining coma was mainly in the thalami rather than the cerebral cortex, as accords with our own experience.)

The *Saikewicz* case dealt with the right of an incompetent individual to refuse treatment that might be indicated (26). Joseph Saikewicz was a 67-year-old ward of the state of Massachusetts who was severely mentally retarded but healthy until he developed acute myelogenous monocytic leukemia. The state school where he lived petitioned the court to appoint a guardian with the intention that the guardian would provide consent for treatment. Medical testimony suggested that the likelihood of benefit of treatment was very small, that the side effects were considerable, and that he would have to be restrained to receive treatment. Employing the substituted judgment theory by which the court hoped to determine what decision Mr. Saikewicz would have made if he were competent, the court concluded that he would have chosen to refuse such treatment. The Supreme Court of Massachusetts indicated that both life-prolonging and life-saving therapy that represented a reasonable therapeutic option could not be withheld from an incompetent individual unless the court sanctioned the decision to withhold. However, the determination of what may represent a "reasonable therapeutic option" would remain with the physician. It is readily conceivable that some physicians caring for an incompetent patient may make a good-faith determination that a certain form of therapy may not be indicated for their patient and so have no need for recourse to the courts.

In the *Dinnerstein* case in Massachusetts, the children of a 67-year-old woman with severe Alzheimer disease and a massive stroke requested that resuscitative efforts be withheld should she suffer a cardiac arrest (27). After the *Saikewicz* decision, there was reluctance to issue "Do Not Resuscitate" (DNR) orders and the matter was brought to the court. The appellate division of the court agreed that resuscitative efforts could properly be withheld in this circumstance and clarified the appropriateness of DNR orders:

> The *Saikewicz* case, if read to apply to the natural death of a terminally-ill patient by cardiac or respiratory arrest, would require attempts to resuscitate dying patients in most cases, without exercise of medical judgment, even when the course of action could be aptly characterized as pointless, even cruel, prolongation of the act of dying. . . . We think it clear that such a result is neither intended nor sanctioned by the Saikewicz case. . . .

The New York State Court of Appeals *In re Eichner* supported a lower court's decision to allow suspension of life support in the case of Brother Fox, an 83-year-old man who remained in a vegetative state after a cardiac arrest (28). Brother Fox had indicated in the past that he would not want to be provided any extraordinary treatment if he were in a condition similar to Karen Quinlan. The court indicated that a competent adult had a right to refuse therapy even if the outcome of that refusal would almost certainly be fatal and that the same standard had to be applied to the incompetent patient. The court saw no need to invoke such doctrines as substituted judgment or constitutional right to privacy. It based its position on the common law right of a competent individual to refuse medical therapy, a right that survives the competency of the individual if the evidence of the refusal is "clear and convincing."

The *Cruzan* case was the first case ever heard by the U.S. Supreme Court on the subject of withholding or withdrawing life support (29,30). The Court declared that both competent and incompetent individuals had the constitutional right to refuse any form of medical therapy. It is important, however, that the laws affecting advance directives and end-of-life care issues in individual states be consulted, because there may be significant differences in the requirements from state to state. For example, New York and Missouri require that surrogate decisions to withdraw support be subject to "clear and convincing evidence" of prognosis and of the patient's previously stated or written preferences regarding removal of life support. In a recent survey of U.S. neurologists, 38% were unnecessarily concerned about being charged with a crime for withdrawing life-sustaining treatment, despite the existing legal protection (12,29). Based on that survey, there appears to be a need for education on end-of-life decision making to bridge the gap between established medical, ethical, and legal guidelines and the current beliefs and practices of many neurologists.

Levels of Treatment

When physicians order termination of treatment, the most aggressive measures are generally withdrawn before the less aggressive ones. Aggressiveness of treatment can be divided into four categories: (a) technology, such as ventilators and dialysis; (b) medications (including vasopressors and antibiotics); (c) hydration and nutrition; and (d) basic care to maintain the comfort, hygiene, and dignity of the patient (19). Do not resuscitate orders exclude a portion of the first category of treatment: endotracheal intubation, mechanical ventilation, and cardiac defibrillation. Vasopressors and antibiotics also may be included in DNR orders. Comfort always must be maintained.

There is an ethical rationale and growing consensus that it is also permissible to withdraw hydration and nutrition in the hopelessly ill patient (5,31,32). Those opposed to classifying hydration and nutrition as medical therapy point out that food and water are essential to life and not providing them is tantamount to killing the patient. Those in favor of classifying hydration and nutrition as medical therapy point out that the provision of food and water to a permanently unconscious patient requires technologies, including implanted feeding gastrostomy tubes and external pumps. The patient would die were it not for the application and vigilant monitoring of these technologies. To some extent, artificial hydration and nutrition remains a controversial issue more because of its symbolic significance than because of any moral distinction between withdrawing hydration and nutrition and withdrawing other therapies of dubious benefit to permanently noncognitive patients. The provision of food and water is psychologically associated with nurturing and caregiving. Fears have been expressed that withdrawing hydration and nutrition from patients may be interpreted as the physician no longer caring for the patient and that society may devalue the lives of its unproductive members (33). These are valid points but should not override the right of a patient to refuse hydration and nutrition as exercised by a proxy decision maker using proper standards of decision making. In the U.S. Supreme Court *Cruzan* decision, the Court found no legal distinction between hydration and nutrition and other medical therapies (29,30).

There now exists wide agreement, although counterintuitive to some, that there is no moral distinction between withholding and withdrawing treatment. Aggressive treatment that was begun with the expectation of recovery may be discontinued when it becomes reasonably certain that the expected recovery will not occur. It can be argued that the discontinuation is the moral equivalent of not initially beginning the therapy because the treatment no longer contributes to the patient's health goal of recovery (3,31,34).

Public Policy

Societal acceptance that it is ethically permissible to withdraw treatment from persistently unconscious patients has been aided by the conclusions of several influential commissions in the United States. In 1983, the President's Commission for the Study of Ethical Problems in Medicine and Biomedical and Behavioral Research published a report concluding that it is both ethical and lawful for physicians to terminate treatment in permanently comatose or vegetative patients provided that the proper decision-making procedures are followed, including clear elucidation of the diagnosis and prognosis, clear identification of the previous wishes of the patient and the present wishes of the family, and local review by the hospital ethics committee (20). The Commission wrote:

> The decisions of patients' families should determine what sort of care permanently unconscious patients receive. Other than requiring appropriate decision making procedures for these patients, the law does not and should not require any particular therapies to be applied or continued, with the exception of basic nursing care that is needed to ensure dignified and respectful treatment of the patient.

In 1989, the American Medical Association Council on Scientific Affairs and Council on Ethical and Judicial Affairs held that it is ethical and lawful to terminate all medical treatment, including the withdrawal of hydration and nutrition, in certain noncognitive patients (16). The Council wrote:

> The social commitment of the physician is to sustain life and relieve suffering. Where the performance of one duty conflicts with the other, the preferences of the patient should prevail. If the patient is incompetent to act in his own behalf and did not previously indicate his preferences, the family or other surrogate decision-maker, in concert with the physician, must act in the best interest of the patient . . . the surrogate decision-maker and physician should consider several factors, including: the possibility for extending life under humane and comfortable conditions; the patient's values about life and the way it should be lived; and the patient's attitudes toward sickness, suffering, medical procedures, and death.
>
> Even if death is not imminent but a patient is beyond doubt permanently unconscious, and

there are adequate safeguards to confirm the accuracy of the diagnosis, it is not unethical to discontinue all means of life-prolonging medical treatment.

> Life-prolonging medical treatment includes medication and artificially or technologically supplied respiration, nutrition, or hydration. In treating a terminally ill permanently unconscious patient, the dignity of the patient should be maintained at all times.

State legislatures and the federal government have enacted laws permitting and regulating termination of medical treatment. One example is The Patient Self Determination Act that went into effect in 1991 increasing the use of advance directives by bringing national attention to this initiative and obliging hospitals and other medical facilities to advise all patients on admission of their right to execute an advance directive. This opportunity for patients to be empowered to limit unwanted care is also a great opportunity for the physician to deal with end-of-life issues as part of the patient's clinical continuum and to be able to discuss those forms of care that the patient may desire or reject. In a recent survey of U.S. neurologists, 95% of respondents reported that advance directives eased the decision-making process regarding withdrawal of life support, but only 30% of their patients had completed such forms (12).

WITHDRAWAL OF TREATMENT: GUIDELINES FOR CLINICIANS

The following general and specific procedural guidelines are offered for physicians faced with decisions to terminate treatment in patients with severe, irreversible brain damage. These guidelines incorporate the aforementioned relevant ethical and legal concepts and the recommendations of several major commissions and study groups that have considered this issue (5,16,35,36). Because these are only guidelines, the particular details of each case must be individually considered before the optimal course of action is chosen.

General

1. *Communicate with the family.* The physician must be compassionate, showing that he or she cares about the family's wishes and feelings and will not abandon the patient. It must be emphasized that to terminate treatment is to allow nature to take its course, and that the physician will do everything within his or her power to ease the passing. Effective communication with families requires frequent conferences and is very time consuming. Communication with families should include answering questions, listening to concerns, and allowing and promoting the grief process.

2. *Communicate with the staff.* Explanations of the basis for treatment decisions must be given to the nursing and house staff, and their input should be requested. The physician should try to develop a staff consensus on the proposed treatment plan because the plan is the ethically correct course of action.

3. *Document decisions carefully.* The medical record should contain a summary of the process by which treatment decisions were made with documentation at each stage.

4. *Follow hospital bylaws.* The physician should learn if his or her hospital has bylaws pertaining to decision making for terminating or limiting treatment. These bylaws should be followed.

5. *Follow state laws.* The physician should learn if his or her state has statutory or case laws pertaining to decision making in terminating treatment. Hospital attorneys usually can provide such information and advice.

Specific

1. *Establish diagnosis.* The physician should distinguish brain death, persistent vegetative state, and other states of profound brain damage on the basis of frequent neurological examinations. Brain-dead patients are declared dead according to standard protocols (Chapter 9).

2. *Establish prognosis.* A confident prognosis is essential before any consideration to terminate treatment should be made. Serial careful neurological examinations are usually necessary to provide a firm prognosis. If in doubt, it is prudent to wait. The longer the severe neurological dysfunction is present, the less is the likelihood for recovery of consciousness. The physician should exercise caution in issuing a poor prognosis for young patients and for those with head trauma because both may be associated with delayed good recovery. Reversible causes of central nervous system dysfunction must be excluded carefully. Determination of prognosis and its limitations are discussed in Chapters 9 and 17.

3. *Identify the patient's preferences.* If advance directives exist through living wills, terminal care documents, natural death acts, or durable power of attorney appointments, these directives can inform the physician of the patient's wishes. In the absence of an advance directive, a proxy decision should be made by the next of kin or a court-appointed guardian. The proxy should be asked to decide using a substituted judgment standard. The physician should support, comfort, and reassure the proxy that he or she has made the right decision and is carrying out the patient's wishes. The best interest standard should be used only if there is no reliable evidence of the patient's wishes or system of values.

4. *Identify the family's preference.* Careful and sensitive explanations of the diagnosis and prognosis must precede identification of the family's preference. The family should be allowed sufficient time to assimilate the tragedy and begin the grieving process before a decision is requested. If the decision is to terminate treatment, reduction of guilt will be a major task. If there is no consensus of the family's pref-

erence, the physician should try to develop one by family meetings. If no consensus can be reached despite the assistance of the ethics committee, social workers, nurses, or chaplains, the case should be referred to court for judicial review and formal guardianship appointment.

5. *Choose level of treatment.* The physician can order the termination of technology, medications, hydration, and nutrition based on his or her assessment, the patient's prior wishes, and the decision of the family. Measures to maintain the patient's comfort, dignity, and hygiene should be maintained. Orders should be written explicitly, and the staff should understand them and concur.

6. *Request oversight by the hospital ethics committee.* The committee should convene and review the decision-making process for the patient in whom the physician plans to discontinue treatment, who is noncognitive but not terminally ill. The function of the committee is to inspect the decision-making process, not to judge the merits of the available options or make the decision. The decision-making power rests with the responsible physician, with inputs from the proxy and family. A brief chart note signifying the committee's approval of the decision-making process will help protect both the patient and physician. If the committee believes that the decision-making process has been improper, it should recommend that the physician's decision to terminate treatment be reversed until the process issue can be resolved. This is a crucial step because it should allow the hospital to avoid formal judicial review in all but a very few cases. In the absence of a hospital ethics committee, the decision-making process should be reviewed by at least one other physician.

7. *Refer to court for judicial review.* Although judicial review should be necessary only rarely, it is advisable if urged by the hospital attorney, if there is an intractable disagreement within the family or evidence that a proxy is deciding selfishly, if there is an uncertain prognosis, or if there is neither advance directive nor proxy available to guide the physician (37).

OTHER ETHICAL ISSUES IN THE NEUROLOGICAL INTENSIVE CARE UNIT

Non–Heart-Beating Organ Donation

Non–heart-beating donation (NHBD) is defined as the surgical recovery of organs after pronouncement of death based on cessation of cardiopulmonary function. Prior to the acceptance of brain death criteria in the 1970s, all organ donations were performed after cardiopulmonary death. Currently though, over 95% of organ donations occur after brain death. Non–heart-beating donation may increase the number of organs (particularly kidneys) available for transplant by 30% and there is no difference in long-term outcome between kidneys obtained from donors with and without a heartbeat (38). Patients who may be evaluated for NHBD have sustained an irreversible brain injury, have not met the criteria for brain death, and a family decision has already been made to withdraw life support. It also should be determined that cardiopulmonary function would likely cease within 1 hour of withdrawal of ventilatory and hemodynamic support. The decision to withdraw treatment should be made independently of and prior to any discussion of organ donation. Death pronouncement should be made by one of the patient's physicians who is not associated with the transplant team. The family must be given the option to be present during the withdrawal of life support and death of the patient. Withdrawal of support ideally occurs in the operating room or the postanesthesia care unit so that surgical recovery of the organs may occur quickly following 5 minutes of asystole as measured by electrocardiograph and arterial pulse monitoring. The family should be supported and prepared for what they will see, what will happen, and that they will need to leave the room shortly after death or organ donation may not occur. Involvement of an ethics consultant is reasonable to assess the family's understanding of NHBD. The organ procurement organization is responsible for all costs related to the evaluation and recovery of organs and tissues for transplantation.

Because there is no ethical or legal distinction between death certified using brain criteria and death certified using cardiopulmonary criteria, there should be no ethical or legal distinction between organ procurement in either case (39). However, there still has been considerable controversy over the ethical issues involved in NHBD. The Institute of Medicine, commissioned by the U.S. Department of Health and Human Services, published a report in 1997 on the considerable variation among organ procurement organizations and hospitals in such areas as criteria for declaration of death and premortem medical interventions to preserve organs (cannulation, anticoagulants, and vasodilators) (40). They recommended a consistent approach to support patients and their families and sustain the integrity and public confidence in the organ transplantation system. Specific guidelines for NHBD policy included having locally approved NHBD protocols open to the public, making case-by-case decisions in conjunction with the family about the premortem administration of medications, requiring family consent for premortem cannulation, having conflict-of-interest safeguards (separate times and personnel for decisions on withdrawal of care and decisions on organ donation), and having a 5-minute observation period after cessation of cardiopulmonary function before determination of death. The Ethics Committee of the American College of Critical Care Medicine in a position statement in 2001 agreed with the Institute of Medicine except that they shortened the recommended observation period for death pronouncement to between 2 and 5 minutes and they also stated that medications that do not harm the patient and are required to improve chances of suc-

cessful donation are ethically acceptable (39). Non–heart-beating donation is an additional donation option that can provide comfort to families who have made the difficult decision to discontinue support. Even though there have been some misperceptions about the ethical issues involved with non–heart-beating donation; education for physicians, nurses, and other hospital staff; combined with a consistent, clearly defined protocol will be important in allowing this option to be more available in the future.

Euthanasia

The term "euthanasia" means a good or happy death, but it has more recently become equated with physician-assisted suicide or an act intended to cause the death of another person. Some have used the term "passive euthanasia" for the withholding or withdrawal of treatment that results in a person's death. This term is not correct, though, unless the intent of the action is that the patient will die. The application of the ethical principle of double effect is illustrated in the aforementioned case of Karen Quinlan. The fact that she lived for nearly a decade after the ventilator was removed demonstrates that the intended result (removal of a burdensome treatment) did not require or depend on the unintended effect (her death) (41). Although physicians have an ethical obligation to honor a competent patient's refusal of therapy, they have no obligation to fulfill a patient's request for physician-assisted suicide or any intervention intended to do harm to the patient. The authors agree with the position statement of the Ethics and Humanities Subcommittee of the American Academy of Neurology (41) that opposes

> physician-assisted suicide, euthanasia, and any other actions by neurologists that are directly intended to cause the death of patients. Even if such actions become legally acceptable, the Academy emphasizes that this will not make them morally or ethically acceptable ipso facto. . . . The Academy does not accept the conclusion that the failures of society and of modern medicine to provide adequate compas-

sionate care for the dying can be used as justification for permitting physicians to hasten, or assist in hastening, the deaths of persons in their care.

In summary, deciding to forgo life-prolonging medical treatment is one of the most difficult decisions neurologists and neurosurgeons must make when caring for their patients. Before making a decision, a diagnosis and prognosis must be made with the highest level of certainty possible. Knowledge of the existing medical, ethical, and legal guidelines will facilitate this process for the physician. Ethical clinical decisions are founded on compassionate and effective open communication between the physician and the patient's family, taking into account both the medical facts and the patient's wishes.

ACKNOWLEDGMENT

The authors gratefully acknowledge the use of material from Dr. James Bernat taken in part from the prior edition of this text.

REFERENCES

1. *Arato v. Avedon,* 5 Cal. 4th 1172, 858 P.2d 598 (Cal. Supreme Court, in bank, 1973).
2. Brody BA. Ethical issues raised by the clinical use of prognostic information. In: Evans RW, Baskin DS, Yatsu FM, eds. *Prognosis of neurological disorders,* 2nd ed. New York: Oxford University Press, 2000:3–10.
3. Beauchamp TL, Childress JF. *Principles of biomedical ethics,* 3rd ed. New York: Oxford University Press, 1989:67–306.
4. *Schloendorff v. Society of New York Hospital,* 211 N.Y. 125, 127, 129; 105 N.E. 92, 93 (1914).
5. President's Commission for the Study of Ethical Problems in Medicine and Biomedical and Behavioral Research. *Making health care decisions: the ethical and legal implications of informed consent in the patient-practitioner relationship.* Washington, DC: US Government Printing Office, 1982.
6. Ethics and Humanities Subcommittee of the American Academy of Neurology. Position statement: certain aspects of the care and management of profoundly and irreversibly paralyzed patients with retained consciousness and cognition. *Neurology* 1993;43:222–223.
7. Goldblatt D. Decisions about life support in amyotrophic lateral sclerosis. *Semin Neurol* 1984;4:104–110.
8. *Satz v. Perlmutter,* Florida 362 So. 2d 160 (Fla App 1978), affirmed by Florida Supreme Court 379 So. 2d 359 (1980).
9. Goldblatt D, Greenlaw J. Starting and stopping the ven-

tilator for patients with amyotrophic lateral sclerosis. *Neurol Clin* 1989;7:798–806.
10. Schneiderman LJ, Spragg RC. Ethical decisions in discontinuing mechanical ventilation. *N Engl J Med* 1988; 318:984–988.
11. Bernat JL, Cranford RE, Kittredge FI Jr, et al. Competent patients with advanced states of permanent paralysis have the right to forgo life-sustaining therapy. *Neurology* 1993;43:224–225.
12. Carver AC, Vickrey BG, Bernat JL, et al. End-of-life care: a survey of US neurologists' attitudes, behavior, and knowledge. *Neurology* 1999;53:284–293.
13. Mayer SA, Kossoff SB. Withdrawal of life support in the neurological intensive care unit. *Neurology* 1999;52: 1602–1609.
14. Schneiderman LJ, Arras JD. Counseling patients to counsel physicians on future care in the event of patient incompetence. *Ann Intern Med* 1985;102:693–698.
15. Uhlmann RF, Pearlman RA, Cain KC, et al. Physicians' and spouses' predictions of elderly patients' resuscitation preferences. *J Gerontol* 1988;43:115–121.
16. American Medical Association Council on Scientific Affairs and Council on Ethical and Judicial Affairs. Persistent vegetative state and the decision to withdraw or withhold life support. *JAMA* 1990;263:426–430.
17. Roark JE, Raffin TA, Ambrogi T, et al. Initiating and withdrawing life support: principles and practice in adult medicine. *N Engl J Med* 1988;318:25–30.
18. Wanzer SH, Federman DD, Adelstein SJ, et al. The physician's responsibility toward hopelessly ill patients: a second look. *N Engl J Med* 1989;320:844–849.
19. Cranford RE. Termination of treatment in the persistent vegetative state. *Semin Neurol* 1984;4:36–44.
20. President's Commission for the Study of Ethical Problems in Medicine and Biomedical and Behavioral Research. *Deciding to forego life-sustaining treatment: ethical, medical, and treatment decisions.* Washington, DC: US Government Printing Office, 1983.
21. Schneiderman LS, Jecker N. Futility in practice. *Arch Intern Med* 1993;153:437.
22. Nora RE, Nora LM. Medical legal issues in the prognosis of neurological disorders. In: Evans RW, Baskin DS, Yatsu FM, eds. *Prognosis of neurological disorders,* 2nd ed. New York: Oxford University Press, 2000:28–39.
23. *In re Helga Wanglie,* Fourth Judicial District (Dist. Ct., Probate Ct. Div.). PX-91-283, Minnesota, Hennepin County (1991).
24. *In re Baby K* 832 F. Supp. 1022 (E.D. Va. 1993) aff'd 16 F.3d 590 (4th Cir. 1994).
25. *In the matter of Karen Quinlan,* 70 N.J. 10, 335 A. 2d 647, 1976.
26. *Superintendent of Belchertown State School v. Saikewicz,* 370 N.E. 2d 417, 1977.
27. *In re Dinnerstein,* 380 N.E. 2d 134, 1978.
28. *Eichner v. Dillon,* 426 N.Y.S. 2d 517, 1980.
29. *Cruzan v. Director, Missouri Dept. of Health,* 497 U.S. 261, 1990.
30. Weir RF, Gostin L. Decisions to abate life-sustaining treatment for nonautonomous patients: ethical standards and legal liability for physicians after *Cruzan. JAMA* 1990;264:1846–1853.
31. Wanzer SH, Adelstein SJ, Cranford RE, et al. The physician's responsibility toward hopelessly ill patients. *N Engl J Med* 1984;310:955–959.
32. Micetich KC, Steinecker PH, Thomasma DC. Are intra-

venous fluids morally required for a dying patient? *Arch Intern Med* 1983;143:975–978.

33. Siegler M, Weisbard AJ. Against the emerging stream: should fluids and nutritional support be discontinued? *Arch Intern Med* 1985;145:129–131.

34. Smedira NG, Evans BH, Grais LS, et al. Withholding and withdrawal of life support from the critically ill. *N Engl J Med* 1990;322:309–315.

35. American Academy of Neurology. Position of the American Academy of Neurology on certain aspects of the care and management of the persistent vegetative state patient. *Neurology* 1989;39:125–126.

36. Stanley JM. The Appleton Consensus: suggested international guidelines for decisions to forego medical treatment. *J Med Ethics* 1989;15:129–136.

37. Meyers DW. Legal aspects of withdrawing nourishment from an incurably ill patient. *Arch Intern Med* 1985; 145:125–128.

38. Weber M, Dindo D, Demartines N, et al. Kidney transplantation from donors without a heartbeat. *N Engl J Med* 2002;347:248–255.

39. Ethics Committee, American College of Critical Care Medicine, Society of Critical Care Medicine. Recommendations for nonheartbeating organ donation. *Crit Care Med* 2001;29:1826–1831.

40. Institute of Medicine. *Non-heart-beating organ transplantation: medical and ethical issues in procurement.* Washington, DC: National Academy Press, 1997.

41. The Ethics and Humanities Subcommittee of the American Academy of Neurology. Assisted suicide, euthanasia, and the neurologist [Position Statement]. *Neurology* 1998;50:596–598.

Subject Index

Page numbers followed by *f* indicate figures. Page numbers followed by *t* indicate tables.